The Massachusetts Eye and Ear Infirmary
Review Manual for
Ophthalmology

The Massachusetts Eye and Ear Infirmary
Review Manual for
Ophthalmology

Jeffrey C. Lamkin, M.D.

Former Chief Resident in Ophthalmology, Harvard Medical School, Boston;
Fellow, Retinal Institute, Mt. Sinai Medical Center, Cleveland

Foreword by
Frederick A. Jakobiec, M.D.

Henry Willard Williams Professor and Chairman of Ophthalmology, and
Professor of Pathology, Harvard Medical School;
Chief of Ophthalmology, Massachusetts Eye and Ear Infirmary, Boston

Little, Brown and Company
Boston/Toronto/London

Library of Congress Cataloging-in-Publication Data

Lamkin, Jeffrey C.
        The Massachusetts Eye and Ear Infirmary review manual for
    ophthalmology / Jeffrey C. Lamkin; foreword by Frederick A.
    Jakobiec.
            p.   cm.
        Includes bibliographical references.
        ISBN 0-316-51293-1
        1. Ophthalmology—Examinations, questions, etc.   I. Massachusetts
    Eye and Ear Infirmary. II. Title.
        [DNLM: 1. Eye Diseases—examination questions. 2. Ophthalmology—
    examination questions. 3. Vision disorders—examination questions.
    WW 18 L232m]
    RE49.L35 1992
    617.7'0076--dc20
    DNLM/DLC
    for Library of Congress   92-49469
                                                                  CIP

Printed in the United States of America

MV-NY

To F.A.J. — for unflagging enthusiasm and encouragement

To Barbara, Barbie, and Shirley — without whom this work
could not have been done

Most of all, to Mary and Elliott, the two most understanding and
gracious ladies in this world

Contents

Foreword

It is a great pleasure to write a brief foreword to *The Massachusetts Eye and Ear Infirmary Review Manual for Ophthalmology*. Dr. Jeffrey Lamkin, the primary organizer and executor of this project with the secondary help of the residents of the Massachusetts Eye and Ear Infirmary, initially conceived it as part of his teaching obligation to the residents while serving as Chief Resident. A highly professional and scholarly set of questions was prepared. It became apparent that many other residents and ophthalmologists seeking to identify the strengths and weaknesses in their ophthalmic knowledge could profit from the dissemination of the material.

The past decade witnessed an explosion in ophthalmic knowledge that was truly daunting and unprecedented. We can expect this expansion to accelerate in the future at an exponential rate. How does one keep abreast of new developments, and how does one form judgments as to what is clinically relevant knowledge and what is of more theoretical or marginal interest at the moment? Most of us are highly specialized in either the knowledge industry or in our clinical practice patterns. If we wish to stay in touch with other specialties of ophthalmology, we tend to need help. Self-assessment and continuing medical education should by now be cornerstones of our professional lives, but these tasks will also be progressively shared with others! We will be increasingly held to higher quality assurance standards, and recertification examinations are about to be put in place. Furthermore, the ability to practice medicine in the future may become aligned with profiles of the clinical outcomes of the patients we treat, as could be mandated by federal agencies and insurance payors. Sound and constantly remodelled knowledge will thus be the best basis for protecting and advancing our clinical practices.

The questions in this publication have been prepared with great care, in order to achieve balance among the various subspecialties of our field and to highlight clinically significant subjects and basic science concepts and findings that undergird them. No effort has been made to reconstruct questions from Board or OKAP examinations; rather, the questions have been created in a way that proceeds from what one group of people has determined to be an essential database for the practicing ophthalmologist who wishes to be informed of recent scientific discoveries and the refashioned foundations of clinical science. As they say in the movies, any resemblance to questions that appear on formal examinations is completely coincidental and reflects the fact that people who are serious students of the subject have independently identified topics that should be within the purview and common fund of knowledge of a contemporary clinician. The questions themselves are less important than the subjects they represent. A well-positioned cadre that can serve as an arbiter for this fund of knowledge is residents-in-training who are eager to equip themselves for their impending clinical professional lives, and who daily critically assess and internalize the rivulets of information that are flowing toward them from their teachers and clinical preceptors.

This textbook is the distinctive product of a unique mind and constellation of talents possessed by Jeffrey Lamkin. I can think of nobody better suited to shepherd this project than Jeffrey because he is guided by an insightful and retentive mind, a capacity for detail and global integration, and an ardent love of knowledge and its transmission to those around him. Due to the depth of his commitment to resident education and that of other colleagues, he has made a tremendous gift of his energies and time to our entire field.

Frederick A. Jakobiec, M.D.

Preface

Many experts in medical education contend that objective examination styles, like those now administered by nearly every medical specialty, are inaccurate and misleading indices of professional competence and ability. Certainly, they are incomplete and will never be capable of judging insight, economy of thought and action, interpersonal skills, or honesty. However, no one can impugn the importance of a solid base of objective knowledge acting as a foundation for the practice of excellence in medicine. *The Massachusetts Eye and Ear Infirmary Review Manual for Ophthalmology* has a single, simple purpose — to act as an aid in assessing one's base of ophthalmic knowledge — for anyone who considers herself or himself a student of ophthalmology. The question-and-answer format was selected because of its accessibility and popularity. A natural and healthy by-product of this assessment should be in-depth, targeted study of areas of apparent weakness.

There are two purposes for which this book was never intended. First, it should not be used as original source material. It is, in every sense of the word, a *review* manual that presumes prior reading and clinical experience. Each question is answered in sufficient detail only to cover the salient points of the question itself, not the entire topic it addresses. Each chapter is referenced to the source materials from which the questions were written and answered. These references should be considered the ultimate authorities.

Second, this book is in no way intended to simulate the Written Qualifying Examination or Ophthalmology Knowledge Assessment Program given annually by the American Board of Ophthalmology (ABO). It should not be used as a means of *practicing* for these examinations, since the majority of questions in this work are presented in formats not used by the ABO. Rather, we have attempted to write and answer a series of questions that thoughtfully address nearly every topic of current clinical and scientific importance in an engaging and meaningful way. The chapter contributors and I have emphasized factual accuracy, fairness, and relevance; please forgive any liberties we took with standard objective question formatting or style.

The residents of the Massachusetts Eye and Ear Infirmary are delighted to welcome you to the pursuit of ophthalmic trivia. Actually, this is no trivial pursuit. We have dedicated the past year to writing and carefully editing more than 2200 questions. Furthermore, the subjects addressed in this work were included only after meeting strict standards for relevancy and fairness. I would like to extend my deepest gratitude to Dr. M. Ronan Conlan, Dr. Deborah S. Jacobs, and Dr. Frederick A. Jakobiec for contributing illustrations.

Any overlap or repetition of topics has been judged appropriate for the subject matter. I hope any reader with concerns or suggestions regarding any of our questions or answers will contact me. Enjoy!

J. C. L.

Contributors

The following residents at the Massachusetts Eye and Ear Infirmary
helped with the compilation of this text.

The Myrmidons:
John S. Berestka, M.D., *Chapter 5*
Vikas K. Jain, M.D., *Chapter 10*
Stephen Y. Lee, M.D., *Chapter 9*
James J. McMillan, M.D., *Chapter 6*
Eric A. Pierce, M.D., Ph.D., *Chapter 7*
Roberto Pineda III, M.D., *Chapter 3*
Chander N. Samy, M.D., *Chapter 1*
Scott D. Smith, M.D., *Chapter 2*

and

Eddy Anglade, M.D., *Chapter 8*
Cynthia Grosskreutz, M.D., Ph.D., *Chapter 11*
Vera O. Kowal, M.D., *Chapter 7*
Leonard A. Levin, M.D., Ph.D., *Chapter 4*
Dennis M. Marcus, M.D., *Chapter 3*
M. Lisa McHam, M.D., *Chapter 9*
Monte D. Mills, M.D., *Chapter 5*
Samuel E. Navon, M.D., Ph.D., *Chapter 6*
Elias Reichel, M.D., *Chapter 10*
Nicholas J. Volpe, M.D., *Chapter 4*

How to Use This Book

As is apparent, the questions in this book are divided into eleven chapters on the basis of relevant topics. The first three are of general importance (Fundamentals, Optics, Pathology); the remainder focus on the various subspecialties that compose modern ophthalmology. Each chapter is divided into two parts: The first consists of all the questions, while the second part contains all the answers — the correct letter/number choice(s), as well as a brief, directed explanation.

There are four question formats used:

1. True or false. These always start with "T or F —."
2. Matching. In many questions of this variety, there may be more than one correct answer for options in either column.
3. Type A multiple choice. In this type, there is one, and only one, correct completion to the question, to be selected from options *a* through *e*.
4. Type K multiple choice. In this format, the stem of the question may have up to four correct completions (options 1–4). The correct answer, to be chosen from options *a* through *e*, is always a predictable combination of the numbered completions. For example:

Regarding the presidency of the United States, which of the following is/are true?

1. Washington was the first U.S. president.
2. Lincoln was the first president to be assassinated.
3. Wilson created the League of Nations.
4. Nixon defeated Kennedy in 1960.

a. 1, 2, and 3.
b. 1 and 3.
c. 2 and 4.
d. 4 only.
e. 1, 2, 3, and 4.

Here, the answer is *a*. Statements 1, 2, and 3 are all correct answers to the question. Notice that for all type K questions, options *a* through *e* are the same — that is, *a* is always 1, 2, and 3; *b* is always 1 and 3; *c* is always 2 and 4; *d* is always 4 only; and *e* is always 1, 2, 3, and 4.

A blank answer sheet for each chapter is provided at the end of the manual. These are perforated and can be removed for recording and comparing answers with the answer key. The authors recommend completing each chapter's questions in their entirety before consulting the answer key.

The Massachusetts Eye and Ear Infirmary
Review Manual for
Ophthalmology

1: Fundamentals of Ophthalmology

1. Which one of the following bones does not form part of the orbit?

   a. palatine.
   b. frontal.
   c. zygomatic.
   d. nasal.
   e. ethmoid.

2. What is the average volume of the human orbit?

   a. 30 cc.
   b. 35 cc.
   c. 40 cc.
   d. 45 cc.
   e. 50 cc.

3. Which of the following is <u>not</u> a part of the medial orbital wall?

   a. ethmoid.
   b. frontal.
   c. lacrimal.
   d. palatine.
   e. maxillary.

4. How many bones compose the lacrimal sac fossa?

   a. 1.
   b. 2.
   c. 3.
   d. 4.
   e. none -- a fossa is a hole.

5. In which bone does the lacrimal gland fossa lie?

   a. frontal.
   b. lacrimal.
   c. maxillary.
   d. zygomatic.
   e. ethmoid.

6. Which orbital wall is the strongest?

   a. medial.
   b. inferior.
   c. lateral.
   d. roof.
   e. All are equally strong.

7. Which one of the following structures does not insert into the lateral orbital tubercle?

   a. check ligament of the lateral rectus.
   b. suspensory ligament of the eyeball (Lockwood's ligament).
   c. lateral canthal tendon.
   d. aponeurosis of the levator muscle.
   e. Whitnall's ligament.

8. Which of the following is/are not transmitted in the optic canal?

   1. optic nerve.
   2. ophthalmic artery.
   3. sympathetic plexus.
   4. central retinal artery.

   a. 1, 2, and 3.
   b. 1 and 3.
   c. 2 and 4.
   d. 4 only.
   e. 1, 2, 3, and 4.

9. How many axons compose a healthy adult optic nerve?

   a. 100,000.
   b. 300,000.
   c. 600,000.
   d. 1,200,000.
   e. 2,400,000.

10. Upon entry to the orbit, the ophthalmic artery runs in what relationship relative to the optic nerve?

    a. inferior.
    b. lateral.
    c. superior.
    d. medial.
    e. variable.

11. The ciliary ganglion:

   a. has three roots, is located 1 cm behind the globe, and is medial to the optic nerve.
   b. has four roots, is located 1 cm behind the globe, and is lateral to the optic nerve.
   c. has four roots, is located 1 cm anterior to the orbital apex, and is medial to the optic nerve.
   d. has three roots, is located 1 cm behind the globe, and is lateral to the optic nerve.
   e. has three roots, is located 1 cm anterior to the orbital apex, and is lateral to the optic nerve.

12. T or F -- There is dual sympathetic innervation to the eye.

13. Which of the following regarding ocular glands is/are true?

   1. The glands of Wolfring and Krause are cytologically similar to the lacrimal gland.
   2. The accessory lacrimal glands produce primarily reflex tear secretion.
   3. The glands of Moll are of the apocrine type.
   4. The meibomian glands are holocrine oil glands that are associated with cilia.

   a. 1, 2, and 3.
   b. 1 and 3.
   c. 2 and 4.
   d. 4 only.
   e. 1, 2, 3, and 4.

14. T or F -- The tarsal plates consist of cartilage.

15. T or F -- The smaller orbital lobe of the lacrimal gland is located posterior to the larger palpebral lobe.

16. T or F -- The canaliculi and lacrimal sac are lined by identical epithelia.

17. What are average adult corneal diameters?

   a. 11 mm horizontally and vertically.
   b. 12 mm horizontally and vertically.
   c. 12 mm horizontally and 11 mm vertically.
   d. 11 mm horizontally and 12 mm vertically.
   e. 10 mm horizontally and vertically.

18. T or F -- The corneal endothelium reacts to injuries or cellular loss with hyperplasia.

19. T or F -- The sclera is highly vascularized.

20. The correct order of angle structures, from central to peripheral, is:

    a. scleral spur (SS), pigmented trabecular meshwork (TM), nonpigmented TM, Schwalbe's line (SL), ciliary body band (CBB).
    b. SL, pigmented TM, nonpigmented TM, CBB, SS.
    c. SL, pigmented TM, nonpigmented TM, SS, CBB.
    d. SL, SS, pigmented TM, nonpigmented TM, CBB.
    e. SL, nonpigmented TM, pigmented TM, SS, CBB.

21. The "filtration" portion of trabecular meshwork (TM) is the:

    a. uveal meshwork.
    b. corneoscleral meshwork.
    c. anterior, nonpigmented TM.
    d. posterior, pigmented TM.
    e. juxtacanalicular TM.

22. T or F -- The trabecular meshwork (TM) is lined by a bilayered endothelium.

23. The site of greatest resistance to aqueous outflow is the:

    a. uveal meshwork.
    b. corneoscleral meshwork.
    c. anterior, non-pigmented trabecular meshwork (TM).
    d. posterior, pigmented TM.
    e. juxtacanalicular TM.

24. The average anteroposterior diameter of a 40-year-old lens is:

    a. 2 to 3 mm.
    b. 3 to 4 mm.
    c. 4 to 5 mm.
    d. 5 to 6 mm.
    e. 6 to 7 mm.

25. The average equatorial diameter of a 40-year-old lens is:

    a. 6 to 7 mm.
    b. 7 to 8 mm.
    c. 8 to 9 mm.
    d. 9 to 10 mm.
    e. 10 to 11 mm.

26. T or F -- The anteroposterior lens diameter does not change throughout life.

27. T or F -- The horizontal diameter of the lens does not change throughout life.

28. T or F -- The posterior capsule is thicker than the anterior capsule.

29. T or F -- The anterior iris surface is lined by a single-layered endothelium.

30. T or F -- The posterior pigment epithelial layer of the iris consists of the pigmented myoepithelial cells of the dilator muscle.

31. Select the correct description of autonomic innervation to the eye:

    a. The iris sphincter muscle receives sympathetic innervation via the short ciliary nerves; the iris dilator muscle receives parasympathetic innervation via the short ciliary nerves.

    b. The iris sphincter muscle receives parasympathetic innervation via the short ciliary nerves; the iris dilator muscle receives sympathetic innervation by the short ciliary nerves.

    c. The iris sphincter muscle receives parasympathetic innervation via the short ciliary nerves; the iris dilator muscle receives sympathetic innervation via the long ciliary nerves.

    d. The iris sphincter muscle receives parasympathetic innervation via the long ciliary nerves; the iris dilator muscle receives sympathetic innervation via long ciliary nerves.

    e. The iris sphincter muscle receives sympathetic innervation via the short ciliary nerves; the iris dilator muscle receives parasympathetic innervation via the long ciliary nerves.

32. T or F -- The choriocapillaris is a continuous vascular system with virtually limitless anastomoses between its different regions.

33. T or F -- The degree of pigmentation observed ophthalmoscopically in the human fundus is dependent on the amount of pigmentation of the retinal pigment epithelium (RPE).

34. T or F -- Retinal pigment epithelial (RPE) cells in the fundus periphery are taller, thinner, and contain more and larger melanosomes than those in the posterior fundus.

35. T or F -- The retinal pigment epithelium (RPE) is a mitotically active structure in the normal human eye.

36. Which one of the following concerning retinal photoreceptors is correct?

    a. Rods contain photopigment discs that are not attached to the cell membrane and synapse with bipolar cells at a rod pedicle.
    b. Cones contain photopigment discs that are not connected to the cell membrane and synapse with bipolar cells at a cone pedicle.
    c. Rods contain photopigment discs that are attached to the cell membrane and synapse with bipolar cells at the rod spherule.
    d. Cones contain photopigment discs that are attached to the cell membrane and synapse with bipolar cells at a cone pedicle.
    e. None of the above.

37. Select the correct neuronal sequence for intraretinal processing:

    a. photoreceptor to Müller cell to ganglion cell.
    b. photoreceptor to bipolar cell to ganglion cell.
    c. photoreceptor to horizontal cell to amacrine cell.
    d. photoreceptor cell to horizontal cell to ganglion cell.
    e. photoreceptor to amacrine cell to bipolar cell.

38. In the entire retina, rods outnumber cones by a ratio of approximately:

    a. 2:1.
    b. 5:1.
    c. 8:1.
    d. 20:1.
    e. 50:1.

39. Which one of the following is correct?

    a. The external and internal limiting membranes of the retina are basement membranes of Müller cells.
    b. The external and internal limiting membranes are basement membranes of the bipolar cells.
    c. The external limiting membrane is the basement membrane of the Müller cell, while the internal limiting membrane is not a true membrane.
    d. The internal limiting membrane is the true basement membrane of the Müller cell, while the external limiting membrane is not a true membrane.
    e. None of the above.

40. A cilioretinal artery contributes to some portion of the macular circulation in approximately:

    a. 5% of individuals.
    b. 15%.
    c. 25%.
    d. 40%.
    e. 50%.

41. The inner retinal circulation's deepest level of penetration is the:

    a. ganglion cell layer.
    b. inner plexiform layer.
    c. inner nuclear layer.
    d. outer plexiform layer.
    e. outer nuclear layer.

42. Select the correct association of retinal layer and synaptic connections:

    a. outer plexiform layer: bipolar and ganglion cells.
    b. inner plexiform layer: bipolar and ganglion cells.
    c. outer plexiform layer: photoreceptor and ganglion cells.
    d. inner plexiform layer: photoreceptor and ganglion cells.
    e. inner plexiform layer: photoreceptor and bipolar cells.

43. Which of the following sites provide <u>firm</u> uveoscleral attachment?

                 1. optic nerve.
                 2. vortex veins.
                 3. scleral spur.
                 4. ora serrata.

    a. 1, 2 and 3.
    b. 1 and 3.
    c. 2 and 4.
    d. 4 only.
    e. 1, 2, 3, and 4.

44. In what quadrant is the ora serrata farthest from the limbus?

    a. superotemporal.
    b. inferotemporal.
    c. inferonasal.
    d. inferotemporal.
    e. nasal.

45. T or F -- The ora is smoother (i.e., fewer serrations, or teeth) nasally then temporally.

46. T or F -- Myelinated nerve fibers in the retina result when Schwann cells migrate beyond the lamina cribrosa to form a myelin sheath around ganglion cell axons.

47. Upon entering the cranial cavity, the optic nerve runs:

    a. lateral to the internal carotid artery and inferior to the anterior cerebral artery.
    b. medial to the internal carotid artery and inferior to the anterior cerebral artery.
    c. medial to the internal carotid artery and superior to the anterior cerebral artery.
    d. lateral to the internal carotid artery and superior to the anterior cerebral artery.
    e. lateral to the internal carotid artery and lateral to the anterior cerebral artery.

48. Which of the following concerning ganglion axon decussation is true?

   a. More ganglion cells cross in the chiasm than do not cross.
   b. Equal numbers of ganglion cells cross in the chiasm as do not cross.
   c. Fewer numbers of ganglion cells cross than do not cross in the chiasm.
   d. A greater proportion of macular fibers cross than peripheral fibers.
   e. A greater portion of peripheral fibers cross than macular fibers.

49. Which one of the extraocular muscles is served by a single nucleus that is shared by both oculomotor nerve nuclei?

   a. superior rectus.
   b. medial rectus.
   c. inferior oblique.
   d. levator palpebrae superioris.
   e. inferior rectus.

50. Which is the only muscle supplied by the oculomotor nerve that receives <u>crossed</u> innervation?

   a. superior rectus.
   b. medial rectus.
   c. inferior oblique.
   d. levator palpebrae superioris.
   e. inferior rectus.

51. Which one of the following concerning the pupillomotor fibers of the third cranial nerve is true?

   a. They run central in the nerve, in the superior division.
   b. They run central in the nerve, in the inferior division.
   c. They run peripheral in the nerve, in the superior division.
   d. They run peripheral in the nerve, in the inferior division.
   e. They are distributed evenly throughout the superior division.

52. T or F -- The fifth cranial nerve has both motor and sensory components.

53. Which of the following structures do <u>not</u> travel in the wall of the cavernous sinus?

   a. third and fourth cranial nerves.
   b. fourth and fifth cranial nerves.
   c. fifth and sixth cranial nerves.
   d. sixth cranial nerve and the internal carotid artery.
   e. the internal carotid artery.

54. T or F -- Ocular colobomas arise from failure of fusion of the lips of the optic cup, most typically superotemporally.

55. T or F -- The retinal pigment epithelial (RPE) cells are the first cells in the body to produce melanin.

56. T or F -- Myelination of optic nerve axons to the lamina cribrosa is rarely completed before 6 months of age.

57. T or F -- The lens of the eye develops from neurectoderm.

58. Mesenchymal structures of the head, including the eye, are all derived from:

    a. mesoderm.
    b. neural crest cells.
    c. a combination of mesoderm and ectoderm.
    d. a combination of neural crest cells and ectoderm.
    e. a combination of neural crest cells and mesoderm.

59. Neural crest cells give rise to the following structures:

    a. corneal epithelium, stroma, endothelium, and ciliary muscle.
    b. the entire sclera, optic nerve sheath, uveal melanocytes, entire choroid.
    c. orbital bones, fat, trochlear cartilage, extraocular muscles, and orbital connective tissues.
    d. ciliary body, ciliary epithelium, iris stroma, orbital bones, and orbital connective tissues.
    e. optic nerve sheath, uveal melanocytes, choroidal stroma, ciliary muscle, and iris stroma.

60. The mesoderm gives rise to:

    a. the pupillomotor muscles, ciliary muscle, and extraocular muscles.
    b. all vascular endothelia, extraocular muscles, and the trochlea.
    c. all vascular endothelia, pupillomotor muscles, and all blood vessels.
    d. all vascular endothelia, all extraocular muscles, and temporal sclera.
    e. ciliary muscle, extraocular muscles, all orbital blood vessels, and some orbital connective tissue.

61. The surface ectoderm supplies all of the following structures except:

    a. the lacrimal gland.
    b. the eyelid glandular systems.
    c. the eyelid skin.
    d. the corneal epithelium.
    e. the substantia propria of the conjunctiva.

62. T or F -- The primary vitreous is slowly displaced peripherally as secondary vitreous develops centrally.

63. What factor distinguishes anophthalmia from microphthalmia?

    a. the size of the globe.
    b. the presence or absence of a globe.
    c. the presence or absence of lid fusion.
    d. the presence or absence of organic abnormalities of globe.
    e. the presence or absence of nervous system disorders.

64. What factor distinguishes microphthalmia from nanophthalmia?

    a. the size of the globe.
    b. the presence or absence of a globe.
    c. the presence or absence of lid fusion.
    d. the presence or absence of organic abnormalities of globe.
    e. the presence or absence of nervous system disorders.

65. All of the following conditions may present as a cystic bulge within the palpebral fissure except:

    a. cystic coloboma.
    b. orbital encephalocele.
    c. microphthalmos.
    d. nanophthalmos.
    e. congenital rhabdomyosarcoma.

66. Which one of the following concerning dermoids is false?

    a. They represent hamartomatous arrests of epidermal and connective tissues.
    b. They may be found in the conjunctiva and/or in the orbit.
    c. The solid variety is most frequently found at the limbus.
    d. Dermolipomas are usually solid, consisting entirely of fatty and fibrous tissue, most commonly between the lateral and superior rectus muscles.
    e. Epibulbar dermoids are associated with the Goldenhar syndrome.

67. Which one of the following concerning anterior segment dysgenesis is false?

    a. All varieties may be inherited as autosomal dominant traits and may be either unilateral or bilateral.
    b. Posterior embryotoxon is the most mild of the peripheral varieties.
    c. Rieger's anomaly consists of Axenfeld's anomaly plus iris atrophy.
    d. Rieger's syndrome is Rieger's anomaly plus facial and musculoskeletal anomalies.
    e. In Peter's anomaly, the central cornea is always opacified, and the lens is always densely adherent to the posterior corneal surface.

68. Which one of the following concerning aniridia is false?

    a. Generally, no iris tissue is present on histopathology.
    b. Aniridia may be either familial or sporadic.
    c. Aniridia is not associated with the autosomal dominant forms of Wilms' tumor.
    d. There is an association of aniridia with Wilms' tumor, genitourinary anomalies and mental retardation.
    e. In aniridia associated with Wilms' tumor, there is frequently a deletion on the short arm of chromosome 11.

69. Which one of the following concerning pediatric lenticular disorders is true?

    a. Spherophakia is associated with both Marfan's and the Weill-Marchesani syndromes, and differentiation of these two syndromes is frequently difficult.
    b. In Lowe's syndrome, there are typically cataracts, glaucoma, and aminoaciduria, and women are affected more frequently than men.
    c. Cataracts in the congenital rubella syndrome are generally dense nuclear cataracts.
    d. Defects in the rubella syndrome are typically isolated (that is, there are no other systemic abnormalities).
    e. Glaucoma and cataract are frequently coincident in the congenital rubella syndrome.

70. Which one of the following concerning persistent hyperplastic primary vitreous (PHPV) is false?

    a. It is generally unilateral.
    b. Visual prognosis is usually good.
    c. It is most easily differentiated from retinoblastoma by the coincidence of microphthalmos or cataract.
    d. It may calcify.
    e. It is almost always sporadic.

71. Which one of the following concerning tear secretion is false?

    a. The basal, continual tear secretion is maintained by the accessory lacrimal glands of Krause and Wolfring.
    b. The glands of Wolfring are located along the orbital margin of each tarsus, with the glands of Krause in the conjunctival fornix.
    c. Basal tear secretion is maintained by parasympathetic innervation.
    d. Both sympathetic and parasympathetic nerve stimuli are important for reflex tear secretion.
    e. Conjunctiva and meibomian glands also contribute to the tear film.

72. Which one of the following concerning corneal metabolism is false?

    a. Oxygen is provided to the cornea by both tears and aqueous humor.
    b. Most of the metabolic fuel for the cornea is derived from aqueous humor.
    c. Penetration of molecules through corneal epithelium and stroma is most facilitated with charged ionic species.
    d. Mature corneal stromal fibers are composed of type 1 collagen.
    e. Glycosaminoglycan type and distribution in the cornea are critical for corneal clarity.

73. Which one of the following concerning Descemet's membrane and corneal endothelium is false?

    a. Descemet's membrane consists of type IV collagen.
    b. Posterior keratoconus can be differentiated from Peter's anomaly by the presence of fetal Descemet's membrane.
    c. Fetal Descemet's membrane can be differentiated from adult Descemet's membrane by its banding pattern.
    d. The number of endothelial cells increases with age.
    e. The corneal endothelium actively maintains corneal deturgescence via a pump system dependent on Na^+/K^+-ATPase function and carbonic anhydrase.

74. Aqueous humor enters the posterior chamber from the ciliary processes via:

    a. diffusion.
    b. ultrafiltration.
    c. active secretion.
    d. b and c.
    e. a, b, and c.

75. Which one of the following concerning prostaglandins is false?

    a. The cyclo-oxygenase reaction culminates in the production of prostaglandins, prostacyclin, and thromboxane.
    b. In general, prostaglandins cause mydriasis.
    c. Corticosteroids block both cyclo-oxygenase and lipoxygenase.
    d. The effect of prostaglandins on intraocular pressure is complex, with low doses lowering intraocular pressure and high doses raising intraocular pressure.
    e. Prostacyclin is a vasodilator found primarily in endothelial cells, while thromboxane is a vasoconstrictor found primarily in platelets.

76. For each of the following substances, indicate whether their aqueous humor concentrations are higher than, similar to, or lower than plasma:

    a. sodium.   1. higher.
    b. potassium.   2. lower.
    c. calcium.   3. similar.
    d. iron.
    e. lactate.
    f. ascorbate.
    g. glucose.

77. Which of the following enzymes are normally present at functioning levels in aqueous humor?

                1. carbonic anhydrase.
                2. lysozyme.
                3. hyaluronidase.
                4. lactate dehydrogenase.

    a. 1, 2, and 3.
    b. 1 and 3.
    c. 2 and 4.
    d. 4 only.
    e. 1, 2, 3, and 4.

78. The partial pressure of oxygen in aqueous humor is:

    a. 40 mm Hg.
    b. 55 mm Hg.
    c. 75 mm Hg.
    d. 85 mm Hg.
    e. 100 mm Hg.

79. The most mitotically active lens epithelial cells are located:

    a. at the anterior pole.
    b. at the posterior pole.
    c. at the equator.
    d. in a ring around the anterior lens.
    e. in a ring around the posterior lens.

80. Which one of the following statements concerning the protein fractions of the lens is false?

    a. Lens fiber proteins are separated into two major groups, water soluble and water insoluble.
    b. The water-insoluble fraction is further divided into three types of crystallin proteins.
    c. Alpha crystallin is the largest of the lens proteins.
    d. Beta crystallin is the most abundant of the lens proteins.
    e. The water-insoluble fraction increases with age and is present in much higher concentrations in nuclear cataracts.

81. T or F -- There is an active pump mechanism in the lens that drives ionic movements across the lens, both anteroposteriorly and posteroanteriorly.

82. T or F -- The lens will become translucent or opaque, if deprived of glucose.

83. T or F -- The lens will become translucent or opaque, if deprived of oxygen.

84. The syneresis of aging is due to:

   a. diffuse decreases in hyaluronic acid concentration.
   b. diffuse decreases in collagen concentration.
   c. focal decreases in collagen concentration.
   d. motion-induced collagen damage.
   e. light-induced collagen damage.

85. Which of the following conditions are associated with significant decreases in <u>both</u> collagen and hyaluronic acid concentrations in human vitreous?

   a. myopia.
   b. aphakia.
   c. diabetes mellitus.
   d. a and b.
   e. a and c.

86. T or F -- Whether vitreous hemorrhage clots depends on the degree of vitreous liquefaction.

87. T or F -- Vitamin A is delivered to the eye entirely as all-*trans* retinol.

88. T or F -- To regenerate 11-*cis* retinaldehyde, the *cis* confirmation must be regenerated at the retinal pigment epithelium (RPE).

89. T or F -- The final step in regeneration of 11-*cis* retinaldehyde takes place in the photoreceptor outer segment.

90. Which one of the following concerning the effects of light on rod outer segment metabolism is false?

   a. In the dark, high cyclic guanosine monophosphate (cGMP) levels keep sodium channels open and rod outer segments depolarized.
   b. Light absorption leads to configurational changes in rhodopsin and activation of transducin.
   c. Transducin, through an amplification cascade, activates phosphodiesterase (PDE).
   d. Phosphodiesterase (PDE) causes a fall in cGMP levels.
   e. Falling intracellular cGMP leads to closure of sodium channels, with subsequent further depolarization of the rod outer segment.

91. T or F -- Like the lens, the retina is primarily dependent on anaerobic metabolism (glycolysis).

92. All of the following are effective methods of increasing ocular absorption of topically applied materials (without increasing systemic absorption) except:

    a. adding a second eye drop immediately after the first.
    b. waiting 10 minutes between different medications.
    c. nasolacrimal sac compression.
    d. closing the eyes quietly for 3 to 5 minutes after administration.
    e. addition of topical anesthetic immediately prior to administration.

93. All of the following factors increase the amount of medication penetrating the cornea except:

    a. higher concentration of the drug.
    b. higher viscosity of the vehicle.
    c. higher pH of the drug.
    d. higher lipid solubility of the drug.
    e. addition of benzalkonium chloride.

94. All of the following ocular structures have physiologically important cholinergic receptors except:

    a. extraocular muscles.
    b. ciliary body muscle.
    c. lacrimal gland tissue.
    d. iris dilator muscle.
    e. meibomian glands.

95. T or F -- In a patient with open-angle glaucoma, direct-acting cholinergic agents act to lower intraocular pressure by decreasing relative pupillary block.

96. Unwanted side effects of direct cholinergic agonists include all of the following except:

    a. poor dark adaptation.
    b. decreased vision in older patients.
    c. headache in younger patients.
    d. possible aggravation or induction of angle-closure glaucoma.
    e. induced hyperopia.

97. Rank the following from 1 to 5 in order of decreasing cycloplegic duration.

    a. homatropine.   1.
    b. cyclopentolate.   2.
    c. atropine.   3.
    d. tropicamide.   4.
    e. scopolamine.   5.

98. T or F -- Cocaine 4% is used to establish the presence of Horner's syndrome, and hydroxyamphetamine is used to localize the lesion.

99. Following a unilateral dose of apraclonidine, it is easy to identify the eye that received the medication by its:

   a. lid retraction.
   b. increased conjunctival injection.
   c. miosis.
   d. all of the above.
   e. none of the above.

100. Adrenergic agonists generally:

   a. increase aqueous humor production, decrease outflow facility, and increase intraocular pressure.
   b. increase aqueous humor production, increase outflow facility, and increase intraocular pressure.
   c. increase aqueous humor production, increase outflow facility, and decrease intraocular pressure.
   d. decrease aqueous humor production, decrease outflow facility, and decrease intraocular pressure.
   e. decrease aqueous humor production, increase outflow facility, and decrease intraocular pressure.

101. T or F -- The mechanisms by which apraclonidine and timolol lower intraocular pressure (IOP) are related.

102. Dipivalyl epinephrine (dipivefrin [Propine]) is converted to epinephrine in the:

   a. tears.
   b. conjunctiva.
   c. cornea.
   d. aqueous humor.
   e. iris stroma.

103. Which would be the best single medication for treatment of primary open-angle glaucoma (POAG) in a 69-year-old patient with chronic bronchitis, labile hypertension, and chronic depression treated with monoamine oxidase (MAO) inhibitors, who is 5 years' status post-intracapsular cataract extraction with no implant?

   a. epinephrine.
   b. dipivefrin.
   c. pilocarpine.
   d. timolol.
   e. acetazolamide (Diamox).

104. T or F -- Aqueous humor secretion is exquisitely sensitive to the administration of carbonic anhydrase inhibitors.

105. T or F -- Part of methazolamide's increased efficacy relative to acetazolamide is due to its ability to induce a greater degree of metabolic acidosis.

106. Carbonic anhydrase inhibitors (CAIs) should be used with great caution in all of the following types of patients except:

    a. patients with a remote history of nephrolithiasis.
    b. patients with chronic liver failure.
    c. patients on thiazide diuretics.
    d. patients on digoxin.
    e. chronic schizophrenics.

107. Which one of the following concerning glucocorticoid effects is false?

    a. They inhibit neovascularization.
    b. They do not affect immunoglobulin titers.
    c. They act through impairing the efferent limb of the immune response.
    d. They impair epithelial healing.
    e. They act via blocking release of arachidonic acid from phospholipids.

108. T or F -- If a patient on chronic topical steroid therapy fails to show a rise in intraocular pressure in 6 weeks, it is very unlikely to occur.

109. T or F -- Aspirin use may be associated with asthma attacks and hypersensitivity reactions due to shunting of products from the lipoxygenase pathway to the cyclo-oxygenase pathway.

110. T or F -- Cromolyn sodium is most effective when used prophylactically; however, symptomatic relief may be obtained with intensive administration.

111. Which one of the following concerning the penicillins and cephalosporins is false?

    a. Both act by inhibiting bacterial cell wall synthesis.
    b. Both contain beta-lactam bonds.
    c. These antibiotics have greater activity against gram-positive organisms due to the oligopolysaccharide (OPS) coat of many gram-negative bacteria.
    d. Probenecid counteracts resistance mechanisms by inactivating the beta-lactamase of bacteria.
    e. The most prominent mode of bacterial resistance to this group of antibiotics is the production of beta-lactamase enzymes.

112. In the following question, select the description in the right-hand column that matches the group of antibiotics in the left-hand column.

a. penicillin G, penicillin V.
b. nafcillin, dicloxacillin.
c. ampicillin, amoxicillin.
d. ticarcillin, mezlocillin.

1. highly effective against most gram-positive and gram-negative cocci, including anaerobes.
2. antimicrobial activity extended to gram-negative species, most notably *Pseudomonas*.
3. less potent against susceptible organisms than penicillin G, but more effective against beta-lactamase-producing organisms.
4. moderate gram-negative activity, including some *Hemophilus* and *Proteus* species.

113. Given a history of a hypersensitivity reaction to a penicillin, the probability of a similar reaction to a cephalosporin is approximately:

a. 1%.
b. 5%.
c. 10%.
d. 15%.
e. 20%.

114. Which one of the following concerning antibiotic mechanisms is false?

a. Sulfonamides act by inhibiting bacterial DNA synthesis.
b. Tetracycline is poorly water soluble but may be dissolved in eye drops containing mineral oil.
c. Chloramphenicol use is most strongly associated with aplastic anemia when used orally.
d. Aminoglycoside efficacy is strictly dependent on anaerobically supported antibiotic uptake.
e. Erythromycin acts by inhibiting bacterial protein synthesis.

115. Which one of the aminoglycosides is <u>most</u> resistant to bacterial enzymatic inactivation?

a. gentamicin.
b. tobramycin.
c. kanamycin.
d. amikacin.
e. neomycin.

116. The aminoglycoside that most frequently induces a topical hypersensitivity reaction is:

   a. gentamicin.
   b. tobramycin.
   c. kanamycin.
   d. amikacin.
   e. neomycin.

117. Which one of the following concerning vancomycin is false?

   a. It inhibits bacterial replication by blocking cell wall synthesis.
   b. It is generally bactericidal against all *Streptococcus* species.
   c. It is the gram-positive drug of choice in filtering bleb-related endophthalmitis.
   d. Because of its poor gastrointestinal uptake, it is an excellent drug for pseudomembranous colitis.
   e. The nephrotoxicity of vancomycin is generally potentiated by concomitant use of aminoglycosides.

118. Which one of the following concerning the ocular antiviral agents is false?

   a. Vidarabine (ara-A) is an analog of adenine, while idoxuridine (Stoxil) and trifluridine (Viroptic) are analogs of thymidine.
   b. Trifluridine is more soluble than vidarabine or idoxuridine.
   c. Trifluridine is the most effective of the three.
   d. Cross-resistance to different agents is commonly seen.
   e. Trifluridine has the least corneal toxicity.

119. Which one of the following concerning trisomy 13 (Patau's syndrome) is false?

   a. Fewer than 5% will survive to 3 years of age.
   b. The central nervous system is typically severely affected.
   c. A clenched fist deformity is characteristic.
   d. Cardiovascular and renal defects are very common.
   e. The syndrome has been seen only in complete trisomy of chromosome 13.

120. Which one of the following concerning trisomy 18 (Edward's syndrome) is false?

   a. It is the second most common chromosomal nondisjunction syndrome.
   b. Survival in trisomy 18 tends to be shorter than in trisomy 13.
   c. Outstanding features include mental retardation and numerous musculoskeletal abnormalities.
   d. The effect of maternal age is important in this trisomy.
   e. Glaucoma is more likely with trisomy 18 than with trisomy 13.

121. Which one of the following concerning Down's syndrome is false?

    a. Ninety-five percent are due to meiotic nondisjunction, while the remaining 5% are translocation errors.
    b. A specific region of the long arm of chromosome 21 is responsible for its pathogenesis.
    c. Classic findings include the simian crease, hypoplasia of the middle phalanx of the fifth finger, and congenital heart disease.
    d. Patients with Down's syndrome frequently have low serum purine levels.
    e. The composition of amyloid protein in the central nervous system of patients with Down's syndrome is remarkably similar to that seen in patients with Alzheimer's disease.

122. Which one of the following concerning Turner's syndrome is false?

    a. It is the only disorder of sex chromosomes with characteristic eye findings.
    b. Physical findings include short stature, webbing of the neck, nonpitting edema, and coarctation of the aorta.
    c. The incidence of dyschromatopsia in this syndrome is identical to that of normal women.
    d. Classic eye findings include prominent epicanthal folds, ptosis, and blue sclera.
    e. Patients with Turner's syndrome are always sterile.

123. Increasing paternal age has been associated with all of the following disorders except:

    a. the craniosynostoses.
    b. Treacher Collins syndrome.
    c. neurofibromatosis.
    d. Klinefelter's syndrome.
    e. Waardenburg's syndrome.

124. Chromosomal fragility is associated with each of the following disorders except:

    a. neurofibromatosis.
    b. ataxia-telangiectasia.
    c. Fanconi's anemia.
    d. Bloom's syndrome.
    e. xeroderma pigmentosum.

125. Concerning the long-arm thirteen (13q) deletion syndrome:

    a. the larger the deletion, the more severe the syndrome.
    b. retinoblastoma, part of the syndrome, is inherited in an autosomal dominant fashion.
    c. the defect is recessive at the cellular level.
    d. tumorogenesis requires a second insult ("hit") in this syndrome.
    e. the chance of a carrier's offspring developing retinoblastoma is 50%.

126. Which one of the following concerning the genetics of aniridia is true?

    a. The autosomal dominant form is the only form to feature aniridia with <u>no</u> other ocular abnormalities.
    b. The aniridia associated with Wilms' tumors is most often isolated.
    c. The genitourinary anomalies in patients with this syndrome are of equal severity in both sexes.
    d. When confronted with a patient with newly diagnosed aniridia, the first step the ophthalmologist should take is a careful examination of family members.
    e. Computed tomography (CT scanning) is the most sensitive method of detecting an early Wilms' tumor.

127. In Marfan's syndrome, the presence of ectopia lentis, arachnodactyly, aortic aneurysm, and tall habitus is an example of genetic:

    a. penetrance.
    b. variable expressivity.
    c. dominant inheritance.
    d. phenocopying.
    e. pleiotropism.

128. From the following list, select the racial predilection that is <u>incorrect</u>:

    a. Riley-Day syndrome -- Ashkenazi Jews.
    b. Glucose-6-phosphate dehydrogenase deficiency -- Mediterraneans.
    c. Oguchi's disease -- Chinese.
    d. polydactyly -- African Americans.
    e. diabetes mellitus, type 2 -- Pima Indians.

129. Which one of the following concerning the normal curve and distribution is false?

    a. The graph of this distribution forms a bell-shaped curve.
    b. The mean, the median, and mode have the same values.
    c. The mean plus or minus one standard deviation includes approximately 68% of all observations.
    d. The mean plus or minus two standard deviations includes 99% of all observations.
    e. The formula for standard deviation (S.D.) in a normal distribution of n samples, a_1-a_n, is:

$$S.D. = \sqrt{\frac{\{\Sigma(\bar{a} - a_n)^2\}}{n-1}}$$

130. An investigator attempts to show that a new topical medication is effective in reducing intraocular pressure (IOP). He states that patients who took his medication had IOP that was significantly lower than patients given placebo and says his p value is equal to 0.01. Which one of the following concerning this situation is false?

a. He is willing to reject the null hypothesis with a significance level greater than 0.01.
b. If the difference in intraocular pressure between his treatment and placebo groups was actually due to chance, he is falling victim to type 1 statistical error.
c. There is a 1% chance that the results that occurred were due to chance alone.
d. If he chooses to accept the null hypothesis because he feels his probability level is too high, when in fact there was a true treatment difference, then he is falling victim to type 2 statistical error.
e. The power of his test is 0.99, or 1 minus his type 1 error.

131. Which of the following structures is/are transmitted in the inferior orbital fissure or infraorbital groove/canal?

1. infraorbital nerve.
2. inferior division of the oculomotor nerve.
3. nerve from the pterygopalatine ganglion.
4. superior ophthalmic vein.

a. 1, 2, and 3.
b. 1 and 3.
c. 2 and 4.
d. 4 only.
e. 1, 2, 3, and 4.

132. Which of the following bones do not form part of the orbital floor?

1. zygomatic.
2. sphenoid.
3. maxillary.
4. ethmoid.

a. 1, 2, and 3.
b. 1 and 3.
c. 2 and 4.
d. 4 only.
e. 1, 2, 3, and 4.

133. Match the optic nerve segments listed on the right with their appropriate lengths and/or characteristics listed on the left.

a. longest segment.
b. shortest segment.
c. segment with most variable length.
d. divided into three subsegments.
e. most vulnerable to indirect trauma.
f. most redundant segment.
g. only segment not bathed in cerebrospinal fluid.

1. intraocular.
2. intraorbital.
3. intracanalicular.
4. intracranial.

134. Which of the following muscles is/are supplied by the superior division of the oculomotor nerve?

1. iris sphincter.
2. iris dilator.
3. inferior rectus.
4. levator palpebrae superioris.

a. 1, 2, and 3.
b. 1 and 3.
c. 2 and 4.
d. 4 only.
e. 1, 2, 3, and 4.

135. T or F -- The ptosis associated with third nerve palsy is generally moderate to severe.

136. T or F -- The ptosis associated with Horner's syndrome is generally moderate to severe.

137. With which of the following nerves does parasympathetic innervation to the iris sphincter travel?

a. nerve to the inferior rectus.
b. nerve to the inferior oblique.
c. nerve to the superior rectus.
d. nerve to the superior oblique.
e. long ciliary nerves.

138. Which of the following are innervated by cranial nerve V (trigeminal nerve)?

        1. corneal sensation.
        2. pterygoid muscles.
        3. masseter muscles.
        4. orbicularis oculi.

    a. 1, 2, and 3.
    b. 1 and 3.
    c. 2 and 4.
    d. 4 only.
    e. 1, 2, 3, and 4.

139. T or F -- The facial nerve does not have a branch within the orbit.

140. Which one of the following sets of nerve fibers synapses in the ciliary ganglion?

    a. sympathetic fibers to iris dilator.
    b. sympathetic fibers to choroid and ciliary body.
    c. parasympathetic fibers to iris sphincter.
    d. parasympathetic fibers to choroid and ciliary body.
    e. sensory fibers from the anterior globe (cornea, iris, ciliary body).

141. Match the distances from limbus to tendinous insertion for each of the rectus muscles:

    a. superior rectus.   1. 5.5 mm.
    b. medial rectus.   2. 6.9 mm.
    c. inferior rectus.   3. 7.7 mm.
    d. lateral rectus.   4. 6.5 mm.

142. Which of the following extraocular muscles does not originate anatomically from the orbital apex?

        1. superior rectus.
        2. superior oblique.
        3. inferior rectus.
        4. inferior oblique.

    a. 1, 2, and 3.
    b. 1 and 3.
    c. 2 and 4.
    d. 4 only.
    e. 1, 2, 3, and 4.

143. Which of the following extraocular muscles does not originate mechanically from the orbital apex?

           1. superior rectus.
           2. superior oblique.
           3. inferior rectus.
           4. inferior oblique.

  a. 1, 2, and 3.
  b. 1 and 3.
  c. 2 and 4.
  d. 4 only.
  e. 1, 2, 3, and 4.

144. Which of the following structures is <u>not</u> transmitted within the superior orbital fissure?

  a. superior ophthalmic vein.
  b. superior division of the third cranial nerve.
  c. ophthalmic artery.
  d. inferior division of the third cranial nerve.
  e. fourth cranial nerve.

145. Which of the following structures enter(s) the orbit outside the annulus of Zinn?

           1. nasociliary nerve.
           2. lacrimal nerve.
           3. inferior division of the third cranial nerve.
           4. fourth cranial nerve.

  a. 1, 2, and 3.
  b. 1 and 3.
  c. 2 and 4.
  d. 4 only.
  e. 1, 2, 3, and 4.

146. In general, the last muscle to be rendered akinetic with a retrobulbar anesthetic block is the:

  a. superior rectus.
  b. superior oblique.
  c. inferior rectus.
  d. inferior oblique.
  e. levator palpebrae superioris.

147. Which is the only extraocular muscle typically supplied by one anterior ciliary artery?

  a. superior rectus.
  b. medial rectus.
  c. inferior rectus.
  d. lateral rectus.
  e. superior oblique.

148. T or F -- The anterior ciliary arteries usually terminate in rectus muscles as muscular feeder branches.

149. T or F -- The motor units of the extraocular muscles are significantly larger than those of other striated muscles.

150. Which upper eyelid structure is considered analogous to the capsulopalpebral fascia of the lower eyelid?

    a. Müller's muscle.
    b. levator muscle.
    c. levator aponeurosis.
    d. Whitnall's ligament.
    e. orbital septum.

151. The suspensory ligament of the globe is also known as:

    a. Whitnall's ligament.
    b. Lockwood's ligament.
    c. levator aponeurosis.
    d. capsulopalpebral fascia.
    e. lateral rectus check ligament.

152. Which one of the following statements regarding the arterial supply to the globe is correct?

    a. There are 2 long posterior ciliary arteries (LPCA), and they enter the sclera posteriorly near the optic nerve at 3 and 9 o'clock.
    b. There are 10 to 12 LPCA, and they enter the sclera posteriorly in a circle around the optic nerve.
    c. There are 7 LPCA, and they terminate in the rectus muscles.
    d. There are 7 LPCA, and they terminate in the major arterial circle of the iris after providing feeders to the rectus muscles.
    e. There are 2 LPCA, and they enter the sclera posteriorly near the optic nerve at 6 and 12 o'clock.

153. T or F -- Bowman's membrane is the basement membrane of the corneal epithelium.

154. T or F -- Bowman's membrane is continuously produced throughout life.

155. T or F -- Descemet's membrane is the basement membrane of the corneal endothelium.

156. Match the structures, functions, or characteristics listed in the right column with their appropriate retinal layers listed on the left:

a. cell bodies whose processes project into the lateral geniculate and pretectal nuclei.
b. Müller cell bodies.
c. horizontal and bipolar cell synapses.
d. storage of dietary vitamin A.
e. cell bodies whose processes form spherules and pedicles.
f. high baseline cGMP levels and membrane depolarization.
g. amacrine and bipolar cell synapses.
h. flame-shaped retinal hemorrhages.

1. inner nuclear layer.
2. photoreceptor layer.
3. ganglion cell layer.
4. nerve fiber layer.
5. retinal pigment epithelium.
6 outer plexiform layer.
7. inner plexiform layer.
8. outer nuclear layer.

157. T or F -- Descemet's membrane is continuously produced throughout life.

158. T or F -- The capsule of the crystalline lens is the basement membrane of the lens epithelium.

159. The volume of the average human vitreous cavity is:

a. 1 ml.
b. 2 ml.
c. 4 ml.
d. 8 ml.
e. 12 ml.

160. The first retinal cells to differentiate to a recognizable level are:

a. photoreceptor cells.
b. bipolar cells.
c. ganglion cells.
d. Müller cells.
e. horizontal cells.

161. Which one of the following concerning photoreceptors is false?

a. Outer segment membranes are very rigid (semisolid).
b. The major protein isolated from rod outer segments is rhodopsin.
c. The chromophore for all the visual pigments is 11-*cis* retinaldehyde.
d. Differences in spectral absorption are due to different interactions between the chromophore and the protein (opsin) to which it is bound.
e. The four visual pigment proteins have considerable sequence homology, implying a common ancestry.

162. Which one of the following concerning photoreceptor dynamics is false?

a. Rods shed their outer segments shortly after dawn.
b. Steady, constant dark adaptation will ablate rod outer segment shedding.
c. Only the *cis* configuration of 11-retinaldehyde can initiate the light absorption cascade.
d. The first step in regeneration of the chromophore is the formation of all-*trans* retinol.
e. The chromophore is aligned parallel to the outer segment disc to enhance light capture.

163. Indirect-acting miotics (e.g., phospholine iodide) may dangerously increase systemic sensitivity to which of the following medications?

1. ester-type local anesthetics (tetracaine).
2. monoamine oxidase inhibitors.
3. depolarizing paralytic agents.
4. amide-type local anesthetics (lidocaine).

a. 1, 2, and 3.
b. 1 and 3.
c. 2 and 4.
d. 4 only.
e. 1, 2, 3, and 4.

164. Which one of the following concerning local anesthetics is false?

a. Amide-type agents are preferred to ester-type agents because of their longer duration of action and lower systemic toxicity.
b. Patients who are deficient in serum cholinesterase are susceptible to prolonged toxic effects of all local anesthetics.
c. Topical anesthetics disrupt intercellular tight junctions, resulting in increased epithelial permeability to topical agents that are subsequently administered.
d. Lidocaine is the agent of choice in conjunctival biopsy.
e. Proparacaine is the agent of choice for obtaining corneal cultures.

165. The cell most commonly used for karyotypic analysis is the:

a. erythryocyte.
b. platelet.
c. neutrophil.
d. B-lymphocyte.
e. T-lymphocyte.

166. T or F -- The short arm of any human chromosome is labeled "p" for the French word "petite."

28

167. What is the diameter of the human fovea?

    a. 0.5 mm (500 microns).
    b. 1.0 mm (1000 microns).
    c. 1.5 mm (1500 microns).
    d. 2.0 mm (2000 microns).
    e. 2.5 mm (2500 microns).

168. Which one of the following extraocular muscles is served by a contralateral brainstem subnucleus?

    a. superior rectus.
    b. medial rectus.
    c. inferior oblique.
    d. levator palpebrae superioris.
    e. inferior rectus.

Answers

1.   d.   The nasal bone lies medial to the orbit. The zygomatic, frontal, and ethmoid bones form parts of the lateral, superior, and medial bony orbit, respectively. The palatine bone forms a small portion of the posterior orbital floor.

2.   a.   Thirty cubic centimeters (cc, or ml for liquid measures) is approximately 2 tablespoons.

3.   d.   The orbital plate of the ethmoid bone composes most of the medial orbital wall. The lacrimal bone lies just anterior and forms part of the lacrimal sac fossa. The frontal and maxillary bones contribute to the superior and inferior medial orbit, respectively. The palatine bone forms part of the posterior orbital <u>floor</u>.

4.   b.   The lacrimal sac fossa is formed by the frontal process of the maxilla and the lacrimal bone. It cradles the lacrimal sac and is continuous with the nasolacrimal canal.

5.   a.   The lacrimal gland fossa lies in the anterolateral orbital roof within the zygomatic process of the frontal bone.

6.   c.   The lateral wall of the orbit is the thickest and strongest aspect of the bony orbit. It is formed by the zygoma and the greater wing of the sphenoid.

7.   e.   The lateral orbital tubercle of Whitnall is a small elevation in the orbital margin of the zygoma. It lies 11 mm below the frontal zygomatic suture. The tubercle is an important attachment site for all of the structures listed in question 7 except (ironically) Whitnall's ligament. This is a condensation of fascia in the superior orbit that inserts 10 mm <u>above</u> Whitnall's tubercle.

8.   d.   The central retinal artery arises from the ophthalmic artery <u>after</u> the latter passes through the optic canal. The central retinal artery then dives into the center of the optic nerve where it travels until it exits from the optic nerve head.

9.   d.   Approximately 1.2 million axons form a normal optic nerve. Each axon originates from the ganglion cell layer of the retina and extends to the lateral geniculate body. Fetal optic nerves contain a greater number, some of which regress by birth. Fewer axons may be a feature of certain optic nerve diseases (e.g., glaucoma).

10.   a.   The ophthalmic artery enters the orbit through the optic canal just inferior to the optic nerve. Within the orbit, it then courses lateral, superior, and finally medial to the optic nerve, until it forms the supraorbital, anterior, and posterior ethmoidal arteries.

11. e. The ciliary ganglion receives three roots:

1. A long sensory root that contains sensory fibers from the cornea, iris, and ciliary body. This root delivers sensation to the central nervous system (CNS) via the nasociliary nerve (V1).
2. A short motor root that carries preganglionic parasympathetic axons to the iris sphincter. This root arises from the lower division of the oculomotor nerve. These are the only fibers that synapse here.
3. A sympathetic root that innervates the blood vessels of the uvea. This root arises from a plexus around the internal carotid artery and passes through the optic foramen (with the ophthalmic artery).

12. True. All of the third-order sympathetic neurons to the eye begin in the superior cervical ganglion and travel along the internal carotid artery into the cavernous sinus. The pupillomotor fibers then join the ophthalmic division of the trigeminal nerve (V1), the nasociliary nerve, and, finally, the long ciliary nerves. The orbital and uveal vasomotor nerves and sympathetic nerves to the lacrimal gland and Müller's muscles enter the orbit with the ophthalmic artery, form the sympathetic root of the ciliary ganglion, and are distributed with the short ciliary nerves.

13. b. The accessory lacrimal glands are the glands of Krause and Wolfring, which produce primarily basal tear secretion. The meibomian glands can have aberrant cilia grow through their orifices in acquired and congenital distichiasis but normally have no associated appendages. The glands of Zeis are modified sebaceous glands associated with cilia.

14. False. The substance of the tarsus feels like cartilage but, microscopically, consists of densely packed type I collagen without hyalocytes.

15. False. The palpebral lobe is the smaller lobe and lies in the superolateral conjunctival fornix. (The larger orbital lobe does lie posterior to the smaller palpebral lobe.)

16. False. The canaliculi are lined with stratified, squamous epithelium. The lacrimal sac consists of a bilayer -- a superficial columnar layer and a deep, flattened layer.

17. c.

18. False. Mitosis of the endothelium rarely occurs. However, corneal endothelial cells will spread out and enlarge (polymegathism).

19. False. The sclera, like the cornea, is virtually avascular except for two areas: (1) the superficial vessels of the episclera, and (2) the intrascleral vascular plexus located immediately posterior to the limbus.

20. e.

21. d. The brunt of aqueous outflow passes through the posterior TM, accounting for its heavier pigmentation.

22. False. The trabecular meshwork consists of thin, perforated connective tissue sheets arranged in a sheet-like pattern. The connective tissue "beams" are lined by a monolayered endothelium.

23. e. Animal outflow studies have shown that the TM immediately proximal to Schlemm's canal (juxtacanalicular TM) is the limiting factor for outflow facility.

24. c.

25. d.

26. False. The anteroposterior lens diameter gradually increases throughout life as lens epithelial cells replicate and migrate centrally into the nucleus. An elderly person's lens is considerably thicker than a young person's lens.

27. True.

28. False. The anterior capsule is almost twice as thick as the posterior capsule and increases in thickness throughout life.

29. False. Only the posterior surface of the iris is covered by a continuous layer of cells. The anterior surface consists of (unlined) stroma.

30. False. The anterior layer of iris pigment is composed of myoepithelial cells. The posterior layer consists of pigmented cells with their basal surfaces oriented toward the posterior chamber. The anterior layer is continuous with retinal pigment epithelium (RPE), while the posterior layer is continuous with the neurosensory retina.

31. c. Parasympathetic fibers originate from the Edinger-Westphal subnucleus in the midbrain, follow the inferior division of the oculomotor nerve as it bifurcates in the cavernous sinus, continue with the branch supplying the inferior oblique muscle, and synapse in the ciliary ganglion. Postganglionic fibers are transmitted via the short ciliary nerves to the iris sphincter. Sympathetic fibers originate in the ipsilateral posterolateral hypothalamus and pass through the brain stem to synapse in the intermediolateral gray matter of the spinal cord between the levels of C8-T2 (ciliospinal center of Budge). The second-order neurons exit the spinal cord, pass over the lung apex, and synapse in the superior cervical ganglion. Third-order neurons travel with the internal carotid plexus, enter the cavernous sinus, and travel with the ophthalmic division of the trigeminal nerve to the orbit. Thereafter, the fibers travel within the nasociliary nerve and then the long ciliary nerves to the iris. (Whew!)

32. False. Fluorescein angiography demonstrates that the choriocapillaris is arranged in a lobular pattern, especially in the posterior pole. Functionally, the choriocapillaris is an end-arteriole system.

33. False. It is primarily dependent on the number of pigmented melanocytes in the choroid. RPE pigmentation contributes to a lesser degree.

34. False. RPE cells in foveal area are taller, more closely packed, and have more and larger melanosomes, contributing to decreased fluorescence of this area during fluorescein angiography.

35. False. In the human infant eye, approximately 4 to 6 million RPE cells are present. Although the surface area of the eye increases, only a small increase in the number of RPE cells occurs, and mitotic figures are not usually observed. In disease states, however, the RPE may become actively mitotic (hyperplastic).

36. d.   Rods and cones are characterized by three components: synaptic body, inner segment, and outer segment. The synaptic body of a rod is called a spherule, whereas that of the cone is called a pedicle. Rod discs are not attached to the cell membrane, but cone discs are continuous with it.

37. b.   Intraretinal processing occurs from photoreceptors to bipolar cells to ganglion cells with modulation by horizontal (outer plexiform layer) and amacrine (inner plexiform layer) cells.

38. d.   Approximately 120 million rods and 6 million cones interact with 1.2 million ganglion cells in an eye. Therefore, the ratio of rods to cones is approximately 20:1. (Some studies cite a ratio as low as 12:1.)

39. e.   The external limiting membrane (ELM) is highly fenestrated and composed of attachment sites of adjacent photoreceptors and Müller cells. The internal limiting membrane (ILM) is formed by footplates of Müller cells and attachments to the basal lamina of retinal astrocytes. Neither "membrane" should be thought of as a true basement membrane.

40. b.   A cilioretinal artery contributes to the vascular supply of the retina in approximately 50% of individuals and 30% of eyes. Also, in 15% of individuals, it contributes to macular circulation.

41. c.   Retinal blood vessels usually do not extend beyond the inner third of the inner nuclear layer.

42. b.   The outer plexiform layer is composed of interconnections between photoreceptor synaptic bodies, horizontal, and bipolar cells. The inner plexiform layer is composed of connections between bipolar cells, amacrine cells, and ganglion cells.

43. a.   The ora serrata is an anatomic landmark for retinal topography but has no significance regarding uveoscleral anatomy.

44. b.   The distance from the ora serrata to Schwalbe's line varies from 5.75 mm nasally to 6.50 mm inferotemporally. (This is where vitrectomy infusion ports are placed.)

45. False.   The ora is smooth temporally but appears serrated nasally.

46. False.   Normally, axons of ganglion cells do not become myelinated until after they pass through lamina cribrosa, as part of the intraorbital optic nerve. When myelinated fibers are visible ophthalmoscopically, oligodendroglia have migrated anteriorly.

47. b.   After exiting the optic foramen, the optic nerve is bounded by the anterior cerebral artery superiorly, the internal carotid artery laterally, and the ophthalmic artery inferiorly.

48. a.   Approximately 53% of optic nerve fibers are crossed and 47% uncrossed.

49. d. Only the levator is served by a single subnucleus. It sits dorsal, central, and at the inferior end of the group of subnuclei that compose the two third cranial nerve nuclei. The superior recti have two subnuclei, each controlling the <u>contralateral</u> nerve. In contrast, the inferior obliques and the medial recti each have individual subnuclei that control the <u>ipsilateral</u> nerves. The superior oblique is served by the fourth nerve.

50. a. See answer 49.

51. d. The pupillomotor fibers of the third cranial nerve run in the inferior division, which carries them to the ciliary ganglion. They are among the axons in the periphery of the nerve, making them easily susceptible to compression.

52. True. The fifth cranial nerve is responsible for facial sensation and supplies motor fibers to the muscles of mastication (temporalis, masseter, pterygoids), as well as the tensor veli palatini, tensor tympani, anterior belly of the digastric, and mylohyoid muscles.

53. d. The third, fourth, and fifth cranial nerves travel within the walls of the cavernous sinus. The sixth nerve and the internal carotid artery travel through the sinus itself, and are thus more susceptible to injury by sinus lesions, such as meningioma and aneurysm.

54. False. While ocular colobomas do form as the result of failure of optic cup fusion, they most commonly are found in an inferior and somewhat nasal location. Normal fusion usually starts near the equator and runs anteriorly and posteriorly.

55. True. The production of melanin in the developing retinal pigment epithelium starts at the posterior pole and progresses anteriorly, usually reaching completion by the sixth week of embryonic development. This is the first melanin production known to take place in the body.

56. False. Some studies have documented completion of myelination by as early as 36 weeks' gestation. By 1 month postpartum, myelination is almost always complete (although sheaths may thicken with time).

57. False. The lens is derived from surface ectoderm.

58. e. Neural crest cells and mesoderm both contribute to the mesenchymal structures of the head. (Mesenchyme is the embryonic tissue that gives rise to connective tissue.) The stroma of the iris and the muscular layer of orbital vessels are examples of neural crest contributions. The endothelium of those same vessels is of mesodermal origin.

59. e. Neural crest gives rise to ciliary musculature, corneal stroma, endothelium (but <u>not</u> epithelium), most of the sclera (excepting a temporal portion, of mesodermal origin), choroidal stroma, some of the orbital bones, orbital cartilage, orbital connective tissue, nerve sheaths, and uveal melanocytes.

60. d. Blood vessel endothelia, extraocular muscles, and temporal sclera are all mesodermal in origin. The pupillomotor muscles are neuroectodermal in orgin.

61. e. Conjunctival epithelium is derived from surface ectoderm, but the substantia propria is derived from neural crest.

62. False. The primary vitreous is actually displaced centrally to become Cloquet's canal.

63. b.   Anophthalmia is the absence of an identifiable eye. Microphthalmia describes the presence of a small, disorganized eye. In nanophthalmia, the eye is smaller than normal, but otherwise unremarkable.

64. d.   See answer 63.

65. d.   Nanophthalmos is, by definition, a small, but otherwise normal eye. Cysts are not seen in association with it.

66. a.   Dermoids are choristomas, that is, normal cells and/or tissue present in abnormal locations.

67. e.   In Peter's anomaly, the central cornea is always opacified because of the central defect in Descemet's membrane and the absence of endothelium. The lens may be adherent to the cornea, but this is not always seen.

68. a.   There is nearly always some rudimentary iris tissue present, although it may be difficult to see clinically. Sporadic aniridia is associated with Wilms' tumor, but aniridia is not found in patients with autosomal dominant Wilms' tumor. When aniridia is associated with mental retardation, Wilms' tumor, ambiguous genitalia, or other genitourinary anomalies, there is usually a small deletion in the short arm of chromosome 11 (11p minus).

69. c.   Patients with Marfan's syndrome are usually tall and lean, in contrast to patients with Weill-Marchesani syndrome who are short and stocky. Lowe's syndrome is inherited in an X-linked fashion and is thus found almost exclusively in men. Any organ in the body may be damaged by rubella, and the rubella syndrome is characterized by the triad of cataracts, deafness, and cardiac defects. Juvenile glaucoma and cataract rarely coincide with congenital rubella infection.

70. b.   The visual prognosis in PHPV is poor. An eye with leukocoria that is small is unlikely to harbor retinoblastoma. Likewise, retinoblastoma does not typically cause cataract.

71. c.   The glands of Krause and Wolfring, which produce the basal tear secretion, are not innervated. The lacrimal gland is responsible for reflex tear secretion and receives both sympathetic and parasympathetic innervation.

72. c.   Aqueous humor provides the majority of the glucose needed by the endothelium, stroma, and epithelium. Hydrophobic molecules penetrate the epithelium most easily, while hydrophilic molecules penetrate stroma more easily.

73. d.   Endothelial cells do not divide. As endothelial cells are damaged or die, the number of endothelial cells on a given cornea decreases, and the cells enlarge and spread out.

74. e.   Diffusion, ultrafiltration, and active secretion all occur at the ciliary processes. The majority of aqueous appears to be produced by active, energy-dependent secretion from the inner, nonpigmented ciliary epithelium.

75. b.   Topical administration of type E and F prostaglandins, as well as arachidonic acid causes miosis. High doses of prostaglandins will cause an increase in intraocular pressure. Low doses of some prostaglandins, in contrast, appear to lower intraocular pressure in some animal species. By blocking phospholipase, corticosteroids effectively inhibit both the lipoxygenase and cyclooxygenase pathways.

76. a. 3.
    b. 3.
    c. 2.
    d. 3.
    e. 1.
    f. 1.
    g. 2.

77. a.   Carbonic anhydrase, although present in only trace amounts in the aqueous, has a high enough turnover that it is felt to be functionally significant. Hyaluronidase is present in aqueous and may participate in regulation of resistance to aqueous outflow. Lysozyme is present and may function bacteriocidally. Lactate dehydrogenase, not normally detectable in aqueous, may be a marker for retinoblastoma.

78. b.   This is approximately one-third the concentration found in the earth's atmosphere and is entirely derived from anterior chamber blood flow.

79. d.   Lens epithelial cells are located anteriorly underneath the lens capsule. Epithelial cells in a ring around the anterior lens, or the germinative zone, exhibit the highest level of DNA synthesis. Newly formed cells migrate toward the lens equator, where they differentiate into lens fiber cells.

80. b.   The water-<u>soluble</u> proteins are divided into three types of crystallins that are fractionated into four electrophoretic groups. Alpha crystallins are the largest, with molecular weights over 500,000 daltons. Beta crystallins are the most abundant, making up about 55% of the water-soluble protein. Gamma crystallins are the smallest.

81. True. Na^+/K^+-dependent ATPases move sodium from posterior to anterior and potassium from anterior to posterior.

82. True.   Unlike the retina, the lens can function without oxygen, but not without glucose.

83. False.   See answer 82.

84. c.   When focal collagen concentration drops, vitreous becomes more liquid and collapses.

85. a.   In aphakia, the concentration of hyaluronate drops. In diabetes mellitus, the amount of vitreous collagen is low. Only in myopia are both substances present at abnormally low levels.

86. True.   When bleeding occurs in a region of formed vitreous, a smaller, tighter clot that is more resistant to degradation is formed. In liquid vitreous, blood disperses and is cleared quickly.

87. True.   Vitamin A, stored hepatically, is transported in serum as all-*trans* retinol.

88. True.   Conversion between aldehyde and alcohol (and vice versa) occurs in the photoreceptors, while the *trans* to *cis* conversion takes place in the RPE.

89. True.   The final step is isomerization of 11-*cis* retinol to 11-*cis* retinaldehyde.

90. e. Photoreceptors are more active electrically (depolarized) in the dark! With light absorption, transducin (via PDE) lowers cGMP, which <u>hyper</u>polarizes the cell and <u>decreases</u> synaptic exchange with bipolar cells.

91. False. The retina is strictly oxygen dependent (unlike the lens; see answer 82).

92. a. Adding a second drop will increase systemic absorption as well. Local anesthetic disrupts corneal epithelial barrier functions, enhancing local uptake.

93. c. pH extremes trigger reflex tearing, with subsequent dilution of the drug. Benzalkonium chloride, like local anesthetics, disrupts the corneal epithelium.

94. d. <u>Adrenergic</u> receptors are found in the cell membranes of the iris dilator muscle. Nicotinic cholinergic receptors mediate extraocular muscle contraction. Muscarinic receptors mediate autonomic responses (accommodation, secretions).

95. False. Although relative pupillary block may be diminished, ciliary body contraction "opens" the trabecular meshwork by pulling on the scleral spur, thus increasing outflow.

96. e. Miosis and induced <u>myopia</u> are generally problematic in younger patients. In the elderly, aggravation of cataractous visual loss may be important.

97. 1. c (1-2 weeks).
     2. e (1 week).
     3. a (1-3 days).
     4. b (12-24 hours).
     5. d (2-4 hours).

98. True. Cocaine blocks the reuptake of norepinephrine into presynaptic vesicles. This will cause the secondary accumulation of norephinephrine, resulting in pupillary dilation. In Horner's syndrome, there is less neurotransmitter release, less accumulation, and thus less dilation. Hydroxyamphetamine (Paredrine) causes release of norepinephrine and results in dilation. If the lesion is postganglionic, there will be less norepinephrine and less dilation. If the lesion is preganglionic, there will be normal or supranormal dilation (if there is upregulation of receptors) because the postganglionic fibers synthesize and store norepinephrine in a normal fashion.

99. a. Side effects of apraclonidine (Iopidine) that have been reported include lid retraction, conjunctival <u>blanching</u>, mydriasis, lethargy, xerostomia, and allergic reactions. The first three are directly attributable to its adrenergic activity.

100. c. Beta-adrenergic agonists (e.g., epinephrine) are thought to decrease intraocular pressure, despite their tendency to <u>increase</u> aqueous humor production, by increasing uveoscleral outflow.

101. True. Timolol maleate decreases intraocular pressure by reducing aqueous humor production via cyclic adenosine monophosphate mediated mechanisms. Apraclonidine is thought to decrease intraocular pressure by inhibiting aqueous humor secretion through the same cAMP final common pathway.

102. c. Dipivalyl epinephrine is a prodrug of epinephrine that contains two pivalyl residues. Epinephrine is released into the anterior chamber when the pivalyl groups are cleaved by corneal esterases.

103. c.   Since epinephrine has been associated with a reversible cystoid maculopathy (approximately 25% of chronically treated aphakic eyes), both epinephrine and the prodrug dipivefrin would be relatively contraindicated in this case. Furthermore, alpha agonists (epinephrine is an alpha and beta-agonist) are contraindicated in patients who may have an abnormally increased sensitivity to their cardiovascular effects due to the use of drugs such as MAO inhibitors, tricylic antidepressants, cocaine or reserpine. In general, depression may be a side effect of beta blockers and a relative contraindication to acetazolamide therapy. Thus, the best single alternative drug in this case would be pilocarpine.

104. False.   Clinically, carbonic anhydrase must be more than 99% inhibited to decrease aqueous humor secretion significantly.

105. False.   Unlike acetazolamide, methazolamide is not actively secreted into the renal tubules, and metabolic acidosis is less pronounced. It is also less effective for reducing intraocular pressure.

106. a.   A remote history of spontaneous nephrolithiasis (> 5 years earlier) is not thought to be a contraindication for starting CAI therapy. Recent stones (< 5 years earlier) may be. CAIs potentiate hepatic encephalopathy and the potassium-wasting effects of thiazides. Sensitivity to digoxin is increased by hypokalemia. Psychiatric disturbances may also be exacerbated by CAIs.

107. d.   At the tissue level, glucocorticoids suppress early inflammatory responses such as local vascular congestion, edema, and hyperthermia as well as late inflammatory responses such as capillary and fibroblast proliferation and deposition of collagen. Glucocorticoids do not affect immunoglobulin titers or the afferent limb of cell-mediated immunity, nor do they significantly deter epithelial healing (stromal healing and collagen synthesis are affected).

108. False.   Late steroid-induced intraocular pressure rises are common, and intraocular pressure should be monitored during the entire course of therapy.

109. False.   Aspirin causes inhibition of cyclo-oxygenase, and thus arachidonic acid is diverted to the lipoxygenase pathway. This is thought to be the underlying mechanism for the asthma attacks and hypersensitivity reactions (via increased production of leukotrienes).

110. False.   Cromolyn sodium has no direct antihistaminic effect (receptor blockade) and can only be effective if used prophylactically.

111. d.   Probenecid competitively inhibits penicillin excretion by the kidney.

112. 1. a.
    2. d.
    3. b.
    4. c.

113. c.   Approximately 10% of patients with a history of a hypersensitivity reaction to penicillin will have cross-reactivity to the cephalosporins.

114. d.   Sulfonamides indirectly inhibit bacterial DNA synthesis by blocking the synthesis of folic acid (folic acid is a cofactor in nucleic acid synthesis). Only <u>aerobic</u> bacteria are susceptible to aminoglycosides. Anaerobic organisms are resistant because the mechanism by which the drugs are taken up by microorganisms is driven by aerobic metabolism.

115. d.   The most important clinical cause of acquired bacterial resistance to aminoglycosides is the production of microbial enzymes that inactivate the drug. These enzymes are genetically transmitted by bacterial plasmids. Of the aminoglycosides, amikacin is the least sensitive to inactivation by this mechanism.

116. e.   Hypersensitivity reactions may occur following topical administration of any of the aminoglycosides but occur most frequently with neomycin. Such reactions occur in 6 to 8% of patients. Other important adverse reactions common to aminoglycosides include ototoxicity and nephrotoxicity.

117. b.   Vancomycin acts by the inhibition of cell wall synthesis. It is primarily active against gram-positive bacteria including methicillin-resistant strains of *Staphylococcus*. It is not considered to be bactericidal against *Streptococcus faecalis* but is effective against this species in combination with gentamicin.

118. d.   Trifluridine and idoxuridine are thymidine analogs, while vidarabine is an adenine analog. All of these agents inhibit DNA synthesis and are effective in treating herpes simplex. Trifluridine is more effective than the other two. Cross-resistance to these agents has not yet been seen.

119. e.   Since the phenotypic expression of trisomy 13 (Patau's syndrome) is caused by presence of three copies of a portion of the long arm of chromosome 13, the syndrome can be caused by trisomy of the entire chromosome or any portion that includes the segment from 13q14 to the q terminus.

120. b.   There is slightly higher mortality in trisomy 13 than in trisomy 18. About 75% of babies with trisomy 13 die by 6 months of age, while about 50% of babies with trisomy 18 die by that age.

121. d.   Serum purine levels in Down's syndrome patients are typically <u>elevated</u>. The enzymes required for the biosynthesis of purines are coded by genes present on the long arm of chromosome 21. The presence of a third set of these genes presumably results in the elevation of serum purine levels.

122. c.   Turner's syndrome is caused by monosomy of the X chromosome in all cells, monosomy X mosaicism, or structural abnormalities of the X chromosome. Approximately 60% of affected individuals have monosomy X in all body cells. The absence of a second X chromosome can result in the full expression of X-linked recessive disorders with the same frequency as that found in normal <u>men</u>.

123. d.   Individuals with genotype 47XXY have the phenotype known as Klinefelter's syndrome. This is caused by meiotic nondisjunction of the two X chromosomes in oogenesis and has been associated with increased <u>maternal</u> age.

124. a.   Although neurofibromatosis (von Recklinghausen's disease) has been associated with increased paternal age, no association with chromosome fragility has been observed.

125. e.   Hereditary retinoblastoma, part of the long-arm 13 deletion syndrome, is inherited as an autosomal dominant trait, as determined by pedigree analysis. The inherited factor is actually the <u>absence</u> of a functional gene at the 13q14 locus. Both genes at this locus must be dysfunctional to permit tumorogenesis; thus, the trait is recessive at the cellular level. Since the first "hit" is inherited, only one postfertilization hit is required for tumorogenesis in hereditary retinoblastoma. The natural de novo mutation rate is high enough, however, that the probability that at least one retinal precursor cell will take a second hit during development is very high. Still, penetrance is incomplete (80%). Thus offspring of a carrier have a <u>40%</u> chance of developing a tumor (80% of 50%).

126. d.   Sporadic aniridia (i.e., nonfamilial), often associated with glaucoma or cataract, can be caused by a new deletion of an interstitial segment of chromosome 11 (11p13). This deletion also results in genitourinary malformations (which may be <u>subtle in females</u>), mental retardation, and Wilms' tumor. Hereditary aniridia can occur with autosomal dominant or autosomal recessive inheritance patterns and is associated with other ocular anomalies including nystagmus, cataract, glaucoma, corneal abnormalities, and hypoplasia of the optic nerve. Examination of family members may differentiate sporadic from hereditary aniridia. Chromosome analysis is also helpful. Intravenous pyelography (IVP) is probably more sensitive than CT scanning for early detection of Wilms' tumor.

127. e.   The expression of multiple discrete anomalies in various organs caused by a single gene mutation is termed genetic pleiotropism. Alterations in the connective tissues throughout the body result in the characteristic manifestations of Marfan's syndrome.

128. c.   Oguchi's disease, a form of congenital stationary night blindness, is seen primarily in Japanese individuals.

129. d.   The mean ± 2 standard deviations includes approximately 95% of observations. The mean ± 3 standard deviations includes greater than 99% of observations.

130. e.   The power of a statistical test is a measure of its ability to detect a difference between the treatment and control groups when a true difference exists. The power is defined as 1 - (type 2 error). The power of a statistical test to detect a difference between the groups in a clinical trial is increased by a larger sample size and by a greater actual difference caused by the intervention.

131. b.   The infraorbital nerve is a branch of the maxillary division of the trigeminal nerve, carrying sensory fibers from the cheek. It enters the orbit via the infraorbital foramen and exits through the inferior orbital fissure. The nerve from the pterygopalatine ganglion, carrying post-ganglionic secretory fibers for the lacrimal gland, is also transmitted through the inferior orbital fissure. The inferior division of the oculomotor nerve, as well as the superior ophthalmic vein, enter the orbit through the superior orbital fissure.

132. c.   The orbital floor is formed by the zygomatic, maxillary, and palatine bones. The sphenoid contributes to the orbital roof, while the ethmoid contributes to the medial wall of the orbit.

133. a. 2.
    b. 1.
    c. 4.
    d. 1.
    e. 3.
    f. 2.
    g. 1.

134. d.   The iris sphincter receives parasympathetic innervation via the inferior division of the oculomotor nerve. The inferior rectus is also supplied by the inferior division. The iris dilator is supplied by sympathetic fibers running with the nasociliary and long ciliary nerves, branches of the first division of the trigeminal nerve.

135. True.   The oculomotor nerve supplies the levator palpebrae superioris, and interruption of this supply results in profound ptosis.

136. False.   Müller's muscle is sympathetically innervated and provides 2 to 3 mm of eyelid "lift." Thus, ptosis associated with Horner's syndrome is typically mild.

137. b.   See answer 134.

138. a.   The orbicularis oculi muscle, responsible for reflex as well as willful eyelid closure, is supplied by the facial (VII) nerve. The fifth cranial nerve is responsible for facial sensation and supplies motor fibers to the muscles of mastication (temporalis, masseter, pterygoids), as well as the tensor veli palatini, tensor tympani, anterior belly of the digastric, and mylohyoid muscles.

139. False.   Parasympathetic secretory innervation to the lacrimal gland originates in the superior salivatory nucleus (pons) and travels within the nervus intermedius as part of the facial nerve. After branching off as the greater superficial petrosal nerve within the fallopian canal, they synapse at the pterygopalatine ganglion. Postganglionic fibers run superiorly into the orbit through the inferior orbital fissure, joining the zygomaticotemporal nerve. A branch of this nerve then runs into the lacrimal gland to stimulate reflex tearing.

140. c.   See answer 134.

141. a. 3.
    b. 1.
    c. 4.
    d. 2.

142. d.   The inferior oblique is unique among the seven extraocular muscles in its anterior anatomic origin (from the orbital floor, just posterolateral to the lacrimal sac fossa).

143. c.   While the superior oblique has its anatomic origin at the orbital apex, it acts mechanically as if its origin were at the trochlea. Thus, like the inferior oblique, the superior oblique generates a "pull" that is directed toward the front of the orbit.

144. c.   The ophthalmic artery travels within the optic foramen.

145. c.   The lacrimal, frontal, and trochlear nerves all enter outside the annulus of Zinn. The nasociliary, oculomotor, and abducens nerves enter through the annulus.

146. b.　Because it is the only extraocular motor nerve to enter the orbit outside the muscle cone, the trochlear nerve is the last to be affected by an appropriately administered retrobulbar block.

147. d.　Each of the rectus muscles, except the lateral, receives branches from two anterior ciliary arteries. The lateral rectus receives one. Thus, there are a total of seven anterior ciliary arteries.

148. False.　The anterior ciliary arteries supply the rectus muscles and then continue on, terminating anteriorly in the major arterial circle of the iris.

149. False.　Motor units, defined as one terminal motor nerve branch and all the muscle fibers it serves, are smaller in the extraocular muscles than anywhere else in the body. This permits the finest control of force generation and muscle action possible.

150. c.　The capsulopalpebral fascia is a condensation of noncontractile fascia from the sheaths of the inferior oblique and inferior rectus muscles. Like the aponeurosis of the levator muscle, it retracts the tarsus.

151. b.　Lockwood's ligament is a condensation of connective tissue in the inferior orbit and acts as a "sling" for the globe.

152. a.　There are 10 to 12 short posterior ciliary arteries, which enter the sclera in a circle around the optic nerve. There are 7 anterior ciliary arteries, which provide muscular feeding branches and terminate in the major arterial circle of the iris.

153. False.　Bowman's "membrane" is an acellular condensation of corneal stroma immediately beneath the basement membrane of the corneal epithelium. The term Bowman's zone is more appropriate.

154. False.　Once violated or destroyed by inflammatory pannus, Bowman's zone is permanently disturbed, leaving a corneal scar.

155. True.

156. a. 3.　Note that the outer plexiform layer is the region of photoreceptor-bipolar
　　b. 1.　synapses as well as bipolar-horizontal interactions. The inner plexiform
　　c. 6.　layer is the region of bipolar-ganglion cell synapses, as well as bipolar-amacrine
　　d. 5.　interactions.
　　e. 8.
　　f. 2.
　　g. 7.
　　h. 4.

157. True.　Descemet's membrane becomes progressively thickened with age and with endothelial disease states.

158. True.

159. c.　This is about the same as 1 teaspoon.

160. c.

161. a.   The consistency of rod outer segments is more liquid, like olive oil. Spectral absorption peaks reflect different opsin structures and, subsequently, different interactions with the chromophore, which is 11-*cis* retinaldehyde for all photoreceptors.

162. b.   Rod outer segment shedding in animal models will persist even after several days in the dark. On the contrary, dark <u>deprivation</u> (i.e., constant light adaptation) will rapidly ablate normal rod disc shedding.

163. b.   Systemic anesthetic toxicity can be seen with coadministration of indirect miotics and ester-type local anesthetics. This occurs because ester-type anesthetics are inactivated systemically by serum cholinesterase, which is blocked by the indirect miotics. Amide anesthetics are hepatically inactivated and, thus, are not affected. Inactivation of systemic muscular depolarizing agents also depends on serum cholinesterase activity. Prolonged paralysis can result from coadministration with indirect miotics.

164. b.   Ester-type anesthetics generate hypersensitivity reactions more commonly than amide types. Patients with congenital or iatrogenic (indirect miotics, pesticides) cholinesterase deficiencies will only have difficulty with the ester class of anesthetics, since the amide types are hepatically inactivated.

165. e.

166. True.   (True trivia.)

167. c.   Note that the diameter of the fovea and that of the optic nerve head are roughly equal.

168. a.   Thus, nuclear third nerve palsy may feature contralateral upgaze palsy!

References

1. Moses, Robert A., and Hart, William M. (eds.). <u>Adler's Physiology of the Eye</u> (8th ed.). St. Louis: C.V. Mosby Company, 1987.

2. Newell, Frank W. <u>Ophthalmology: Principles and Concepts</u> (6th ed.). St. Louis: C.V. Mosby Company, 1986.

3. Weingeist, Thomas. "Section 2: Fundamentals and Principles of Ophthalmology." in F.M.Wilson (ed.). <u>Basic and Clinical Science Course</u>. San Francisco: American Academy of Ophthalmology, 1991-1992.

2: Optics and Refraction

1. Which of the following regarding the wave properties of light is/are true?

    1. Light energy is proportional to its wavelength.
    2. When light enters a medium of higher index of refraction, it slows down.
    3. When light enters a medium of higher index of refraction, its frequency diminishes.
    4. The index of refraction of any material varies with the wavelength of incident light.

    a. 1, 2, and 3.
    b. 1 and 3.
    c. 2 and 4.
    d. 4 only.
    e. 1, 2, 3, and 4.

2. T or F -- A photon of blue light has greater energy than a photon of red light.

3. The laser interferometer utilizes the principles of:

    1. constructive interference.
    2. destructive interference.
    3. high coherence.
    4. low coherence.

    a. 1, 2, and 3.
    b. 1 and 3.
    c. 2 and 4.
    d. 4 only.
    e. 1, 2, 3, and 4.

4. The Haidinger brush phenomenon is due to which special characteristic of light transmission?

    a. interference.
    b. polarization.
    c. diffraction.
    d. scattering.
    e. reflection.

5. Which of the following concerning diffraction is/are true?

   1. It is responsible for a limit on pinhole acuity of approximately 20/25.
   2. It is a limiting factor for visual acuity with pupils smaller than about 2 mm.
   3. Long wavelengths are diffracted more than short wavelengths.
   4. Diffraction is responsible for the blue color of the sky.

   a. 1, 2, and 3.
   b. 1 and 3.
   c. 2 and 4.
   d. 4 only.
   e. 1, 2, 3, and 4.

6. The features of laser light that enhance its intensity or brightness include:

   1. directionality.
   2. coherence.
   3. polarization.
   4. polychromaticity.

   a. 1, 2, and 3.
   b. 1 and 3.
   c. 2 and 4.
   d. 4 only.
   e. 1, 2, 3, and 4.

7. T or F -- The material for which each laser is named corresponds to the substance that is actually emitting the amplified light.

8. Which of the following are means of increasing laser power per delivery?

   1. increasing energy per delivery.
   2. Q-switching.
   3. mode locking.
   4. increasing time of exposure at a set energy.

   a. 1, 2, and 3.
   b. 1 and 3.
   c. 2 and 4.
   d. 4 only.
   e. 1, 2, 3, and 4.

9. Which of the following concerning refraction of light at interfaces is/are true?

     1. Light will bend toward the normal as it enters a medium of higher index of refraction.
     2. The index of refraction of any given substance is greater for longer wavelengths.
     3. Total internal reflection renders the anterior chamber angle invisible by a slit lamp.
     4. Tight traversing a plane parallel plate at any incident angle is not refracted.

   a. 1, 2, and 3.
   b. 1 and 3.
   c. 2 and 4.
   d. 4 only.
   e. 1, 2, 3, and 4.

10. T or F -- The minimum angle of deviation produced by a prism occurs when incident light strikes the prism perpendicular to its anterior face.

11. Which of the following concerning prisms and their units and calibration is/are true?

     1. The power in prism diopters is the number of centimeters light is displaced for every centimeter the light travels.
     2. Glass prisms are calibrated while held in the angle of minimum deviation.
     3. The Prentice position may be most closely approximated by placing a prism in the frontal plane.
     4. Real images created by prisms are deviated toward the prism base.

   a. 1, 2, and 3.
   b. 1 and 3.
   c. 2 and 4.
   d. 4 only.
   e. 1, 2, 3, and 4.

12. T or F -- Any real image can be focused on a screen or photographic film.

13. Which of the following concerning linear magnification is/are true?

> 1. Magnification is equal to the ratio of object size to image size.
> 2. A magnification value less than zero implies inversion of the image relative to the object.
> 3. Magnification is equal to the image vergence divided by the object vergence.
> 4. A magnification value less than one implies that the image is smaller than the object.

a. 1, 2, and 3.
b. 1 and 3.
c. 2 and 4.
d. 4 only.
e. 1, 2, 3, and 4.

14. T or F -- For media other than air, the reduced vergence is less than the vergence.

15. If the average eye's power is 60 D, and its average (internal) index of refraction is 1.33, what is its approximate primary focal length in air?

a. 17 cm.
b. 17 mm.
c. 22 cm.
d. 22 mm.
e. none of the above.

16. What is this average eye's approximate secondary focal length?

a. 17 cm.
b. 17 mm.
c. 22 cm.
d. 22 mm.
e. none of the above.

17. In a thick lens, refraction may be considered to take place at the:

> 1. primary focal plane.
> 2. primary principal plane.
> 3. secondary focal plane.
> 4. secondary principal plane.

a. 1, 2, and 3.
b. 1 and 3.
c. 2 and 4.
d. 4 only.
e. 1, 2, 3, and 4.

18. Which of the following concerning the cardinal planes of a thick lens is/are true?

 1. In optical systems with the same refractive medium on both sides, the nodal points and principal points coincide.
 2. If the media on either side have different indices of refraction, the nodal points are displaced toward the medium with the higher index of refraction.
 3. In the human eye, the principal planes may be considered to be superimposed.
 4. In the human eye, the nodal points may be considered to be superimposed.

 a. 1, 2, and 3.
 b. 1 and 3.
 c. 2 and 4.
 d. 4 only.
 e. 1, 2, 3, and 4.

19. T or F -- The absolute value of the back vertex power of a meniscus spectacle lens is always greater than that of the front vertex power.

20. The angular magnification of a retinal image afforded by direct ophthalmoscopy in an emmetrope is approximately:

 a. 5X.
 b. 10X.
 c. 15X.
 d. 20X.
 e. 25X.

21. Which of the following concerning surgical loupes and telescopic low-vision aids is/are true?

 1. These devices are basically small astronomic telescopes.
 2. These devices generally feature an "add" lens.
 3. The total magnification of any loupe is equal to the power of the eyepiece divided by the power of the objective.
 4. Image size is determined in part by the working distance of the loupes.

 a. 1, 2, and 3.
 b. 1 and 3.
 c. 2 and 4.
 d. 4 only.
 e. 1, 2, 3, and 4.

22. Which of the following concerning optical aberrations of spherical lenses is/are true?

1. The cornea's steeper peripheral curvature tends to counteract spherical aberration.
2. The typical interval of chromatic aberration in the human eye is approximately 2.5 D.
3. Tilting a lens along the horizontal axis will induce sphere of the same sign and cylinder of opposite sign along that axis.
4. In an emmetrope, blue light is focused more anterior to the retina than red light is focused posterior to it.

   a. 1, 2, and 3.
   b. 1 and 3.
   c. 2 and 4.
   d. 4 only.
   e. 1, 2, 3, and 4.

23. T or F -- The image perceived when looking through a Maddox rod is virtual and perpendicular to the real image formed by the rod.

24. If a point source of light is placed a great distance to the left of a +2.00 +2.00 x 180 lens, what shape will an image located 37.5 cm to the right of the lens have?

   a. a vertical line.
   b. a vertical oval.
   c. a circle.
   d. a horizontal oval.
   e. a horizontal line.

25. Which of the following is/are cross-cylinders?

1. +0.50 x 90, +0.50 x 180.
2. +1.00 -0.50 x 90.
3. +0.50 -0.50 x 180.
4. +0.50 -1.00 x 90.

   a. 1, 2, and 3.
   b. 1 and 3.
   c. 2 and 4.
   d. 4 only.
   e. 1, 2, 3, and 4.

26. T or F -- The field of view for an observer looking at a plane mirror may be increased by backing away from the mirror.

27. A patient with a corneal scar is carefully refracted. Best corrected acuity is 20/40. With a pinhole over his correction, his acuity improves to 20/25. The best explanation for this is:

   a. spherical aberration.
   b. myopic astigmatism.
   c. cataract.
   d. irregular astigmatism.
   e. malingering.

28. Vernier acuity is important in taking measurements with which of the following ophthalmic instruments?

   1. keratometry.
   2. lensometry.
   3. applanation tonometry.
   4. automated refractors.

   a. 1, 2, and 3.
   b. 1 and 3.
   c. 2 and 4.
   d. 4 only.
   e. 1, 2, 3, and 4.

29. In each of the following situations, which of the following pairs represent(s) conjugate planes?

   1. Indirect ophthalmoscopy: the patient's retina and the observer's retina.
   2. The uncorrected nonaccommodating ametrope: the retina and the far point of the eye.
   3. Neutralization in retinoscopy: the patient's retina and the peephole of the retinoscope.
   4. Indirect ophthalmoscopy: the patient's pupil and the examiner's pupils.

   a. 1, 2, and 3.
   b. 1 and 3.
   c. 2 and 4.
   d. 4 only.
   e. 1, 2, 3, and 4.

30. T or F -- The binocular amplitude of accommodation is generally the same as the monocular amplitude of accommodation.

31. T or F -- The duration of the mydriatic effect of cycloplegic agents is generally greater than that of the cycloplegic effect.

32. The accommodative amplitude of a 60-year-old healthy person is approximately:

    a. 14.0 D.
    b. 10.0 D.
    c. 6.0 D.
    d. 1.5 D.
    e. 0.5 D.

33. In a group of healthy American adults, the average refractive error is approximately:

    a. -1.00 D.
    b. -0.50 D.
    c. plano.
    d. +0.50 D.
    e. +1.00 D.

34. Methods of reducing cylinder-induced distortion and asthenopia include:

    1. plus cylinder lenses.
    2. minimizing vertex distance.
    3. use of Jackson cross-cylinders of lowest possible power.
    4. rotation of the cylinder axis toward 90 or 180 degrees.

    a. 1, 2, and 3.
    b. 1 and 3.
    c. 2 and 4.
    d. 4 only.
    e. 1, 2, 3, and 4.

35. Which of the following is/are problems with aphakic spectacle lenses?

    1. barrel distortion.
    2. ring scotoma.
    3. image minification.
    4. jack-in-the-box phenomenon.

    a. 1, 2, and 3.
    b. 1 and 3.
    c. 2 and 4.
    d. 4 only.
    e. 1, 2, 3, and 4.

36. T or F --Posterior chamber intraocular lenses (IOLs) cause no image magnification.

37. A patient undergoing extracapsular cataract extraction with posterior chamber intraocular lens implantation (ECCE/PCIOL) has an average preoperative keratometry measurement of 44.5 D. By mistake, the surgeon enters 43.5 D in her lens calculator, which recommends +18.00 D for distance emmetropia. This lens is subsequently implanted. Which of the following regarding this situation is/are true?

    1. The implant used is "too strong" for this eye.
    2. An similar error in axial length measurement (1.0 mm) would result in a larger postoperative refractive error than this 1.0 D error.
    3. The patient will require minus spectacle correction for distance emmetropia.
    4. The miscalculation will not affect the choice of an appropriate anterior chamber IOL.

    a. 1, 2, and 3.
    b. 1 and 3.
    c. 2 and 4.
    d. 4 only.
    e. 1, 2, 3, and 4.

38. The most important factor in determining the A-constant of an intraocular lens (IOL) is the:

    a. number of haptics.
    b. chemical nature of the haptics.
    c. configuration of the lens (e.g., biconvex, planoconvex).
    d. use of surface passivation.
    e. final lens position in the eye.

39. T or F -- Enhancement of the retinoscopic reflex is obtained by fully rotating the handle.

40. Which of the following concerning retinoscopic neutralization of refractive error is/are true?

    1. As neutralization is approached, the streak moves faster.
    2. As neutralization is approached, the streak becomes brighter.
    3. As neutralization is approached, the streak becomes wider.
    4. As neutralization is approached, the streak becomes narrower.

    a. 1, 2, and 3.
    b. 1 and 3.
    c. 2 and 4.
    d. 4 only.
    e. 1, 2, 3, and 4.

41. An examiner sits 50 cm from a patient being refracted by retinoscopy. While sweeping the streak at axis 45 degrees, a +3.00 D sphere neutralizes the reflex; with the streak at axis 135 degrees, +5.00 D sphere neutralizes the reflex. What is the patient's final retinoscopic refraction?

    a. +1.00 +4.00 x 135.
    b. +5.00 -2.00 x 45.
    c. +1.00 +2.00 x 135.
    d. +3.00 +2.00 x 135.
    e. +3.00 -2.00 x 135.

42. Which of the following retinoscopic reflex phenomena is/are useful for approximating the axis of small cylindrical errors?

    1. intensity.
    2. break.
    3. skew.
    4. thickness.

    a. 1, 2, and 3.
    b. 1 and 3.
    c. 2 and 4.
    d. 4 only.
    e. 1, 2, 3, and 4.

43. T or F -- Astigmatic dial refraction is designed for use with plus cylinders.

44. T or F -- Cross-cylinder estimation of cylinder axis and power is best performed with the patient fogged.

45. T or F -- The red-green duochrome test is best introduced with the patient fogged.

46. T or F -- The binocular balancing test is best performed with the patient fogged.

47. A 5-year-old child is noted to have a 20 prism diopter esotropia that increases to 45 prism diopters while reading at 20 cm. The patient's pupillary distance is 50 mm. With the child reading through his distance correction, a +3.00 D lens placed over each eye decreases the esotropia at near to 20 prism diopters. The patient's accommodative convergence to accommodation (AC/A) ratio, as determined by the gradient method, is:

    a. 3:1.
    b. 5:1.
    c. 8:1.
    d. 10:1.
    e. 15:1.

48. For the child described in question 47, the AC/A ratio as determined by the heterophoria method is:

    a. 3:1.
    b. 5:1.
    c. 8:1.
    d. 10:1.
    e. 15:1.

49. A 35-year-old myope presents to an ophthalmologist complaining of difficulty reading. She recently started wearing soft contact lenses to enhance her career as a television newscaster. Potential reasons for her new difficulty is/are most likely:

    1. dry eyes.
    2. increased convergence demand.
    3. increase in relative magnification.
    4. increased accommodative demand.

    a. 1, 2, and 3.
    b. 1 and 3.
    c. 2 and 4.
    d. 4 only.
    e. 1, 2, 3, and 4.

50. A patient is refracted to 20/20 visual acuity (at distance). +3.00 D spheres are added to this correction, and he is asked to read a 20/30 near target, which is brought progressively closer. He is able to read the target at distances between 20 and 40 cm. His comfortable working distance is approximately 40 cm. What is the correct power add for this man's bifocals?

    a. +0.75 D.
    b. +1.25 D.
    c. +1.75 D.
    d. +2.50 D.
    e. +3.00 D.

51. The age of the patient in question 50 is approximately:

    a. 36 years.
    b. 40 years.
    c. 44 years.
    d. 48 years.
    e. 52 years.

52. The distance refraction in question 50 must be:

    a. incorrect by +1.00 D (i.e., 1.00 D extra plus).
    b. incorrect by +0.50 D.
    c. appropriate.
    d. incorrect by -0.50 D (i.e., 0.50 D extra minus).
    e. incorrect by -1.00 D.

53. A 64 year-old architect presents to an ophthalmologist complaining of difficulty reading at work. His current correction is +5.00 D OU with a +2.00 D add. His range of clear vision with this current prescription includes:

        1. infinity to 100 cm.
        2. 20 to 15 cm.
        3. 50 to 33 cm.
        4. infinity to 15 cm.

    a. 1, 2, and 3.
    b. 1 and 3.
    c. 2 and 4.
    d. 4 only.
    e. 1, 2, 3, and 4.

54. The architect in question 53 would like to be able to read the blueprints at approximately 25 cm, as well as work on a drafting board at a distance of 50 cm to 60 cm. His corrected distance acuity is 20/20. The best prescription to address his needs might be:

    a. + 5.00 D with a + 3.50 D add.
    b. + 6.00 D with a + 3.50 D add.
    c. + 5.00 D with a + 2.00 D near add and a + 1.00 D intermediate add.
    d. + 5.00 D with a + 3.50 D near add and a + 1.50 D intermediate add.
    e. a referral to your least favorite partner.

55. T or F -- Image jump is primarily a problem for presbyopes with significant anisometropia.

56. T or F -- Image displacement is primarily a problem for presbyopes with significant anisometropia.

57. T or F -- For the anisometrope, image displacement is generally more troublesome than image jump.

58. A patient wearing new glasses comes in complaining of diplopia. The prescription is OD: +3.00 -1.00 x 180 with a +2.00 D add, and OS: -2.50 -1.00 x 90 with a +2.00 D add. A tropia is present when the patient is reading at a comfortable distance. While reading, the visual axis is 2 cm nasal and 2 cm inferior to the distance optical center and 0.5 cm nasal and 1.2 cm above the optical center of the add in each lens. What is the induced prismatic effect for this patient?

    a. 3Δ base up and 1Δ base out OD.
    b. 3Δ base up and 1Δ base in OD.
    c. 9Δ base down OD and 13Δ base out OD.
    d. 9Δ base up OD and 13Δ base out OD.
    e. 9Δ base up OD and 1Δ base out OD.

59. Alternate cover testing at near of the patient in question 58 probably revealed:

    a. right hyper and exo deviation.
    b. left hyper and exo deviation.
    c. left hyper and eso deviation.
    d. right hyper and eso deviation.
    e. you can't tell because you are thoroughly confused.

60. T or F -- The complaints of the patient in question 58 are due strictly to image jump.

61. Suitable methods for correcting the problem in question 58 might include:

    1. press-on prisms.
    2. "slab-off" grinding.
    3. dissimilar segments.
    4. contact lenses with reading glasses.

    a. 1, 2, and 3.
    b. 1 and 3.
    c. 2 and 4.
    d. 4 only.
    e. 1, 2, 3, and 4.

62. Image jump is most troublesome for bifocals of the:

    a. fused type.
    b. round top type.
    c. flat top type.
    d. ribbon type.
    e. progressive add type.

63. T or F -- UV-A light contains longer wavelengths than UV-C light.

64. A 72-year-old patient with bilateral macular degeneration has a distance acuity of 20/100. The add required for this patient to read newspaper print is:

    a. +1.00 D.
    b. +3.00 D.
    c. +4.00 D.
    d. +5.00 D.
    e. +10.00 D.

65. The patient in question 64 should be informed that his working distance will be approximately:

   a. 10 cm.
   b. 20 cm.
   c. 25 cm.
   d. 35 cm.
   e. 100 cm.

66. A 32-year-old patient with Stargardt's disease has a distance acuity of 20/200. The add required for this patient to read newspaper print comfortably is:

   a. +1.00 D.
   b. +3.00 D.
   c. +4.00 D.
   d. +6.00 D.
   e. +10.00 D.

67. The patient in question 66 should be informed that his working distance will be approximately:

   a. 10 cm.
   b. 20 cm.
   c. 25 cm.
   d. 33 cm.
   e. 100 cm.

68. The advantages of hand-held magnifiers as low-vision aids include which of the following?

   1. greater working distance.
   2. greater ease of use for patients with poor manual dexterity.
   3. wider range of available magnifying powers.
   4. wider field of view.

   a. 1, 2, and 3.
   b. 1 and 3.
   c. 2 and 4.
   d. 4 only.
   e. 1, 2, 3, and 4.

69. The main advantage of telescopic aids for near work is:

   a. decreased convergence requirement.
   b. wider field of view.
   c. greater depth of focus.
   d. greater working distance.
   e. greater flexibility regarding head position.

70. Which of the following is/are important in determining the oxygen flux across a contact lens?

      1. the diffusion coefficient for oxygen in the lens.
      2. the thickness of the central portion of the lens.
      3. the partial pressure gradient of oxygen across the lens.
      4. the solubility of oxygen in the lens.

    a. 1, 2, and 3.
    b. 1 and 3.
    c. 2 and 4.
    d. 4 only.
    e. 1, 2, 3, and 4.

71. T or F -- As the diameter of a rigid contact lens increases (with a fixed radius of curvature), the lens becomes effectively steeper.

72. T or F -- As the radius of curvature of a rigid contact lens increases (with a constant diameter), the lens becomes steeper.

73. Which of the following patients has/have significant lenticular astigmatism?

      1. refraction: -1.00 -1.00 x 180;
         keratometry: 43.0 D at 90 degrees, 42.0 D at 180 degrees.
      2. refraction: -5.00 -3.00 x 90;
         keratometry: 44.0 D at 90 degrees, 42.0 D at 180 degrees.
      3. refraction: -1.00 -2.00 x 90;
         keratometry: 42.0 D at 90 degrees, 44.0 D at 180 degrees.
      4. refraction: -4.00 -1.00 x 180;
         keratometry: 42.0 D at 90 degrees, 42.0 D at 180 degrees.

    a. 1, 2, and 3.
    b. 1 and 3.
    c. 2 and 4.
    d. 4 only.
    e. 1, 2, 3, and 4.

74. A patient requesting rigid gas-permeable contact lens has a best refraction OD of -4.00 +1.25 x 90. Keratometry OD is 44.0 D at 90 degrees and 42.5 D at 180 degrees. The conversion to radius of curvature is 7.70 mm at 90 degrees, 7.95 mm at 180 degrees. The only posterior curve available is 7.80 mm. The power for best vision is:

    a. -2.00 D.
    b. -2.75 D.
    c. -3.00 D.
    d. -3.50 D
    e. -4.00 D.

75. With rigid gas-permeable lenses, what percentage of corneal oxygen requirements are met by trans-contact lens oxygen movement?

    a. 10%.
    b. 25%.
    c. 50%.
    d. 75%.
    e. 90%.

76. T or F -- Diameter variations are more important in soft contact lens fitting than in rigid gas-permeable (RGP) contact lens fitting.

77. A patient requesting soft contact lens has a spectacle correction of -6.00 +1.00 x 90 (vertex distance = 15 mm) and keratometry OD of 44.0 D (7.70 mm) at 90 degrees, and 42.5 D (7.95 mm) at 180 degrees. A lens with base curve 8.6 mm and diameter 14.5 mm is selected. The lens power for best acuity is:

    a. -5.00 D.
    b. -5.50 D.
    c. -6.00 D.
    d. -6.50 D.
    e. -7.00 D.

78. Which of the following factors is/are important for increasing oxygen transmission across extended-wear contact lenses?

    1. decreased lens thickness.
    2. a minus carrier.
    3. increased lens water content.
    4. ballasting.

    a. 1, 2, and 3.
    b. 1 and 3.
    c. 2 and 4.
    d. 4 only.
    e. 1, 2, 3, and 4.

79. T or F -- Images generated in fundus biomicrocopy using the Goldmann contact lens and +90 D lenses are real inverted images.

80. Applanation tonometry measures the amount of force required to flatten an area of cornea with a diameter equal to:

    a. 3.06 mm.
    b. 6.12 mm.
    c. 1.53 mm.
    d. 0.06 mm ^{2}.
    e. 3.06 cm.

81. T or F -- For every 4 D of corneal astigmatism, applanation tonometry will be incorrect by 1 mm Hg.

82. Which one of the following concerning direct ophthalmoscopy is false?

   a. The linear magnification is 15X.
   b. A myope's disc appears larger than an emmetrope's.
   c. The image is a virtual, upright image.
   d. The dial on an direct ophthalmoscope is intended to neutralize both the examiner's and patient's refractive error.
   e. A hyperope's disc appears smaller than an emmetrope's.

83. Which one of the following regarding indirect ophthalmoscopy of an emmetropic eye is false?

   a. The image the examiner observes is a real, inverted image in the focal plane of the condensing lens.
   b. Conjugate planes include the patient's and the examiner's retinas and the patient's and examiner's pupils.
   c. If the examiner uses a 20 D condensing lens, the lateral magnification is approximately 3X and the axial magnification approximately 2.25X.
   d. A 30 D condensing lens provides greater magnification and a larger field of view than a 20 D condensing lens.
   e. Aspheric condensing lenses are preferred for indirect ophthalmoscopy.

84. Which one of the following concerning keratometry is false?

   a. Corneal curvature is measured by using the cornea's power as a convex mirror.
   b. A central image is doubled to negate the effect of eye movement.
   c. Conventional keratometry measures the curvature of the central 6 mm of the cornea.
   d. The refractive power of the average cornea equals 337.5 divided by its radius of curvature (in mm).
   e. Manual keratometry may be misleading following radial keratotomy or corneal transplantation.

85. A slide is placed 25 cm to the left of a lens. The image is in perfect focus on a screen 1 m to the right of the lens. What is the power of the lens?

   a. +0.25 D.
   b. -3.00 D.
   c. +4.00 D.
   d. +5.00 D.
   e. +3.00 D.

86. How far from a +24 D camera lens should an object be placed to be focused onto film 5 cm to the right of the lens?

   a. 25 cm to the left of the lens.
   b. 50 cm to the right of the lens.
   c. 50 cm to the left of the lens.
   d. 25 cm to the right of the lens.
   e. 20 cm to the left of the lens.

87. Where should a +8.00 D lens be placed to form an image 0.5 m from a real object (assuming light travels from left to right)?

   a. 50 cm to the left of the object.
   b. 25 cm to the right of the object and 25 cm to the left of the image.
   c. 100 cm to the right of the object and 50 cm to the right of the image.
   d. 75 cm to the right of the object and 25 cm to the left of the image.
   e. 12.5 cm to the right of the object and 37.5 cm to the left of the image.

88. A patient wears a -10 D spectacle lens at a vertex distance of 20 mm for distance correction. What power contact lens will be required for proper distance correction?

   a. -8.25 D.
   b. -9.00 D.
   c. -12.50 D.
   d. -11.50 D.
   e. -10.00 D.

89. Where is the far point of an eye with a +4.00 D "error lens"?

   a. 17 mm in front of the cornea.
   b. 25 cm in front of the cornea.
   c. 5.5 mm inside the cornea.
   d. 25 cm behind the cornea.
   e. at the retina.

90. Where is the far point of the eye ~~corrected~~ *THAT NEEDS CORRECTION* with a +4.00 D lens?

   a. 17 mm in front of the cornea.
   b. 25 cm in front of the cornea.
   c. 5.5 mm inside the cornea.
   d. 25 cm behind the cornea.
   e. at the retina.

91. An aphake wears a spectacle correction of +10.0 D at vertex distance of 20 mm. Where should a +3.0 D lens be placed to correct this patient for distance?

    a. 10 cm in front of the eye.
    b. 25 cm in front of the eye.
    c. 33 cm in front of the eye.
    d. 35 cm in front of the eye.
    e. 50 cm in front of the eye.

92. A crystal ball with an opaque rear surface sits on a pedestal. Its internal radius of curvature is 50 cm. Its index of refraction is 3.00. Which of the following concerning this "lens" are correct (considering only the front surface of the crystal ball)?

    1. Its refractive power is +8.00 D.
    2. Its primary focal length is 25 cm.
    3. Its secondary focal length is 25 cm.
    4. Light originating at infinity will come to focus inside the crystal ball.

    a. 1, 2, and 3.
    b. 1 and 3.
    c. 2 and 4.
    d. 4 only.
    e. 1, 2, 3, and 4.

93. If the crystal ball's radius is the same (50 cm) but its index of refraction is 1.50, which of the following is/are true?

    1. Its refractive power is +1.00 D.
    2. Primary focal length is 1 m.
    3. Its secondary focal length is 1.5 m.
    4. Light from infinity would come to focus inside this crystal ball.

    a. 1, 2, and 3.
    b. 1 and 3.
    c. 2 and 4.
    d. 4 only.
    e. 1, 2, 3, and 4.

94. Consider another crystal ball with index of refraction of 1.50 and internal radius of curvature of 10 cm. Which of the following is/are true?

        1. Its primary focal length is 20 cm.
        2. Its power is +15.0 D.
        3. Its secondary focal length is 30 cm.
        4. Light from infinity would come to focus inside this crystal ball.

    a. 1, 2, and 3.
    b. 1 and 3.
    c. 2 and 4.
    d. 4 only.
    e. 1, 2, 3, and 4.

95. T or F -- If the center of curvature of a spherical refractive surface lies on the same side as object light, the radius of curvature of the surface is positive.

96. T or F -- If the center of curvature of a spherical refractive surface lies on the same side as the medium of higher index of refraction, the net power of the surface is greater than zero.

97. A child is watching her goldfish swim inside a tank with internal radius of curvature of 1/3 m. If the goldfish swims up to her and returns her gaze at a distance of 1/3 m from the tank wall, where will the child believe the fish to be (assume the index of refraction of water is 4/3)?

    a. 1/5 m inside the tank.
    b. 4/15 m inside the tank.
    c. 1/2 m inside the tank.
    d. 4/9 m inside the tank.
    e. 1/3 m inside the tank.

98. A penlight is dropped into a rectangular aquarium filled with water so that the bulb burns 1/2 m from the aquarium side it faces. To an observer looking in, where will the bulb appear to be burning?

    a. 1/2 m inside the tank.
    b. 1/2 m outside the tank.
    c. at the tank surface.
    d. 3/8 m outside the tank.
    e. 3/8 m inside the tank.

99. Concerning the reduced schematic eye, if the effective power is assumed to be +60 D, and the internal index of refraction is assumed to be 1.33, which of the following is/are true?

> 1. The primary focal point is approximately 17 mm in front of the cornea.
> 2. The secondary focal point is approximately 17 mm inside the cornea.
> 3. The nodal point of the eye can be located with this information.
> 4. The eye acts as a simple magnifier with power 4X.

a. 1, 2, and 3.
b. 1 and 3.
c. 2 and 4.
d. 4 only.
e. 1, 2, 3, and 4.

100. If a biconvex thin lens has a front surface with a radius of curvature of 10 cm, a back surface with a radius of curvature of 5 cm, and an index of refraction of 1.50, what is its total power in air?

a. +5 D.
b. +10 D.
c. +15 D.
d. -5 D.
e. -10 D.

101. An intraocular lens implant (IOL) is labeled as +18.0 D. Its specifications list an index of refraction of 1.50. Which one of the following concerning the IOL power is correct?

a. It is +18.0 D in air and +54.0 D in the eye.
b. It is +18.0 D in air and +6.0 D in the eye.
c. It is +18.0 D in the eye and +6.0 D in air.
d. It is +18.0 D in the eye and +54.0 D in air.
e. It is +18.0 D in both the eye and air.

102. In the following image ray diagram, which of the following is/are true (assume all light travels left to right)?

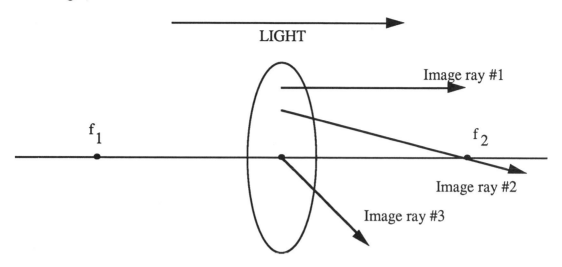

LIGHT

Image ray #1

f_1

f_2

Image ray #2

Image ray #3

1. Object ray #1 must have passed through the lens's secondary focal point.
2. Object ray #2 must have been traveling parallel to the lens axis.
3. This lens must be negative in power.
4. Object ray #3 must have passed through the lens undeviated.

a. 1, 2, and 3.
b. 1 and 3.
c. 2 and 4.
d. 4 only.
e. 1, 2, 3, and 4.

103. T or F -- The true power of a meniscus lens is always greater than the back vertex power.

104. T or F -- The true power of a meniscus lens is always greater than the front vertex power.

105. An afocal telescope is constructed with -10 D and +4 D lenses. What is the distance between the lenses?

a. 5 cm.
b. 15 cm.
c. 20 cm.
d. 25 cm.
e. 30 cm.

106. Concerning the image formed by this afocal telescope of an object at infinity, which of the following is/are true (assuming an emmetropic user)?

    1. If the -10 D lens is held closer to the eye, the image is magnified by a factor of 2.5X.
    2. The image is upright.
    3. The image is virtual.
    4. No accommodation is required for viewing this image.

    a. 1, 2, and 3.
    b. 1 and 3.
    c. 2 and 4.
    d. 4 only.
    e. 1, 2, 3, and 4.

107. An afocal telescope is constructed from +10 D and +4 D lenses. What is the distance between the lenses?

    a. 10 cm.
    b. 15 cm.
    c. 20 cm.
    d. 25 cm.
    e. 35 cm.

108. Concerning the image formed by the afocal telescope in question 107, of an object 1 m away, which of the following are true (assuming an emmotropic user)?

    1. If the +10 D lens is held near the eye, the image is magnified by a factor of 2.5X.
    2. The image is upright.
    3. The image is virtual.
    4. No accommodation is required to view the the image.

    a. 1, 2, and 3.
    b. 1 and 3.
    c. 2 and 4.
    d. 4 only.
    e. 1, 2, 3, and 4.

109. Afocal surgical loupes are constructed with an eyepiece of -20 D and an objective of +10 D. A +4 D add is placed immediately adjacent to the objective lens. Assume that the vertex distance (from eyepiece to eye) is zero. What is the accommodation required for viewing an object 30 cm from the eye?

    a. 0 D.
    b. 1 D.
    c. 3.5 D.
    d. 10 D.
    e. 12 D.

110. Using the loupes from question 109, approximately what accommodation is required to view an object 15 cm from the eye?

    a. 0 D.
    b. 1 D.
    c. 3.5 D.
    d. 10 D.
    e. 15 D.

111. What is the magnification of the loupes in question 109?

    a. 1X.
    b. 2X.
    c. 4X.
    d. 8X.
    e. 16X.

112. An aphake uses a +12.5 D contact lens for distance correction. How much image size change is generated with this correction?

    a. 0%.
    b. 7% magnification.
    c. 7% minification.
    d. 7X magnification.
    e. 7X minification.

113. What is the appropriate spectacle to give the patient in question 112 for distance correction (assume vertex distance is 20 mm)?

    a. +3.5 D.
    b. +8.0 D.
    c. +10 D.
    d. +12.5 D.
    e. +16.5 D.

114. How much image size change will be generated by the spectacle correction in question 113?

    a. 0%.
    b. 33% magnification.
    c. 33% minification.
    d. 33X magnification.
    e. 33X minification.

115. A high myope is corrected with a -10 D contact lens. How much image size change is generated with this correction?

a. 0%.
b. 5% magnification.
c. 5% minification.
d. 5X magnification.
e. 5X minification.

116. What would be the correct spectacle correction for distance for the patient in question 115 (assume vertex distance is 20 mm)?

a. -8.50 D.
b. -9.50 D.
c. -11.0 D.
d. -12.5 D.
e. -15.0 D.

117. What will be the image size change generated by the spectacle correction in question 116?

a. 0%.
b. 24% magnification.
c. 24% minification.
d. 24X magnification.
e. 24X minification.

118. A man stands 1 m in front of a plane mirror. Which of the following is/are true concerning the image?

1. The image is 50 cm in back of the mirror.
2. The image is real.
3. The man could see more of himself by moving farther away from the mirror.
4. The image is upright.

a. 1, 2, and 3.
b. 1 and 3.
c. 2 and 4.
d. 4 only.
e. 1, 2, 3, and 4.

119. Where is the image of a real object located 50 cm in front of a convex mirror with radius of curvature equal to 20 cm?

a. The image is 8.33 cm in front of the mirror.
b. The image is 12.5 mm in front of the mirror.
c. The image is 8.33 cm in back of the mirror.
d. The image is 12.5 cm in back of the mirror.
e. The image is 12.5 mm in back of the mirror.

120. T or F -- The image created in question 119 is virtual.

121. T or F -- The image created in question 119 is magnified by a factor of 6X.

122. T or F -- The image created in question 119 is upright.

123. Assume that the cornea has an index of refraction equal to 1.38, that its front surface has a radius of curvature 7.7 mm, and that its rear surface has a radius of curvature equal to 7.6 mm. Also assume that the index of refraction of aqueous humor is 1.33. Which one of the following is false?

    a. The posterior refractive surface of the cornea has negative power.
    b. The total refractive power of the cornea is +42.8 D.
    c. The anterior reflecting surface of the cornea has negative power.
    d. The total reflecting power of the anterior corneal surface is -42.75 D.
    e. The net refractive power of the cornea may be represented by one spherical surface with a reduced radius of curvature of 7.9 mm and an index of refraction of 1.3375.

124. An underworked ophthalmology resident decides to verify the size of an anterior chamber intraocular lens implant in a new patient whose implant card records an optic diameter of 6.0 mm. Assuming that the patient's cornea is identical to that described in question 123, and that the implant rests on the iris 3 mm posterior to the anterior corneal surface, what will the resident record as the optic diameter with his slit lamp calipers?

    a. 4.4 mm.
    b. 5.5 mm.
    c. 6.0 mm.
    d. 6.7 mm.
    e. 7.8 mm.

125. A patient's pupillary reflex (reflection) is checked with a penlight held 40 cm away from her cornea. Where is the image of the penlight located (using the average corneal parameters given in question 123)?

    a. 3.8 mm outside the eye.
    b. 3.8 mm inside the eye.
    c. 2.5 mm outside the eye.
    d. 2.5 mm inside the eye.
    e. at the anterior corneal surface.

126. To ease indirect opthalmoscopy through a small pupil, an examiner might:

    a. move the condensing lens closer to the patient.
    b. move the condensing lens away from the patient.
    c. move his/her head toward the lens.
    d. move his/her head away from the lens.
    e. increase illumination of the patient's fundus.

127. Novices at indirect ophthalmoscopy tend to move closer to the patient than the optimal examining distance to:

    a. enhance image depth.
    b. enhance image size and detail.
    c. ease examination through small pupils.
    d. rest their arms.
    e. increase illumination of the patient's fundus.

128. Annoying reflexes during indirect ophthalmoscopy may be moved out of the line of visualization if the examiner:

    a. moves the condensing lens closer to the patient.
    b. moves the condensing lens away from the patient.
    c. moves his/her head toward the lens.
    d. moves his/her head away from the lens.
    e. tilts the lens obliquely.

129. In retinoscopy with plano-mirror technique, which of the following are true?

    1. The image of the streak is between the examiner and patient.
    2. "With" motion is neutralized using plus lenses.
    3. With a Copeland retinoscope, the handle must be down.
    4. "Against" motion implies that the patient's far point is between the examiner and the patient.

    a. 1, 2, and 3.
    b. 1 and 3.
    c. 2 and 4.
    d. 4 only.
    e. 1, 2, 3, and 4.

130. T or F -- By Knapp's rule, correction of any anisometropia with a lens at the primary focal point of the eye will result in no disparity in retinal image sizes.

Answers

1. c. Light energy is proportional to its <u>frequency</u>. When light enters a medium of higher refractive index, its velocity decreases; its frequency remains the same, but its wavelength decreases. The index of refraction decreases with increasing wavelength (i.e., shorter wavelengths are refracted <u>more</u>).

2. True. The energy of a photon of light is proportional to its frequency as given by the equation:

   Energy E = h x frequency

   where h = Planck's constant. Blue light is of higher frequency than red light and therefore has greater energy per photon.

3. a. The laser interferometer uses the highly coherent light of the laser to create an interference pattern on the retina. The pattern seen by the patient consists of light and dark bands created by constructive and destructive interference, respectively.

4. b. The Haidinger brush phenomenon is useful in sensory testing of the fovea. The phenomenon is created by rotating a polarizer continuously in front of a uniform blue field. The normal subject will see a rotating figure that looks like a double-ended brush. The effect is created because Henle's layer of the macula (outer plexiform layer) is oriented in such a way as to polarize incoming light.

5. a. Because of diffractive effects, pinhole vision is rarely better than 20/25 even with an optimal pinhole aperture of 1.2 mm. Pupil sizes less than about 2.5 mm will create diffractive effects that limit acuity. The sky is blue because light of higher frequency is <u>scattered</u> more than light of lower frequency. This has nothing to do with diffraction.

6. a. A laser beam's high directionality, coherence, and linear polarization enhance its intensity. Laser light is <u>mono</u>chromatic.

7. True. The active medium is the chemical environment (e.g., argon, krypton) that supports stimulated emission of coherent light.

8. a. Power is defined as energy per unit time. Increasing energy while keeping exposure time constant increases power. Decreasing the time over which an amount of energy is delivered also increases power. Q-switching and mode locking are means of increasing the peak power a laser is able to generate.

9. b. The index of refraction for any medium is greater for shorter wavelengths. Refraction will occur at any interface between media with different indices of refraction. According to Snell's law, light rays striking the interface <u>perpendicular</u> to the interface will <u>not</u> be bent. Light traversing a plane parallel plate is refracted twice (at the front and back surfaces).

10. False. The angle of minimum deviation is produced by a prism when light undergoes equal bending at the two faces. When light strikes the prism perpendicular to one of its surfaces (Prentice position), the angle of deviation is greater.

11. d. One prism diopter is defined as a 1 cm displacement over a <u>100 cm</u> distance. Glass prisms are calibrated in the Prentice position, in which one face is perpendicular to the incident light. When measuring strabismus with glass prisms, they must be held in this position to be accurate; that is, glass prisms must be held with one surface perpendicular to the visual axis. Real images are deviated toward the prism base. <u>Virtual</u> images are deviated toward the apex.

12. False. Real images can <u>usually</u> be formed on a screen. One exception is the real image of the retina formed by an indirect ophthalmoscope. This real image cannot be formed on a screen because the screen would block the illumination system of the ophthalmoscope.

13. c. Magnification is equal to the ratio of image <u>size</u> to object <u>size</u> (i/o) or object <u>vergence</u> to image <u>vergence</u> (U/V) (since size and vergence are reciprocally related). Magnification less than zero (i.e., negative) implies an inverted image. Magnification less than one implies an image smaller than the object (minification).

14. False. Reduced vergence is equal to the index of refraction divided by the reference distance. The reduced vergence is greater than the vergence because for media other than air, the refractive index is greater than one.

15. b. The primary focal length (in meters) of any lens system equals the index of refraction of the object space divided by the lens power ($f_1 = n_1/P$). In air, $n_1 = 1$, so $f_1 = 1/P$. The reciprocal of 60 D (the power of the average eye) is 0.017 m, or 17 mm.

16. d. The secondary focal length (in meters) of any lens system equals the index of refraction of the image space divided by the lens power ($f_2 = n_2/P$). The refractive index of the ocular media is 1.33. $f_2 = 1.33/60$ D $= 0.0222$ m, or 22.2 mm.

17. c. In a thick lens system, the primary principal plane acts as an infinitely thin refracting surface at which object light originating from the primary focal plane is converted into parallel light rays. The secondary principal plane acts as an infinitely thin refracting surface at which incoming parallel light is made to converge toward the secondary focal point. No refraction is considered to occur at the primary or secondary focal planes.

18. e. One should also remember that if the refractive media on the two sides are different, the principal points are displaced toward the medium of lower index of refraction.

19. True. Since the focal length measured from the "rear" vertex of a meniscus lens is always shorter than the corresponding "front" focal length, the absolute value of the back vertex power ($P = n/f$, where $n = 1$ in air) is always greater than that of the front vertex power. The true power is somewhere between the two.

20. c. The magnification of a simple plus lens is defined as the ratio of the angular size of the image produced by the lens to the angular size of the object viewed at 25 cm. The formula for angular magnification by a simple plus lens of power P is $M = P/4$. Since the average power of an emmetropic eye is + 60 D, magnification $M = 60/4 = 15X$.

21. c. The devices mentioned are usually small <u>Galilean</u> telescopes, since Galilean telescopes are shorter and provide an upright image without additional optical elements. The total magnification is equal to the magnifying power of the "add" (P/4--magnification of a plus lens; see answer 20) multiplied by the power of the Galilean telescope (= [-(power of eyepiece)/power of objective]).

22. d. The flatter (not steeper) peripheral cornea tends to counteract spherical aberration. The total interval of chromatic aberration in the human eye is about 1.25 D. Tilting a lens along its horizontal axis induces sphere of the <u>same</u> (not opposite) sign, as well as cylinder of the same sign and along the same axis. Shorter wavelengths of light are refracted more than longer wavelengths. When yellow light is focused on the retina (as is the case in emmetropia or proper spectacle correction), blue light is 0.87 D anterior to the retina, green light is 0.37 D anterior, and red light is 0.37 D posterior to the retina.

Red + Green light → yellow

23. True. A Maddox line produces two line images of a point light source--a real image that is too close to the eye to be seen, as well as a virtual image running through the light source. The real image is parallel to the cylinders' axes, while the virtual image is perpendicular. This is true for all spherocylindrical lenses (even those with no power in one meridian).

24. b. The power of this lens is +4.00 D at the 90-degree meridian. Therefore, a horizontal focal line will be formed 25 cm from the lens. The power of this lens is +2.00 D at the 180-degree meridian. Therefore, a vertical focal line will be formed 50 cm from the lens. The circle of least confusion is located halfway, <u>diopterically</u>, between the two focal lines (i.e., at the spherical equivalent). In this case the circle of least confusion is at 3.00 D, or 33 cm. The image at 37.5 cm is between the circle and the vertical line. Thus, the image will be a vertical oval.

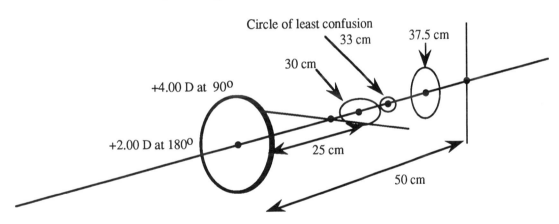

25. d. A cross-cylinder is a lens made of two cylinders of equal but opposite power at right angles to one another. The spherical equivalent of any cross-cylinder is <u>zero</u>. Notice that option 1 is a +0.50 sphere.

26. False. The field of view for an observer looking at a plane mirror stays the same regardless of the observer's position.

27. d. The corneal scar may be producing irregular astigmatism, which cannot be corrected by spherocylindrical spectacle lenses. The pinhole greatly minimizes nonaxial light rays, which require refraction to come into focus on the retina.

Answers

28. a. Vernier acuity refers to the ability of a normal human eye to discriminate between two line segments in the frontal plane separated by as little as 8 seconds of arc (one-third the diameter of a cone). Determination of accurate end points with the keratometer, lensmeter, and applanation tonometer relies on this degree of spatial discrimination.

29. e. Conjugate planes are related by being the object and image of one another.

30. False. The binocular amplitude of accommodation usually exceeds the monocular amplitude of accommodation.

31. False. Believe it or not, this is controversial. Some experts maintain that the duration of the mydriatic effect of cycloplegic agents is shorter than the cycloplegic effect. Other prominent experts disagree (vehemently). All cycloplegic agents produce dilation, but not all dilating agents produce cycloplegia.

So how DARE you give an absolute answer asshole.

32. d. Accommodative amplitude decreases with age with the following approximations:

1. Accommodative amplitude at age 40 = 6.0 D, age 44 = 4.5 D, and at age 48 = 3.0 D.
2. Below age 40, accommodative amplitude increases by 1.0 D for every 4 years.
3. Above age 48, accommodative amplitude decreases by 0.5 D for every 4 years.

Here, the accommodative amplitude for a 60-year-old equals:

$$3.0 \text{ D} - 1.5 \text{ D} = 1.5 \text{ D}$$

(Please note that many expert strabismus and optics experts vociferously object to the use of these accommodative tables since they are approximations and may be incorrect in specific instances. Still, they do provide a helpful guide to the rate of attrition of accommodative capabilities in the average emmetrope).

33. c. Although the development of the refractive state is not thoroughly understood, general trends appear evident. Low-grade hyperopia in infancy and childhood usually drifts toward emmetropia in adult life.

Exophoria is noted in gen population

34. c. Cylindrical lenses produce minor monocular distortions caused by differential meridional magnification, which may produce intolerable binocular spatial distortions. The sources of differential meridional magnification can be minimized by:

1. prescribing the minus cylinder form.
2. minimizing vertex distance.
3. decreasing cylinder power (while maintaining the proper spherical equivalent).
4. rotating the axis of the correcting cylinder toward 90 or 180 degrees.

35. c. The majority of distortions of aphakic spectacle lenses stem from their position anterior to the pupil and include image magnification, ring scotoma, pincushion distortion, and jack-in-the-box phenomenon.

36. False. The magnification associated with any corrective lens diminishes as the lens approaches the eye's nodal point. An IOL, therefore, decreases image magnification to less than 4%, compared to 20 to 30% with aphakic spectacle correction and 7 to 12% with aphakic contact lens correction. Obviously, posterior chamber IOLs yield less magnification than anterior chamber IOLs.

37.   a.   Empiric formulas have been developed that predict proper IOL power for emmetropia (or various refractive errors). The widely used SRK formula is:

$$P = A - 2.5\,L - 0.9\,K$$

          where P = power of the IOL required for emmetropia
                A = a constant determined by the characteristics of the IOL
                L = axial length in mm
                K = average keratometry reading

Keratometry that is underestimated by 1.0 D will lead to an IOL that is stronger than intended by approximately 1.0 D. This is true for any IOL whose power is based on this keratometry, regardless of position. The refractive correction necessary for distance emmetropia will depend on the position of the IOL within the eye. Vergence calculations could be done to determine the actual spectacle correction, but for an IOL that is too strong, the correction would have to be minus. Since the axial length is multiplied by 2.5 (rather than 0.9), a 1 mm error in axial length will have a greater effect on postoperative refraction than a 1.0 D error in keratometry.

38.   e.   The A-constant depends on factors that determine the final lens position in the eye such as anterior versus posterior chamber placement, haptic angulation, and the shape of lens.

39.   False.   Rotating the sleeve rotates the streak itself. By moving the sleeve <u>up or down</u>, the rays can be made convergent or divergent, enhancing the image.

40.   e.   The following characteristics of the streak indicate the approach to neutralization:

    1. The reflex moves faster.
    2. The reflex becomes brighter.
    3. The reflex becomes wider.

If the refractive error is <u>large</u>, the beam will initially become more <u>narrow</u> as neutralization is approached, then widen again near the appropriate correction.

41.   c.   To express the result in minus cylinder form, the "less minus" lens is taken as the spherical correction, and gross retinoscopy is +5.00 - 2.00 x 45. The working distance is 50 cm, so 2.00 D must be subtracted from the spherical portion, giving a net result of +3.00 - 2.00 x 45. To express this in plus cylinder form, the "less positive" lens is taken as the spherical correction, giving a gross retinoscopy of +3.00 +2.00 x 135. Subtracting 2.0 D (the working distance) gives a net result of +1.00 +2.00 x 135.

42.   b.   At the correct axis, the following are true:

    1. The break phenomenon disappears (the intercept and reflex are parallel).
    2. The width of the streak is narrowest.
    3. The intensity is brightest.
    4. Skew motion is no longer observed.

Intensity and skew are primarily useful for small astigmatic errors, while break and width are best judged with an <u>enhanced</u> streak. Astigmatic errors less than 1.0 D do not enhance well, so break and width are not readily appreciable.

43. False. To use an astigmatic dial, the patient is fogged to relax accommodation, and the "sharpest and clearest" line is sought, representing one of the principal meridians. The astigmatism is neutralized by adding <u>minus</u> cyclinder perpendicular to this line until all lines are equally clear. Remember that the axis of this correcting cylinder is the mirror image of the clock-line when placed over the patient. A simple rule for converting from clock hours to trial frame axis is as follows: Take the lower of the two clock hours belonging to the line 90 degrees from the clearest line on the dial. Multiply this number by 30. This represents the axis for the correcting minus cylinder. For example, if the fogged patient reports that the 2 to 8 line is sharpest, the minus cylinder must be placed with its axis parallel to the 11 to 5 line. The lower of the two numbers is 5. Multiplying by 30, the minus cylinder should be placed with its axis at 150 degrees.

44. False. The spherical equivalent is discovered by fogging the eye to relax accommodation, then adding minus sphere until vision is sharpest. At this point, the circle of least confusion is on the retina. Then, the cross-cylinder is introduced to find axis and power. The circle of least confusion must remain on the retina throughout cross-cylinder testing. When fogged, the circle of least confusion is anterior to the retina.

45. True. The sphere end point can be verified by the duochrome test, but this test does not relax accommodation. Therefore, the test should be introduced with the patient slightly fogged, such that the letters on the red side are clearer (the red letters will focus <u>behind</u> the green letters, closer to the retina). Then, minus sphere is added until letters on the green and red sides are equally clear.

46. True. Except during cycloplegic refraction, fogging is needed to remove unequal accommodative influences. If the eyes are not balanced, fogging will degrade vision less in the eye that is more overminused.

47. c. Using the gradient method, AC/A (the ratio of prism diopters of accommodative convergence to diopters of accommodation) is calculated by placing plus lenses in front of each eye and determining the change in the deviation at near. This change, divided by the power of the plus lens used (amount of weakened accommodation), gives the number of prism diopters of accommodative convergence per diopter of accommodation. In this case, 45 -20 = 25, divided by 3 is (approximately) 8:1. Gradient method:

$$AC/A = \frac{\text{deviation with lens - deviation without lens}}{\text{lens power}}$$

In these calculations, esodeviations are positive and exodeviations are negative, by convention.

48. d. The heterophoria method makes use of similar reasoning, while taking into account the effect of interpupillary distance (PD)--i.e., larger PDs require greater convergence for fusion. Heterophoria method:

$$AC/A = \frac{\text{deviation at near - deviation at distance}}{\text{accommodation}} + PD \text{ (cm)}$$

where PD = interpupillary distance in cm. The denominator represents the number of diopters of accomodation required for the near target (the reciprocal of the reading distance in meters). In this case, PD is 5 cm, the deviation at near is 45Δ, and the deviation at distance is 20Δ. Accommodation will be 5 D at 20 cm. Thus,

$$AC/A = 25/5 + 5 = 10:1$$

49. c. There are two factors: the shorter vertex distance of contact lenses results in a greater accommodative demand for myopes and a decreased accommodative demand for hyperopes. More convergence will also be required for near work because the patient will lose the helpful base-in prismatic effect of her myopic spectacles.

50. b. This is the type of measurement that can be made using a Prince rule. After being "fogged" with the +3.00 D adds, the patient is found to have an effective far point of 40 cm (2.5 D) and an effective near point of 20 cm (5.0 D). This patient must have a range of accomodation of 5.0 - 2.5, or 2.5 D. Experience has shown that, in general, about half of this is available without causing strain (accommodative reserve). Our patient would therefore have about 1.25 D of readily available accommodative reserve. His working distance of 40 cm calls for 2.50 D of total accommodation, of which he can comfortably provide 1.25 D. Therefore, an add of +1.25 D (2.50-1.25) would be most appropriate.

51. e. See answer 32.

52. d. The patient's distance correction must be about 0.5 D "overminused," since fogging with +3.00 D brought his far point to 0.40 m (2.5 D), rather than the expected 0.33 m for an appropriately corrected eye.

53. b. A typical 64 year old has a 1.0 D amplitude of accommodation. Assuming proper distance correction, the range of clear vision with distance correction is from infinity (relaxed accommodation) to 100 cm (using his full 1.0 D of accommodation). His +2.00 D add provides clear vision from 50 cm (relaxed accommodation) to 33 cm (using his full 1.0 D of accommodation).

54. d. The only way to fulfill all his visual needs is with a trifocal combination. An add of +1.50/+3.50 gives an intermediate range from 40 to 67 cm (+1.50 D lens coupled with +1.00 D maximal accommodation) and near range from 22 to 30 cm (+3.50 plus 1.0 D of accommodation).

55. False. Image jump is a phenomenon related to encountering the sudden prismatic effect of a reading add as the gaze is moved downward into the add. The sudden addition of the prismatic effect of the add causes images to "jump," typically upward. Image jump can occur in any correction whose add does not have its optical center at the top of the segment.

56. True.   Image displacement occurs in all corrections as gaze moves away from the optical center of the correcting lens; this is unlikely to be significantly distressing unless an imbalanced displacement occurs, as in anisometropia. The other situation where image displacement is troublesome is when an increased demand is made on an already taxed vertical fusional system ability, as in compensated vertical phoria.

57. True.   On the other hand, occupational demands often make image jump more troublesome.

58. e.   Solving this problem is much facilitated by preparing diagrams marked with the <u>powers</u> in the 90 and 180 degree meridians, the visual axes, and the optical axes for the distance corrections and adds. Image displacement in prism diopters is:

(cm from the optical axis in the given meridian) x (power of the lens in diopters)

This needs to be done for both the distance corrections and the adds <u>separately</u>. After this, the results are combined--first for each side, then for a net effect on both eyes.

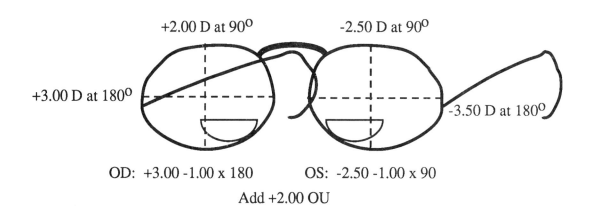

+2.00 D at 90°   -2.50 D at 90°

+3.00 D at 180°   -3.50 D at 180°

OD: +3.00 -1.00 x 180   OS: -2.50 -1.00 x 90

Add +2.00 OU

58. (cont.)

OD:

d = center of distance segment
n = center of add
X = visual axis while reading

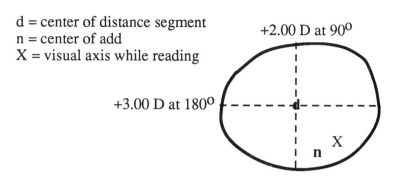

+2.00 D at 90°

+3.00 D at 180°

OD: +3.00 -1.00 x 180
Add +2.00

OD:	Distance	Vertical meridian:	2.0 cm x + 2.00 D = 4Δ base up
		Horizontal meridian:	2.0 cm x + 3.00 D = 6Δ base out
	Add	Vertical meridian:	1.2 cm x + 2.00 D = 2.4Δ base down
		Horizontal meridian:	0.5 cm x + 2.00 D = 1.0Δ base out
Net OD:			1.6Δ base up, 7.0Δ base out

OS:

-2.50 D at 90°

d = center of distance segment
n = center of add
X = visual axis while reading

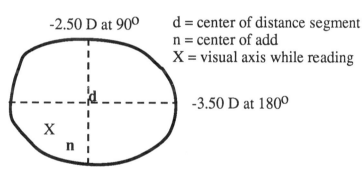

-3.50 D at 180°

OS: -2.50 -1.00 x 90
Add +2.00

OS:	Distance	Vertical meridian:	2.0 cm x - 2.50 D = 5.0Δ base down
		Horizontal meridian:	2.0 cm x - 3.50 D = 7.0Δ base in
	Add	Vertical meridian:	1.2 cm x - 2.00 D = 2.4Δ base down
		Horizontal meridian:	0.5 cm x - 2.00 D = 1.0Δ base out
Net OS:			7.4Δ base down 6.0Δ base in

Net (both eyes): 9Δ base up OD,   1Δ base out OD

58. (cont.) Note that when determining a net prismatic effect for <u>two</u> eyes, vertical prisms of different base orientation (base up plus base down) are additive, while horizontal prisms of same orientation (base in plus base in, or base out plus base out) are additive. For the net effect over <u>one</u> eye, prisms of the same orientation are additive (e.g., base up plus base up, base in plus base in).

59. a. It is easiest to visualize the patient's deviation by considering what correcting prisms would be needed: 9 Δ base up, and 1 Δ base out OD is corrected with 9Δ base down and 1Δ base in OD. Since the gaze deviation is away from the base of any correcting prism, right hyper and right exo deviations must be present.

60. False. This patient's problem with diplopia is due to image displacement-induced phoria/tropia, not image jump. Note that the image displacement is mostly due to the anisometropic distance segments.

61. e. Press-on prisms are occasionally helpful. Slab-off grinding and dissimilar segments act by changing the position of the optical centers of the lenses to lessen the differential prism. Contact lenses obviate the problem entirely. This is true because the visual axis is always through the optical center of a contact lens, regardless of viewing position. Thus, no prismatic effect from anisometropic correction is created.

62. b. Image jump occurs at the segmentation line when the optical center of the add is not at its upper edge. A round top bifocal segment has its optical center farther from its upper edge than other types and therefore causes the greatest image jump. These are commonly used only for aphakic spectacles to minimize image displacement.

63. True. UV-A: 400-320 μm--90% of UV light from sun.
UV-B: 320-280 μm--10% of UV light from sun.
UV-C: less than 280 μm--absorbed by ozone.

64. d. For near vision aids, the reciprocal of the Snellen fraction at distance gives the approximate accommodation needed to read newspaper print. With distance vision of 20/100, accommodation equal to 100/20, or +5.0 D is required. Since a 72-year-old has less than 1.00 D of accommodative amplitude, he will require the entire +5.00 D as an add.

65. b. By Kestenbaum's rule, the reciprocal of the distance acuity is the working distance (in diopters) required for reading newsprint. The working distance in centimeters is equal to 100 divided by this diopter value.

66. d. A 32-year-old has about 8.00 D of accommodative amplitude, 4.00 D of which can be comfortably used (accommodative reserve). Since this patient requires 10.00 D of accommodation to read newsprint (20/200 distance acuity), an add of at least +6.00 D is required for comfortable reading.

67. a. The working distance in diopters is given by Kestenbaum's rule as the reciprocal of the distance acuity. The distance in centimeters is 100 divided by this diopter value. Note that the power of the add has nothing to do with the working distance in younger patients.

68. b. Hand-held magnifiers have a greater working distance (i.e., a greater eye to object distance). They are available in a range of powers from +3.00 to +68.00 D. They do, however, have a smaller field of view than high adds and must be held by hand.

69. d.   Afocal telescopes magnify without decreasing the working distance. Adds may be used to lessen the accommodative demand of these aids. They do, however have a small field of view and small depth of field, so the head must be positioned precisely.

70. e.

$$O_2 \text{ flux} = (D \times K \times P)/L$$

where: D = diffusion coefficient of oxygen in the lens
                                       K = solubility of oxygens in the lens
                                       P = partial pressure gradient of oxygen across the lens
                                       L = central thickness of the lens

71. True.   Holding the radius of curvature constant, larger diameter lenses are effectively steeper.

72. False.   At a given diameter, radius of curvature and lens steepness are inversely proportional.

73. c.   Lenticular astigmatism is defined as astigmatism detected on refraction in excess of the corneal astigmatism. In cases where the refractive cylinder matches the keratometric cylinder, there can be no significant lenticular astigmatism.

74. d.   In fitting rigid contact lenses, if there is a greater than 0.2-mm difference between the radii of the principal corneal meridians, a lens of intermediate curvature, steeper than the flatter meridian by one-third to one-half the difference between meridians, is used. This creates a positive tear film lens, so minus power must be added to the orginal power. The starting power is the <u>sphere</u> of the refraction written in minus cylinder form and corrected for vertex distance if necessary (powers greater than ±4.00 D).

         -4.00 + 1.25 x 90 is equivalent to -2.75 -1.25 x 180. A (+) tear lens of +0.75 is created by the choice of 7.80 mm base curve (0.25 D for every 0.05 mm). Thus, -0.75 D must be added to -2.75 D. (Vertex distance is not important for powers ≤ 4.00 D.)

75. e.   For rigid gas-permeable lenses, 90% of oxygen transfer occurs across the lens, 10% by tear film exchange.

76. False.   Lens diameter is important in fitting both soft and RGP contact lenses. However, diameter is the main factor affecting RGP lens centration.

77. a.   For soft lenses, the spherical equivalent is used, after correction for vertex distance. The spherical equivalent of this correction is -5.50 D. Correcting for the vertex distance of 15 mm, the appropriate contact lens has a power of -5.00 D.

78. b.   Extended wear lenses are currently available as hydrogel soft lenses. Increasing the lens water content and decreasing lens thickness increase oxygen transmission. Minus carriers and ballasting play no role in oxygen transmission.

79. False.   A +90 D aspheric lens produces a real inverted image anterior to the lens, similar to the condensing lens of indirect ophthalmoscopy. Both the Hruby lens (-55 D, plano-concave) and the Goldmann fundus contact lens (-64 D, plano-concave) essentially nullify the refractive power of the cornea and create an <u>upright, virtual</u> image of the fundus approximately 2 cm posterior to the lens.

80. a. The Goldmann applanation tonometer uses a split-field plastic prism to indicate when a corneal area 3.06 mm in diameter has been flattened. The force in dynes required to flatten this area, multiplied by 10, is equal to the IOP in mm Hg.

81. True. Measurement of intraocular pressure (IOP) with applanation can be inaccurate if significant corneal astigmatism is present. An elliptical rather than a circular area will be applanated. Splitting the ellipse at a 43-degree angle to the major axis gives the best results. Alternatively, taking the mean of readings at 90 degrees and 180 degrees can reduce the error. With-the-rule cylinder causes underestimation (1 mm Hg/4 D) and against-the-rule cylinder causes overestimation of IOP.

82. a. The direct ophthalmoscope operates on the optical principle that light emanating from the retina of an emmetropic patient will be focused on the retina of an emmetropic observer. Lenses are used between the patient and observer to correct for nonemmetropic situations. In emmetropia, magnification obtained with the direct ophthalmoscope is approximately 15X, since the patient's eye acts as a simple plus magnifier of power 60 D (angular magnification - M = P/4 or 60 D/4 = 15X). In conditions of ametropia, the interposition of lenses creates a Galilean telescope. Therefore, if the patient is myopic, the retina appears more magnified, and if the patient is hyperopic or aphakic, it appears less magnified. Remember that in afocal systems, magnification must be considered in angular, rather than linear, terms.

83. d. A 30 D lens offers less magnification (2X) but a larger field of view than a 20 D lens. While axial magnification is the square of linear magnification, it must be reduced by a factor of 4 for indirect ophthalmoscopy, since the patient's pupil is expanded by a factor of 4 for delivery to both pupils of the examiner.

84. c. Conventional keratometry measures the curvature of only the central 3 mm of the cornea.

85. d.

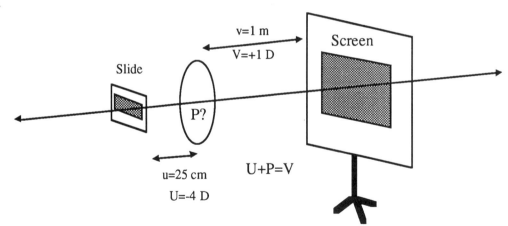

Using the formula U + P = V, the power of the lens to focus the light on the screen can be calculated. We can calculate U and V respectively, because we know the distance of the object to the lens (0.25 m) and the distance from the lens to the screen (1 m). From the formula:
U = -1/(0.25 m) = -4 D and V = 1/1 m = +10 D.
Therefore, P = V-U = 1-(-4) = +5.00.
Note U is negative because it is a real object; therefore light rays must be diverging from it. All real objects are composed of divergent (minus) light. All real images are composed of convergent (plus) light.

86. a.

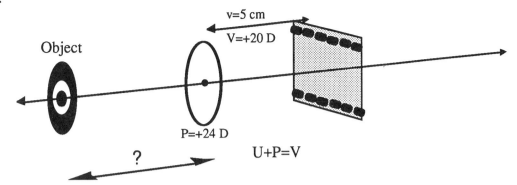

Again we can use the formula U + P = V, where U = vergence of light from the object, P = power of the lens, and V = vergence of light forming the image. Since we know the power of the lens and the distance of the image from the lens we can solve for U and therefore u, the distance from object to lens.

P = +24 D and V = 1/V = 1/.05 m = +20 D (real image)
Thus, U = V - P, U = 20-24 = -4
Finally, U = 1/u or u = 1/U, u = 1/4 m or 25 cm to the left of the lens

87. b.

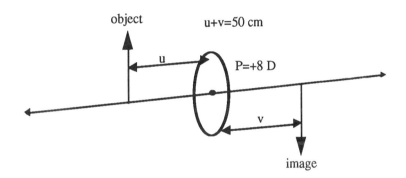

This question is a bit more difficult. If the object and image are 50 cm apart, then u (object-lens distance) + v (lens-image distance) = 0.5 m and U + P = V, where P = 8 D. Since the object is real, u must be negative.

u + v = 0.5 m or
- 1/U + 1/V = 1/2

Multiplying through by -U gives: + 1 + (-U/V) = -1/U
Multiplying through by V:

V - U = -1/2UV

We know U + 8 = V, so:

(8 + U) - U = -1/2 (8 + U) U

reorganizing:

U^2 + 8U + 16 = 0, which is the equivalent to
$(U + 4)^2$ = 0 or U = -4, so u = 1/-4 or 25 cm to the left of the lens

87. (cont.)   Since V = 8 + U = 4
                V = 1/v = 25 cm to the right of the lens

88. a.

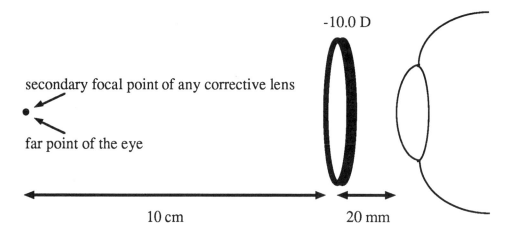

The principle of neutralization of refractive errors is to create an image of infinity at the eye's far point. With accommodation relaxed, the far point and the retina are conjugate, so infinity (moved to the far point by the corrective lens) will be conjugate with the retina. Thus, the corrective lens's secondary focal point must coincide with the eye's far point. Since this eye is corrected with a - 10 D spectacle lens, its far point must be 10 cm in front of the spectacle lens. Given a vertex distance of 2 cm, the far point must be 12 cm from the cornea. Thus, the proper contact lens must have its secondary focal point 12 cm in front of the cornea. $f_2 = n_2/P$, so $P = n_2/f_2 = 1.00/0.12$ m = -8.33 D.

89. b.   The far point is defined as that point in space from which light will focus sharply on the retina, <u>with accommodation fully relaxed</u>. For the emmetropic eye, this point is at optical infinity. The near point is defined as that point in space from which light will focus sharply on the retina, <u>with accommodation fully active</u>. An eye with a +4.00 D "error" lens is 4 D too strong and is corrected (neutralized) with a -4.00 D lens. Myopic eyes can be thought of as having positive error lenses. The far point of a myopic eye (with a positive error lens) is in front of the eye, at a distance in meters equal to the reciprocal of the power of the error lens in diopters. In this case, this is 1/4 of a meter, or 25 cm in front of the eye.

90. d.   Because this eye requires a + 4 D lens for correction, it is hyperopic. A hyperopic eye is too weak.   Thus, for light to fall on the retina of a hyperopic eye, it must be converging. The far point of the hyperopic eye is where the convergent light would intersect (as a virtual object), if it were not bent onto the retina by the refractive power of the hyperopic eye. The far point of any ametropic eye is simply the secondary focal point of the corrective lens or $f_2 = 1/4$ D, 25 cm behind the cornea.

91. b.

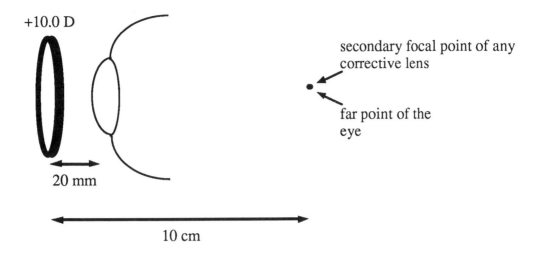

+10.0 D

20 mm

10 cm

secondary focal point of any corrective lens

far point of the eye

Again, the secondary focal point of a corrective lens must coincide with the eye's far point. This eye's far point is 10 cm (100/10 D) <u>behind</u> the spectacle plane. Given a 2-cm vertex distance, the far point is 8 cm behind the cornea. A +3.00 D lens must be placed with its secondary focal point at this same point. Since its secondary focal length is 33 cm, it must be placed 25 cm in front of the cornea.

92. c.

The refracting power of a spherical interface separating two media of different indices of refraction is given by:

$$P = (n_2 - n_1)/r$$

where P = power of the surface, n_1 = refractive index of first medium light travels in, n_2 = refractive index of second medium light travels in, and r = radius of curvature of surface in meters. n_2 = 3.00, n_1 = 1.00 (air), and r = +0.5 m.

The sign of "r" is assigned by convention: "r" is positive if the center of curvature of the surface is on the side opposite the origin of the incident light. If the center of curvature is on the same side of the interface as the origin of light, then r is negative.

Thus,

$$P = 3-1/+0.5 = \underline{+4\ D}$$
Primary focal length = n_1/P = 25 cm
Secondary focal length = n_2/P = 75 cm

Since the <u>diameter</u> of the ball is 100 cm, the secondary focal point (75 cm inside) lies inside the ball.

93. a.

Since P = n_2 - n_1/r, P = 1.50 -1.00/+0.5 = +1 D
Primary focal length = n_1/P = 1 m
Secondary focal length = n_2/P = 1.5 m

Since f_2 = 1.5 m and the diameter of the crystal ball is 1.0 m light coming from infinity could not come to focus inside this crystal ball.

94. b.

Since $P = n_2 - n_1/r$, $P = 1.50-1.00/0.10$ m or +5 D
Primary focal length, $f_1 = n_1/P = 1/5$ m, or 20 cm
Secondary focal length, $f_2 = 1.5/5$ m, or 30 cm

Light from infinity would not come to focus inside this crystal ball because its diameter is 20 cm.

95. False. The radius of curvature of a refractive surface is defined as positive if the center of curvature of the surface is on the side of the surface <u>opposite</u> to the origin of incident (object) light.

96. True. The following is a simple method to determine the sign of the power of a spherical refractive surface: If the center of curvature of the refracting surface is on the same side as the medium of higher index of refraction, the surface is positive, regardless of direction of light propagation.

97. e.

Since $P = n_2 - n_1/r$, $P = 1.33-1.00/0.33$ m or + 1 D

$$U + P = V$$

In this case, reduced vergences, accounting for the index of refraction of the object space (1.33) and the image space (1.00), must be used. So:

$$U = n_1/u, \text{ and } V = n_2/v$$
$$U = -(4/3)/(1/3) = -4$$
$$V = U+P = -4 + 1 = -3 = n_2/v$$
$$n_2 = 1.00 \text{ (air)},$$
so $v = 33$ cm inside the tank

The image is virtual (composed of divergent light) and upright (magnification U/V greater than zero).

98. e.

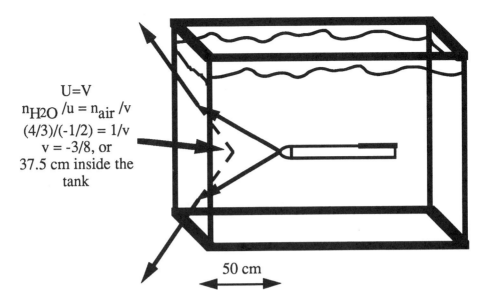

$U = V$
$n_{H2O}/u = n_{air}/v$
$(4/3)/(-1/2) = 1/v$
$v = -3/8$, or
37.5 cm inside the tank

50 cm

The power of a plane sheet of glass is zero, because r is infinite. Since $U + P = V$ and $P = 0$, $U = V$. But, because the index of refraction of the object space($n_{H2O} = 1.33$) is different than that of the image space ($n_{air} = 1.00$), u does not equal v!

$$U = -n_1/u = (4/3)/(-1/2) = -8/3 \text{ D}$$
$$V = n_2/v = U = -8/3 \text{ D}$$
$$\text{Since } n_2 = 1.00, v = -3/8 \text{ m} = 37.5 \text{ cm}$$

Since the light rays are diverging ($V < 0$), the image must be virtual and inside the tank.

99. b.   In the schematic eye, the primary focal point is located approximately 17 mm anterior to the eye ($f_1 = n_1/P = 1/60 \text{ D} = 0.017$ m, or 17 mm). The distance between the secondary focal point and the secondary nodal point is always equal to the primary focal length. The secondary focal point is located approximately 22.5 mm inside the eye ($f_2 = n_2/P = 1.33/60 \text{ D} = 0.0222$ m, or 22.2 mm). Thus, the nodal point must be about 5 mm inside the eye. Because the indices of refraction are different on either side of the cornea, the primary and secondary focal lengths are not equal.

100. c.   The total power of the lens is equal to the sum of the powers of the two refractive surfaces. For the front surface, $P = n_2 - n_1/r_1 = 1.5-1.0/0.10 = +5$ D (the power is positive because the center of curvature is on the same side as the medium with higher index of refraction. For the rear surface, $P = n_1 - n_2/r_2 = 1.0-1.5/-0.05 = +10$ D. The total power is the sum of these two powers, or +15 D. An alternative method for this problem utilizes the formula for total power of two combined spherical refractive surfaces in medium n_1, with medium n_2 between them:

$$P = (n_2-n_1) \times (1/r_1 + 1/r_2)$$

101. d.   IOL powers are generally labeled according to their power immersed in aqueous humor, which has an index of refraction of approximately 1.33. In this case, the power of the IOL would be +18 D in aqueous. The power of the lens in air can be calculated by using a ratio of the difference in the indices of refraction.

$$P(air)/P(eye) = n(IOL)-n(air)/n(IOL)-n(eye)$$
$$\text{Here, } P(air)/P(eye) = 1.50-1.00/1.50-1.33 = 3$$
$$P(air) = 3 \times P(eye) = 3 \times 18 = 54 \text{ D}$$

Note that the len's effective power is greater when the difference in index of refraction between the lens and the surrounding medium is greater.

102. c.   Image ray #1 leaves the lens parallel to the lens axis and therefore must have passed through the <u>primary</u> focal point, not the secondary focal point. Image ray #2 passes through the secondary focal point. Therefore, its object ray must have been traveling parallel to the lens axis. The lens shown is a converging lens with its secondary focal point to the right and, therefore, must be positive in power. Ray #3 is traveling through the nodal point and therefore travels through the lens undeviated.

103. False.   See answer 19. For plus and minus lenses, the absolute value of the powers may be described as follows:

$$/P(back)/ > /P(true)/ > /P(front)/$$

104. True.   As noted in answer 103, the true power of a lens is greater than the front vertex power.

105. b.

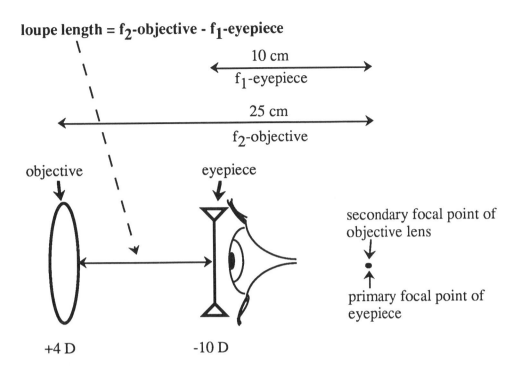

loupe length = f_2-objective - f_1-eyepiece

10 cm
f_1-eyepiece

25 cm
f_2-objective

objective

eyepiece

secondary focal point of objective lens

primary focal point of eyepiece

+4 D

-10 D

In an afocal telescope, the lenses must be placed such that the secondary focal point of the objective lens coincides with the primary focal point of the eyepiece. If both lenses are positive, as in an astronomic telescope, the distance between the lenses is the sum of the focal lengths. If the eyepiece is negative, as in a Galilean telescope, the distance between the lenses is the difference between the focal lengths. In this Galilean telescope, f(objective) = 25 cm, and f(eyepiece) = 10 cm. The difference between the two, 15 cm, is the length of the device.

106. e.   The magnification of an afocal telescope equals:

M = -(eyepiece power)/objective power
In this case, M = -(-10)/4 = +2.5X

The image formed by a Galilean telescope is an upright image (M > 0). No accommodation is required for viewing this image, since the object is at infinity and would require no accommodation to image without the telescope. The image is virtual, since it is composed of parallel light.

107. e.

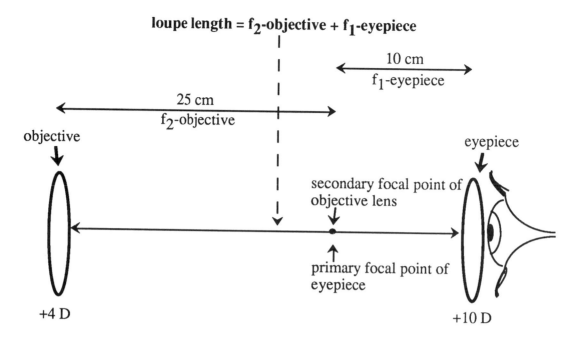

loupe length = f₂-objective + f₁-eyepiece

In an astronomic telescope, both the eyepiece and objective are plus lenses. The distance between the lenses is the sum of the two focal lengths, or 35 cm. (Compare the size of the telescope in question 105 with this telescope.)

108. b.   The magnification of this astronomic telescope also equals:

$$M = -(\text{eyepiece power})/\text{objective power}$$
In this case, $M = -(10)/4 = -5X$

The image formed by any astronomical telescope is inverted (M<0). Accommodation is needed unless the object is at infinity or an add is constructed into the telescope. The image is virtual because it is composed of divergent light (because the object is made of divergent rays).

109. a.   This afocal Galilean telescopic system must be 5 cm long (the difference of the focal lengths of the 2 lenses, 10 cm and 5 cm). The add of +4.00 D is used to decrease the accommodative demand. An object 30 cm from the eye (25 cm from the loupes) will have vergence of -4 D. The +4 D add converts object vergence for the objective to 0 D (U + P = V). Since the objective is +10 D, the image vergence V from the objective is +10 D. The light will come to focus 10 cm from the objective. Since the eyepiece is 5 cm from the objective, this objective image is 5 cm from the eyepiece. Since the light is convergent, the "object" for the eyepiece has vergence of +20 D. V = U + P = +20 + (-20) = 0 D. Thus, light leaves the telescope with zero vergence. Therefore, no accommodation is required for this viewing distance (25 cm from the add).

110. e.   For an object at 10 cm from the loupes (15 cm from the eye):

$$\text{initial } U = -10 \text{ D}$$

For the add:

$$U + P = V, \text{ or } -10 \text{ D} + (+4 \text{ D}) = -6 \text{ D}$$

Since the add and objective are superimposed:

U for the objective = V from the add = -6 D
So for the objective, $U + P = V$, or -6 D + 10 D = +4 D

The objective will create an image about 25 cm (100/4 D) from itself.
The eye piece is 5 cm from the objective, so the objective image (the eyepiece <u>object</u>) is 20 cm from the eyepiece.

So, for the eyepiece, U = +5 D. $U + P = V = +5 + (-20) = V = -15$ D

Since the eyepiece is at a negligible distance from the eye, this is the accommodation needed (+15 D).

111. b.   The angular magnification of loupes with no add equals:

$$M = -(\text{eyepiece power})/\text{objective power}$$

If there is an add to relieve accommodation, this contributes angular magnification as a simple magnifier. The total angular magnification is the <u>product</u> of these two magnification factors, or

$$[P(\text{add})/4] \times [-P(\text{eye piece})/P(\text{objective})]$$

In this case, this is $(+4/4) \times [-(-20)/10] = (+1) \times (+2) = 2X$

112. b.   Image size change can be calculated by considering the eye to have an "error lens" located at the nodal point 5 mm behind the corneal surface. The corrective lens is considered the objective of a Galilean telescope, and the error lens is the eyepiece. Proper distance correction requires that the secondary focal point of the corrective lens be located at the eye's far point, which is the primary focal point of the "error lens."

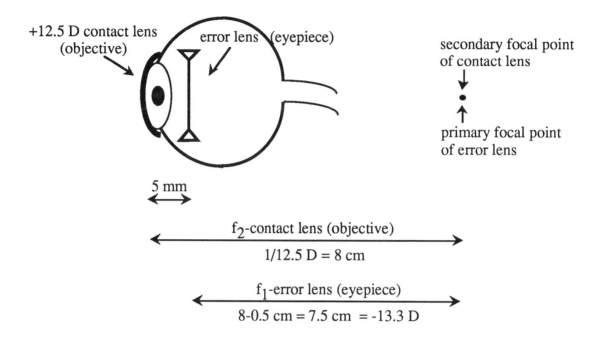

The secondary focal point of the +12.5 D contact lens is located

$$f = 1/12.5D = 0.08 \text{ m (8 cm)}$$

behind the corneal surface. Since the primary focal point of the "error lens" is in the same location, while the error lens is located 0.005 m behind the corneal surface, the power is given by:

$$P_{error} = -1/(0.08 \text{ m} - 0.005 \text{ m}) = -13.3 \text{ D}$$

(The power of the corrective lens and the error lens must be opposite.) If the error lens is thought of as the eyepiece, and the corrective lens as the objective, then magnification of this Galilean telescope is given by:

$$M = -P_{eyepiece}/P_{objective} = -(-13.3 \text{ D})/12.5 \text{ D} = 1.07X$$

That is, the image is 1.07 times the eye of the object, giving 7% magnification (not 7X magnification).

113. c.   With a vertex distance of 20 mm, the corrective lens is located 25 mm in front of the "error lens." The focal length of the corrective lens must be:

$$f = f_{error \, lens} + 0.025 \text{ m} = (1/13.3 \text{ D}) + 0.025 \text{ m} = 0.10 \text{ m}$$
$$P = 1/f = 10.0 \text{ D}$$

114. b.

$$M = -(-13.3 \text{ D})/10.0 \text{ D} = 1.33 = 33\% \text{ magnification}$$
(See questions 108 and 109.)

115. c.

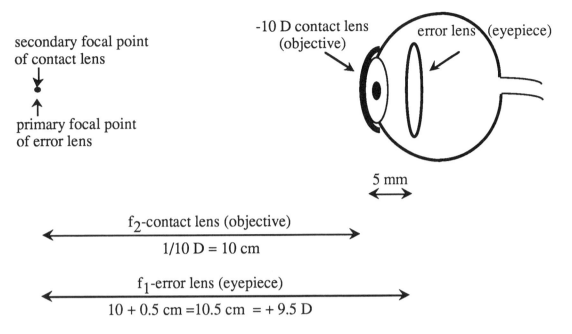

secondary focal point
of contact lens

primary focal point
of error lens

-10 D contact lens
(objective)

error lens (eyepiece)

5 mm

f_2-contact lens (objective)

1/10 D = 10 cm

f_1-error lens (eyepiece)

10 + 0.5 cm =10.5 cm = + 9.5 D

In a myope, the far point is in front of the eye, and the positions of the secondary focal point of the corrective lens and the primary focal point of the error lens must be located in the same place. Since a -10.0 D contact lens located 5 mm in front of the nodal point gives proper correction, the focal length of the error lens is given by

$$f_{error} = -f_{corrective} + 0.005 \text{ m} = -1/P_{corrective} + 0.005 \text{ m}$$
$$f_{error} = -(1/-10.0 \text{ D}) + 0.005 \text{ m} = 0.105 \text{ m}$$

The power is:

$$P_{error} = 1/0.105 \text{ m} = 9.5 \text{ D}$$

The magnification is:

$$M = -P_{eyepiece}/P_{objective} = -9.5 \text{ D}/-10.0 \text{ D} = 0.95$$

This represents 5% minification. Since the power of the eyepiece is positive and the objective negative, this is like looking through a Galilean telescope backward, resulting in minification.

116. d.   With a vertex distance of 20 mm, the distance between the spectacle lens and the "error lens" is 25 mm. The focal length of the corrective lens is therefore:

$$f_{corrective} = f_{error} - 0.025\ m = 0.105\ m - 0.025\ m = 0.08\ m$$

The power is:

$$P = -1/0.08\ m = -12.5\ D$$

117. c. $M = -P_{eyepiece}/P_{objective} = -9.5\ D/-12.5\ D = +0.76 = 24\%$ minification

118. d.   The formula for the power of a mirror is $P = -(2/r)$, where r equals the radius of curvature of the mirror in meters. The vergence formula for mirrors is the same as that for lenses--$U + V = P$. A plane mirror has an infinite radius of curvature and, therefore, no power. It does not change the vergence of light but changes only its direction. Since the object is 1 m in front of the mirror, the object vergence at the mirror is:

$$U = -1/1\ m = -1\ D$$
$$V = U + P = -1\ D + 0\ D = -1\ D$$
$$v = 1/V = -1/1 = -1\ m$$

The image, therefore is located 1 m behind the mirror and is virtual. The magnification for a mirror is the same as for a lens, $M = U/V$:

$$M = U/V = -1\ D/-1\ D = 1X$$

The image and object are the same size, and since the magnification is positive, the image is upright. Since the angle of incidence and the angle of reflection are equal, a mirror half the height of the man will allow him to see his toes, regardless of where he stands.

119. c.   The reflective power of the mirror is:

$$P = -2/r = -2/0.20 \text{ m} = -10 \text{ D}$$

Convex mirror--adds divergence
r > 0

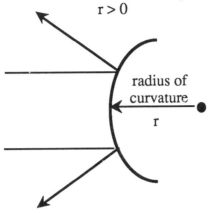

(By definition, a mirror convex toward light has a positive radius of curvature, and a mirror concave toward light has a negative radius of curvature. Therefore, any convex mirror has negative power; any concave mirror has positive power.)

Concave mirror--adds convergence
r < 0

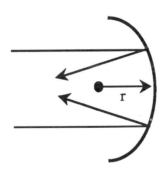

The object is located 50 cm in front of the mirror, so:

$$U = -1/0.5 \text{ m} = -2 \text{ D}$$
$$V = U + P = -2 \text{ D} - 10 \text{ D} = -12 \text{ D}$$

and the image is located:

$$v = 1/V = 1/(-12 \text{ D}) = -0.083 \text{ m} = 8.3 \text{ cm behind the mirror}$$

120. True.   See answer 119. A convex mirror <u>always</u> adds divergence to light. The image light in this question is composed of divergent light. Real images, by definition, are made up of convergent light.

121. False.   Magnification by a mirror is given by the same formula as for a lens, $M = U/V$. Here $M = -2/-12 = 1/6$. The image is 1/6 the size of the object (minified by a factor of 6).

122. True.   If the magnification values is greater than zero, the image is upright (this holds for lenses, as well).

123. d.   The refractive power of the anterior surface of the cornea is given by:

$$P_{front} = (n_2 - n_1)/r = (1.38 - 1)/(0.0077\ m) = +49.4\ D$$

The refractive power of the posterior surface of the cornea is given by:

$$P_{back} = (1.33 - 1.38)/0.0076\ m = -6.6\ D$$

The total refractive power of the cornea, therefore, is:

$$P_{front} + P_{back} = 49.4\ D - 6.6\ D = 42.8\ D$$

The reflecting power of the front surface of the cornea is given by:

$$P = -2/r = -2/0.0077\ mm = -260\ D$$

A single refractive surface at an interface between air and a medium with index of refraction of 1.3375, having a radius of curvature of 7.9 mm, has refractive power of:

$$P = (1.3375 - 1)/0.0079\ m = +42.7\ D$$

which is the same refractive power as the cornea. This is where the formula for conversion from radius of curvature to power is derived:

$$P = 0.3375/r$$
$$r = 0.3375/P$$

124. d.   Consider the implant as the object. The optic diameter measured is a measurement of what we see, namely the image of the optic, not the optic itself. The optic is in aqueous ($n = 1.33$), so its object vergence, U, is:

$$U = -1.33/0.003\ m = -443.3\ D$$
$$P = 42.8\ D$$
$$U + P = V = -443.3\ D + 42.8\ D = -400.5\ D$$
$$M = v/u = U/V = -443.3\ D/-400.5\ D = 1.11X$$

The image of the optic is, therefore, 1.11 times larger than the iris, so if o is the object height and i is the image height:

$$M = i/o = 1.11X$$

$$i = 1.11 \times o = 1.11 \times 6.0\ mm = \underline{6.66\ mm}$$

125. b.   The reflecting power of the corneal surface is given by:

$$P = -2/r = -2/0.0077 \text{ m} = -260 \text{ D}$$

For a penlight held 40 cm (0.40 m) in front of this mirror:

$$U = 1/-0.4 \text{ m} = -2.5 \text{ D}$$
$$U + P = V = -262.5 \text{ D}$$
$$v = 1/V = -1/262.5 \text{ D} = -0.0038 \text{ m} = 3.8 \text{ mm}$$

inside the eye. Light rays reflected off the cornea are <u>divergent</u>, so the virtual image appears to be inside the eye!

126. d.   By moving his/her head away from the condensing lens, a smaller area of the patient's pupil requires illumination, leaving more available for image transmission.

127. b.   Image brightness, clarity, and detail are enhanced by moving closer. This requires a larger pupil, however (see question 126).

128. e.   Higher power condensing lenses have reflexes that require greater tilting of the lens than lower power lenses to shift them out of the viewing axis.

129.   With the retinoscope in the plano-mirror position (handle <u>up</u> on the Copeland model, handle <u>down</u> on the Welch Allyn), the streak image is behind the patient or at infinity. "With" motion indicates the patient's eye is a minus lens system, neutralized with plus lenses. "Against" motion implies the patient's eye is a plus system of sufficient power to cause the new streak image (acted on by the eye) to be located between the patient and the observer.

130. False.   Knapp's rule holds only for axial anisometropia. Most anisometropia is mixed, that is, both refractive and axial.

References

1. Miller, David. "Section 3: Optics, Refraction, and Contact Lenses." in F.M. Wilson (ed.). <u>Basic and Clinical Science Course</u>. San Francisco: American Academy of Ophthalmology, 1991-1992.

2. Rubin, Melvin R. <u>Optics for Clinicians</u> (2nd ed.). Gainesvillle, FL: Triad Scientific, 1977.

3: Ophthalmic Pathology and Intraocular Tumors

1. Match the differentiated cells listed in the left column with each's <u>immediate</u> precursor.

   a. cytotoxic cell.
   b. mast cell.
   c. epithelioid cell.
   d. plasma cell.
   e. giant cell.
   f. macrophage.

   1. basophils.
   2. monocyte.
   3. macrophage.
   4. B-lymphocyte.
   5. T-lymphocyte.

2. Match the conditions listed in the left column with the giant cell type typically seen in each.

   a. lipogranuloma.
   b. sarcoidosis.
   c. juvenile xanthogranuloma.
   d. tuberculosis.
   e. necrobiotic xanthogranuloma.
   f. fungal granuloma.
   g. leprosy.
   h. Erdheim-Chester disease.

   1. Touton.
   2. Langerhans'.
   3. Foreign body.
   4. Langhans'.

3. A Russell body is:

   a. an accumulation of granules within eosinophils.
   b. proteinaceous debris within giant cells.
   c. accumulated lysosomal degradation products within polymorphonuclear leukocytes (PMNs).
   d. proteinaceous antigen debris within macrophages.
   e. concentrated immunoglobulin within plasma cells.

4. T or F -- The hallmark of granulomatous inflammation is the presence of giant cells.

5. Of the following, which inflammation pattern and disease pairing is <u>incorrect</u>?

   a. diffuse granulomatous inflammation -- sympathetic ophthalmia.
   b. discrete granuloma formation -- sarcoidosis.
   c. discrete granulomatous inflammation -- tuberculous leprosy.
   d. diffuse type granulomatous inflammation -- tuberculosis.
   e. zonal type inflammation -- phacoantigenic uveitis.

6. Match the appropriate stain technique with the correct organisms.

   a. Ziehl-Neelsen stain (carbol-fuchsin   1. *Chlamydia.*
      dye with acid decolorization).   2. *Neisseria.*
   b. Giemsa.   3. spirochetes.
   c. Gomori methenamine silver.   4. mycobacteria.
   d. Warthin-Starry.   5. *Candida.*
   e. Hematoxylin-eosin.

7. Which one of the following concerning fungal keratitis is false?

   a. Generally these infections are initiated by trauma involving plant or animal matter.
   b. Topical corticosteroids generally enhance organism replication and penetration.
   c. The actual etiologic agent is dependent on geographic locale.
   d. Most of the important corneal pathogens are molds.
   e. The cornea is an effective barrier to intraocular fungal penetration.

8. Which one of the following concerning chlamydial ocular infections is true?

   a. The cornea is typically spared in chlamydial conjunctivitis.
   b. Disease manifestations are dictated by organism serotype.
   c. The only difference between inclusion conjunctivitis and trachoma is the presence of
      subconjunctival scarring.
   d. Wright's stain is the preferred method of demonstrating the pathognomonic findings.
   e. Typically the inclusion bodies of chlamydial disease are intranuclear.

9. Which one of the following concerning viral ocular disease is false?

   a. The intracytoplasmic inclusions of molluscum contagiosum may cause cellular rupture,
      leading to an adjacent inflammatory reaction.
   b. The host response to herpetic infection is nongranulomatous in primary cases and maybe
      granulomatous in reactivation.
   c. Subacute sclerosing panencephalitis, a chronic central nervous system measles infection,
      may be associated with a retinitis.
   d. Cytomegalovirus (CMV) causes a chorioretinitis that is associated with both
      intracytoplasmic and intranuclear inclusion bodies.
   e. Interferon may be an important host defense mechanism in many viral ocular infections.

10. T or F -- Lepromatous leprosy tends to cause a diffuse granulomatous sclerokeratitis and
    uveitis, while tuberculoid leprosy tends to cause discrete granulomatous disease of the orbit
    and adnexa.

11. Which one of the following concerning intraocular infections is false?

    a. The pork tapeworm *Taenia solium* may cause an intense granulomatous reaction when an intraocular cyst dies.
    b. *Toxocara canis* induces a choroiditis characterized by the eosinophilic abscess.
    c. The cat is the definitive host for *Toxoplasma gondii*.
    d. *Toxoplasma* cyst forms are extracellular, and reactivation requires cyst conversion to a trophozoite.
    e. *Cryptococcus* may cause a meningoencephalitis with optic neuritis and retinitis.

12. T or F -- The hallmark of herpes simplex keratitis and reactivation is multinucleated giant cell infiltration adjacent to Descemet's membrane.

13. Which of the following may present as ocular inflammation (or pseudoinflammation)?

    1. uveal melanoma.
    2. non-Hodgkins lymphoma.
    3. retinoblastoma.
    4. melanocytoma.

    a. 1, 2, and 3.
    b. 1 and 3.
    c. 2 and 4.
    d. 4 only.
    e. 1, 2, 3, and 4.

14. Which one of the following concerning lens-induced uveitis and glaucoma is false?

    a. The term phacoantigenic is preferable to phacoanaphylaxis.
    b. Phacoanaphylactic glaucoma is probably on the same spectrum as phacolytic glaucoma, simply being more severe.
    c. *Proprionibacterium acnes* may be an important contributor to the condition, particularly in pseudophakic eyes.
    d. The classic pattern of inflammation in phacoantigenic glaucoma is the zonal granuloma centered about a site of injury to the lens.
    e. The stimulus for phacoantigenic uveitis appears to be lens cortical protein.

15. All of the following are conditions that may be associated with granulomatous ocular inflammation except:

    a. sarcoidosis.
    b. rheumatoid arthritis.
    c. Behçet's disease.
    d. Vogt-Koyanagi-Harada syndrome (VKH).
    e. syphilis.

16. All of the following are conditions that may be associated with nongranulomatous ocular inflammation except:

   a. choroidal melanoma.
   b. juvenile rheumatoid arthritis.
   c. trauma.
   d. Reiter's syndrome.
   e. cryptococcal endophthalmitis.

17. T or F -- The distinction between Vogt-Koyanagi-Harada syndrome (VKH) and sympathetic ophthalmia (SO) must be made clinically, since there are no distinguishing histologic features.

18. Which one of the following concerning healing in specific ocular tissues is true?

   a. Epithelial migration and ingrowth generally leads to complete replacement of structures lost in full-thickness skin wounds by the sixth week after injury.
   b. Central corneal healing is accomplished only after granulation tissue is extruded from the wound, approximately 4 to 6 weeks after injury.
   c. The most important components in limbal wound healing are scleral vessels and resident cells.
   d. The critical step in healing central and peripheral corneal wounds is metaplasia or migration of endothelial cells to seal the internal defect.
   e. Due to its marked vascularity and rich innervation, the iris generally shows exuberant and rapid wound healing processes.

19. Which one of the following concerning retinal response to injury is true?

   a. Mechanical injury leads to a typical fibrovascular healing response.
   b. Cellular proliferation in retinal healing takes place mainly within the photoreceptor and inner-plexiform layers.
   c. Retinal pigment epithelial (RPE) hyperplasia rarely plays a significant role in retinal healing.
   d. Retinal fibrosis is responsible for the healing strength of a laser or cryotherapy mark.
   e. A rupture of Bruch's membrane will lead to choroidal participation in the human response with subsequent fibrosis.

20. T or F -- The cause of expulsive choroidal hemorrhage is probably distortion of rigid choroidal vessels by high intraocular pressure.

21. T or F -- The histopathologic features of epithelial downgrowth are most consistent with abnormally invasive corneal epithelium.

22. Postoperative sympathetic ophthalmia is most likely to develop following:

    a. uncomplicated intracapsular cataract surgery.
    b. uncomplicated extracapsular cataract surgery.
    c. penetrating keratoplasty in a patient with herpes simplex keratitis and a history of uveitis.
    d. scleral buckling procedure using scleral implants.
    e. filtration procedures on end-stage glaucomatous eyes.

23. Which one of the following concerning the pathology of penetrating keratoplasty is false?

    a. Graft failure implies an immunologic rejection response to the donor cornea.
    b. A graft rejection may be centered on the epithelium, stroma, or endothelium.
    c. Epithelial rejection is generally self-limited and resembles epidemic keratoconjunctivits (EKC).
    d. Stromal rejection most typically presents 2 to 4 weeks postoperatively.
    e. The pathognomonic sign of active corneal graft rejection is the Khoudadoust line, an endothelial precipitate of leukocytes.

24. Select the correct pairing of eponym and pathologic findings:

    a. Elschnig's pearls -- retention of lens fibers in the equatorial area of the capsular fornix.
    b. Elschnig's pearls -- clumps of iris pigment epithelial cells on the anterior lens capsule following trauma.
    c. Vossius' ring -- retention of lens fibers in the equatorial area of the capsular fornix.
    d. Vossius' ring -- clumps of iris pigment epithelial cells on the anterior lens capsule following trauma.
    e. Soemmering's ring -- clumps of iris pigment epithelial cells on the anterior lens capsule following blunt trauma.

25. The earliest accumulations of cystoid macular edema fluid occur in the:

    a. subretinal space.
    b. outer plexiform layer.
    c. inner plexiform layer.
    d. nerve fiber layer.
    e. subinternal limiting membrane space.

26. Which one of the following concerning intraocular hemorrhage is true?

    a. Corneal blood staining is generally the result of pressure-induced displacement of intact red blood cells (RBCs) through a damaged Descemet's membrane.
    b. In hemosiderosis bulbi, hemoglobin accumulation leads to epithelial damage (anterior subcapsular cataract, glaucoma, retinal degeneration).
    c. Ghost cells may be identified by phase contrast microscopy or by stained preparations documenting the presence of Heinz bodies.
    d. Synchysis scintillans is a condition in which hemoglobin breakdown products crystallize in the dependent portion of the vitreous.
    e. An ochre membrane results from vitreous hemorrhage coating the posterior lens capsule.

27. T or F -- A secluded pupil (seclusio pupillae) implies a complete membranous covering of the pupil due to inflammation.

28. Which of the following features are considered necessary to label an eye phthisical?

                1. abnormally small (shrinkage).
                2. disorganization.
                3. atrophy.
                4. calcification.

a. 1, 2, and 3.
b. 1 and 3.
c. 2 and 4.
d. 4 only.
e. 1, 2, 3, and 4.

29. Focal points of scleral weakness or thinning that are significant in blunt ocular trauma include all of the following except:

a. the superficial scleral sulcus.
b. the sclera immediately posterior to the rectus muscle insertions.
c. the sclera immediately adjacent to the superior oblique insertion.
d. the sclera immediately adjacent to the inferior oblique insertion.
e. the lamina cribrosa.

30. Which of the following regarding the phakomatous choristoma is/are true?

                1. It may be associated with ocular colobomata.
                2. Acquired forms have been reported.
                3. There is frequently associated hyperpigmentation.
                4. The most frequent site of involvement is the eyelid.

a. 1, 2, and 3.
b. 1 and 3.
c. 2 and 4.
d. 4 only.
e. 1, 2, 3, and 4.

31. All of the following are histopathologic manifestations of angle recession except:

a. a cleavage plane between longitudinal ciliary body fibers and sclera.
b. atrophy of the ciliary muscle fibers.
c. change in the ciliary body shape from triangular to fusiform.
d. posterolateral displacement of ciliary processes.
e. an epithelial-like membrane covering the trabecular meshwork and angle structures (in some cases).

32. Retinal dialysis is most likely to develop in the

        1. inferotemporal quadrant.
        2. superotemporal quadrant.
        3. superonasal quadrant.
        4. inferonasal quadrant.

  a. 1, 2, and 3.
  b. 1 and 3.
  c. 2 and 4.
  d. 4 only.
  e. 1, 2, 3, and 4.

33. A 44-year-old man is hammering metal on metal and suddenly experiences pain and loss of vision in his right eye. He is examined and noted to have an intravitreal foreign body, which has passed through the cornea and central lens. A correct description of his injury would be:

        1. double perforating injury.
        2. corneal and lenticular perforating injury.
        3. double corneal and lenticular penetrating injury.
        4. ocular penetrating injury.

  a. 1, 2, and 3.
  b. 1 and 3.
  c. 2 and 4.
  d. 4 only.
  e. 1, 2, 3, and 4.

34. Which one of the following concerning intraocular contamination is true?

  a. Siderosis bulbi is generally due to damage to ocular epithelial tissues by ferric (Fe^{+3}) ion.
  b. Copper foreign bodies with greater than 85% elemental copper generally lead to chalcosis, characterized by copper deposits in basement membranes.
  c. Glass, platinum and porcelain are similar in their relative inert status as intraocular foreign bodies.
  d. Sterile vegetable matter will generally elicit no intraocular inflammatory response.
  e. Lead is an inert intraocular foreign body.

35. Which one of the following alkaline solutions constitutes the greatest threat to intraocular chemical injury?

  a. hydrochloric acid.
  b. ammonium hydroxide (ammonia).
  c. calcium hydroxide (lime).
  d. boric acid.
  e. petroleum.

36. All of the following are true concerning the effects of wavelength-specific ocular radiation except:

    a. microwave radiation -- cataract.
    b. infrared radiation -- true lens exfoliation.
    c. UV -- welder's flash.
    d. ionizing radiation -- retinal gliosis.
    e. ionizing radiation -- conjunctival ulceration and atrophy.

37. T or F -- A hamartoma consists of normal tissue in an abnormal location, while a choristoma consists of abnormal tissue in a normal location.

38. T or F -- An in utero insult at the beginning of the first trimester is more likely to lead to glaucoma, while one after the first trimester is more likely to lead to cataract.

39. Which of the following are variations on the hyaloidolenticular vascular system?

                    1. Bergmeister's papilla.
                    2. persistent hyaloid artery.
                    3. Mittendorf's dot.
                    4. persistent pupillary membrane.

    a. 1, 2, and 3.
    b. 1 and 3.
    c. 2 and 4.
    d. 4 only
    e. 1, 2, 3, and 4.

40. Which one of the following concerning common congenital adnexal conditions is true?

    a. Epidermoid and dermoid cysts frequently arise in continuity with boney suture lines and underlying orbital periosteum.
    b. Eyelid hemangiomas are usually of the capillary type and have only cosmetic implications.
    c. Conjunctival dermoids are hamartomatous lesions that may arise as part of Goldenhar's syndrome.
    d. The primary difference between conjunctival dermoid tumors and dermoid cysts of the eyelids and orbit is the presence of pilosebaceous units in the latter.
    e. Dermolipomas of the conjunctiva are related to dermoids and are generally easily surgically removed.

41. Match the gonioscopic and clinical findings with the appropriate eponym.

    a. Prominent, anteriorly placed   1. Rieger's anomaly.
       Schwalbe's line.   2. posterior embryotoxon.
    b. a plus iris processes to Schwalbe's   3. Reiger's syndrome.
       line.   4. Axenfeld's syndrome.
    c. b plus glaucoma.   5. Axenfeld's anomaly.
    d. b plus iris atrophy and corectopia.
    e. d plus dental/facial anomalies.

42. T or F -- The basic feature of the spectrum constituting Peters' anomaly is central absence of Descemet's membrane with a cloudy cornea (leukoma).

43. Which of the following conditions may be associated with <u>congenital</u> ectopia lentis?

        1. Marfan's syndrome.
        2. Ehlers-Danlos syndrome.
        3. congenital glaucoma.
        4. Peters' anomaly.

a. 1, 2, and 3.
b. 1 and 3.
c. 2 and 4.
d. 4 only.
e. 1, 2, 3, and 4.

44. For which of the following disorders is the pattern of inheritance autosomal recessive?

        1. neurofibromatosis.
        2. tuberous sclerosis.
        3. Sturge-Weber syndrome.
        4. ataxia-telangiectasia.

a. 1, 2, and 3.
b. 1 and 3.
c. 2 and 4.
d. 4 only.
e. 1, 2, 3, and 4.

45. Which of the following disorders are <u>commonly</u> associated with congenital or juvenile glaucoma?

        1. von Hippel-Lindau syndrome.
        2. Sturge-Weber syndrome.
        3. ataxia-telangiectasia.
        4. neurofibromatosis.

a. 1, 2, and 3.
b. 1 and 3.
c. 2 and 4.
d. 4 only.
e. 1, 2, 3, and 4.

46. Which of the following disorders commonly have posterior segment findings?

   1. von Hippel-Lindau syndrome.
   2. Sturge-Weber syndrome.
   3. ataxia-telangiectasia.
   4. neurofibromatosis.

   a. 1, 2, and 3.
   b. 1 and 3.
   c. 2 and 4.
   d. 4 only.
   e. 1, 2, 3, and 4.

47. For each of the following phakomatoses, select the correct clinical manifestation. (Note that manifestations may be used more than once, and each disorder may have more than one manifestation!)

   a. von Hippel-Lindau syndrome.   1. pulsating exophthalmos.
   b. Sturge-Weber syndrome.   2. astrocytic hamartoma of the optic
   c. neurofibromatosis.   nerve and retina.
   d. tuberous sclerosis.   3. retinal capillary hemangioma.
   e. ataxia-telangiectasia.   4. choroidal cavernous hemangioma.
                                            5. irregular retinal vessels.

48. All of the following are phakomatoses except:

   a. Sturge-Weber syndrome.
   b. von Recklinghausen's disease.
   c. Bourneville's disease.
   d. Wyburn-Mason syndrome.
   e. Louis-Bar syndrome.

49. Which one of the following concerning persistent hyperplastic primary vitreous (PHPV) is true?

   a. The size of the eye is generally normal.
   b. Angle-closure glaucoma early in life is common.
   c. The retina generally remains attached despite central fibrovascular proliferation.
   d. The visual prognosis is good.
   e. Cataract is rarely seen in this condition.

50. Retinal dysplasia may be seen in association with:

> 1. microphthalmos.
> 2. trisomy 13.
> 3. uveal colobomata.
> 4. maternal LSD abuse.

a. 1, 2, and 3.
b. 1 and 3.
c. 2 and 4.
d. 4 only.
e. 1, 2, 3, and 4.

51. Macular hypoplasia has been associated with:

> 1. aniridia.
> 2. albinism.
> 3. PHPV.
> 4. neurofibromatosis.

a. 1, 2, and 3.
b. 1 and 3.
c. 2 and 4.
d. 4 only.
e. 1, 2, 3, and 4.

52. Congenital cataracts may be associated with which of the following chromosomal disorders?

> 1. trisomy 21 (Down's syndrome).
> 2. trisomy 13 (Patau's syndrome).
> 3. 11p- syndrome.
> 4. trisomy 18 (Edwards' syndrome).

a. 1, 2, and 3.
b. 1 and 3.
c. 2 and 4.
d. 4 only.
e. 1, 2, 3, and 4.

53. PHPV may be associated with which of the following chromosomal abnormalities?

> 1. trisomy 21.
> 2. trisomy 18.
> 3. 11p- syndrome.
> 4. trisomy 13.

a. 1, 2, and 3.
b. 1 and 3.
c. 2 and 4.
d. 4 only.
e. 1, 2, 3, and 4.

54. The fetal alcohol syndrome may be associated with ocular conditions including:

        1. retinal vascular tortuosity.
        2. optic nerve hypoplasia.
        3. esotropia.
        4. ptosis.

    a. 1, 2, and 3.
    b. 1 and 3.
    c. 2 and 4.
    d. 4 only.
    e. 1, 2, 3, and 4.

55. Match the pathologic condition with the potential gland of origin. (Note that each condition may be associated with more than one gland. Glands may be used more than once or not at all.)

    a. Sjögren's syndrome.   1. Moll's glands.
    b. sebaceous carcinoma.   2. glands of Zeis.
    c. external hordeolum.   3. glands of Krause and Wolfring.
    d. sudoriferous cyst.   4. eccrine sweat glands.
    e. syringoma.   5. meibomian glands.

56. T or F -- Preseptal cellulitis may lead to orbital cellulitis in a normal eye.

57. T or F -- Dermal amyloid infiltration is generally a localized phenomenon, while conjunctival amyloid infiltration typically suggests systemic disease.

58. Roughly what percentage of patients with xanthelasma will have a systemic dyslipidemia?

    a. 20%.
    b. 25%.
    c. 33%.
    d. 50%.
    e. 75%.

59. Which one of the following concerning juvenile xanthogranuloma (JXG) is false?

    a. Lesions appear as yellow-orange skin nodules.
    b. Touton giant cells are a prominent feature.
    c. The color of these lesions arises from intercellular lipofuscin deposition.
    d. Tan or orangish nodules on the iris are a common manifestation.
    e. Intraocular JXG may present as a spontaneous hyphema.

60. Which one of the following concerning cystic structures of the eyelids is true?

    a. An epidermoid cyst may be separated from a dermoid cyst at the slit lamp by transillumination characteristics.
    b. The prime feature differentiating an epidermoid cyst from a ductal cyst is the characteristic of the fluid filling the cyst.
    c. Histologically, the lining of a ductal cyst is always a cuboidal eccrine epithelium.
    d. The key histopathologic feature separating epidermoid from dermoid cysts is the nature of the cyst wall.
    e. Dermoid cysts are frequently associated with Goldenhar's sydrome.

61. Which of the following definitions of epidermal pathologic findings is/are correct?

    1. hyperkeratosis: thickening of the prickle cell layer.
    2. parakeratosis: thickening of the keratin layer.
    3. acantholysis: loss of the normal keratin layer.
    4. dyskeratosis: intraepidermal keratinization.

    a. 1, 2, and 3.
    b. 1 and 3.
    c. 2 and 4.
    d. 4 only.
    e. 1, 2, 3, and 4.

62. T or F -- Collagen with a bluish hue on hematoxylin-eosin staining is frequently a marker for previous ultraviolet radiation damage.

63. T or F -- The main difference between seborrheic and actinic keratoses is the presence of pigmentation in the former.

64. The lesion least likely to be clinically or pathologically mistaken for squamous cell carcinoma of the eyelid is:

    a. actinic keratosis.
    b. keratoacanthoma.
    c. seborrheic keratosis.
    d. pseudoepitheliomatous hyperplasia.
    e. basal cell carcinoma.

65. Which one of the following concerning basal cell carcinoma of the eyelid is false?

    a. It is the second most common malignant tumor of the eyelid.
    b. The lower lid is more frequently involved than the upper lid.
    c. Medial canthal tumors generally carry a poorer prognosis.
    d. Important histologic clues to the basal cell origin of this tumor include nests and cords of epidermal basilar cells with peripheral palisading and cracking artifact.
    e. Cystic basal cell carcinomas frequently present as blue eyelid cysts.

66. Which one of the following concerning sebaceous neoplasms is false?

    a. They may arise from meibomian, Zeis, or caruncular sebaceous glands.
    b. A history of radiation is a risk factor.
    c. Benign sebaceous tumors may be associated with gastrointestinal malignancy.
    d. Histopathologic clues to the diagnosis include pagetoid spread of tumor cells, foamy tumor cells, and cystic necrosis of cell nests.
    e. Typically, hematoxylin-eosin staining is sufficient to make the diagnosis.

67. Which one of the following concerning pigmented eye lesions is false?

    a. Unlike congenital nevi, acquired nevi rarely become malignant.
    b. Most eyelid nevi are acquired.
    c. Acquired nevi typically present around age 10.
    d. Nevi are best described by the location of cellular proliferation.
    e. The degree of elevation of a nevus is directly proportional to the extent of epithelial or junctional involvement.

68. T or F -- The caruncle is a specialized conjunctival structure.

69. Which one of the following concerning ocular amyloidosis is false?

    a. Conjunctival foci most frequently herald primary localized disease.
    b. The deposits, regardless of location, are prone to spontaneous hemorrhage.
    c. The stain of choice is Congo red, which will bring out the deposits' dichroism and birefringence.
    d. Dermal infiltration of amyloid frequently arises in cases of primary localized amyloidosis.
    e. Chronic conjunctival inflammation or irritation may lead to secondary amyloidosis.

70. Which one of the following concerning lymphoid lesions of the conjunctiva is false?

    a. They most frequently occur on the palpebral conjunctiva.
    b. They are typically salmon-pink and soft.
    c. Eyelid skin involvement heralds increased risk for systemic lymphoma.
    d. Russell bodies and Dutcher bodies frequently mark a lymphoid lesion as "reactive" (nonneoplastic).
    e. Approximately 10% of patients with systemic lymphoma will develop conjunctival infiltration.

71. Which one of the following concerning squamous cell lesions of the conjunctiva is false?

    a. They are typically preceded in time by foci of carcinoma in situ (severe epithelial dysplasia).
    b. They typically arise in the interpalpebral fissure near the limbus.
    c. Only specific variants of squamous cell carcinoma will infiltrate the globe.
    d. Hematogenous metastasis is not unusual with squamous cell carcinoma.
    e. Squamous cell lesions may simulate pagetoid sebaceous cell carcinoma.

72. T or F -- Conjunctival melanoma occurs more frequently in patients with ocular melanocytosis and oculodermal melanocytosis.

73. T or F -- The most frequent histopathologic diagnosis for a white patient in his 30s with conjunctival melanosis is junctional nevus.

74. Which of the following is/are true concerning primary acquired melanosis (PAM) of the conjunctiva?

    1. The incidence is highest for middle-aged persons.
    2. Unremitting rapid growth is characteristic.
    3. The risk of progression to conjunctival melanoma is approximately 50% if the melanocytic proliferation appears atypical.
    4. PAM without atypia has been noted to progress to conjunctival melanoma.

    a. 1, 2, and 3.
    b. 1 and 3.
    c. 2 and 4.
    d. 4 only.
    e. 1, 2, 3, and 4.

75. Which of the following is/are true concerning conjunctival melanoma?

    1. Three-quarters of cases arise de novo and one-quarter from PAM with atypia.
    2. The overall mortality is 25%.
    3. Like uveal melanoma, metastases frequently involve the liver.
    4. Prognosis is best assessed by melanocytic atypia and growth pattern.

    a. 1, 2, and 3.
    b. 1 and 3.
    c. 2 and 4.
    d. 4 only.
    e. 1, 2, 3, and 4.

76. The malignant tumor whose histopathology most closely resembles a neoplastic or "transformed" pyogenic granuloma is:

    a. squamous cell carcinoma.
    b. basal cell carcinoma.
    c. Kaposi's sarcoma.
    d. capillary hemangioma.
    e. rhabdomyosarcoma.

77. The differential diagnosis for interstitial keratitis includes:

     1. sarcoidosis.
     2. onchocerciasis.
     3. congenital syphilis.
     4. acanthamoeba.

    a. 1, 2, and 3.
    b. 1 and 3.
    c. 2 and 4.
    d. 4 only.
    e. 1, 2, 3, and 4.

78. Which one of the following regarding "combined hamartomas" of the retina and retinal pigment epithelium (RPE) is false?

    a. They are frequently associated with other developmental ocular anomalies.
    b. They are usually clinically silent until middle age.
    c. One clinical hallmark is retinal vascular tortuosity.
    d. The peripapillary region is most frequently affected.
    e. Vitrectomy with membrane peeling is generally not effective for restoring vision.

79. T or F -- The diagnosis of *Acanthamoeba* keratitis is enhanced by special staining with calcofluor white and culturing on blood agar layered with *Staphylococcus aureus*.

80. Which of the following concerning corneal edema and its common etiologies is/are true?

     1. The presence of guttae and thickened Descemet's membrane is sufficient for the diagnosis of Fuchs' dystrophy.
     2. The differentiating feature between true Fuchs' dystrophy and pseudophakic bullous keratopathy (PBK) is the thickness of Descemet's membrane.
     3. Acute rises in intraocular pressure (IOP) generally cause stromal and epithelial edema.
     4. End-stage histopathology frequently reveals changes identical to map-dot-fingerprint dystrophy.

    a. 1, 2, and 3.
    b. 1 and 3.
    c. 2 and 4.
    d. 4 only.
    e. 1, 2, 3, and 4.

81. Which of the following is/are anterior corneal dystrophies?

    1. map-dot-fingerprint dystrophy.
    2. Reis-Bückler's dystrophy.
    3. Meesman's dystrophy.
    4. granular dystrophy.

    a. 1, 2, and 3.
    b. 1 and 3.
    c. 2 and 4.
    d. 4 only.
    e. 1, 2, 3, and 4.

82. T or F -- The microcystic form of map-dot-fingerprint dystrophy may be difficult to distinguish from Meesman's dystrophy.

83. Which one of the following corneal dystrophies is most likely to be associated with a recurrent erosion syndrome?

    a. granular dystrophy.
    b. Reis-Bückler's dystrophy.
    c. macular dystrophy.
    d. lattice dystrophy.
    e. central cloudy dystrophy.

84. T or F -- Granular dystrophy may be distinguished from macular dystrophy by the clarity of corneal stroma between its deposits.

85. T or F -- Granular dystrophy may be distinguished from macular dystrophy on the basis of a careful family history.

86. Posterior polymorphous dystrophy (PPMD) clinically and/or pathologically may resemble:

    1. Fuchs' dystrophy.
    2. epithelial downgrowth.
    3. congenital hereditary endothelial dystrophy.
    4. the iridocorneal endothelial (ICE) syndromes.

    a. 1, 2, and 3.
    b. 1 and 3.
    c. 2 and 4.
    d. 4 only.
    e. 1, 2, 3, and 4.

87. Which of the following concerning keratoconus is false?

   a. It is associated with atopy, Down's syndrome, and Marfan's syndrome.
   b. The earliest histologic change seen is thinning of the epithelium.
   c. Anterior stromal scarring is typically a late finding, regardless of contact lens use.
   d. Iron deposition in epithelial basal cells is not uncommon.
   e. There may be a hereditary or familial predisposition.

88. Match the eponyms of various iron lines with the appropriate location.

   a. Hudson-Stähli line.   1. at the base of the cone in keratoconus.
   b. Fleischer line.   2. at the base of a filtering bleb.
   c. Stocker line.   3. along the lower lid margin.
   d. Ferry line.   4. along the advancing edge of a pterygium.

89. T or F -- The most sensitive method of detecting an early Kayser-Fleischer ring is with thin beam cross-sectional analysis at the slit lamp.

90. Which of the following concerning the lens capsule is/are true?

   1. Anterior capsular guttae may be seen in aniridia and Lowe's syndrome.
   2. In posterior lenticonus, the primary defect is an abnormally thin posterior capsule.
   3. In any case of hypercupremia, copper may deposit in the lens capsule in a sunflower pattern.
   4. The most common abnormality encountered clinically is the true exfoliation syndrome.

   a. 1, 2, and 3.
   b. 1 and 3.
   c. 2 and 4.
   d. 4 only.
   e. 1, 2, 3, and 4.

91. Which of the following insults may induce lens epithelial replication, degeneration, or metaplasia?

   1. elevated intraocular pressure.
   2. chronic inflammation.
   3. trauma.
   4. atopic dermatitis.

   a. 1, 2, and 3.
   b. 1 and 3.
   c. 2 and 4.
   d. 4 only.
   e. 1, 2, 3, and 4.

92. T or F -- Intralenticular fissures filled with eosinophilic globules are a common artifact due to tissue processing techniques.

93. Which of the following are true concerning the cataract associated with congenital rubella infection?

1. Ocular findings are frequently coincident with abnormalities in the cardiovascular and auditory systems.
2. A distinctive feature of rubella cataracts is the retention of nuclei within central lens fibers.
3. Surgical removal of these cataracts frequently induces aggressive intraocular inflammation.
4. Live virus is present within the lenses of patients with congenital rubella syndrome.

a. 1, 2, and 3.
b. 1 and 3.
c. 2 and 4.
d. 4 only.
e. 1, 2, 3, and 4.

94. The retinal circulation supplies which of the following layers?

1. inner plexiform layer.
2. inner nuclear layer.
3. ganglion cell layer.
4. outer nuclear layer.

a. 1, 2, and 3.
b. 1 and 3.
c. 2 and 4.
d. 4 only.
e. 1, 2, 3, and 4.

95. T or F -- The clinical macula is identical to the histologic macula.

96. Which anatomic features of the fovea contribute to its dark appearance on angiography?

1. changes in RPE melanin.
2. changes in retinal pigmentation.
3. changes in the retinal vascular system.
4. changes in the choroidal melanin.

a. 1, 2, and 3.
b. 1 and 3.
c. 2 and 4.
d. 4 only.
e. 1, 2, 3, and 4.

97. T or F -- Lange's fold is a sensitive indicator of ocular trauma in postmortem ocular examination.

98. Classic macular edema and exudates accumulate in the:

    a. nerve fiber layer.
    b. ganglion cell layer.
    c. inner plexiform layer.
    d. inner nuclear layer.
    e. outer plexiform layer.

99. Microaneurysms are located in the:

    a. nerve fiber layer.
    b. ganglion cell layer.
    c. inner plexiform layer.
    d. inner nuclear layer.
    e. outer plexiform layer.

100. Cotton-wool spots are located in the:

    a. nerve fiber layer.
    b. ganglion cell layer.
    c. inner plexiform layer.
    d. inner nuclear layer.
    e. outer plexiform layer.

101. The preservative/processing technique of choice for biopsy handling in presumed corneal cystinosis involves:

    a. fixation in 10% formalin.
    b. fixation in glutaraldehyde.
    c. frozen sections.
    d. fixation in absolute alcohol.
    e. immediate sectioning after transport in saline-soaked gauze.

102. Which of the following concerning the histopathology of diabetic eye disease is/are true?

    1. There is relative loss of pericytes.
    2. Lacy vacuolization of the iris pigment epithelium is common.
    3. Thickening of the basement membrane of the ciliary epithelium is pathognomonic.
    4. Microaneurysms arise within the ganglion cell layer.

    a. 1, 2, and 3.
    b. 1 and 3.
    c. 2 and 4.
    d. 4 only.
    e. 1, 2, 3, and 4.

103. T or F -- Diabetics are more likely to develop a pigment dispersion syndrome than non-diabetics.

104. Which of the following concerning venous occlusions of the retina is/are true?

1. The inferotemporal quadrant is most frequently involved by branch retinal vein occlusion (BRVO).
2. Between 20 and 25% of BRVO will develop retinal neovascularization.
3. There is no association of BRVO or central retinal vein occlusion (CRVO) with glaucoma.
4. Approximately 50% of patients with untreated BRVO will maintain vision better than 20/40.

a. 1, 2, and 3.
b. 1 and 3.
c. 2 and 4.
d. 4 only.
e. 1, 2, 3, and 4.

105. Which of the following concerning lattice degeneration is/are true?

1. There is usually vitreoretinal fibrosis over the degenerated retina.
2. It may be found in up to 10% of the general population.
3. It is the most common finding associated with retinal detachment.
4. The branching, white lines seen clinically correlate with histopathologically sclerotic retinal vessels.

a. 1, 2, and 3.
b. 1 and 3.
c. 2 and 4.
d. 4 only.
e. 1, 2, 3, and 4.

106. The leading cause of new blindness in the United States is:

a. glaucoma.
b. cataract.
c. age-related macular degeneration.
d. diabetes.
e. retinal detachment.

107. Which of the following concerning drusen of the RPE is/are true?

    1. Calcific drusen are associated with atrophy of surrounding RPE.
    2. Hard drusen are the most common type seen in age-related macular degeneration.
    3. Confluent drusen represent diffuse thickening of the inner layer of Bruch's membrane.
    4. Soft drusen represent microscopic RPE detachments.

    a. 1, 2, and 3.
    b. 1 and 3.
    c. 2 and 4.
    d. 4 only.
    e. 1, 2, 3, and 4.

108. T or F -- Paving stone degeneration represents a disturbance of the inner retinal circulation.

109. T or F -- Peripheral cystoid degeneration is a common risk factor for retinal detachment.

110. Which of the following concerning the genetics of retinoblastoma is/are true?

    1. The pertinent gene is located on the long arm of chromosome 13 (13q).
    2. Retinoblastoma will be expressed in patients who have two abnormal retinoblastoma genes.
    3. Clinically, familial retinoblastoma is transmittted in an autosomal dominant pattern.
    4. New germ cell mutations of 13Q do not increase the risk of nonocular malignancy.

    a. 1, 2, and 3.
    b. 1 and 3.
    c. 2 and 4.
    d. 4 only.
    e. 1, 2, 3, and 4.

111. Which of the following concerning the histopathology of retinoblastoma is/are true?

    1. The tumors are mitotically active with characteristic zones of perivascular proliferation separated by zones of necrosis.
    2. These tumors appear particularly blue microscopically, due to liberated nucleic acid and calcification.
    3. Flexner-Wintersteiner rosettes are extremely specific for retinoblastoma.
    4. Homer Wright rosettes are extremely specific for retinoblastoma.

    a. 1, 2, and 3.
    b. 1 and 3.
    c. 2 and 4.
    d. 4 only.
    e. 1, 2, 3, and 4.

112. Which of the following concerning the prognosis in retinoblastoma is/are true?

   1. The most common route for tumor spread is lymphatic metastasis.
   2. With complete surgical resection, the survival rate exceeds 90%.
   3. The most important prognostic factor for survival is the extent of choroidal invasion.
   4. Bilaterality may increase mortality.

   a. 1, 2, and 3.
   b. 1 and 3.
   c. 2 and 4.
   d. 4 only.
   e. 1, 2, 3, and 4.

113. Which of the following concerning medulloepithelioma is/are true?

   1. The pattern of distribution is similar to that of colobomata.
   2. The cellular characteristics are strikingly similar to retinoblastoma.
   3. Typically, the cells align themselves in a stratified ribbon distribution.
   4. Heteroplastic tissue such as cartilage or smooth muscle may be found within their substance.

   a. 1, 2, and 3.
   b. 1 and 3.
   c. 2 and 4.
   d. 4 only.
   e. 1, 2, 3, and 4.

114. In malignant melanoma of the choroid, the most important prognostic factors are:

   1. sex.
   2. dimensions at the base of the tumor.
   3. degree of pigmentation.
   4. cell type.

   a. 1, 2, and 3.
   b. 1 and 3.
   c. 2 and 4.
   d. 4 only.
   e. 1, 2, 3, and 4.

115. The most common site for metastasis in or around the eye in adults is the:

   a. orbit.
   b. choroid.
   c. retina.
   d. optic nerve.
   e. iris.

116. T or F -- Intraocular lymphoma is likely to involve the central nervous system (CNS) when the choroid is diffusely involved.

117. T or F -- The myositis of idiopathic orbital inflammation (pseudotumor) is characterized by its cellular homogeneity.

118. T or F -- The orbit contains no resident lymphocytes.

119. T or F -- Orbital lymphomas are nearly always B-cell proliferations.

120. Systemic lymphoma is most likely to be associated with ocular adnexal disease characterized by:

    a. large tumor size.
    b. monoclonality.
    c. high degree of cytologic atypia.
    d. follicular pattern of growth.
    e. eyelid involvement.

121. T or F -- Primary orbital tumors are more common than secondary orbital tumors.

122. The most common intraconal orbital tumor is the:

    a. meningioma.
    b. rhabdomyosarcoma.
    c. cavernous hemangioma.
    d. fibrous histiocytoma.
    e. neurofibroma.

123. Which of the following concerning rhabdomyosarcoma is false?

    a. It is one of the most common primary solid malignancies in children.
    b. The clinical presentation is typically acute.
    c. Spontaneous lid ecchymosis is a specific sign.
    d. The embryonal histologic pattern is the most common.
    e. The alveolar pattern has the worst prognosis.

124. Which of the following concerning neurofibromas and schwannomas is/are true?

       1. Unlike schwannomas, neurofibromas are encapsulated.
       2. Both tumors are found in increased frequency in patients with neurofibromatosis type I.
       3. Nodular neurofibroma is classic in neurofibromatosis.
       4. Verocay bodies are seen in Antoni-A type schwannomas.

    a. 1, 2, and 3.
    b. 1 and 3.
    c. 2 and 4.
    d. 4 only.
    e. 1, 2, 3, and 4.

125. Which one of the following concerning lacrimal gland lesions is false?

    a. Roughly 80% are inflammatory or lymphoid lesions, and 20% are epithelial cell tumors.
    b. Among epithelial cell tumors, 50% are benign.
    c. The most common malignant epithelial tumor of the lacrimal gland is the adenoid cystic carcinoma.
    d. Pain as a presenting finding indicates either an inflammatory or malignant lesion.
    e. The most common epithelial tumor, the pleomorphic adenoma, is encapsulated and may be shelled out easily.

126. T or F -- The melanocytoma of the optic nerve head has not been associated with malignant melanoma of the choroid.

127. Which of the following concerning optic nerve glioma is/are true?

       1. Glioma may involve any part of the visual pathway.
       2. The typical age of presentation is between 10 and 20 years.
       3. Rosenthal fibers are not unique to optic nerve glioma.
       4. The prognosis is directly related to histopathologic cell type.

    a. 1, 2, and 3.
    b. 1 and 3.
    c. 2 and 4.
    d. 4 only.
    e. 1, 2, 3, and 4.

128. Which of the following concerning orbital meningioma is/are true?

   1. Primary orbital meningioma is more common than secondary orbital meningioma.
   2. The mean age of patients with primary orbital meningioma is lower than in patients with secondary orbital meningioma.
   3. The prognosis is most closely related to cell type.
   4. Meningioma in the pediatric population have a poorer prognosis.

   a. 1, 2, and 3.
   b. 1 and 3.
   c. 2 and 4.
   d. 4 only.
   e. 1, 2, 3, and 4.

129. Which of the following concerning the histopathology of glaucoma is/are true?

   1. Cavernous atrophy of Schnabel is commonly seen in primary open-angle glaucoma.
   2. Disc pallor noted clinically reflects decreased vascularity of the optic nerve head.
   3. With special stains and careful review of optic nerve specimens, the specific etiology of several types of glaucoma may be determined.
   4. The retina shows ganglion cell dropout and nerve fiber layer atrophy in cases of long-standing glaucoma.

   a. 1, 2, and 3.
   b. 1 and 3.
   c. 2 and 4.
   d. 4 only.
   e. 1, 2, 3, and 4.

130. Which of the following concerning the particulate glaucomas is/are true?

   1. Excessive pigment in the trabecular meshwork is specific for pigment dispersion syndrome.
   2. Pseudoexfoliation is characterized by its bilateral symmetry.
   3. Pseudoexfoliation material is found only within the eye.
   4. After lens extraction, the synthesis of pseudoexfoliation material typically continues.

   a. 1, 2, and 3.
   b. 1 and 3.
   c. 2 and 4.
   d. 4 only.
   e. 1, 2, 3, and 4.

131. T or F -- The lifetime risk of glaucoma in an eye with greater than 180 degrees of angle recession is 5 to 10%.

132. T or F -- The sine qua non of the iridocorneal endothelial syndromes is abnormal corneal endothelial proliferation.

133. Clinical findings indicative of prior attacks of acute angle-closure glaucoma include:

    1. White anterior lenticular opacities.
    2. Segmental iris heterochromia with atrophy.
    3. Peripheral anterior synechiae (PAS).
    4. Narrow angles in the contralateral eye.

  a. 1, 2, and 3.
  b. 1 and 3.
  c. 2 and 4.
  d. 4 only.
  e. 1, 2, 3, and 4.

134. Which of the following eyelid tumors may be associated with internal malignancy?

    1. pilomatrixoma.
    2. trichofolliculoma.
    3. trichoepithelioma.
    4. sebaceous adenoma.

  a. 1, 2, and 3.
  b. 1 and 3.
  c. 2 and 4.
  d. 4 only.
  e. 1, 2, 3, and 4.

135. Which one of the following concerning medulloepithelioma is false?

  a. It primarily affects the peidatric age group.
  b. It is typically cystic on its surface.
  c. It may arise at the optic nerve.
  d. It generally arises from the nonpigmented ciliary epithelium.
  e. The metastatic pattern is most often hematogenous.

136. A pigmented lesion of the choroid is likely to be benign if:

    1. Its diameter is less than 10 mm.
    2. There are drusen and associated lipofuscin deposits.
    3. It is less than 2 mm in height.
    4. There is an associated dependent exudative retinal detachment.

  a. 1, 2, and 3.
  b. 1 and 3.
  c. 2 and 4.
  d. 4 only.
  e. 1, 2, 3, and 4.

137. Fluorescein angiography is helpful in distinguishing choroidal melanoma from:

> 1. metastatic tumors.
> 2. choroidal hemangioma.
> 3. large nevi.
> 4. subretinal hemorrhage.

a. 1, 2, and 3.
b. 1 and 3.
c. 2 and 4.
d. 4 only.
e. 1, 2, 3, and 4.

138. T or F -- The internal reflectivity of melanoma on A-scan ultrasonography is typically lower than that of other choroidal masses.

139. Peak mortality rates following enucleation for uveal melanoma occur approximately:

a. 3 to 6 months postenucleation.
b. 6 to 12 months postenucleation.
c. 1 to 3 years postenucleation.
d. 3 to 5 years postenucleation.
e. 5 to 10 years postenucleation.

140. The most sensitive method for detecting hepatic metastasis in uveal melanoma is:

a. liver enzyme testing.
b. abdominal computed tomography (CT) scanning.
c. abdominal ultrasound.
d. radionuclide liver scanning.
e. physical examination.

141. The "tomato-catsup" fundus is a classic finding in which of the phakomatoses?

a. neurofibromatosis.
b. Sturge-Weber syndrome.
c. tuberous sclerosis.
d. ataxia-telangiectasia.
e. von Hippel-Lindau disease.

142. Which of the following concerning choroidal osteoma is/are true?

    1. It is more common in women.
    2. The majority of cases are bilateral.
    3. It most frequently arises in the peripapillary region.
    4. Ultrasonography is of no valve in distinguishing it from amelanotic melanoma.

    a. 1, 2, and 3.
    b. 1 and 3.
    c. 2 and 4.
    d. 4 only.
    e. 1, 2, 3, and 4.

143. Which of the following concerning the genetics of retinoblastoma is/are true?

    1. It is transmitted in an autosomal dominant fashion with approximately 80% penetrance.
    2. Approximately 6% of retinoblastoma patients will have a family history of retinoblastoma.
    3. Fifteen percent of sporadic cases (i.e., no family history) represent a new germinal mutation.
    4. The parent of a patient with unilateral retinoblastoma and no family history has a 1% chance of having another child with retinoblastoma.

    a. 1, 2, and 3.
    b. 1 and 3.
    c. 2 and 4.
    d. 4 only.
    e. 1, 2, 3, and 4.

144. T or F -- Patients with inherited retinoblastoma are at increased risk for other tumors.

145. Common presenting symptoms or signs in retinoblastoma include:

    1. leukocoria.
    2. buphthalmos.
    3. strabismus.
    4. proptosis.

    a. 1, 2, and 3.
    b. 1 and 3.
    c. 2 and 4.
    d. 4 only.
    e. 1, 2, 3, and 4.

146. The common sites of metastasis of retinoblastoma include:

        1. bone.
        2. regional lymph nodes.
        3. CNS.
        4. lung.

    a. 1, 2, and 3.
    b. 1 and 3.
    c. 2 and 4.
    d. 4 only.
    e. 1, 2, 3, and 4.

147. T or F -- The Reese-Ellsworth classification of retinoblastoma gives prognostic information regarding long-term survival.

148. To be correctly termed von Hippel-Lindau syndrome, retinal capillary hemangioma must be associated with:

        1. pancreatic cysts.
        2. renal cell carcinoma.
        3. pheochromocytomas.
        4. cerebellar hemangioblastomas.

    a. 1, 2, and 3.
    b. 1 and 3.
    c. 2 and 4.
    d. 4 only.
    e. 1, 2, 3, and 4.

149. Which of the following concerning metastatic carcinoma involving the eye and adnexa is/are true?

        1. Up to 10% of patients with known metastases will have ocular or orbital involvement.
        2. Ocular involvement is greater than 5 times more likely than orbital involvement.
        3. In men, lung cancer is the most frequently encountered primary tumor, and in women, breast cancer is the most frequently encountered primary tumor.
        4. Gastrointestinal tumors metastasize to the eye or orbit infrequently.

    a. 1, 2, and 3.
    b. 1 and 3.
    c. 2 and 4.
    d. 4 only.
    e. 1, 2, 3, and 4.

150. Which of the following regarding ocular and adnexal metastasis is/are true?

    1. Isolated retinal metastases are common in gastrointestinal cancers.
    2. There is a slight predominance of left-sided involvement in ocular metastasis.
    3. Breast cancer is particularly likely to <u>present</u> as an ocular or orbital mass (metastasis).
    4. If asymptomatic, treatment of ocular or orbital metastasis may be limited to treatment of the systemic cancer.

a. 1, 2, and 3.
b. 1 and 3.
c. 2 and 4.
d. 4 only.
e. 1, 2, 3, and 4.

Answers

Epithelioid
Giant cell
Langhans
FB cell
Langerhans
Touton

Langerhans - Birbeck
- Eosinophilic granuloma
- Letterer Siwe
- Hand, Schuller, Christian

1. a. 5. Note that macrophages can differentiate into both epithelioid and giant cells. Also note that mast cells are tissue-based basophils (i.e., not circulating).
   b. 1.
   c. 3.
   d. 4.
   e. 3.
   f. 2.

FB cell
Lipogranuloma
Fungal

Touton
Erdhime-Chester,
JXG
Necrobiotic xanthogranuloma

Langhans
Sarcoid
MTB/MCP

2. a. 3. Touton giant cells feature vacuolated cytoplasm outside a nuclear ring with eosinophilic cytoplasm inside. Juvenile xanthogranuloma, Erdheim-Chester disease, and necrobiotic xanthogranuloma feature Touton giant cells. Langhans' giant cells have a peripheral, horseshoe-shaped nuclear rim and are characteristic of sarcoidosis and mycobacterial disease. Foreign body giant cells have haphazardly distributed nuclei. Note that Langerhans' cells are dendritic macrophages (antigen-presenting cells) within epithelia.
   b. 4.
   c. 1.
   d. 4.
   e. 1.
   f. 3.
   g. 4.
   h. 1.

3. e. A Russell body is a spherical-shaped intracellular deposit that forms when antibody accumulates and displaces the nucleus of a plasma cell.

4. False. Although giant cells are often present in granulomatous inflammation, the hallmark is the presence of epithelioid cells.

5. d. There are three subtypes of granulomas: diffuse, discrete, and zonal. Tuberculosis, leprosy, and sarcoidosis are characterized by discrete granulomatous inflammation. A zonal reaction consists of palisading epithelioid cells surrounded by granulation tissue. Diffuse granulomatous inflammation is present in sympathetic ophthalmia, fungal infection, and juvenile xanthogranuloma. VKH

Erdhime Chester is discrete?

6. a. 4.
   b. 1. → and for fungal elements, don't play games with me.
   c. 5.
   d. 3.
   e. 2.

7. e. Although Descemet's membrane is a barrier to many organisms, fungi can penetrate Descemet's membrane into the anterior chamber with relative ease. *Candida* and *Cryptococcus* are yeasts; the majority of corneal pathogens are molds.

8. b. There is typically moderate to severe keratitis in trachoma, usually subepithelial. Adult inclusion conjunctivitis is typically worse inferiorly, in distinction to trachoma, which is typically worse superiorly. Giemsa staining is more effective than Wright's stain at revealing intracytoplasmic inclusions. Serotypes A-C cause trachoma, D-K inclusion conjunctivitis, and LGV 1-3 lymphogranuloma venereum.

9. d. CMV infection produces a retinochoroiditis (primary retinitis with secondary choroiditis). Infected retinal cells contain small basophilic intranuclear and large eosinophilic intracytoplasmic inclusion bodies.

10. True.

11. b.   Infection with *Toxocara canis* produces a retinochoroiditis characterized by an eosinophilic abscess. *Taenia solium* causes relatively little inflammation until the cyst ruptures, when an intense granulomatous reaction can result.

12. True.   The host response to initial herpes simplex infection is nongranulomatous inflammation of the conjunctiva, while reactivation may cause granulomatous inflammation adjacent to Descemet's membrane. It is neither totally sensitive nor totally specific.

13. a.   Large cell lymphoma (reticulum cell sarcoma) may present as a pseudovitritis. Retinoblastoma may present as a pseudohypopyon. Aggressive choroidal melanoma may become necrotic or cause necrosis of the overlying retina with secondary uveitis.

14. b.   Although some authors consider phacotoxic uveitis to be a less severe form of phacoantigenic endophthalmitis, phacolytic glaucoma is not true active inflammation. Rather there is a rise in intraocular pressure caused by clogging of the trabecular meshwork by lens protein and macrophages. Also, because mast cells play no role in "phacoanaphylaxis," phacoantigenic is a better descriptor.

15. c.   Behçet's disease is a non-granulomatous vasculitis that causes acute uveitis with hypopyon, aphthous stomatitis, and genital ulceration. Rheumatoid arthritis causes a zonal granuloma centered on scleral collagen. Sarcoidosis produces a discrete granulomatous reaction, while sympathetic ophthalmia and VKH cause diffuse granulomatous inflammation.

16. e.   Juvenile rheumatoid arthritis and Reiter's syndrome are specifically characterized by recurrent or chronic nongranulomatous uveitis, while choroidal melanoma and ocular trauma may incite secondary ocular inflammation, which is nearly always nongranulomatous. (In the case of a retained intraocular foreign body after trauma, there may be a granulomatous component.) Cryptococcal endophthalmitis, like other fungal causes of ocular inflammation, features marked granulomatous inflammation.

17. False.   Finding the choriocapillaris involved with granulomatous inflammation strongly favors the diagnosis of VKH over SO. Note that sparing of the choriocapillaris favors SO but does not rule out VKH.   *& Vice versa. Since c chronic Relapse there is some choriocapilleris involvment in SO.*

18. d.   Perforating wounds of the cornea do not elicit a typical granulation tissue response because there are no native blood vessels. Stromal swelling is important in the very early response phase to prevent ongoing aqueous leakage. The key response for long-term healing is closure of the internal defect with adjacent endothelial cells, via migration or metaplasia (not replication). Note that any dermal appendages lost are relaced by fibrous (scar) tissue. <u>Epi</u>scleral vessels and resident fibrocytes are responsible for limbal healing (the sclera itself is avascular). The iris, despite rich vascularity and innervation, reacts minimally to mechanical injury.

19. e.   The retina contains no true fibrocytes or fibroblasts. Glial (Müller) cells are the reactive component intraretinally, so that purely retinal injury leads to gliosis and proliferation primarily within the inner nuclear layer. The RPE frequently becomes involved in retinal injury, typically with a hyperplastic response. Intraretinal <u>fibrosis</u> implies involvement of the choroid in the repair process.

20. False.   Expulsive choroidal hemorrhage occurs because rigid choroidal vessels rupture during periods of ocular <u>hypotony</u>.

21. False. Ultrastructual studies reveal that this epithelium resembles conjunctiva more closely than cornea.

22. e. Sympathetic ophthalmia most often occurs after accidental trauma. Most post-operative cases follow filtering procedures on blind, glaucomatous eyes.

23. a. Graft failure is a nonspecific term referring to opacification of the donor cornea. This may occur secondary to endothelial damage, inadequate donor tissue, or postoperative infection.

24. d. Elschnig's pearls are residual lens epithelial cells that proliferate to form small globular, opaque fibers following cataract extraction or surgery. Soemmering's ring is retention of equatorial lens cortical material following extracapsular cataract extraction.

25. b. Because of the oblique orientation of the axons in this layer of the fovea, fluid accumulates more easily here than in retinal layers where the neural and glial elements are oriented radially.

26. c. Corneal blood staining results from displacement of hemoglobin (not RBCs) through a traumatized endothelium but intact Descemet's membrane. In hemosiderosis bulbi, hemosiderin (a hemoglobin breakdown product) accumulation leads to epithelial damage. Synchysis scintillans results from the accumulation of red cell membrane breakdown products (cholesterol) in the vitreous. An ochre membrane is the organization of posterior segment hemorrhage on the posterior surface of a detached vitreous.

27. False. An occluded pupil (occlusio pupillae) satisfies this definition. In contrast, a secluded pupil implies complete (360 degree) lens-pupil apposition, due to severe posterior synechiae.

28. a. Calcification may be seen in atrophic eyes but is not necessary for the diagnosis. The other three, in combination, constitute the diagnosis of phthisis bulbi.

29. d. The insertion of the inferior oblique tendon does not represent an especially weak point of the sclera (this is directly over the center of the macula).

30. d. The phakomatous choristoma represents a congenital developmental anomaly (choristoma) with lens-like tissue forming a mass within the eyelid, usually lower. Such a growth has been reported nowhere else in or on the body. The lesion is rare and has no reported ocular associations.

31. a. A cleavage plane between the longitudinal ciliary body fibers and sclera represents cyclodialysis. In angle recession, the plane of cleavage is between circular and longitudinal fibers of the ciliary muscle.

32. b. Spontaneous dialyses, often in patients with a family history of retinal dialysis, occur most commonly in the inferotemporal quadrant. Traumatic dialyses, on the other hand, occur most frequently in the superonasal quadrant, probably as a contrecoup effect from inferotemporal blunt trauma.

33. c. Passage into (but not through) a structure is called penetrating injury. Passage through a structure is called perforating injury. This patient perforated his cornea and lens but penetrated his eye. Had the foreign body passed through the posterior sclera, he would have suffered what is clumsily termed a double penetrating injury.

34. c. Siderosis bulbi is due to epithelial damage caused by ferrous (Fe^{+2}) iron. Copper foreign bodies with greater than 85% elemental copper lead to a suppurative noninfectious endophthalmitis. Chalcosis occurs when the copper concentration is between 70 and 85%. Vegetable matter is rarely sterile; in addition, it elicits a severe granulomatous reaction. Lead does elicit an inflammatory reaction, albeit not as severe as copper or iron.

35. b. Ammonium hydroxide has the greatest capability to penetrate into the anterior chamber. Petroleum products cause damage from detergent-like actions.

36. d. Radiation primarily affects the retinal vasculature and may cause neovascularization, vitreous hemorrhage, and neovascular glaucoma. Primary retinal gliosis, however, does not occur because the retina itself is relatively radioresistant.

37. False. A hamartoma consists of aberrant tissue elements in their normal location (e.g., astrocytoma of the optic nerve head), while a choristoma consists of normal tissue in an abnormal location (e.g., dermoid cyst of the orbit or eyelid).

38. False. On the contrary, an in utero insult at beginning of the first trimester is likely to lead to cataract, since this is when the lens placode is forming.

39. e. Persistent pupillary membrane is an incomplete regression of the anterior tunica vasculosa lentis. Bergmeister's papilla is a nonpatent hyaloid artery remnant extending from the optic disc. If this structure is patent, it is called persistent hyaloid artery. Mittendorf's dot is an opacity on the inferonasal posterior lens capsule from connective tissue associated with the central hyaloid vasculature and posterior tunica vasculosa.

40. a. Eyelid hemangiomas can have further implications such as astigmatism and amblyopia. Conjunctival dermoids are choristomas, not hamartomas (see answer 37). Dermoid cysts of the eyelids have pilosebaceous units in their walls, while epidermoid cysts do not. Conjunctival dermoids are solid tumors of the conjunctiva. Dermolipomas can have significant morbidity associated with attempts at surgical removal--ptosis, dry eye, and lateral rectus paresis.

41. a. 2.
    b. 5.
    c. 4.
    d. 1.
    e. 3.

42. True. Although highly variable, the basic features of Peter's anomaly are central corneal opacification associated with absence of Descemet's membrane. Iris stroma and/or lens may attach to this defect in cornea.

43. e. Most congenital ectopia lentis is associated with homocystinuria and Marfan's syndrome. However, numerous other conditions--Peters' anomaly, Weill-Marchesani syndrome, oxycephaly, aniridia, coloboma, congenital glaucoma, and megalocornea--can also be associated with ectopia lentis.

44. d.   Five diseases characterized by disseminated hamartomas are known as phakomatoses -- von Hippel-Lindau disease (angiomatosis retinae), Sturge-Weber syndrome (encephalotrigeminal angiomatosis), neurofibromatosis (von Recklinghausen's disease), tuberous sclerosis (Bourneville's disease), and ataxia-telangiactasia (Louis-Bar syndrome). Of these, only ataxia-telangiectasia is inherited on an autosomal recessive basis. The others are autosomal dominant or sporadic.

45. c.   Juvenile glaucoma has been reported with Sturge-Weber syndrome and neurofibromatosis. (Rubeotic glaucoma may be seen as a late sequela of the von Hippel-Lindau syndrome.)

46. e.   All of these may have fundus findings. von Hippel-Lindau syndrome features hemangioblastoma of the retina. Sturge-Weber syndrome is associated with diffuse and focal choroidal hemangiomas, and ataxia-telangiectasia with retinal vascular telangiectasias. Neurofibromatosis patients may have astrocytic hamartomas in the retina or optic nerve head.

47. a. 3.   Although not as common as in tuberous sclerosis, astrocytic hamartoma of the
    b. 4.   retina and optic disc may be seen in neurofibromatosis.
    c. 1, 2.
    d. 2.
    e. 5.

48. d.   Although it is frequently discussed as a phakomatosis, the vascular anomalies in Wyburn-Mason syndrome are malformations, not true hamartomas.

49. b.   In PHPV, the fibrovascular proliferation behind the lens is associated with a small eye, and angle-closure glaucoma is common. In addition, cataract and retinal detachment can occur, and macular and/or optic nerve hypoplasia usually portends a poor visual prognosis.

50. e.   Retinal dysplasia is an abnormal proliferation of the developing retina and can occur in all of the entities listed, in addition to Peters' anomaly, congenital glaucoma, cyclopia, and synophthalmia.

51. a.

52. e.

53. d.

54. e.   The amount of, duration of, and stage of pregnancy for teratogenic alcohol exposure have not been defined. Other ocular features of this syndrome include blepharophimosis, epicanthal skin folds, strabismus, and ptosis.

55. a. 3.
    b. 2, 5.
    c. 2.
    d. 1, 4.
    e. 4.

56. True. One of the causes of orbital cellulitis is extension of infection from adjacent tissue including preseptal cellulitis. With a normal orbital septum (i.e., no prior surgery or trauma), this should only occur with delayed or inappropriate treatment.

57. False. The location of the amyloid deposit is important, since conjunctival nodular amyloid is usually a local phenomenon, whereas subcutaneous amyloid suggests a systemic amyloidosis.

58. c. These benign lesions are caused by collections of subepithelial cells containing cholesterol and other lipids (called "foam cells" because of their appearance in histologic preparations). Most patients with xanthelasma do not have a systemic hyperlipidemia.

59. c. Juvenile xanthogranulomata are small, benign, histiocytic tumors that are usually multiple and can be found in the iris. They are highly vascular, which, along with the lipid content, contributes to their characterisitic orange tint. Their rich vascularity also accounts for a propensity for spontaneous ecchymosis (when in the skin) or hyphema (when in the iris).

60. d. Epidermoid and dermoid cysts are both filled with dense secretions, mostly keratin, and thus do not transilluminate like clear fluid-filled ductal cysts. While epidermoid and dermoid cysts both contain keratinizing squamous epithelial linings, dermoids cysts also include other (dermal) structures such as hair follicles and sebaceous glands. Goldenhar's syndrome is associated with epibulbar, solid dermoids.

61. d. Besides thickening of the keratin layer, parakeratosis also implies retention of nuclei in the keratin layer. Hyperkeratosis is a thickening of the keratin layer, not the "prickle cell" layer (the latter is known as acanthosis). Acantholysis occurs in the "prickle cell" layer with breakdown of the desmosomal intercellular connections, which give it its name and characteristic histologic appearance.

62. True. Hematoxylin-eosin staining of ultraviolet light-damaged collagen may reveal a characteristic bluish tint (basophilia) instead of the customary red (eosinophilia). This reflects a chemical alteration in the collagen structure, referred to as elastosis, because of its histologic similarity to elastin.

63. False. Seborrheic keratosis is a benign epidermal lesion featuring thickening of the "prickle cell" layer (acanthosis) and keratin layer (hyperkeratosis). Actinic keratosis is considered a premalignant lesion, which has features that may include hyperkeratosis, but also elastosis or dysplasia. While seborrheic keratosis is often pigmented, this is not a distinguishing feature.

64. c. Seborrheic keratoses have a characteristic "stuck-on" superficial look that should help prevent them from being mistaken for carcinoma. The others can all easily mimic squamous cell carcinoma in clinical or histologic appearance.

65. a. Basal cell carcinoma is, by a large margin, the most common malignant tumor of the eyelid. Medial canthal tumors carry a worse prognosis due to their tendency to infiltrate more deeply (especially if the lacrimal drainage system or sinuses become involved). The cystic variant can appear blue secondary to the accumulation of blood breakdown products inside.

66. e. Fat staining is often needed to help conclusively identify sebaceous cell carcinoma, as the spreading pattern can easily mimic epithelial dysplasia, carcinoma-in-situ, as well as basal cell or squamous cell carcinoma.

67. e. Elevation is the result of migration of nevus cells into the dermis. Junctional nevi are flat.

68. False. The caruncle is specialized in that it has accessory lacrimal glands as well as hair follicles--structures not found elsewhere in the otherwise similar nonkeratinized, stratified squamous epithelium of the conjunctiva. Pilosebaceous units render the caruncle more "skin-like" than conjunctival.

69. d. Dermal amyloid infiltration is an ominous herald of systemic amyloidosis, usually associated with multiple myeloma.

70. a. Conjunctival lymphoid proliferations, both benign and malignant, occur most commonly in the fornices. Approximately 65 to 70% (2/3) of eyelid lymphomas will be associated with systemic lymphoma.

71. d. Hematogenous metastasis of conjunctival squamous cell carcinoma is rare. Spindle cell and mucoepidermoid carcinomas are forms of squamous cell carcinoma with the potential for intraocular invasion.

72. False. Ocular melanocytosis is more common in whites; oculodermal melanocytosis (nevus of Ota) is essentially the same condition, but with abnormally increased pigmentation of the eyelid skin as well. It is more often found in darker skinned races. There is an increased risk of uveal, not conjunctival melanoma in whites with oculodermal melanocytosis.

73. False. The junctional nevus is felt to represent a stage in the maturation of conjunctival nevi that is not commonly seen in histopathologic specimens. It is likely that most progessed to become subepithelial nevi by the age of 30 years. The diagnosis of junctional nevus in someone over the age of 30 years should raise suspicion of primary acquired melanosis (PAM) of the conjunctiva.

74. b. Primary acquired melanosis of the conjunctiva is felt to be a premalignant condition only in cases with melanocytic atypia. They do occur mostly in people of middle age and change size or grow slowly over many years.

75. c. Three-quarters (75%) of conjunctival melanomas arise from preexistent PAM with atypia, and the overall mortality rate is about 25%. The growth pattern (pagetoid spread) and depth of tumor penetration (greater than 0.75 mm) are important prognostic factors. Unlike uveal melanoma, conjunctival melanoma usually metastasizes to the preauricular and submandibular nodes first.

76. c. The cellular elements present in pyogenic granuloma include fibroblasts and endothelial cells. Kaposi's sarcoma is a neoplastic proliferation of endothelium in a background of spindle cells. Benign areas within the tumor look similar to pyogenic granuloma.

77. a.   Interstitial keratitis (IK) is a nonulcerating inflammation of the corneal stroma leading to vascularization and scarring. Causes include congenital syphilis, herpes simplex, herpes zoster, leprosy, Lyme disease, tuberculosis, onchocerciasis, sarcoidosis, and Cogan's syndrome (IK and vestibuloauditory dysfunction associated with polyarteritis). Acanthamoeba is typically ulcerative.

78. b.   These rare, fascinating hamartomatous lesions typically present with visual loss, strabismus, or leukocoria in children or adolescents. Colobomata, optic nerve pits, retinoschisis, and other hamartomas have been reported in association with these lesions. Three features are considered essential to the diagnosis: (1) pigmentary disturbance, (2) gliosis, and (3) retinal vascular irregularities, including leakage on angiography. The lesion is usually too extensive to be successfully addressed with membrane peeling.

79. False.   Calcofluor white staining will enhance identification of Acanthamoeba in corneal tissue. Nonnutrient blood agar layered with *Escherichia coli* is required to grow Acanthamoeba in culture.

80. d.   In order to diagnose Fuchs' dystrophy, corneal edema must be present. In Fuchs' dystrophy, endothelial cells are reduced in number or absent. In PBK, endothelial count may be near normal. Descemet's membrane is thickened in both disorders. Acute rises in IOP will typically cause only epithelial edema, provided the endothelium is otherwise healthy. Intraepithelial cysts of degenerating epithelial cells, similar to map-dot-fingerprint dystrophy, can be seen in resolved or chronic corneal edema.

81. a.   Granular dystrophy is a stromal dystrophy, Meesman's dystrophy and map-dot-fingerprint dystrophy are epithelial. Reis-Bückler's dystrophy is localized to Bowman's zone.

82. False.   Three kinds of lesions are seen within the epithelium and its basement membrane in map-dot-fingerprint dystrophy--map lines, dots, and microcysts. In Meesman's dystrophy, tiny gray or transparent epithelial vesicles that extend to the limbus are seen. These differ in appearance from the microcysts of map-dot-fingerprint dystrophy, which are usually white-gray and have distinct edges.

83. b.   Erosions are rare in macular and granular dystrophy; the predominant symptom of macular dystrophy is visual loss.

84. True.   Discrete, focal, white "granular" deposits in the anterior stroma are noted in granular dystrophy. The cornea between deposits is clear. In macular dystrophy, the gray-white stromal opacities have indistinct edges, and the intervening stroma is hazy.

85. True.   Transmission of granular dystrophy is autosomal dominant. Macular dystrophy is inherited in an autosomal recessive pattern.

86. c.   Posterior polymorphous dystrophy has a variable clinical spectrum. Findings on the posterior cornea include vesicles, stromal edema, gray lesions, bands with scalloped edges, and iridocorneal adhesions. Although variable, it is distinct from other dystrophies. Pathologically, the abnormal endothelial proliferation can be strikingly similar to that seen in the iridocorneal endothelial syndromes, as well as epithelial downgrowth.

87. b. The earliest histologic changes in keratoconus are breaks in the epithelial basement membrane and Bowman's layer. Corneal topography may reveal subclinical keratoconus in family members of affected patients.

88. a. 3. Each of these iron lines represents basal epithelial uptake of iron.
    b. 1.
    c. 4.
    d. 2.

89. False. The best examination technique for detecting early Kayser-Fleisher rings is gonioscopy, since the deposits are first detectable in the most peripheral Descemet's membrane.

90. a. True exfoliation refers to a characteristic "scrolling" of the anterior lens capsule following excessive infrared radiation exposure (glassblowers are typically affected). It is far less common than pseudoexfoliation.

91. e. Increased intraocular pressure will cause degeneration and death of lens epithelial cells, forming characteristic white patches under the anterior capsule (glaukomflecken). Chronic anterior uveitis may also cause degeneration and necrosis of the anterior lens epithelium. Chronic inflammation may also cause epithelial metaplasia (posterior subcapsular cataract), which can also be caused by trauma. Posterior subcapsular cataract is also a variable feature of atopic dermatitis.

92. False. Morgagnian globules, or eosinophilic globules in slit-like spaces between lens fibers, are considered a reliable sign of cortical degeneration. Empty fissures within cortex are a common processing artifact.

93. e.

94. a. The retinal circulation supplies the nerve fiber layer, the ganglion cell layer and the inner one-third of the inner nuclear layer. The choroidal circulation supplies the remainder of the neurosensory retina and RPE.

95. False. The clinical macula is a circular region 1 to 2 disc diameters centered around the foveola. The histologic macula is the central region of the retina with a ganglion cell layer greater than one cell thick.

96. a. There are three main features to explain the dark appearance of the fovea on fluorescein angiography. First, the RPE cells are taller, narrower, and filled with greater numbers of more pigmented melanosomes. Second, yellow xanthophyll pigment located in the ganglion and bipolar cells block fluorescence. Finally, the center of the fovea is avascular, so contributes no overlying fluorescence.

97. False. During fixation of normal infant eyes, the sclera shrinks considerably. This leads to redundancy of the retina, manifest as Lange's fold.

98. e.

99. d.

100. a.

101. d. Only absolute alcohol preserves the crystalline deposits for microscopy.

102. a.   Microaneurysms are located in the inner nuclear layer.

103. True.   Due to glycogen accumulation, pigment epithelia in diabetics are easily displaced.

104. c.   CRVO is clearly associated with primary open-angle glaucoma (POAG). A reputed association of BRVO with POAG is less well established. The superotemporal arcade is most frequently involved with BRVO.

105. c.   The vitreous over lattice lesions is liquefied but firmly attached at the margins of the affected retina. Myopia is associated with 40% of rhegmatogenous retinal detachment (RRD), while lattice has been estimated to be associated with 25 to 30% of RRD.

106. c.   Age-related macular degeneration is the leading cause of new blindness in the United States. Cataract and trachoma are leading causes of blindness worldwide.

107. e.

108. False. Occlusion of the choriocapillaris (outer retinal circulation) causes focal, sharply demarcated areas of RPE and retinal atrophy recognized as "paving stones" or "cobblestones."

109. False. Peripheral degenerative cystoid degeneration is extraordinarily common in the elderly and does not increase the risk of rhegmatogenous retinal detachment.

110. a.   The "retinoblastoma gene" is a tumor suppressor gene; that is, the normal gene suppresses the development of retinoblastoma. If both suppressors are lost, neoplasms develop. In "familial retinoblastoma," the patient inherits one defective gene from a parent, which is present throughout all cell lines. Subsequent somatic mutations inactivate the fellow (normal) gene and lead to tumor development. When new germ cell mutations occur early in embryogenesis, the gene will be distributed throughout all cell lines. This explains bilateral retinoblastoma in patients with no family history. This situation mimics familial retinoblastoma, but there is no family history (a new mutation).

111. a.   Homer Wright rosettes are seen in neuroblastoma (primary tumors only) and medulloblastoma, as well as retinoblastoma.

112. c.   Direct extension into the central nervous system is, by far, the most common route of spread. Hematogenous dissemination may also be seen.

113. e.   Medulloepitheliomas (diktyomas) probably arise from primitive neuroepithelium, generally along the line of closure of the embryonic ocular fissure. Mucinous cysts are common.

114. c.   The two independent prognostic factors seem to be basal diameter and cell type. Other features, particularly tumor location, have been shown to correlate, less predictably, with survival.

115. b.   In children, the orbit is more commonly involved.

116. False. Intraocular lymphoma associated with CNS disease has a tendency to infiltrate the neurosensory retina and/or between the RPE and Bruch's membrane. Choroidal lymphoma is not associated with CNS lymphoma.

117. **False.** The cellular infiltrate seen in idiopathic myositis may include neutrophils, eosinophils (particularly in children), and even giant cells, in addition to plasma cells and lymphocytes.

118. **True.** Neither lymph nodes nor lymphocytes are normally present within the orbit. This often makes the classification of lymphomas as well as the distinction between benign proliferations and lymphomas difficult.

119. **True.** The majority of lymphomas are B-cell lymphomas of the non-Hodgkin's type.

120. **e.** The location of the tumor is the most powerful prognostic indicator of biologic behavior. Preseptal lid infiltrates are thought to signal a higher probability of systemic lymphoma than either orbital (intermediate risk) or conjunctival (lowest risk) lymphomas. It is now known that monoclonality is not definitely predictive of progression to systemic disease. Both benign reactive hyperplasia and malignant lymphoma may show a follicular growth pattern. Tumor size and the degree of cellular atypia are not effective for prognostication.

121. **False.** Secondary orbital neoplasms (local extension or metastasis) are far more common than primary neoplasms.

122. **c.**

123. **c.** Rhabdomyosarcoma and Wilms' tumor are the two most common primary solid malignancies in children. Typically, there is sudden and rapidly progressive proptosis that requires emergency treatment. The three histologic variants of rhabomyosarcoma include the embryonal, which is the most common type, the alveolar, and the rare adult differentiated pleomorphic type. The alveolar type has the least favorable prognosis. Spontaneous lid ecchymoses are seen in rhabdomyosarcoma but are not specific for this condition, as they may occur in metastatic neuroblastoma and Ewing's sarcoma.

124. **c.** Neurofibromas are not encapsulated but may be circumscribed. Both neurofibromas and Schwannomas (neurilemmoma) are found in increased frequency in patients with neurofibromatosis type I. Isolated neurofibromas do not necessarily indicate systemic involvement. Verocay bodies are groups of cells that resemble sensory corpuscles.

125. **e.** For the general ophthalmologist, approximately 20% of lacrimal gland lesions are epithelial cell tumors and 80% are lymphoid or inflammatory lesions. Benign mixed tumor (pleomorphic adenoma) constitutes approximately 50% of epithelial tumors of the lacrimal gland. Although the pleomorphic adenoma may appear encapsulated, microscopic lobules of tumor may prolapse through the capsule. Furthermore, incomplete excision is clearly associated with multiple recurrences and malignant degeneration.

126. **False.** Melanocytoma of the optic nerve head is a benign, deeply pigmented melanocytic tumor but has been associated with adjacent choroidal melanoma in rare cases.

127. **b.** These tumors most often present in the first decade of life. Rosenthal fibers are enlarged, eosinophilic cell processes and are not unique to optic nerve gliomas. All visual pathway gliomas are of the relatively indolent pilocytic variety.

128. c.　The majority of orbital meningiomas are secondary (extensions of intracranial meningiomas). The mean age of presentation of primary optic nerve sheath meningioma is lower than in the secondary type (20% are seen at age < 10). Nearly all meningioma of the orbit are of the meningothelial cell type. Pediatric meningioma are particularly aggressive, with rapid infiltration of the central nervous system.

129. d.　Disc pallor is thought to correspond to limited reorganization and proliferation of glial cells and not to decreased vascularity. Although changes in the optic nerve head may be diagnostic of glaucoma, they often convey no information as to the etiology of the specific mechanism of glaucoma. Damage from glaucoma to the optic nerve head is manifested in the retina as atrophy of both the nerve fiber and ganglion cell layers. Cavernous (Schnabel's) optic atrophy is also seen occasionally in nonglaucomatous eyes and consists of cystoid spaces posterior to the lamina cribrosa.

130. d.　Excessive pigment in the trabecular meshwork may be seen in the pigment dispersion syndrome and the pseudoexfoliation syndrome, as well as after surgery, uveitis, or trauma. Pseudoexfoliation glaucoma is characterized by its asymmetry. Pseudoexfoliation material is thought to be closely associated with elements of the elastic system (oxytalan and small elastic fibers) and has been detected within the conjunctival substantia propria. Although pseudoexfoliation material is found adjacent to the lens epithelium and on the lens capsule, it continues to be deposited after cataract extraction.

131. True.　Angle recession is a tear between the longitudinal and circular muscles of the ciliary body. Approximately 5 to 10% of patients with greater than 180 degrees of angle recession will eventually develop glaucoma.

132. True.　The iridocorneal endothelial syndromes are all characterized by abnormal proliferation of corneal endothelium affecting the cornea, angle structures, and the iris.

133. e.　Acute angle-closure glaucoma can result in lens epithelial necrosis (glaukomflecken), sectoral iris ischemia with atrophy, and PAS after iridotomy. If the fellow eye has a narrow angle, this suggests primary angle closure, since the condition is typically symmetric.

134. c.　The combination of sebaceous adenomas and gastrointestinal malignancy is the Muir-Torre syndrome. Trichofolliculoma may be associated with breast and thyroid neoplasms, both benign and malignant.

135. e.　Medulloepithelioma may show either benign or malignant histologic characteristics. Even when cytologically malignant, this tumor is rarely metastatic.

136. a.　Pigmented choroidal lesions less than 10 mm in greatest diameter and less than 1 mm in height are nearly always benign. Tumors greater than 3 mm in height are nearly always melanomas. Overlying RPE degeneration and drusen are frequently associated with choroidal nevi, although these may be seen in melanoma. An associated serous retinal detachment is common with choroidal melanoma but may be seen (rarely) with nevi.

137. d.   There are no fluorescein angiographic signs that are specific for choroidal melanoma. Subretinal hemorrhage (most frequently from choroidal neovascularization) can be differentiated from melanoma by the absence of late hyperfluorescence characteristic of melanoma.

138. True.   A-scan ultrasonography of choroidal melanoma shows low internal reflectivity, particularly compared to choroidal hemangioma, which has strikingly <u>high</u> internal reflectivity.

139. c.   Mortality from systemic metastasis of choroidal melanoma peaks during the second year after diagnosis. It falls off steadily afterwards.

140. a.   The liver is the predominant site of metastasis of uveal melanoma.

141. b.   Sturge Weber disease is associated with a distinctive, diffuse choroidal hemangioma which causes a reddish, thickened appearance of large areas of the fundus which has been likened to tomato catsup.

142. b.   Choroidal osteomas are benign bony tumors that are more common in the peripapillary region of young women. Approximately 25% are bilateral. Ultrasonography demonstrates a highly reflective surface due to the presence of a bony plate, which also results in the loss of normal orbital echoes behind the tumor.

143. e.   Approximately 94% of retinoblastoma cases are sporadic. About 15% of these cases represent mutations involving the germ cell line, and patients are therefore capable of transmitting the gene to offspring. A patient with unilateral involvement and no family history of retinoblastoma is very likely a sporadic case, and the likelihood that the parents will have another affected child is only about 1%. The inherited form of retinoblastoma is transmitted as an autosomal dominant trait with incomplete penetrance (about 80-90%) according to pedigree analysis.

144. True.   Children with inherited retinoblastoma are at increased risk of other malignancies, most commonly osteogenic sarcoma. Other associated malignancies include rhabdomyosarcoma, brain tumors, fibrosarcoma, and other soft-tissue sarcomas.

145. b.   The most common presenting signs in retinoblastoma are leukocoria and strabismus. Rare presenting signs include iris heterochromia, spontaneous hyphema, and fixed pupil. Proptosis generally occurs only in advanced disease.

146. a.   Retinoblastoma can metastasize either hematogenously or, in advanced cases, via conjunctival lymphatics. The lung is not a common site of metastasis of retinoblastoma, except by extension of tumor from an adjacent bony metastasis.

147. False.   The Reese-Ellsworth classification provides prognostic information regarding visual outcome following therapy for retinoblastoma. It does not provide prognostic information regarding survival.

148. d.   Retinal capillary hemangiomatosis associated with cerebellar hemangioblastoma is termed von Hippel-Lindau syndrome. Other lesions, including renal cell carcinoma and pheochromocytoma, are associated but are not a part of the definition of the syndrome. Multiple retinal angiomas without cerebellar tumors is referred to as von Hippel disease.

149. e.   Autopsy studies have shown that up to 10% of patients with known metastatic disease will have ocular or orbital involvement. Orbital metastases are much less common than ocular metastases at autopsy. As noted, gastrointestinal primary tumors are a relatively infrequent source of metastasis to the eye and orbit, although colon primaries have been reported.

150. c.   The choroid is the typical site of involvement by metastatic tumors. The retina is rarely the first ocular tissue involved. Due to the different branching patterns of the right and left carotid system, the left eye seems more susceptible to metastasis (several studies have reported a ratio of about 1.5:1 of left-sided to right-sided ocular metastasis). Breast metastases typically present months or years <u>after</u> treatment of the primary tumor. Ocular radiation therapy is generally reserved for symptomatic ocular metastasis. Ocular metastases are most commonly choroidal. Isolated retinal metastasis is rare.

References

1. Spencer, William H. (ed.). <u>Ophthalmic Pathology, An Atlas and Textbook</u> (3rd ed.). Philadelphia: W.B. Saunders Company, 1985.

2. Folberg, Robert. "Section 4: Ophthalmic Pathology and Intraocular Tumors." in F.M. Wilson (ed.). <u>Basic and Clinical Science Course</u>. San Francisco: American Academy of Ophthalmology, 1991-1992.

4: Neuro-Ophthalmology

1. T or F -- The photostress recovery test may be useful in an eye with decreased vision to differentiate between macular and optic nerve disease.

2. Which one of the following concerning the visual evoked response (VER) is <u>false</u>?

   a. The VER is an electrical signal that must be extracted from the simultaneously generated electroencephalogram (EEG).
   b. The stimulus may consist of either a flash of white light or a pattern, presented either transiently or continuously via pattern reversal.
   c. The two critical parameters used for functional evaluation include the height of the first positive or upward wave and the amount of time between stimulus presentation and the appearance of this wave.
   d. VER is not useful for distinguishing optic neuropathy from retinal disorders.
   e. Uses of the flash VER include visual acuity assessment in preverbal children, assessment of optic nerve function in suspected multiple sclerosis, and reliable establishment of factitious visual loss.

3. A patient presents complaining of decreased vision in the left eye. His acuities are 20/20 OD and 20/100 OS. The examination is entirely unremarkable, and the diagnosis of factitious visual loss is considered. Tests that would be particularly useful in establishing this diagnosis include:

   1. optokinetic nystagmus testing.
   2. gently rocking a large mirror in front of the patient with the good eye occluded.
   3. introducing a prism base up in front of the left eye while the patient is reading binocularly.
   4. performing a fogging refraction.

   a. 1, 2, and 3.
   b. 1 and 3.
   c. 2 and 4.
   d. 4 only.
   e. 1, 2, 3, and 4.

4. A patient comes in complaining of decreased vision in the left eye. His acuities are 20/20 OD and light perception OS. The examination is entirely unremarkable, and the diagnosis of factitious visual loss appears in the differential. Tests that would be particularly useful in establishing this diagnosis include:

      1. optokinetic nystagmus testing.
      2. gently rocking a large mirror in front of the patient with the good eye occluded.
      3. introducing a prism base up in front of the left eye while the patient is reading binocularly.
      4. performing a fogging retraction.

    a. 1, 2, and 3.
    b. 1 and 3.
    c. 2 and 4.
    d. 4 only.
    e. 1, 2, 3, and 4.

5. Lesions affecting the optic tract may be associated with:

      1. unilateral decreased visual acuity.
      2. ipsilateral afferent pupillary defect.
      3. contralateral afferent pupillary defect.
      4. homonymous hemianopsia.

    a. 1, 2, and 3.
    b. 1 and 3.
    c. 2 and 4.
    d. 4 only.
    e. 1, 2, 3, and 4.

6. T or F -- Impairment of oculovestibular caloric reflexes suggests supranuclear disturbance of eye movements.

7. T or F -- In the setting of an upgaze paresis, upturning of the eyes upon forceful opening of closed eyelids implies a supranuclear lesion.

8. Which of the following concerning magnetic resonance imaging (MRI) is/are true?

    1. Short repetition times (TR) and short echo times (TE) are used to generate T1-weighted images.
    2. On a T1-weighted image, vitreous is dark, and on a T2-weighted image, vitreous is bright.
    3. Air and cortical bone give a dark (hypointense) signal on MRI.
    4. T1-weighted images tend to show anatomy well, while T2-weighted images tend to show pathology well.

    a. 1, 2, and 3.
    b. 1 and 3.
    c. 2 and 4.
    d. 4 only.
    e. 1, 2, 3, and 4.

9. Which one of the following concerning the intracranial portion of the optic nerve is false?

    a. It is typically 10 to 17 mm in length.
    b. It enters the intracranial cavity inferior to the frontal lobe and anterior cerebral artery.
    c. It enters the intracranial cavity medial to the internal carotid artery.
    d. Within the cranial cavity, it runs parallel to the hypophyseal stalk at a 45-degree incline.
    e. There is generally some redundancy within the intracranial optic nerve.

10. Which of the following concerning the optic chiasm is/are true?

    1. As many fibers cross as do not cross.
    2. The posterior portion of the chiasm has a high density of macular fibers.
    3. The chiasm typically lies 1 mm above the anterior pituitary gland.
    4. Inferonasal retinal fibers cross in the anterior portion of the chiasm.

    a. 1, 2, and 3.
    b. 1 and 3.
    c. 2 and 4.
    d. 4 only.
    e. 1, 2, 3, and 4.

11. T or F -- Segregation of retinal ganglion cell terminals into the six layers of the lateral geniculate body is a function of the cells' receptive fields.

12. T or F -- Superior fibers of the optic radiations, carrying information from the inferior visual field, run in close relationship to the internal capsule.

13. At which retrochiasmal location(s) can a single lesion induce a monocular visual field defect?

   1. lateral geniculate body.
   2. parietal lobe.
   3. temporal lobe.
   4. occipital lobe.

   a. 1, 2, and 3.
   b. 1 and 3.
   c. 2 and 4.
   d. 4 only.
   e. 1, 2, 3, and 4.

14. Match each of the various disorders listed below with its most likely visual field defect.

   a. ischemic optic neuropathy.
   b. optic nerve pit with serous retinal detachment.
   c. toxic/nutritional optic neuropathy.

   d glaucoma.
   e. hereditary optic neuropathy.
   f. optic neuritis.

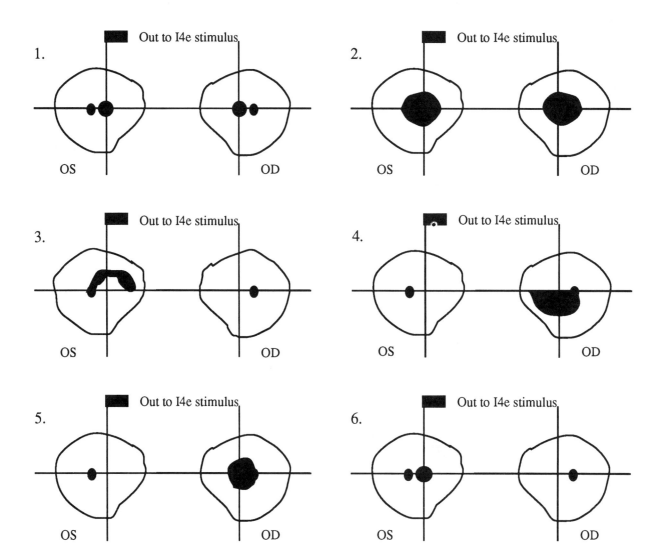

15. Match each of the visual pathway locations listed below with its appropriate visual field defect(s).

   a. posterior chiasm.
   b. anterior chiasm.
   c. optic nerve.
   d. thalamus.
   e. mid-chiasm.

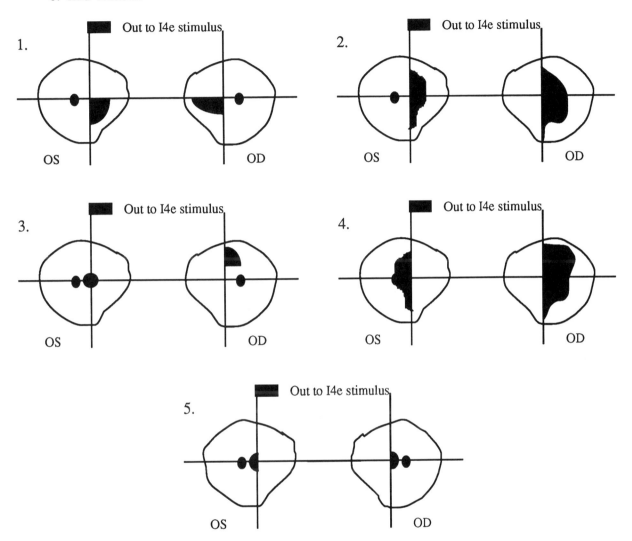

16. Which of the following features is/are consistent with a temporal lobe lesion?

   1. seizures.
   2. optokinetic nystagmus (OKN) abnormalities.
   3. formed visual hallucinations.
   4. high congruity of visual field deficits.

   a. 1, 2, and 3.
   b. 1 and 3.
   c. 2 and 4.
   d. 4 only.
   e. 1, 2, 3, and 4.

Questions

17. Which of the following features is/are consistent with a parietal lobe lesion?

> 1. agnosia.
> 2. right-left confusion.
> 3. OKN abnormalities.
> 4. homonymous hemianopia denser inferiorly.

a. 1, 2, and 3.
b. 1 and 3.
c. 2 and 4.
d. 4 only.
e. 1, 2, 3, and 4.

18. Which of the following features is/are consistent with an occipital lobe lesion?

> 1. unformed hallucinations.
> 2. macular sparing.
> 3. sparing of the temporal crescent.
> 4. OKN abnormalities.

a. 1, 2, and 3.
b. 1 and 3.
c. 2 and 4.
d. 4 only.
e. 1, 2, 3, and 4.

19. Causative events in the pathophysiology of optic disc edema include:

> 1. swollen axons.
> 2. extracellular fluid accumulation.
> 3. cessation of axonal transport.
> 4. breakdown of the blood retinal barrier.

a. 1, 2, and 3.
b. 1 and 3.
c. 2 and 4.
d. 4 only.
e. 1, 2, 3, and 4.

20. Which of the following concerning papilledema is/are true?

        1. Loss of venous pulsations is a particularly specific finding.
        2. Symptoms accompanying papilledema may include visual loss and diplopia.
        3. The most typical visual field finding in chronic papilledema is an enlarged blind spot.
        4. Papilledema may be unilateral.

    a. 1, 2, and 3.
    b. 1 and 3.
    c. 2 and 4.
    d. 4 only.
    e. 1, 2, 3, and 4.

21. Which of the following are universal findings in patients with pseudotumor cerebri?

        1. papilledema.
        2. increased intracranial pressure.
        3. normal neurologic examination.
        4. normal neuro-imaging studies.

    a. 1, 2, and 3.
    b. 1 and 3.
    c. 2 and 4.
    d. 4 only.
    e. 1, 2, 3, and 4.

22. The indications for treatment of pseudotumor cerebri include:

        1. papilledema.
        2. severe headache.
        3. obesity.
        4. visual field loss.

    a. 1, 2, and 3.
    b. 1 and 3.
    c. 2 and 4.
    d. 4 only.
    e. 1, 2, 3, and 4.

23. All of the following are included in the differential diagnosis with nonarteritic (idiopathic) anterior ischemic optic neuropathy except:

    a. demyelinative optic neuritis.
    b. systemic lupus erythematosus (SLE).
    c. syphilis.
    d. pseudotumor cerebri.
    e. giant cell arteritis.

24. Which of following concerning giant cell arteritis is/are true?

1. It is exceedingly rare in patients less than 50 years old.
2. Forty percent of untreated patients will develop some form of permanent visual loss.
3. Sixty-five percent of untreated patients will have contralateral involvement after permanent visual loss in one eye.
4. In a patient with anterior ischemic optic neuropathy but no other localizing signs or symptoms, a normal erythrocyte sedimentation rate (ESR) rules out the diagnosis of giant cell arteritis.

a. 1, 2, and 3.
b. 1 and 3.
c. 2 and 4.
d. 4 only.
e. 1, 2, 3, and 4.

25. Which one of the following concerning nonarteritic anterior ischemic optic neuropathy is false?

a. Visual loss is generally less severe than in the arteritic variety.
b. The condition most frequently associated with it is hypertension.
c. Life expectancy is considerably shorter than for patients who suffer a central retinal artery occlusion.
d. There is a 25% chance of subsequent occurence in the contralateral eye.
e. The presence of a large cup in the contralateral unaffected optic disc makes the diagnosis unlikely.

26. Approximately what percentage of patients with multiple sclerosis (MS) will develop clinical optic neuritis?

a. 1%.
b. 10%.
c. 25%.
d. 55%.
e. 100%.

27. What percentage of patients with severe multiple sclerosis (MS) will, on autopsy examination, have demyelinative lesions of the optic nerves?

a. 10%.
b. 25%.
c. 50%.
d. 75%.
e. 100%.

28. Which of the following concerning optic nerve glioma is/are true?

    1. It primarily affects children.
    2. The majority of patients will have associated neurofibromatosis.
    3. Presenting findings include visual loss, strabismus, proptosis, or hypothalamic abnormalities.
    4. These tumors are more likely to be aggressively malignant in children than in adults.

    a. 1, 2, and 3.
    b. 1 and 3.
    c. 2 and 4.
    d. 4 only.
    e. 1, 2, 3, and 4.

29. T or F -- Collateral vessels at the optic disc are highly specific for optic nerve meningioma.

30. Which of the following concerning optic nerve meningiomas is/are true?

    1. It primarily affects children.
    2. The majority of patients will have associated neurofibromatosis.
    3. On computed tomography (CT) scanning, affected optic nerves have a "kinked" appearance.
    4. These tumors are more likely to be aggressively malignant in children than in adults.

    a. 1, 2, and 3.
    b. 1 and 3.
    c. 2 and 4.
    d. 4 only.
    e. 1, 2, 3, and 4.

31. T or F -- Dominant optic atrophy is usually slowly progressive throughout life.

32. Which of the following concerning Leber's hereditary optic neuropathy is/are true?

    1. All offspring of a female carrier are either affected or carriers.
    2. Ten percent of female carriers will be affected.
    3. There is generally sequential asymmetric bilateral involvement.
    4. A small percentage of patients will enjoy partial or complete recovery late in their course.

    a. 1, 2, and 3.
    b. 1 and 3.
    c. 2 and 4.
    d. 4 only.
    e. 1, 2, 3, and 4.

33. A 23-year-old man presents complaining of sudden loss of vision in his right eye. His acuities are 20/200 OD and 20/20 OS. Examination is normal with exception of a swollen optic nerve, dilated retinal veins, and scattered dense retinal hemorrhages. The factor that most convincingly argues against the diagnosis of papillophlebitis is the patient's:

    a. age.
    b. sex.
    c. visual acuity.
    d. absence of cotton-wool spots.
    e. retinal hemorrhages.

34. Which one of the following concerning optic nerve drusen is false?

    a. They are generally silent clinically.
    b. They are generally bilateral.
    c. They are common in African Americans and Orientals.
    d. Associated visual field defects may resemble those of glaucoma.
    e. Associated loss of acuity is very unusual.

35. T or F -- Morning glory disc syndrome is more common in women than in men.

36. The work-up for optic nerve hypoplasia might include:

                   1. a careful history of maternal drug use.
                   2. a careful history of maternal medical disorders.
                   3. endocrinologic evaluation.
                   4. neuro-imaging.

    a. 1, 2, and 3.
    b. 1 and 3.
    c. 2 and 4.
    d. 4 only.
    e. 1, 2, 3, and 4.

37. T or F -- Concerning pituitary tumors, the secreting variety is more likely to present with visual loss than the nonsecreting variety.

38. T or F -- Bitemporal macular hemianopia (bitemporal central scotomas) may be a false-localizing sign.

39. In the left column are listed various retrochiasmal visual disorders. Match each defect with its correct anatomic locus.

    a. alexia with agraphia.
    b. alexia without agraphia.
    c. cerebral dyschromatopsia.
    d. prosopagnosia.
    e. unformed hallucinations.

    1. bilateral inferior occipitotemporal junction.
    2. unilateral occipital lobe.
    3. dominant angular gyrus.
    4. unilateral or bilateral inferior occipitotemporal junction.
    5. occipital lobe and corpus callosum.

40. In the left column are listed neurologic deficits that may be associated with a fascicular third nerve palsy. Match each deficit with its correct anatomic locus.

    a. contralateral coarse tremor.
    b. contralateral hemiparesis.
    c. contralateral ataxia.

    1. superior cerebellar peduncle.
    2. red nucleus.
    3. cerebral peduncle.

41. The most common location for a cerebral aneurysm associated with acute third nerve palsy is:

    a. the junction of posterior communicating and posterior cerebral arteries.
    b. the junction of the vertebral and superior cerebellar arteries.
    c. the posterior communicating artery.
    d. the junction of posterior communicating artery and the internal carotid artery.
    e. the junction of the internal carotid artery and the anterior communicating artery.

42. T or F -- A third nerve palsy associated with a cerebral aneurysm is always painful.

43. A 42-year-old diabetic man presents with a painful partial third nerve palsy. On his first follow-up visit, you notice that, when looking down, his upper eyelid appears to retract or lag. This finding essentially rules out the possibility of:

    a. diabetic third nerve palsy.
    b. aneurysm.
    c. meningioma.
    d. syphilitic gumma.
    e. trauma.

44. The most common cause of acquired fourth nerve palsy in adults is:

    a. tumor.
    b. trauma.
    c. vascular.
    d. idiopathic.
    e. aneurysm.

45. The best method for detecting a decompensated congenital fourth nerve palsy is:

    a. the three-step (Bielschowsky head tilt) test.
    b. distance and near prismatic measurements.
    c. double Maddox rod testing.
    d. vertical fusional amplitude measurements.
    e. the Lancaster red-green test.

46. A 35-year-old Chinese man presents with right ptosis, right elevation weakness, facial hypesthesia, and keratoconjunctivitis sicca OD. This picture is highly suggestive of:

    a. meningioma.
    b. chordoma.
    c. diabetic vascular neuropathies.
    d. nasopharyngeal carcinoma.
    e. aneurysm.

47. T or F -- Sixth nerve palsy due to an intracavernous lesion may present as abduction palsy plus miosis.

48. The finding that all three types of Duane's syndrome share is:

    a. a deficit of abduction.
    b. a deficit of adduction.
    c. retraction with adduction.
    d. esotropia.
    e. exotropia.

49. T or F -- The sixth nerve is more resistant to damage within the cavernous sinus, since it runs within its substance, rather than within its lateral wall.

50. T or F -- Damage to the right frontal eye field will result in permanent, complete inability to generate a leftward saccade.

51. Which one of the following concerning oculomotor apraxia is false?

    a. Both congenital and acquired forms may be observed.
    b. Pursuits are generally affected more than saccades.
    c. Horizontal movements are generally affected much more than vertical movements.
    d. In the acquired form, blinks are frequently utilized to break fixation.
    e. In the congenital form, children frequently use compensatory exaggerated head turns to refixate.

52. Which of the following ocular motor disorders is associated with malignancy?

   a. square-wave jerks.
   b. ocular flutter.
   c. opsoclonus.
   d. dysmetria.
   e. ocular bobbing.

53. Typically, the first saccadic movement to be affected in progressive supranuclear palsy (PSP) is:

   a. upward.
   b. downward.
   c. leftward.
   d. rightward.
   e. saccades are equally affected in all directions.

54. T or F -- The latency in generating a pursuit movement is shorter than that for a saccade.

55. Hypertropia associated with ipsilateral adduction weakness is most suggestive of:

   a. decompensated congenital fourth nerve palsy.
   b. dorsal midbrain syndrome.
   c. "one-and-a-half" syndrome.
   d. skew deviation with internuclear ophthalmoplegia (INO).
   e. progressive supranuclear palsy (PSP).

56. The dorsal midbrain syndrome is associated with all of the following except:

   a. upward gaze paresis.
   b. accommodative abnormalities.
   c. light-near dissociation.
   d. lid retraction.
   e. paradoxic OKN.

57. All of the following are features of congenital motor nystagmus except:

   a. oscillopsia.
   b. normal visual acuity.
   c. paradoxic OKN.
   d. amplitude dampened by convergence.
   e. amplitude increased by fixation.

58. Monocular nystagmus in a toddler raises the specter of:

    a. optic nerve meningioma.
    b. craniopharyngioma.
    c. rhabdomyosarcoma.
    d. chiasmal glioma.
    e. metastatic neuroblastoma.

59. According to Alexander's law, in which position should upbeat nystagmus be most prominent?

    a. upgaze.
    b. downgaze.
    c. left gaze.
    d. right gaze.
    e. convergence.

60. Which pattern of nystagmus is most localizing?

    a. upbeat nystagmus.
    b. periodic alternating nystagmus.
    c. vestibular nystagmus.
    d. downbeat nystagmus.
    e. see-saw nystagmus.

61. Which visual field defect is most likely to be associated with see-saw nystagmus?

    a. central scotoma.
    b. bitemporal hemianopia.
    c. incongruous hemianopia.
    d. congruous hemianopia.
    e. a visual field defect should not be associated with see-saw nystagmus.

62. T or F -- Saccades, pursuits, and vergence eye movements all utilize the same pathways for eye movement generation.

63. T or F -- Upper motor neuron facial nerve paralysis usually leaves voluntary eyelid closure intact.

64. T or F -- Orbicularis weakness may be seen with lower brainstem lesions.

65. T or F -- In Parkinson's disease, volitional eyelid movements are impaired, while reflex and emotional movements are intact.

66. Which one of the following concerning the facial nerve is false?

   a. The sensory innervation of the tongue terminates in the nucleus solitarius, and the motor innervation to the lacrimal gland arises in the superior salivatory nucleus.
   b. The first branch of the facial nerve is the greater superficial petrosal nerve, which synapses in the geniculate ganglion.
   c. Within the fallopian canal, the facial nerve gives off a motor branch to the stapedius muscle and sensory branches for the skin behind the ear.
   d. The chorda tympani continues on past the geniculate ganglion, carrying sensory innervation to the tongue and motor innovation to the salivary glands.
   e. The motor branches to the intrinsic facial muscles branch within the parotid gland.

67. T or F -- The Marcus Gunn "jaw-wink" reflex is an example of aberrant regeneration.

68. Bell's palsy may be associated with:

   1. diabetes.
   2. hypertension.
   3. pregnancy.
   4. herpes zoster infections.

   a. 1, 2, and 3.
   b. 1 and 3.
   c. 2 and 4.
   d. 4 only.
   e. 1, 2, 3, and 4.

69. What percentage of patients with Bell's palsy will experience complete spontaneous recovery?

   a. 5%.
   b. 25%.
   c. 50%.
   d. 75%.
   e. 100%.

70. T or F -- The facial nerve is the most frequently involved cranial nerve in neurosarcoidosis.

71. T or F -- Hemifacial spasm is probably a disorder of the basal ganglia.

72. Facial myokymia in a child is frequently associated with:

   a. chiasmal glioma.
   b. nasopharyngeal carcinoma.
   c. cerebellar hemangioblastoma.
   d. pontine glioma.
   e. spasmus nutans.

73. Which of the following may be confused with essential blepharospasm?

    1. severe dry eye.
    2. retained conjunctival foreign body.
    3. hemifacial spasm.
    4. tardive dyskinesia.

a. 1, 2, and 3.
b. 1 and 3.
c. 2 and 4.
d. 4 only.
e. 1, 2, 3, and 4.

74. Which of the following regarding the pupillary reflex is/are true?

    1. The pupil pathway terminates in pretectal nuclei after passing, without synapsing, through the lateral geniculate body (LGB).
    2. The decussation at the chiasm is responsible for a normal consensual pupillary response.
    3. Sympathetic pupillary fibers originate in the superior cervical ganglion, travel in the cranial vault with the internal carotid artery, and enter the orbit with the ophthalmic artery through the optic foramen.
    4. The pathway for accommodative miosis enters the Edinger-Westphal nucleus anterior to the pathway for light-induced miosis.

a. 1, 2, and 3.
b. 1 and 3.
c. 2 and 4.
d. 4 only.
e. 1, 2, 3, and 4.

75. Which of the following concerning light-near dissociation is/are true?

    1. A key finding in the diagnosis of Argyll Robertson pupils is the presence of miosis.
    2. Argyll Robertson pupils are the most common manifestation of neurosyphilis.
    3. The most common etiology of the dorsal midbrain syndrome in a child under 10 years of age is a pineal gland tumor.
    4. The most common etiology for the dorsal midbrain syndrome in a patient over the age of 60 is multiple sclerosis.

a. 1, 2, and 3.
b. 1 and 3.
c. 2 and 4.
d. 4 only.
e. 1, 2, 3, and 4.

76. Pupillary dilation may be the only sign of oculomotor nerve palsy in which of the following disorders?

        1. uncal herniation.
        2. diabetic microvascular disease.
        3. basilar meningitis.
        4. cerebral aneurysm.

    a. 1, 2, and 3.
    b. 1 and 3.
    c. 2 and 4.
    d. 4 only.
    e. 1, 2, 3, and 4.

77. Which one of the following concerning Adie's tonic pupil is false?

    a. Most patients will manifest Adie's syndrome.
    b. The majority of affected patients will have unilateral involvement.
    c. Pupillary size generally diminishes <u>after</u> accommodative symptoms abate.
    d. Pupillary constriction in response to pilocarpine 1/8% is conclusive evidence of denervation hypersensitivity.
    e. The differential diagnosis of a tonic pupil includes herpes zoster, syphilis, and giant cell arteritis.

78. Which of the following concerning Horner's syndrome is/are true?

        1. The distribution of anhidrosis is helpful in locating the lesion.
        2. Cocaine 4% will dilate the pupil of the patient with Horner's syndrome, whereas it will leave a normal pupil unchanged.
        3. The evaluation of a patient whose miotic pupil dilates in response to hydroxyamphetamine consists of chest x-ray and careful neurologic examination.
        4. A Horner's syndrome with coincident ipsilateral headache is indicative of spontaneous carotid dissection, even in the setting of a normal carotid angiogram.

    a. 1, 2, and 3.
    b. 1 and 3.
    c. 2 and 4.
    d. 4 only.
    e. 1, 2, 3, and 4.

79. The first step in evaluating a patient with anisocoria is:

    a. the swinging flashlight test.
    b. testing of extraocular movements.
    c. OKN testing in the vertical direction.
    d. slit-lamp examination.
    e. pharmacologic testing.

80. T or F -- The lifetime risk of developing multiple sclerosis after an initial bout of optic neuritis is higher for women than for men.

81. T or F -- The most common cranial mononeuropathy seen in multiple sclerosis is an isolated oculomotor palsy.

82. T or F -- Five to 10% of patients with multiple sclerosis will have findings of posterior uveitis, including pars planitis and/or retinal periphlebitis.

83. Pheochromocytoma may be seen as part of:

    1. neurofibromatosis.
    2. tuberous sclerosis.
    3. angiomatosis retinae.
    4. ataxia-telangiectasia.

    a. 1, 2, and 3.
    b. 1 and 3.
    c. 2 and 4.
    d. 4 only.
    e. 1, 2, 3, and 4.

84. Astrocytic hamartomas of the retina or optic nerve head may be seen in:

    1. Sturge-Weber syndrome.
    2. neurofibromatosis.
    3. ataxia-telangiectasia.
    4. tuberous sclerosis.

    a. 1, 2, and 3.
    b. 1 and 3.
    c. 2 and 4.
    d. 4 only.
    e. 1, 2, 3, and 4.

85. The triad of adenoma sebaceum, mental retardation, and seizures is considered pathognomonic for:

    a. neurofibromatosis.
    b. Sturge-Weber syndrome.
    c. ataxia-telangiectasia.
    d. tuberous sclerosis.
    e. angiomatosis retinae.

86. Seizures are often seen in patients with:

       1. neurofibromatosis.
       2. tuberous sclerosis.
       3. ataxia-telangiectasia.
       4. Sturge-Weber syndrome.

  a. 1, 2, and 3.
  b. 1 and 3.
  c. 2 and 4.
  d. 4 only.
  e. 1, 2, 3, and 4.

87. Infantile or juvenile glaucoma may be seen in:

       1. neurofibromatosis.
       2. tuberous sclerosis.
       3. Sturge-Weber syndrome.
       4. ataxia-telangiectasia.

  a. 1, 2, and 3.
  b. 1 and 3.
  c. 2 and 4.
  d. 4 only.
  e. 1, 2, 3, and 4.

88. T or F -- The histopathology of the retinal tumor of von Hippel's disease is most consistent with cavernous hemangioma.

89. Chronic sinopulmonary infections may be seen as part of:

       1. neurofibromatosis.
       2. tuberous sclerosis.
       3. angiomatosis retinae.
       4. ataxia-telangiectasia.

  a. 1, 2, and 3.
  b. 1 and 3.
  c. 2 and 4.
  d. 4 only.
  e. 1, 2, 3, and 4.

90. Which one of the following concerning Kearns-Sayre syndrome is false?

   a. The complete syndrome has an onset of symptoms or signs before age 20 years.
   b. The pigmentary retinopathy is generally associated with good visual function throughout life.
   c. The progressive external ophthalmoplegia associated with the syndrome typically presents as diplopia.
   d. Heart block develops late in the course of the syndrome.
   e. Elevated cerebrospinal fluid (CSF) protein may predict patients at risk of developing heart block.

91. T or F -- The presence of polychromatic cataract ("Christmas tree" cataract) in association with progressive external ophthalmoplegia (PEO) suggests the diagnosis of Wilson's disease.

92. The most specific sign in Graves' ophthalmopathy is:

   a. lid retraction with lag in downgaze.
   b. conjunctival injection over the horizontal rectus muscles.
   c. superficial punctate keratitis.
   d. proptosis.
   e. diplopia in upgaze.

93. The second most frequently involved extraocular muscle in Graves' ophthalmopathy is the:

   a. inferior rectus.
   b. lateral rectus.
   c. superior rectus.
   d. medial rectus.
   e. inferior oblique.

94. The least frequently involved muscle in Graves' opthalmopathy is the:

   a. inferior rectus.
   b. lateral rectus.
   c. superior rectus.
   d. medial rectus.
   e. inferior oblique.

95. What percentage of patients with myasthenia gravis (MG) present with ocular findings only?

   a. 5%.
   b. 10%.
   c. 25%.
   d. 50%.
   e. 75%.

96. What percentage of patients with myasthenia gravis will develop Graves' disease?

    a. 5%.
    b. 10%.
    c. 15%.
    d. 20%.
    e. 25%.

97. What percentage of patients with myasthenia gravis will develop thymoma?

    a. 1%.
    b. 10%.
    c. 25%.
    d. 50%.
    e. 75%.

98. For a patient to be reassured that systemic disease is unlikely, ocular myasthenia should remain localized for what length of time?

    a. 3 months.
    b. 6 months.
    c. 1 year.
    d. 2 years.
    e. 5 years.

99. Animal studies show that irreversible ischemic retinal damage occurs after what duration of retinal vascular occlusion?

    a. 30 minutes.
    b. 50 to 60 minutes.
    c. 90 to 100 minutes.
    d. 3 hours.
    e. 12 hours.

100. T or F -- The major cause of mortality in patients with embolic central retinal artery occlusion (CRAO) is massive cerebral infarction.

101. Clues to the presence of high-grade carotid stenosis include:

    1. low-grade anterior segment inflammation.
    2. cataract.
    3. hypotony.
    4. contralateral corneal arcus.

    a. 1, 2, and 3.
    b. 1 and 3.
    c. 2 and 4.
    d. 4 only.
    e. 1, 2, 3, and 4.

102. Typical symptoms in vertebrobasilar insufficiency include:

        1. ataxia.
        2. hemiparesis.
        3. vertigo.
        4. monocular blurring or loss of vision with phosphenes.

a. 1, 2, and 3.
b. 1 and 3.
c. 2 and 4.
d. 4 only.
e. 1, 2, 3, and 4.

103. A 29-year-old woman presents to an ophthalmologist complaining of pain on eye movements and blurry vision in her right eye. Review of systems documents a 3-week history of paresthesias in the right lower leg approximately 6 months prior to the onset of her visual disturbance. The patient reports that she noticed her visual disturbance develop over the 2 or 3 days prior to presentation. Examination discloses a visual acuity of 20/60 OD and 20/20 OS. She is able to interpret correctly 4 of 11 Ishihara plates with her right eye and 10 of 11 plates with her left eye. Visual fields disclose a central scotoma in the right eye and are normal for the left eye. There is no afferent pupillary defect (APD) noted. Which one of the following is true?

a. The patient probably has an acute maculopathy.
b. The patient probably has factitious visual loss.
c. The patient probably had a similar episode affect her left eye sometime in the past.
d. The patient probably has a hereditary optic neuropathy.
e. A neutral density filter placed over her left eye might elicit an afferent pupillary defect.

104. The only recognized neurologic association with Coats' disease is:

a. facioscapulohumeral dystrophy.
b. myotonic dystrophy.
c. cerebral angiitis.
d. cerebrovascular congophilic angiopathy.
e. progressive external ophthalmoplegia.

105. A 14-year-old girl is brought to the ophthalmologist by her parents after complaining that "the page swims when I try to read." The examination is normal with the exception of pronounced downbeat nystagmus. A careful review of systems documents the presence of intermittent headaches in the occipital region, which are intensified with anger or sudden head movement. The patient denies any use of prescription or illicit drugs, including alcohol. Her CT scan is most likely to resemble:

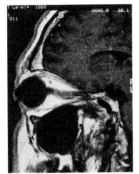

a.

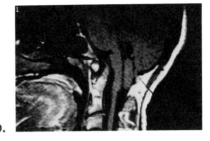

b.

c.

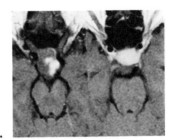

d.

e.

106. Modalities likely to relieve the patient's reading difficulties successfully include:

    1. clonazepam (Klonopin).
    2. carbamazepine (Tegretol).
    3. basilar craniectomy.
    4. psychotherapy.

a. 1, 2, and 3.
b. 1 and 3.
c. 2 and 4.
d. 4 only.
e. 1, 2, 3, and 4.

107. A 9-year-old boy presents to the ophthalmologist complaining that he has lost his position on the school basketball team because he cannot see the basket. He notes occasional morning headaches but denies any nausea or vomiting. Examination reveals visual acuity of 20/40 OD and 20/25 OS. The patient has marked symmetric weakness of upgaze bilaterally. His pupils are 7 mm and poorly reactive to light with better reaction to a near target. There is approximately 2 mm of superior scleral show bilaterally. Fundus examination suggests optic atrophy OU. Visual field testing discloses a bitemporal hemianopia. Review of systems documents increased consumption of water with frequent urination at night. The most likely diagnosis is:

a. pinealoma.
b. pontine glioma.
c. cerebellar astrocytoma.
d. chiasmal glioma.
e. hereditary optic atrophy.

108. After neuro-imaging, an important step in diagnostic evaluation of the patient in question 107 would be:

a. visual evoked responses.
b. EEG.
c. Farnsworth D-15 color vision testing.
d. lumbar puncture.
e. electromyograms.

109. Which of the following concerning optic neuritis in childhood is/are true?

1. It is more commonly bilateral than unilateral.
2. The visual prognosis is very poor.
3. The pathophysiology is believed to be related to autoimmune demyelination.
4. Enlargement of optic nerves on neuro-imaging implies another, more ominous, diagnosis.

a. 1, 2, and 3.
b. 1 and 3.
c. 2 and 4.
d. 4 only.
e. 1, 2, 3, and 4.

110. The differential diagnosis for presumed posterior ischemic optic neuropathy includes:

1. radiation optic neuropathy.
2. post-coronary artery bypass graft surgery.
3. giant cell arteritis.
4. essential hypertension.

a. 1, 2, and 3.
b. 1 and 3.
c. 2 and 4.
d. 4 only.
e. 1, 2, 3, and 4.

111. In a patient complaining of headache and transient visual obscurations whose examination reveals bilateral disc edema, the first diagnostic intervention to be undertaken is:

    a. lumbar puncture.
    b. automated perimetry.
    c. emergent CT scanning.
    d. measurement of blood pressure.
    e. measurement of sedimentation rate.

112. Which of the following disorders is clearly associated with optic nerve drusen?

    a. migraines.
    b. pseudotumor cerebri.
    c. giant cell arteritis.
    d. retinitis pigmentosa.
    e. normal tension glaucoma.

113. T or F -- Most meningiomas causing an optic neuropathy arise from outside the orbit.

114. Which histopathologic variety of meningioma is most commonly seen within the orbit?

    a. angioblastic.
    b. transitional.
    c. meningothelial.
    d. fibroblastic.
    e. pilocytic.

115. A meningioma arising in which location is most likely to lead to optic disc edema?

    a. sphenoid wing.
    b. olfactory groove.
    c. planum sphenoidale.
    d. optic nerve sheath.
    e. cavernous sinus.

116. T or F -- Heavy consumption of alcohol and cigarettes together is sufficient for the development of tobacco/alcohol amblyopia.

117. Important blood tests in the evaluation of patient with bilateral optic atrophy and cecocentral scotomas include:

> 1. serum B_{12} level.
> 2. FTA-Abs.
> 3. serum folate level.
> 4. serum cyanide level.

a. 1, 2, and 3.
b. 1 and 3.
c. 2 and 4.
d. 4 only.
e. 1, 2, 3, and 4.

118. The most common fundus finding in a patient with acute traumatic optic neuropathy is:

a. disc edema.
b. disc pallor.
c. disc hemorrhage.
d. choroidal ruptures.
e. none of the above.

119. Which of the following concerning diabetic papillopathy is/are true?

> 1. It is typically a disorder affecting older, type II diabetics.
> 2. Visual loss is generally severe.
> 3. The papillopathy is generally followed by the development of florid neovascularization.
> 4. Development of the disorder seems to be independent of the degree of blood sugar control.

a. 1, 2, and 3.
b. 1 and 3.
c. 2 and 4.
d. 4 only.
e. 1, 2, 3, and 4.

120. Modalities useful in the treatment of optic neuropathy secondary to Graves' disease include:

> 1. subtotal thyroidectomy.
> 2. orbital radiation.
> 3. chronic (greater than 4 weeks) oral prednisone therapy.
> 4. two- or three-wall orbital decompression.

a. 1, 2, and 3.
b. 1 and 3.
c. 2 and 4.
d. 4 only.
e. 1, 2, 3, and 4.

121. Bromocriptine treatment may be indicated in the management of a patient with a pituitary tumor that is secreting:

a. prolactin.
b. growth hormone.
c. thyrotropin.
d. nonsecreting.
e. Bromocryptine is useful in the management of all pituitary tumors.

122. The development of sudden severe headache with accompanying acute visual loss is a well-recognized complication of:

1. meningioma.
2. intracavernous carotid artery aneurysm.
3. hypothalamic glioma.
4. pituitary adenoma.

a. 1, 2, and 3.
b. 1 and 3.
c. 2 and 4.
d. 4 only.
e. 1, 2, 3, and 4.

123. Match each symptom complex listed in the left column with its appropriate name.

a. severe throbbing headache with associated nausea and photophobia.
b. severe throbbing headache preceded by scintillating scotoma and followed by nausea and photophobia.
c. scintillating scotoma, followed by nausea and photophobia.

1. migraine equivalent.
2. common migraine.
3. classic migraine.

124. Which of the following features favor the diagnosis of cerebral arteriovenous malformation rather than migraine?

1. fortification spectra that are more fleeting and less well defined.
2. family history of headaches.
3. fixed visual field defect.
4. nausea associated with visual disturbances.

a. 1, 2, and 3.
b. 1 and 3.
c. 2 and 4.
d. 4 only.
e. 1, 2, 3, and 4.

125. A 34-year-old woman presents complaining of double vision while reading. The examination is normal with the exception of a small-angle left hypertropia in downgaze and poor elevation of the left eye as well. Review of systems is normal, and she denies any history of antecedent trauma. The next step in diagnosis should be:

a. tensilon test.
b. CT scanning.
c. MRI scanning.
d. orbital ultrasound.
e. forced duction testing.

126. A 40-year-old man presents to an ophthalmologist complaining of diagonal binocular diplopia following a motor vehicle accident. Findings consistent with a bilateral fourth nerve palsy include:

1. a right hypertropia with right head tilt.
2. a left hypertropia with left head tilt.
3. excyclodeviation greater than 10 degrees on double Maddox rod testing.
4. a V pattern esotropia.

a. 1, 2, and 3.
b. 1 and 3.
c. 2 and 4.
d. 4 only.
e. 1, 2, 3, and 4.

127. Which features are necessary to conclude a motility disturbance is a skew deviation?

1. a vertical component.
2. noncomitance.
3. pattern of motility inconsistent with a single muscle or nerve dysfunction.
4. other obvious brainstem abnormalities.

a. 1, 2, and 3.
b. 1 and 3.
c. 2 and 4.
d. 4 only.
e. 1, 2, 3, and 4.

128. Brainstem nuclei critical for the generation of normal vertical eye movements include:

    1. paramedian pontine reticular formation.
    2. the rostral interstitial nucleus of medial longitudinal fasciculus.
    3. the abducens nucleus.
    4. the interstitial nucleus of Cajal.

    a. 1, 2, and 3.
    b. 1 and 3.
    c. 2 and 4.
    d. 4 only.
    e. 1, 2, 3, and 4.

129. T or F -- The most common etiology for bilateral sixth nerve palsy is small vessel disease causing infarction of the nerve trunks.

130. T or F -- The most common etiology of unilateral sixth nerve palsy in children is postviral inflammation.

131. What finding in a child with isolated abduction deficit most strongly argues for the diagnosis of Duane's retraction syndrome rather than a congenital sixth nerve palsy?

    a. inability to fully abduct the eye volitionally.
    b. normal abduction on oculocephalic rotational testing.
    c. orthotropia in primary gaze.
    d. normal adduction.
    e. involvement of the left eye only.

132. Features found in all cases of internuclear ophthalmoplegia (INO) include:

    1. ipsilateral adduction slowing or weakness.
    2. exotropia.
    3. contralateral abduction nystagmus.
    4. skew deviation.

    a. 1, 2, and 3.
    b. 1 and 3.
    c. 2 and 4.
    d. 4 only.
    e. 1, 2, 3, and 4.

133. Features frequently found coincidentally with internuclear ophthalmoplegia (INO) include:

> 1. rotary nystagmus.
> 2. vertical nystagmus.
> 3. convergence-retraction nystagmus.
> 4. skew deviation.

a. 1, 2, and 3.
b. 1 and 3.
c. 2 and 4.
d. 4 only.
e. 1, 2, 3, and 4.

134. T or F -- Bilateral INO is more commonly seen in cerebrovascular disease than in demyelinative disease.

135. A brainstem lesion that involves the medial longitudinal fasciculus at its junction with the abducens nucleus will most likely cause:

a. INO with skew.
b. Foville's syndrome.
c. walleyed bilateral INO.
d. Fisher syndrome.
e. "One-and-a-half" syndrome.

136. A lesion that involves both medial longitudinal fasciculi near their junctions with the third nerve nuclei may cause:

a. INO with skew.
b. Foville's syndrome.
c. walleyed bilateral INO.
d. Fisher syndrome.
e. "One-and-a-half" syndrome.

137. A variant of the Guillain-Barré syndrome that only involves only the brainstem and cranial nerves is known as:

a. INO skew.
b. Foville's syndrome.
c. walleyed bilateral INO.
d. Fisher syndrome.
e. "One-and-a-half" syndrome.

138. T or F -- The clinical distinction between a cavernous sinus syndrome and an orbital apex syndrome is best made by the presence of proptosis in the latter.

139. A healthy patient presents complaining of a painful double vision. Examination reveals normal visual acuity, diminished corneal sensation, and global impairment of ocular motility in the left eye, with no proptosis. There is pain with eye movements, and the globe and orbit are slightly tender. CT and MRI scanning are both normal, and the patient rapidly responds to 60 mg of oral prednisone a day. The probable diagnosis is:

a. intracavernous carotid artery aneurysm.
b. sphenoid wing meningioma.
c. orbital pseudotumor.
d. Tolosa-Hunt syndrome.
e. cavernous sinus thrombosis.

140. Potential complications of carotid-cavernous fistulae include:

1. retinal neovascularization.
2. cataract.
3. glaucomatous optic nerve damage.
4. corneal ulceration.

a. 1, 2, and 3.
b. 1 and 3.
c. 2 and 4.
d. 4 only.
e. 1, 2, 3, and 4.

141. T or F -- Both high-flow and low-flow carotid-cavernous fistulae may be associated with a history of head trauma.

142. A 59-year-old man presents to the emergency room complaining of sudden-onset oscillopsia and diplopia. Examination reveals an alcohol smell on his breath, normal acuity, bilateral abduction deficits, and coarse binocular nystagmus. Appropriate intervention should include:

a. intravenous glucose.
b. intravenous naloxone (Narcan).
c. intravenous chlordiazepoxide (Librium).
d. intravenous thiamine.
e. coffee.

143. Which of the following optic disc lesions are distinguished by autofluorescence?

1. myelinated nerve fibers.
2. astrocytic hamartomas.
3. optic nerve pits.
4. optic nerve drusen.

a. 1, 2, and 3.
b. 2 and 4.
c. 1 and 3.
d. 4 only.
e. 1, 2, 3, and 4.

144. Match the ganglia in the right column with the appropriate characteristics listed in the left column (note that each ganglion may be assigned to more than one characteristic).

a. cell bodies with processes providing facial sensation.
b. origin of postganglionic fibers to the iris dilator muscle.
c. origin of the greater superficial petrosal nerve.
d. located in Meckel's cavity.
e. origin of postganglionic fibers to iris sphincter.
f. located in fallopian canal.
g. origin of postganglionic fibers to lacrimal gland.
h. located near the angle of the mandible.
i. located lateral to the intraorbital optic nerve.

1. pterygopalatine ganglion.
2. geniculate ganglion.
3. gasserian ganglion.
4. ciliary ganglion.
5. superior cervical ganglion.

145. The approximate prevalence of giant cell arteritis in the population over the age of 50 is 1 in:

a. 75.
b. 750.
c. 7500.
d. 75,000.
e. 750,000.

146. The approximate prevalence of polymyalgia rheumatica (PMR) in the population over the age of 50 is 1 in:

a. 20.
b. 200.
c. 2000.
d. 10,000.
e. 20,000.

147. Clinical characteristics that may be seen with chiasmal compression include:

1. field abnormalities more notable centrally with fainter test objects.
2. postfixation blindness.
3. temporal color desaturation.
4. diplopia.

a. 1, 2, and 3.
b. 2 and 4.
c. 1 and 3.
d. 4 only.
e. 1, 2, 3, and 4.

148. Diagnostic modalities useful in confirming the presence of suspected optic disc drusen include:

      1. CT scanning.
      2. fundus photos with standard fluorescein angiography filters.
      3. ophthalmic ultrasound.
      4. MRI scanning.

  a. 1, 2, and 3.
  b. 2 and 4.
  c. 1 and 3.
  d. 4 only.
  e. 1, 2, 3, and 4.

149. A woman with known multiple sclerosis presents to an ophthalmologist complaining of "a tiny blind spot in my right eye." Examination discloses a right afferent pupillary defect and slight ocular tenderness OD. The examiner attempts to confirm diagnostic suspicions by eliciting the Pulfrich phenomenon. To do this, the examiner:

  a. asks her to glance quickly back and forth horizontally and report any photopsias.
  b. asks the patient to climb briskly several flights of stairs and report any visual loss.
  c. asks the patient to watch the pendulum on the grandfather clock across the room and report any three-dimensional movement.
  d. spins the examining chair while the patient fixates her outstretched thumb, watching for any nystagmus.
  e. carefully observes optic disc vasculature and color during digital pressure on the globe.

150. The test that best correlates with the pathophysiology underlying the Pulfrich phenomenon is:

  a. electroculography (EOG).
  b. visual evoked response (VER).
  c. electroretinography (ERG).
  d. calorics and electronystagmography.
  e. fluorescein angiography.

151. A 44-year-old woman presents to an ophthalmologist complaining that "my friends say my eyes look funny." The patient's external appearance is shown in color plate 1. Which one of the following regarding this condition is true?

  a. The most likely etiology in this woman is multiple sclerosis.
  b. The patient might admit to using thyroid hormones for weight control.
  c. An associated bilateral deficit in upgaze will be accompanied by convergence-retraction nystagmus.
  d. Cranial MRI is the diagnostic evaluation of choice.
  e. Bilateral levator recessions should be performed now, if the patient desires.

152. Which one of the following clinical features is not associated with the biopsy findings shown in color plate 2?

a. asynchronous bilateral visual loss.
b. fever.
c. amaurosis fugax.
d. headache.
e. age less than 50 years old.

153. A 28-year-old man undergoes routine eye examination. There are no positive findings, except for those shown in color plate 3. Which of the following are true?

1. The findings are probably congenital.
2. There may be associated neovascularization.
3. There may be an associated retinal detachment.
4. These lesions may communicate with the subarachnoid space.

a. 1, 2, and 3.
b. 1 and 3.
c. 2 and 4.
d. 4 only.
e. 1, 2, 3, and 4.

154. A 31-year-old woman presents complaining of 2 days of blurry, washed-out vision in her left eye. On closer questioning, she admits that moving her eyes is slightly painful. She also describes intermittent tingling in her right foot, which usually occurs as she showers. Acuity is 20/25 OD and 20/100 OS. There is no relative afferent pupillary defect on either side, but she can only read 2 of 12 Ishihara plates with her left eye (after correctly reading 11 of 12 with her right eye). The right fundus is normal, and the left fundus is shown in color plates 4 and 5. Which one of the following regarding this young woman is false?

a. The disc findings are unrelated to the pigmented lesion.
b. The disc findings are related to her pain with eye movement.
c. Oral prednisone has been found to be beneficial in the treatment of this disorder.
d. The patient might also notice poorer vision in her right eye while she showers.
e. Careful examination might disclose anterior chamber cells.

155. A 23-year-old obese woman is seen for routine ophthalmologic examination. The examination is entirely normal with the exception of bilaterally elevated discs with indistint margins. The right optic nerve is shown in color in color plate 6. Plate 7 is a pre-injection photo from fluorescein angiography. Which one of the following regarding this patient is true?

a. The condition depicted is typically associated with mild to moderate visual loss.
b. The filters on the fluorescein camera must be of poor quality.
c. The clinical and histologic findings reflect axoplasmic stasis and congestion.
d. There may be an associated arcuate field defect.
e. The findings in plate 7 are pathognomonic for her condition.

156. Select the CT scan that is most likely to create the visual field disturbance shown in Figure 4-1 below.

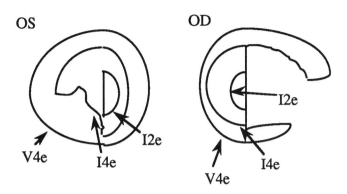

Figure 4-1

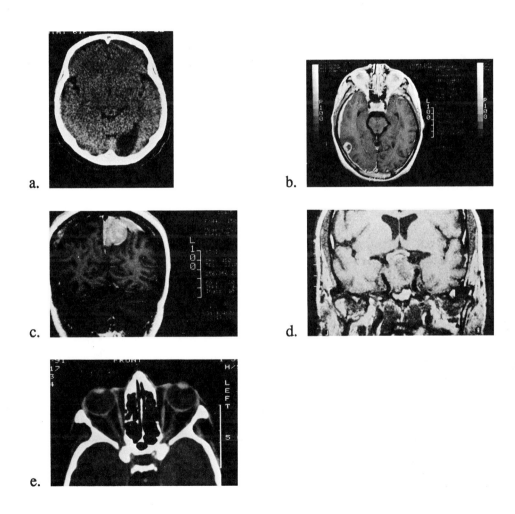

157. A 43-year-old man presents complaining of persistent red eye OS, present ever since a car accident 6 weeks earlier. Besides redness, he has noted intermittent horizontal diplopia without pain. His examination is normal, except for 4 mm of proptosis on the left, a mild deficit in abduction, and prominent conjunctival vessels. His right eye is entirely normal. Figure 4-2 depicts his clinical appearance. Which one of the following radiographic studies is most likely to belong to this patient?

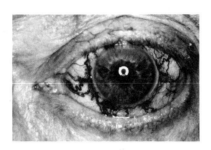

Figure 4-2

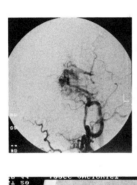

a.

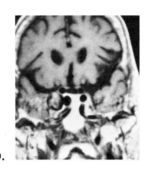

b.

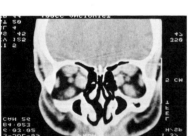

c.

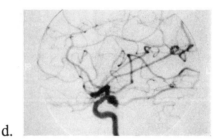

d.

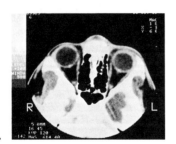

e.

158. Which one of the following abnormalities might be expected in a young child with bilaterally poor vision and the CT scan shown in Figure 4-3?

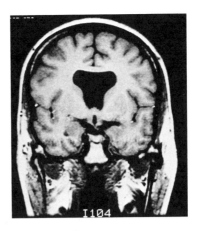

Figure 4-3

a. precocious puberty.
b. mental retardation and lacunar peripheral retinopathy.
c. ash-leaf macules.
d. panhypopituitarism.
e. pheochromocytoma.

159. A unilateral brainstem lesion at the level of the central nervous system shown in Figure 4-4 is most likely to produce which one of the following neurologic deficits?

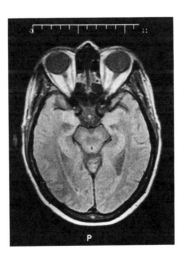

Figure 4-4

a. alexia without agraphia.
b. combined abducens and facial palsies.
c. "one-and-a-half" syndrome.
d. corneal hypesthesia.
e. third nerve palsy and contralateral hemiplegia.

Answers

1. **True.** Patients who have a maculopathy will take longer (90-180 seconds) to recover pretest vision after looking into a bright light for 10 seconds. Patients with optic nerve disease will have a normal recovery time (less than 60 seconds). The test is probably only valid for patients with vision better than 20/80.

2. **e.** A pattern VER (as opposed to a flash VER) is required for visual acuity assessment in preverbal children. Although the VER is useful in establishing factitious visual loss, its reliability is limited by the fact that patients can produce false readings by using accommodation to fog their vision. Abnormalities in VER latency and amplitude have been reported in various maculopathies and retinopathies and thus cannot distinguish optic neuropathy from retinal disorders with complete reliability.

3. **d.** Although optokinetic nystagmus, the rocking mirror test, and the base-up prism test can help discover factitious monocular blindness, they are not sensitive enough to diagnose factitious visual deficit at the 20/100 level. For such mild visual deficits, a fogging refraction, stereo acuity, and red-green glasses may be useful in diagnosing factitious visual loss.

4. **e.** See answer 3. A fogging refraction is probably the most useful tool to master for this problem, since it can be applied to any level of factitious visual loss.

5. **e.** An optic tract lesion may cause unilateral decreased visual acuity if the lesion is not complete or if the optic nerve or chiasm is also involved. If the optic nerve or chiasm is involved, the afferent pupillary defect is typically ipsilateral. Pure optic tract lesions will produce a <u>contra</u>lateral afferent pupillary defect (since more than one-half of afferent fibers cross) as well as a complete homonymous hemianopia.

6. **False.** To the contrary, <u>intact</u> oculovestibular reflexes in a patient with a gaze palsy implies a supranuclear disturbance. If the vestibular system can drive the eyes in the direction of the paretic field of gaze, the gaze paresis must be supranuclear in nature. Impaired oculocephalic responses indicate that the infranuclear, end-organ function is responsible for the motor disturbance.

7. **True.** Upturning of the eyes upon forceful opening of closed eyelids is known as the Bell's phenomenon. If forcefully opening closed eyelids stimulates upgaze, the final common pathway (infranuclear) for upgaze must be intact.

8. **e.** MRI is based on applying a radiofrequency pulse to tissue and measuring the change in tissue's nuclear spin and magnetic vector. The longitudinal relaxation time is termed T1. Fat is bright and water is dark on T1-weighted images. In contrast, fat is dark and water is bright on T2-weighted images. Some tissues such as cortical bone, rapidly flowing fluid (blood), and air give no signal at all on MRI.

9. **e.** While there is some redundancy of the optic nerve within the orbit, the intracranial optic nerve has little "slack." The dimensional characteristics of the optic nerve can be remembered with the mnemonic phone number 125-1017, which stands for the lengths of the intraocular (1), intraorbital (25), intracanalicular (10), and intracranial (17) portions of the optic nerve.

10.   c.   Fifty-three percent of the retinal ganglion cells cross in the chiasm (this difference is occasionally important clinically). The macular fibers constitute a large portion of the optic chiasm and most decussate in the posterior chiasm. The chiasm lies approximately 1 <u>cm</u> (not 1 mm) above the anterior pituitary gland. The inferior nasal retinal fibers cross in the anterior chiasm and loop anteriorly in the contralateral optic nerve before traveling posterior. This loop is called Wilbrand's knee.

11.   False.   The retinal ganglion cell terminals are segregated by eye (ipsilateral versus contralateral) rather than on the basis of which receptive field the ganglion cells serve. The ipsilateral ganglion cells synapse in layers 2, 3, and 5 while the contralateral ganglion cells synapse in layers 1, 4, and 6.

12.   False.   In fact, the <u>inferior</u> fibers of the optic radiations pass extremely close to the internal capsule. The combination of a superior hemianopic contralateral visual field defect and a contralateral hemiparesis can be produced by a small infarct in this region.

13.   d.   The temporal 30 degrees of a binocular visual field is perceived by the nasal-most retina of the ipsilateral eye only. These "temporal crescents" are represented in the anterior-most visual cortex. A lesion in this area will produce a monocular visual field defect in the far temporal periphery, the so-called temporal crescent syndrome.

14.   a. 4.   Ischemic optic neuropathy typically produces an altitudinal (inferior more often than
       b. 5.   superior) or, less commonly, an arcuate visual field defect. A cecocentral scotoma
       c. 2.   involves fixation as well as the blind spot and can be produced by toxic neuropathies
       d. 3.   (always bilateral), as well as an optic pit with serous retinal detachment (usually
       e. 1.   unilateral). Optic neuritis typically produces a unilateral central scotoma, as well.
       f. 6.   However, virtually any pattern of monocular field loss may be seen. Glaucoma classically causes arcuate field loss and/or nasal steps.

15.   a. 5.   Binasal hemianopsia is almost never due to chiasmal compression and is
       b. 3.   usually the result of glaucoma. Incongruous homonymous hemianopias can be
       c. 1.   caused by thalamic lesions that compress the optic tracts. A bitemporal
       d. 2.   hemianopic central scotoma is produced by a lesion compressing the macular
       e. 4.   fibers of the posterior chiasm.

16.   b.   OKN abnormalities indicate lesions of the parietoccipital (slow-phase pursuit abnormalities) or the frontal lobe (fast-phase recovery abnormalities). High congruity of visual field deficits indicates a lesion in the occipital lobe. Both partial complex seizures and formed visual hallucinations may be seen with temporal lobe lesions.

17.   e.   Parietal lobe lesions are associated with agnosia and right-left confusion. A parietal lobe lesion will also affect slow-phase pursuit movements toward the ipsilateral side. Unlike temporal lobe lesions, which produce hemianopias that are denser superiorly, parietal lobe lesions produce hemianopias that are denser inferiorly.

18.   a.   Formed hallucinations occur with temporal lobe pathology. Depending on the location of the occipital lobe lesion, the temporal crescent, the representation of which is located in the most anterior visual cortex, may be either spared (more common) or affected. While OKN asymmetry may rarely occur with occipital lesions, this finding is generally indicative of a parietal locus of disease.

19. b.   Key events in the development of true disc edema include cessation of axonal transport with swelling of axons. The increase in disc volume is due to enlargement of axons, rather than increased extracellular fluid, as seen in edema of other tissues. Breakdown of the blood-retinal barrier does occur, detected as leakage on fluorescein angiography, but this is not important in the development of disc edema.

20. c.   While loss of spontaneous venous pulsations is an early sign of papilledema, remember that about 20% of normal patients lack venous pulsations. Transient obscurations of vision (TOV) often accompany papilledema and are episodes of unilateral or bilateral visual loss lasting only a few seconds. The most typical visual field finding in acute papilledema is an enlarged blind spot; in chronic papilledema, the most common visual field loss occurs in the inferonasal quadrant. Although rare, unilateral papilledema may occur. For example, if contralateral optic atrophy exists, papilledema will occur only in the viable disc.

21. c.   Pseudotumor cerebri is characterized by (1) increased intracranial pressure on lumbar puncture, (2) normal neuro-imaging studies (although the ventricles may be small), and (3) normal cerebrospinal fluid. Papilledema need not be present for the diagnosis. While the neurologic examination is usually normal, sixth nerve palsy may occur with increased intracranial pressure of any etiology.

22. c.   Obesity is not an indication for treatment, although weight loss often improves the condition.

23. d.   Bilateral disc edema with minimally decreased or normal acuity distinguishes pseudotumor cerebri from anterior ischemic optic neuropathy.

24. a.   "Occult" giant cell arteritis is a recently recognized entity in which atypical clinical findings are present (malaise, anorexia). Despite a normal ESR, biopsy is positive and steroids are effective.

25. c.   Although patients with nonarteritic anterior ischemic optic neuropathy (NAION) may have a slightly higher incidence of cardiac and cerebrovascular disease, life expectancy is not significantly diminished. Patients with central retinal artery occlusion are at significant risk of fatal myocardial infarction or stroke.

26. d.   In a retrospective review of autopsy findings, nearly 100% of patients dying of MS had some degree of optic nerve demyelination, but only 55% (approximately) of all MS patients develop clinical optic neuritis.

27. e.   See answer 26.

28. b.   Ninety percent of optic gliomas occur in the first two decades of life. Twelve to 38% of patients will have associated neurofibromatosis (NF-1). Malignant gliomas of the visual pathways, although rare, occur more frequently in adults than in children. Survival averages 6 to 9 months after diagnosis.

29. False.   Collateral vessels at the disc connecting the retinal and choroidal vascular systems may also be secondary to vascular occlusive disease of the retina, long-standing primary open-angle glaucoma, or (rarely) optic nerve glioma.

30. d. In contrast to optic nerve gliomas, meningiomas occur primarily in adults. While persons with NF-1 have a higher incidence of meningiomas than the general population, a minority of persons with meningiomas have NF-1. With contrast CT scanning, the peripheral part of the involved optic nerve may show enhancement, resulting in the "railroad track" sign ("kinking" is specific for optic nerve glioma).

31. False. Dominant (Kjer) optic neuropathy manifests between age 5 and 10 years. Visual loss may progress until the midteens, at which point it usually stabilizes.

32. e. The incidence of spontaneous recovery has been reported to be as high as 10%, although most experts feel it is probably considerably less than this.

33. c. Patients with "papillophlebitis" have normal or near normal visual acuity. Whether this is different from a nonischemic central retinal vein occlusion (CRVO) in a young person is hotly disputed. An inflammatory etiology has been proposed but not substantiated.

34. c. Optic nerve drusen occur almost exclusively in whites.

35. True. Morning glory disc syndrome is characterized by a mass of glial tissue with radiating blood vessels, peripapillary atrophy, and pigmentation of chorioretinal tissue. It is usually unilateral and is more common in women (2:1). Visual acuity is usually poor.

36. e. Optic nerve hypoplasia is seen with greater incidence in children of diabetic mothers and following fetal exposure to antiepileptic medications, quinine, or LSD. Optic nerve hypoplasia, particularly bilateral involvement, has been associated with other midline developmental anomalies--absence of the septum pellucidum and hypothalamic-pituitary abnormalities. Endocrine dysfunction is manifest as hypoglycemic seizures and growth retardation. This combination of clinical findings is known as DeMorsier's syndrome.

Look at Basal encephalocele for cause of Optic N Hypoplasia

37. False. Nonsecreting tumors often present with visual field loss, whereas secreting tumors present with endocrine dysfunction. An exception is prolactin-secreting tumor in males.

38. True. When the causative lesion is not located at the site responsible for a clinical sign, it is described as false-localizing. Bitemporal macular hemianopia can only arise from compression of the posterior chiasm. While most lesions responsible for this compression are parasellar, a lesion distant from this site--for example, a tumor at the base of the brainstem--may also lead to chiasmal compression. This occurs if the lesion causes obstructive hydrocephalus, which enlarges the third ventricle, compressing the chiasm.

39. a. 3. The pathways for visual processing are not yet entirely characterized but appear
    b. 5. to depend heavily on the dominant parietal lobe, usually the left. Right
    c. 4. homonymous hemifields transmit information to the left occipital lobe,
    d. 1. then to the angular gyrus of the left parietal lobe. Left homonymous hemifields
    e. 2. are perceived by the right occipital lobe. Higher functions require processing
    through the splenium of the corpus callosum to the angular gyrus. This pathway
    may explain some of the following clinical observations. A left parietal lesion
    involving the angular gyrus results in complete inability to analyze visual
    information--alexia with agraphia. A lesion of the corpus callosum results in
    inability to process information from the left homonymous hemifield (right occipital
    cortex). A left occipital lesion prevents processing of the right homonymous
    hemifields. However, if the left parietal lobe remains intact, reading and writing
    ability are not affected. The inferior occipitotemporal junction subserves color
    sensation for the entire contralateral hemifield. For complete (both right and left
    hemifields) cerebral dyschromatopsia, bilateral lesions are necessary.

40. a. 2. Oculomotor neurons leave their nuclear complex, then pass through the red
    b. 3. nucleus and the medial portion of the cerebral peduncle. Therefore,
    c. 1. involvement of adjacent structures will have additional clinical characteristics.
    Involvement of the red nucleus produces a contralateral "rubral" tremor, and
    cerebral peduncle involvement produces contralateral hemiparesis. Finally, superior
    cerebellar peduncle involvement may produce ataxia.

41. d. The most common location for a cerebral aneurysm with third nerve palsy is the
    junction of posterior communicating artery and internal carotid artery.

42. False. Precipitous aneurysmal distention due to hemorrhage of the posterior communicating
    artery at its junction with the internal carotid artery may occur, creating a third nerve
    palsy. Ninety-five percent include pupillary involvement, and pain is nearly always
    present, but not universally.

43. a. Third nerve regeneration does not occur with diabetic oculomotor neuropathy.
    Aberrant regeneration of the third nerve implies another etiology, such as aneurysm,
    tumor, or trauma.

44. b. The long intracranial course of the trochlear nerve leaves it especially susceptible to
    damage from closed head trauma. This occurs due to contrecoup injury from the
    free tentorial edge. Ischemic damage, usually due to diabetes mellitis, is second, and
    idiopathic palsies are third. Hydrocephalus, vascular loops, or tumor can compress
    the trochlear nerve as well.

45. d. The three-step test is useful for diagnosis but does not differentiate between
    congenital and acquired trochlear nerve palsy. Large vertical fusional amplitudes
    (greater than 5 prism diopters) suggest a decompensated congenital lesion.

46. d. Nasopharyngeal carcinoma can involve numerous cranial nerves because of its
    proximity to the prepontine basal cistern. Most frequently, the trigeminal nerve is
    involved, causing facial hypesthesia. The abducens nerve is the second most
    common. The hallmark of nasopharyngeal carcinoma is its propensity to involve
    multiple cranial nerves noncontiguously. The neoplasm is most common in Chinese
    men. The least differentiated forms are also known as Schmincke and Regaud
    tumors.

47. True. Within the cavernous sinus, sympathetic branches of the paracarotid plexus joins the sixth nerve briefly. Occasionally, an intracavernous lesion can produce sixth nerve palsy with postganglionic Horner's syndrome, producing pupillary miosis.

48. c. Duane's syndrome may be secondary to hypoplasia or aplasia of the abducens nucleus, with lateral rectus innervation via the oculomotor nerve. It has various presentations, but retraction of the adducted globe appears most consistently. The three types of Duane's syndrome are distinguished by the relative ability to adduct or abduct:

   type 1 - limited abduction but full adduction
   type 2 - normal abduction but limited adduction
   type 3 - both abduction and adduction are limited

49. False. In the cavernous sinus, cranial nerves III, IV, and V are relatively protected <u>within</u> the walls of the sinus, but cranial nerve VI runs in the middle of the sinus and is more <u>prone</u> to injury.

50. False. Horizontal saccades originate in the contralateral frontal lobe, but either hemisphere can produce ipsilateral saccades if the other hemisphere is damaged. Appropriate stimulation of the parietal or occipital cortex can also produce contralateral saccades.

51. b. Oculomotor apraxia is an inability to initiate voluntary horizontal saccades. Congenital oculomotor apraxia is characterized by striking compensatory head movements, and acquired lesions usually produce defects in initiation of bidirectional saccades, with use of the blink to break the fixation reflex. Pursuits remain relatively unaffected.

52. c. Opsoclonus consists of nonstop, random, directionally unpredictable saccades and may be seen in the presence of neuroblastoma, as well as some types of visceral carcinomas. In contrast, <u>square-wave jerks are a microsaccadic fixation disturbance associated with cerebellar disease of various kinds.</u> Ocular flutter consists of spontaneous groups of back-and-forth horizontal saccades that may occur during fixation or at the end of a normal horizontal saccade; they are not associated with any malignancies. Ocular motor dysmetria is a back-and-forth saccadic motion about the point of fixation that occurs following an otherwise normal saccade. It is felt to represent "overshooting" of the intended fixation point. <u>Ocular bobbing is most commonly seen in comatose and/or quadriplegic patients with large infarcts or brainstem hemorrhages.</u>

53. b. In PSP, downward gaze is generally affected first, becoming smaller and slower. Saccades are affected more than pursuits.

54. True. The time period between detection of movement and the beginning of smooth pursuit (for tracking) is between 125 and 135 milliseconds. Initiation of saccadic movement requires from 150 to 200 milliseconds from the first perception of a target.

55. d. Skew deviation is, by definition, a vertical misalignment of gaze that cannot be assigned to a single nerve or muscle weakness. In the presence of an INO, the hypertropic eye is often on the same side as the adduction deficit (medial rectus dysfunction). Fourth nerve palsy does not produce difficulty with adduction. The "one-and-a-half" syndrome results in, among other things, complete horizontal paralysis of one eye and limitation of the other to abduction only. PSP, as discussed in answer 53, is a disorder of movement that does not produce a resting vertical gaze deviation. Dorsal midbrain syndrome (Parinaud's syndrome) does not feature an adduction deficit (see answer 56).

56. e. Upward gaze paresis, light-near dissociation, lid retraction, accommodative abnormalities, and convergence-retraction nystagmus are all features of the dorsal midbrain (Parinaud's) syndrome. Furthermore, skew deviation and papilledema may be seen, depending on the etiology. The lid retraction--Collier's sign--may worsen with attempted upgaze. Convergence-retraction nystagmus is also a response to an effort at upgaze that triggers medial rectus contractions. Hence, this form of "nystagmus" is worsened by upward OKN testing. Paradoxic OKN is not a feature (see answer 57).

57. a. Congenital motor nystagmus has several features including normal visual acuity, paradoxic OKN (caused by the abnormal movements of nystagmus appearing "slow" and against the expected direction of target tracking), dampening by convergence, and aggravated by fixation. Fortunately, oscillopsia is not normally a problem.

58. d. Monocular nystagmus has been associated with chiasmal and hypothalamic gliomas. It is also seen in blind eyes, multiple sclerosis, and spasmus nutans--a transient, fast-beating but low-amplitude nystagmus found during the first 5 years of life.

59. a. Alexander's law describes the increased frequency and amplitude of nystagmus movements accompanying gaze in the direction of the fast component. Of the various forms of nystagmus, downbeat nystagmus most frequently violates Alexander's law.

60. e. Upbeat nystagmus can be due to lesions of the anterior vermis and lower brainstem, as well as drugs and Wernicke's encephalopathy. Downbeat nystagmus may be localized to anatomic structures at the craniocervical junction and may be seen in certain intoxications (alcohol, lithium). Vestibular nystagmus has its etiology within the vestibular system. Periodic alternating nystagmus can also localize to the craniocervical junction but may be seen in other forms of posterior fossa disease. See-saw nystagmus results from third ventricle tumors or diencephalic lesions involving the connections to the interstitial nucleus of Cajal and is thus the most localizing of those mentioned.

61. b. Bitemporal hemianopia may be seen in acquired see-saw nystagmus, since the posterior chiasm is most vulnerable to diencephalic lesions, which may provoke it.

62. False. Vergence eye movements are felt to have a pathway of their own for stimulating the brainstem motor nuclei; the actual pathway remains undetermined. Saccades originate in the contralateral frontal lobe, while pursuits arise in the ipsilateral parietal lobe.

63. True. Because of bilateral supranuclear input to upper facial muscles (orbicularis), voluntary eye closure is preserved in upper motor neuron seventh nerve palsy.

64. True. Pontine disease can produce orbicularis weakness.

65. False. Spontaneous or reflexive blinking requires normal function of the basal ganglia--as do other nonvolitional facial expressions. Thus, these are commonly affected in Parkinson's disease. Volitional movements, in distinction, are generally not adversely influenced.

66. b. The greater superficial petrosal nerve synapses in the pterygopalatine ganglion, not the geniculate ganglion. Actually, there are no synapses at the geniculate ganglion.

67. False. The Marcus Gunn "jaw-wink" reflex is an example of synkinesis (abnormal innervation connecting two groups of normally unrelated muscles, such that they contract together), but it is not synkinesis as a result of aberrant regeneration, which usually follows a peripheral neuropathy or trauma to nerve. The "jaw-wink" is a congenital/neurogenic phenomenon.

68. e. Idiopathic self-limited facial nerve palsy has been associated with diabetes, hypertension, and pregnancy. Herpes zoster virus can produce a facial palsy identical to Bell's (the Ramsay Hunt syndrome). Since Bell's palsy is by definition idiopathic, herpes zoster should be considered separately.

69. d. About 75% can be expected spontaneously to recover "completely," although some will have some degree of aberrant regeneration.

70. True. The parotid gland can become infiltrated with granulomas, and the facial nerve is involved at this site. Facial nerve involvement in sarcoidosis is frequently bilateral, although asymmetric. The second most commonly involved cranial nerve is the optic nerve.

71. False. Of the three most common causes of facial nerve overactivity, only essential blepharospasm is believed to be related to basal ganglia dysfunction. Compression of the facial nerve in the cerebellopontine angle by anomalous vessels has been demonstrated in 90% of cases of hemifacial spasm. Tumors in the cerebellopontine angle can also cause hemifacial spasm. Facial myokomia is caused by disease in the pons involving the facial nucleus or fascicle. The most common causes include multiple sclerosis in adults and pontine glioma in children.

72. d. See answer 71. Optic nerve gliomas are associated with compressive optic neuropathy; chiasmal gliomas may cause hypothalamic dysfunction. Spasmus nutans is a monocular nystagmus that usually occurs in the first year of life.

73. e. Tardive dyskinesia can produce facial grimacing and blepharospasm, similar to Meige's syndrome. Hemifacial spasm is distinct from essential blepharospasm in that multiple facial muscles are involved. Like blepharospasm, hemifacial spasm is more often unilateral. Reflex blepharospasm can be caused by a number of disorders, including severe dry eye, intraocular inflammation, and foreign bodies.

74. d. The afferent pupillomotor fibers exit the optic tracts just before the lateral geniculate body (LGB); they do <u>not</u> pass through the LGB. While postganglionic pupillomotor fibers in the sympathetic pathway do arise from the superior cervical ganglion, the sympathetic pathway leading to these fibers is thought to originate in the posterior hypothalamus. In addition, postganglionic sympathetic fibers enter the orbit with the ophthalmic division of the trigeminal nerve through the superior orbital fissure. The consensual pupillary response is seen because of decussation at the prectectal nuclei. Were the chiasm split in half, consensual responses would be preserved.

75. b. Argyll Robertson pupils are miotic, irregular, do not react to light, but have a normal near response. This is a rare finding in some patients with tertiary syphilis. In the light-near dissociation of Parinaud's dorsal midbrain syndrome, the pupils are larger. In young children, the most common cause of this syndrome is a tumor in the region of the pineal gland. In young adults, head trauma and multiple sclerosis are frequently seen. In patients over 60, stroke is most commonly to blame.

76. b. Oculomotor nerve palsy usually includes ptosis, limitation of ocular motility, and pupillary abnormalities. In uncal herniation and basilar meningitis, pupil dilation may be the only sign of third nerve palsy. In cases of carotid aneurysm, the pupil is usually involved, along with other functions of the third nerve. If the pupil is not involved, it is less likely that an aneurysm is the cause of the palsy. Total oculomotor palsy with a spared pupil in elderly patients usually suggests a microvascular etiology.

77. d. While 1/8% pilocarpine is very dilute, some patients with normal pupils will respond to this dose. Thus, a weaker preparation (0.05%) is recommended. The majority of patients affected will have unilateral pupillary involvement and depressed tendon reflexes. After many months or years, an Adie's pupil will become miotic.

78. b. Horner's syndrome is defined as ipsilateral ptosis and miosis. Ptosis is secondary to lack of Müller's muscle function. Anhidrosis may or may not be present. Localization of the lesion in Horner's syndrome is part of the clinical work-up and may be guided by the extent of anhidrosis. First-order lesions (CNS) cause ipsilateral anhidrosis of the entire body. Second-order lesions (Pancoast's tumor, neck trauma) cause ipsilateral facial anhidrosis. Third-order lesions cause anhidrosis only around the affected eye or none at all. In response to 4% cocaine, a normal pupil will dilate, but a Horner's pupil will dilate poorly. Hydroxyamphetamine (Paredrine) will cause a similar response in preganglionic Horner's syndrome only. Painful Horner's syndrome may be caused by many disorders (neck trauma, migraine, cluster headaches), but spontaneous dissection of the common carotid artery must be ruled out.

79. d. The majority of patients with nonphysiologic anisocoria have sphincter muscle dysfunction visible at the slit lamp. Trauma is most common, followed by Adie's pupil.

80. True. Fifteen years following an initial episode of optic neuritis, roughly 80% of women and 60% of men will have developed multiple sclerosis (MS).

81. False. The most common cranial mononeuropathy in MS is optic neuritis. The most frequently affected motor nerve is the sixth nerve.

82. True. Retinal vascular infiltration (lymphocytic) and vitreous cells may be seen in a small percentage of active MS cases.

83. b. Pheochromocytomas produce, secrete, and store catecholamines. They are most often derived from the adrenal medulla but may arise in the sympathetic ganglia. Two phakomatoses, neurofibromatosis and von Hippel-Lindau disease, are associated with the tumor.

84. c.

85. d.

86. c. Seizures are part of the classic triad in tuberous sclerosis. Patients with Sturge-Weber syndrome and meningeal hemangioma may have seizure disorders.

87. b. Unilateral congenital glaucoma is seen in 25% of cases of Sturge-Weber syndrome, often associated with an angioma on the upper lid. Likewise, a plexiform neurofibroma of the upper lid is closely associated with juvenile glaucoma in von Recklinghausen's disease.

88. False. The characteristic ocular lesion of angiomatosis retinae, or von Hippel's disease, is a retinal angioblastoma. This is a retinal capillary hemangioma (hemangioblastoma). The cavernous hemangioma of the retina is a rare lesion that can be associated with similar skin and central nervous system lesions.

89. d. Patients with ataxia-telangiectasia may have associated IgA (secretory immunoglobulin) deficiency, with severe respiratory infections.

90. c. Four signs constitute complete Kearns-Sayre syndrome: (1) progressive external ophthalmoplegia, (2) mild pigmentary retinal degeneration, (3) onset before age 20, and (4) heart block, potentially lethal and among the last signs to develop. Some studies indicate that elevated CSF protein correlates with the presence of heart block.

91. False. Many systemic syndromes include PEO, which is a nondescriptive term for chronically progressive loss of eye movements. One such syndrome is myotonic dystrophy. A diagnostic feature of myotonic dystrophy is the presence of polychromatic ("Christmas tree") cataracts, which may present even in the "amyotonic" forms. Wilson's disease is associated with the sunflower cataract.

92. a. Conjunctival injection and superficial punctate keratitis are nonspecific, as is proptosis. Diplopia in upgaze is also seen in orbital floor fractures. The lid retraction and lag are probably the most specific.

93. d. The most frequently involved muscle in dysthyroid orbitopathy is the inferior rectus. The medial rectus is the second most frequently affected muscle and may simulate a sixth nerve palsy.

94. b.

95. d. While 75% of all myasthenics will have eye findings at presentation, only 33 to 50% will have ocular myasthenia only. A higher percentage (90%) of patients with MG will develop ocular symptoms during the course of the disease. Ptosis is the most common.

96. a. A tiny fraction of patients with Graves' disease will develop MG as well.

97. b.   Radiologic investigation is mandatory for all myasthemics in order to discover thymic enlargement. Thymomas are most common in older male patients with MG. Thymectomy may be curative in this setting.

98. d.

99. c.   Studies of central retinal artery ligation in rhesus monkeys established this value.

100. False.   Patients with embolic CRAO are at great risk of myocardial infarction. Stroke is also more likely after CRAO, but the most common cause of death is heart disease.

101. e.   Intraocular pressure may be low (due to ciliary hypoperfusion), normal, or elevated (due to neovascularization of the iris and angle). Unilateral arcus is highly suggestive of carotid disease on the side without corneal arcus. Carotid stenosis protects the ipsilateral cornea from serum lipid deposition.

102. a.   Transient monocular blindness is the hallmark of carotid (anterior) disease. Vertebrobasilar insufficiency typically causes binocular visual blurring or oculomotor symptoms.

103. c.   The patient's ocular signs and symptoms clinically suggest the diagnosis of demyelinative optic neuritis. With a history of paresthesias in her right legs, the diagnosis of multiple sclerosis should be entertained. An afferent pupillary defect almost invariably occurs in the acute phase. This patient most likely had a subclinical contralateral episode of optic neuritis in the past and therefore no detectable APD. APDs are always relative--that is, comparing one optic nerve to the contralateral nerve.

104. a.   The etiology of Coats' disease is unknown, and there does not appear to be any genetic, familiar, racial, or ethnic predisposition. However, Coats'-type retinal vascular changes have been noted in patients with facioscapulohumeral muscular dystrophy, Turner's syndrome, Senior-Loken syndrome, and one variant of the epidermal nevus syndrome. In addition, Coats'-like retinopathy has been noted in up to 3.6% of patients with retinitis pigmentosa.   *DRUSEN seen in 2-3% of pts c̄ RP.*

105. b.   Downbeat nystagmus in primary position is localized to the craniocervical junction (or certain intoxications). This patient's clinical symptoms of intermittent occipital headaches with sudden head movements or anger suggest the diagnosis of Arnold-Chiari malformation.

106. b.   Clonazepam and suboccipital craniotomy have been used in the treatment of downbeat nystagmus in patients with Arnold-Chiari malformation. On the other hand, carbamazepine toxicity has been associated with downbeat nystagmus.

107. a.   This patient appears to have Parinaud's dorsal midbrain syndrome, which may include the following findings: pupillary light-near dissociation, lid retraction (Collier's sign), upgaze paresis, convergence-retraction nystagmus, fixation instability, small-amplitude skew deviation, and papilledema (if ventricular outflow has been compromised). The most common cause in this age group would be a pinealoma. Other causes include stroke, hydrocephalus, and multiple sclerosis.

108. d.   After neuro-imaging has been obtained, a lumbar puncture would be an important step in the diagnostic evaluation of this patient because pinealoma classically sheds cells into the CSF.

109. b. Optic neuritis in childhood is more commonly bilateral. Visual prognosis is generally good, with near complete recovery over several weeks. Diffuse enlargement of the optic nerve on CT scan may be seen in this condition, mimicking a neoplasm of the optic nerve sheath.

110. a. The differential diagnosis for posterior ischemic optic neuropathy should include radiation optic neuropathy, status post-coronary artery bypass graft, giant cell arteritis, and syphilis. Well-controlled essential hypertension is associated with anterior ischemic optic neuropathy but not posterior ischemic optic neuropathy.

111. d. Bilateral disc edema and headache may be caused by several things, but malignant hypertension should be first on the list to be excluded, since it is quite easy to do so. After checking blood pressure, a neuro-image should be obtained emergently.

112. d.

113. True. Most clinically important orbital meningiomas originate in the intracranial cavity.

114. c. Meningothelial (syncytial) meningioma is virtually the only histopathologic type of meningioma seen within the orbit.

115. d. In general, optic nerve compression greater than 1 cm from the globe does not cause disc edema.

116. False. So called tobacco-alcohol amblyopia seems to be seen only in heavy smokers/drinkers with poor nutrition. This has lead many to believe that a combination of toxic plus nutritional insults must be necessary for the development of the disorder.

117. a. The most common etiologies of bilateral central or cecocentral scotomas include hereditary optic neuropathy and nutritional optic neuropathy (vitamin B12 and folate deficiency), drug toxicity, tobacco-alcohol amblyopia, and infiltrative disorders such as syphilis and tuberculosis. Cyanide levels are not helpful in suspected tobacco-alcohol amblyopia.

118. e. Although disc edema, disc hemorrhages, and choroidal rupture may be seen in acute traumatic optic neuropathy, the most common finding is a normal fundus. Disc pallor would be unusual in the acute setting but present in all cases after several weeks.

119. d. The development of diabetic papillopathy appears to be independent of serum glucose levels. Diabetic papillopathy is classically seen in young adults with type I diabetes and moderate to severe retinopathy. Associated visual loss is generally mild. The disorder generally resolves spontaneously.

120. c.   Thyroid optic neuropathy is considered to be a compressive optic neuropathy due to enlargement of extraocular muscles at the orbital apex. Treatment of thyroid optic neuropathy may include orbital radiation (usually 1500-2500 rads over a 10-day period) and orbital decompression, which provides the most potential for decompression of the optic nerve. Systemic corticosteroids are thought to be effective only in the acute congestive phase and not in the fibrotic period. Thus, if no response is noted within 3 weeks, systemic steroids should be tapered and another modality should be considered. Although a subtotal thyroidectomy may provide primary treatment of dysthyroid state, it will have no effect on the eye findings (except, perhaps, lid retraction).

121. a.   Bromocryptine has been shown to be effective primarily in the management of prolactin-secreting pituitary tumors and is less effective or ineffective with other types of pituitary tumors.

122. d.   The symptoms presented in this question are indicative of pituitary apoplexy, in which there is a hemorrhage into a pituitary tumor. A sudden severe headache is a common presenting symptom; other manifestations depend on the direction of the expansion of pituitary gland. Acute painful visual loss is uncommon with the other disorders.

123. a. 2.   A migraine equivalent is a scintillating scotoma that may be followed by nausea
     b. 3.   and photophobia but is not associated with a headache. A common migraine is a
     c. 1.   severe throbbing headache associated with nausea and photophobia but with no other neurologic or visual disturbance. A classic migraine is a severe throbbing headache preceded by scintillating scotoma or other auras and followed by nausea and photophobia.

124. b.   Symptoms that suggest a cerebral arteriovenous malformation include fortification spectra that are less well defined and fleeting and a fixed visual defect. A family history of headaches and nausea associated with visual disturbances are more suggestive of a migraine. Field defects may be found during acute migraine headaches, but those present interictally suggest another diagnosis.

125. e.   The patient described has limitation of upgaze and downgaze in the affected eye. Making the distinction between a restrictive and a paralytic process by doing forced duction testing would be the best way to further narrow the differential diagnosis.

126. e.   These findings, as well as right hypertropia in left gaze and left hypertropia in right gaze, are typical features of a bilateral fourth nerve palsy.

127. b.   A skew deviation is a motility disturbance with a vertical component that does not have a pattern consistent with a discrete muscle underaction or nerve palsy. They are generally due to supranuclear or vestibulo-ocular dysfunction and generally reflect brainstem disease. They are typically comitant, but not always.

128. c.   Although transient changes in vertical eye movements and slowing of vertical saccades can result from lesions of the paramedian pontine reticular formation, nuclei critical for the initiation of vertical eye movements are the rostral interstitial nucleus of the medial longitudinal fasciculus (riMLF) and the interstitial nucleus of Cajal (INC).

129. False. Small vessel disease is the most common cause of <u>unilateral</u> sixth nerve palsy. More common causes of bilateral sixth nerve palsy include increased intracranial pressure, head trauma, and tumors of the ventral brainstem.

130. True. An isolated sixth nerve palsy in children is most commonly attributable to postviral inflammation occurring 1 to 3 weeks following a nonspecific viral illness of the upper respiratory tract. Recovery is generally complete and occurs within 10 to 12 weeks.

131. c. Medial rectus contracture is distinctly uncommon in Duane's syndrome. In congenital sixth nerve palsy, it is quite common and results in esotropia in primary position. Although the left eye is more commonly involved in Duane's syndrome, this does not help in distinguishing from a congenital sixth nerve palsy. The other findings would be present in both conditions.

132. b. Disruption of the medial longitudinal fasciculus (MLF), which carries projections of interneurons from the contralateral sixth nerve nucleus to the ipsilateral medial rectus subnucleus, results in ipsilateral absence or slowing of adduction and contralateral abduction nystagmus. This combination of findings is termed internuclear ophthalmoplegia. Vertical nystagmus and skew deviations are frequently found in association with internuclear ophthalmoplegia but are not universal.

133. c.

134. False. Bilateral INO is more frequent in demyelinating disease than in cerebrovascular disease. This is because the brainstem blood supply is lateralized--right and left circulations are usually discrete and end at the midline. Demyelinization does not respect the midline.

135. e. A lesion of the abducens nucleus results in an ipsilateral gaze paresis due to disruption of the motor neurons and interneurons to the contralateral medial rectus mediating gaze conjugacy via the contralateral MLF. A lesion that disrupts both the abducens nucleus and the ipsilateral MLF will result in the combination of an ipsilateral gaze palsy and internuclear ophthalmoplegia. This combination has been termed the "one-and-a-half" syndrome. The only horizontal eye movement that remains is contralateral abduction.

136. c. Exotropia in primary position can occasionally occur in association with a bilateral INO, resulting in a syndrome called walleyed bilateral INO.

137. d. Fisher syndrome is generally considered a variant of Guillain-Barré syndrome that results in ophthalmoplegia, ataxia, and areflexia. Elevated CSF protein may be present. Complete recovery is common.

138. False. The presence of optic nerve dysfunction, manifested by decreased vision, an afferent pupillary defect, and/or dyschromatopsia, distinguishes an orbital apex syndrome from a cavernous sinus syndrome, since the optic nerve passes through the optic canal and does not enter the cavernous sinus.

139. d.   Tolosa-Hunt syndrome is felt to be caused by a nonspecific inflammatory process of the cavernous sinus. Findings include painful ophthalmoplegia, sensory deficits of the trigeminal nerve, most commonly the ophthalmic division, and a dramatic response to systemic corticosteroid therapy. Remissions may be spontaneous, with partial or complete reversal of deficits. Episodic recurrence can also occur. Aneurysms of the circle of Willis can produce a similar picture, including steroid responsiveness. A normal MRI makes this unlikely but not impossible.

140. e.   Iris and posterior segment neovascularization, as well as rapidly progressive cataract, may all be seen as complications of the ischemic oculopathy these fistulae generate. Corneal exposure due to proptosis is another potential complication of carotid-cavernous fistula.

141. True.   In the "low-flow" fistulae, the head trauma may be only minor. More significant head trauma is the most frequent cause of high-flow carotid-cavernous fistulae and is present in up to 75% of cases. Spontaneous rupture due to hypertension or atherosclerosis is the cause in most of the remaining cases.

142. d.   Acute thiamine deficiency can result in central scotomas as well as ophthalmoplegia, primarily affecting cranial nerves III and VI. It can be precipitated in nutritionally depleted alcoholics given intravenous glucose alone, due to sudden consumption of systemic thiamine stores.

143. c.   Autofluorescence is produced when certain tissues/material are stimulated with monochromatic blue light and emit in the yellow-green range, as fluorescein does. The two optic nerve lesions that may autofluoresce are astrocytic hamartomas and drusen. Large accumulations of lipofuscin may also autofluoresce . To demonstrate this, fundus photographs should be obtained through the standard fluorescein setup, but without fluorescein injection. Lesions will appear bright, as if they had absorbed fluorescein, even though none was injected. Note that this is NOT the same as a "red-free" photograph. These are produced with a green filter that does not provide sufficient blue light to stimulate autofluorescence.

144. a. 3.   The geniculate ganglion is a condensation of nerve fibers without any true
     b. 5.   synapses. At this "ganglion," the greater superficial petrosal nerve branches
     c. 2.   off the facial nerve carrying preganglionic secretory fibers for the lacrimal
     d. 3.   gland. These fibers synapse in the pterygopalatine ganglion. The gasserian
     e. 4.   ganglion is synonymous with the trigeminal ganglion.
     f. 2.
     g. 1.
     h. 5.
     i. 4.

145. d.   The prevalence increases further with age, approaching 1% in persons over 90 years old.

146. b.   PMR is a surprisingly common disorder.

Answers

147. e.   Chiasmal field defects are characterized by <u>greater loss centrally</u>. <u>Postfixation blindness is a necessary concomitant of bitemporal hemianopia</u>. Objects behind the point of fixation are in the temporal hemifeld of each eye. <u>With loss of these fields, nothing beyond the point of fixation is visible!</u> <u>Reds and greens often appear "washed out" in the temporal hemifield of affected patients</u>. "Hemifield slip" refers to the diplopia these patients may also notice. <u>By mechanisms that are not</u> entirely elucidated, <u>binocular input at the vertical midline</u> seems necessary for motor fusion. When a substantial portion of the vertical midline <u>is not overlapped by both</u> <u>visual fields, there may be loss of motor fusion with resultant diplopia</u>.

148. a.   The calcium that is contained in optic nerve drusen is visible on CT scanning and ultrasound. Since MRI does not image calcium, this modality is not useful. As described above in answer 143, fundus photography through standard fluorescein filters will detect autofluorescence if the drusen are sufficiently near the surface of the nerve head.

149. c.   The Pulfrich phenomenon probably reflects delayed conduction in the demyelinated nerve. Oscillating objects perceived by the affected eye appear to be <u>behind</u> the image seen with the healthy eye, simulating three-dimensional movement where there is only movement within one plane.

150. b.   The delayed implicit time is the electrophysiologic correlate of the bizarre perception known as the Pulfrich phenomenon (see answer 149).

151. b.   Certainly, the most common etiology of bilateral lid retraction in an adult woman is Graves' disease. Lid retraction may also be seen in the setting of iatrogenic thyroid hormone overdosage or abuse. The lid retraction seen in the dorsal midbrain syndrome is often accompanied by upgaze deficits and convergence-retraction nystagmus. However, thyroid disease more commonly produces the combination of upgaze deficit (inferior rectus restriction) and lid retraction. Orbital CT scanning may show fusiform enlargement of multiple extraocular muscles. Cranial MRI offers little. With adequate eyelid closure, the issues for this patient are cosmetic. Still, since the ophthalmopathy may change in nature and severity, lid surgery should be deferred until all eye findings are stable for 6 months.

152. e.   The biopsy shown is from a severely inflamed temporal artery. Copious giant cells may be seen in the arterial media, with partial occlusion of the lumen (some neuro-ophthalmologists feel that thrombosis induced by partial occlusion may be the primary mechanism for the ocular ischemic events that occur in giant cell arteritis [GCA]). Systemic symptoms (fever, malaise, weight loss) have been increasingly recognized as common findings in GCA. Unilateral, new headache is a more specific symptom, along with jaw claudications. Amaurosis fugax is a relatively uncommon, but well-recognized visual symptom in GCA. Only one case of GCA in a patient less than 50 years old has been reported.

153. e.   The appearance of the photograph is suggestive of an optic nerve head pit. These represent congenital herniations of glial and malformed neural tissue through a focal defect in the lamina cribrosa. Some authorities consider these to be localized colobomata. The associated retinopathy may include serous detachment of the macula or peripapillary choroidal neovascularization with subretinal hemorrhage. Intrathecal injection of metrizamide in dogs with optic nerve pits leads to detectable levels of the dye in the subretinal space and vitreous!

154. c.   The clinical history is classic for idiopathic (demyelinative) optic neuritis. The sensory symptoms in her extremity raise the possibility of associated multiple sclerosis. The pigmented lesion superonasal to the disc is probably congenital hypertrophy of the retinal pigment epithelium, with no known relationship to optic neuritis. Optic nerve sheath inflammation is postulated to cause reactive inflammation in the rectus muscle sheaths at the orbital apex, accounting for pain with eye movement. Uhthoff's symptom, worsening of vision with exercise or heat (hot showers), is typical of demyelinating disorders and can be expressed with a variety of motor and sensory findings. A small subset of patients with optic neuritis and multiple sclerosis will have mild anterior or peripheral uveitis (pars planitis). The Optic Neuritis Treatment Trial compared intravenous and oral corticosteroid regimens to placebo. The treated patients enjoyed more rapid rehabilitation, but the group treated with oral prednisone had significantly more recurrences. This treatment is now felt to be unwise. The role of intravenous steroids is still uncertain.

155. d.   Bilaterally elevated discs with indistinct margins raise the possibility of papilledema, particularly in an obese young woman (pseudotumor cerebri). The photo demonstrates two findings arguing against this diagnosis. First, the vessels are clearly visible, with no obscuration of their borders. This is a sensitive finding in true papilledema. Second, two or three tiny excrescences with a crystalline appearance within the neural rim are visible. Plate 7 reveals either auto- or pseudofluorescence (hyperfluorescence despite no injection of fluorescein). The clinical findings are consistent with a lesion known to be associated with autofluorescence, optic nerve drusen. Typically, visual acuity is normal, although there may be associated field defects. Axoplasmic stasis is a feature of true papilledema, rather than pseudopapilledema, which is present here. Autofluorescence is well-described for both optic nerve drusen and astrocytic hamartomas of the optic nerve head. Both lesions may appear quite similar clinically. A distinguishing feature is the hypervascularity of astrocytomas, best revealed with fluorescein angiography.

156. d.   The visual fields reflect a bitemporal hemianopia. This indicates chiasmal compression. While this may occur with severe hydrocephalus of any cause, the primary lesion is usually parasellar. In this case, there is a huge pituitary tumor, probably nonsecreting; the chiasm can be seen riding on top of this impressive mass. Option (a) is a large occipital infarct, (b) is a parietal lobe metastasis, (c) is a meningioma of the falx cerebri, and (e) is a left optic nerve glioma.

157. a.   The corkscrewed conjunctival vessels, all the way to the limbus, are highly suggestive of arterialization of the orbital venous system. With a history of recent trauma, carotid-cavernous fistula is likely. All his clinical findings are consistent with this, as well. Option (b) represents a large intracavernous right carotid artery aneurysm, (c) shows severe bilateral Graves' disease, (d) is a "berry" aneurysm of the posterior communicating artery, and (e) shows bilateral optic disc drusen.

158. d.   The CT scan reveals absence of the septum pellucidum, a thin layer of serous connective tissue separating the two lateral ventricles. This is definitely associated wtih bilateral optic nerve hypoplasia and hypothalamic-pituitary disturbances, typically underfunctioning. Aicardi's sydrome features mental retardation, lacunar retinopathy, and congenital absence of the corpus callosum. Precocious puberty may be a part of polyostotic fibrous dysplasia (Albright's syndrome). Ash-leaf macules and pheochromocytoma are parts of various phakomatoses (tuberous sclerosis, neurofibromatosis, and von Hippel-Lindau syndromes).

159. e.   This MRI cut is a beautiful view of central nervous system anatomy at the level of the midbrain. A unilateral brainstem lesion here could result in numerous defects. Weber's syndrome refers to an intramedullary III nerve lesion within the substance of the cerebral peduncle where descending fibers of the corticospinal tract run. This results in third nerve palsy and contralateral hemiplegia (the motor fibers within the corticospinal tract decussate at the caudal medulla, distal to the lesion of Weber's syndrome).

References

1. Miller, Neil R. (ed.). Walsh and Hoyt's Clinical Neuro-Ophthalmology (4th ed.). Baltimore: Williams and Wilkins, 1988.

2. Feldon, Steven. "Section 5: Neuro-ophthalmology." in F.M. Wilson (ed.). Basic and Clinical Science Course. San Francisco: American Academy of Ophthalmology, 1991-1992.

3. Beck, Roy, and Smith, Craig. Neuro-Ophthalmology: A Problem-oriented Approach. Boston: Little, Brown and Company, 1988.

5: Pediatric Ophthalmology

1. At birth, the length of the average infant human eye is:

   a. 8 to 9 mm.
   b. 12 to 13 mm.
   c. 16 to 17 mm.
   d. 20 to 21 mm.
   e. 23 to 24 mm.

2. The factor primarily responsible for the shallow anterior chamber in a normal infant eye is:

   a. the infant cornea is flatter than the adult cornea.
   b. the infant iris is relatively thicker than the adult iris.
   c. the infant lens is relatively thicker than the adult lens.
   d. there is more positive vitreous pressure in the infant eye than in the adult eye.
   e. the anterior chamber is as deep in infants as it is in adults.

3. T or F -- The corneal diameter of the average normal human infant eye is 10 mm (9.5 - 10.5 mm).

4. The reasons for relatively miotic pupils in infancy include:

   1. relative delay in sympathetic innervation of the eye.
   2. excessive supranuclear input to the Edinger-Westphal nucleus.
   3. increased sensitivity of the light-induced miosis reflex.
   4. immaturity of the dilator pupillae muscle.

   a. 1, 2, and 3.
   b. 1 and 3.
   c. 2 and 4.
   d. 4 only.
   e. 1, 2, 3, and 4.

5. T or F -- The completion of optic nerve myelinization and that of foveal maturation coincide postnatally.

6. Reliable methods of estimating visual acuity in the preverbal child include:

        1. optokinetic nystagmus testing (OKN).
        2. preferential looking testing (PLT).
        3. visual evoked potentials (VEP).
        4. electroretinography (ERG).

    a. 1, 2, and 3.
    b. 1 and 3.
    c. 2 and 4.
    d. 4 only.
    e. 1, 2, 3, and 4.

7. T or F -- Acuity estimates generated by preferential looking testing (PLT) and visual evoked potentials (VEP) generally coincide quite closely.

8. T or F -- In cryptophthalmos, there is a failure of development of normal lid structures over an otherwise normal globe.

9. Congenital colobomas of the eyelids are associated with which systemic syndrome?

    a. Goldenhar's syndrome.
    b. Pierre Robin syndrome.
    c. Hallermann-Streiff syndrome.
    d. Stickler's syndrome.
    e. Trisomy 18.

10. T or F -- Both congenital ectropion and entropion involve the upper lid more frequently than the lower lid.

11. T or F -- Like congenital entropion, distichiasis generally does not cause significant keratopathy.

12. T or F -- There are three varieties of epicanthus: palpebralis, tarsalis, and inversus.

13. T or F -- Telecanthus is synonymous with hypertelorism.

14. Findings seen as part of the blepharophimosis syndrome include:

        1. simple epicanthus (palpebralis).
        2. blepharoptosis.
        3. hypertelorism.
        4. blepharophimosis.

  a. 1, 2, and 3.
  b. 1 and 3.
  c. 2 and 4.
  d. 4 only.
  e. 1, 2, 3, and 4.

15. Which of the following concerning congenital toxoplasmosis is/are true?

        1. Most cases of ocular toxoplasmosis represent congenital infection.
        2. Seroconversion during pregnancy, marking new infection of a mother, is rarely associated with placental transfer of the organism.
        3. A majority of pregnant women are seronegative (i.e., susceptible to infection).
        4. When placental transfer occurs, the infant nearly always develops some obvious manifestation of the infection.

  a. 1, 2, and 3.
  b. 1 and 3.
  c. 2 and 4.
  d. 4 only.
  e. 1, 2, 3, and 4.

16. T or F -- The incidence of congenital toxoplasmosis, both symptomatic and asymptomatic, is approximately 1 in 1000 live births.

17. Signs and symptoms typical of congenital toxoplasmosis include:

        1. hepatosplenomegaly.
        2. seizures with intracranial calcifications.
        3. vomiting and diarrhea.
        4. diffuse pigmentary ("salt-and-pepper") retinopathy.

  a. 1, 2, and 3.
  b. 1 and 3.
  c. 2 and 4.
  d. 4 only.
  e. 1, 2, 3, and 4.

18. Which test results from an infant would support the diagnosis of congenital toxoplasma infection?

    1. Antitoxoplasma IgG antibody.
    2. Antitoxoplasma IgM antibody.
    3. Maternal antitoxoplasma IgM antibody.
    4. Computed tomography (CT) scan revealing intracranial calcifications.

    a. 1, 2, and 3.
    b. 1 and 3.
    c. 2 and 4.
    d. 4 only.
    e. 1, 2, 3, and 4.

19. Medications important in the control of ocular toxoplasmosis include:

    1. pyrimethamine.
    2. sulfadiazine.
    3. prednisone.
    4. folinic acid.

    a. 1, 2, and 3.
    b. 1 and 3.
    c. 2 and 4.
    d. 4 only.
    e. 1, 2, 3, and 4.

20. Which of the following concerning the epidemiology of congenital rubella infection is/are true?

    1. The majority of pregnant women are seronegative (susceptible to rubella infection).
    2. Seroconversion of a mother from negative to positive nearly guarantees infection of the fetus.
    3. Symptomatic fetal defects are uncommon, even with viremia.
    4. Maternal infection during the third trimester rarely leads to fetal infection.

    a. 1, 2, and 3.
    b. 1 and 3.
    c. 2 and 4.
    d. 4 only.
    e. 1, 2, 3, and 4.

21. The most common clinical finding in infants with congenital rubella syndrome is:

    a. pigmentary retinopathy.
    b. patent ductus arteriosus.
    c. sensorineural hearing loss.
    d. mental retardation.
    e. cataract.

22. Which two signs of congenital rubella infection are unlikely to be found simultaneously?

    a. microphthalmia and congenital cataract.
    b. microphthalmia and congenital glaucoma.
    c. congenital cataract and glaucoma.
    d. congenital cataract and a poorly dilating iris.
    e. pigmentary retinopathy and congenital cataract.

23. Live rubella virus may be recovered from an infected infant from which of the following sources?

                        1. conjunctival swabs.
                        2. urine cultures.
                        3. pharyngeal swabs.
                        4. lens aspirates.

    a. 1, 2, and 3.
    b. 1 and 3.
    c. 2 and 4.
    d. 4 only.
    e. 1, 2, 3, and 4.

24. The postoperative course following extraction of infantile cataract associated with the congenital rubella syndrome is distinguished by:

    a. a higher incidence of retinal detachment.
    b. a higher incidence of glaucoma.
    c. poor wound healing.
    d. severe inflammation.
    e. difficulty tolerating aphakic contact lenses.

25. The most common congenital infection in humans is:

    a. toxoplasmosis.
    b. rubella.
    c. cytomegalovirus (CMV).
    d. herpes simplex virus.
    e. syphilis.

26. The most common ocular manifestation of congenital CMV infection is:

    a. cataract.
    b. microphthalmia.
    c. retinochoroiditis.
    d. Peters' anomaly.
    e. strabismus.

27. T or F -- Most cases of congenital herpes simplex infection are due to episodic viremia during gestation.

28. T or F -- Most cases of congenital CMV infection are due to maternal viremia during gestation.

29. T or F -- Like congenital CMV infection, congenital herpes simplex virus infection is frequently asymptomatic.

30. T or F -- The ocular manifestations of congenital herpes simplex infection resemble those of acquired infections in adolescence and adulthood.

31. Transplacental spread of which of the following microorganisms is important in the spread of congenital infection?

                1. Toxoplasma.
                2. CMV.
                3. Treponema pallidum.
                4. herpes simplex.

    a. 1, 2, and 3.
    b. 1 and 3.
    c. 2 and 4.
    d. 4 only.
    e. 1, 2, 3, and 4.

32. Ocular manifestations of congenital syphilis infection frequently include:

                1. salt-and-pepper retinitis.
                2. pseudoretinitis pigmentosa.
                3. interstitial keratitis.
                4. microphthalmia.

    a. 1, 2, and 3.
    b. 1 and 3.
    c. 2 and 4.
    d. 4 only.
    e. 1, 2, 3, and 4.

33. Hutchinson's triad, considered diagnostic of congenital syphilis infection, includes:

   a. peg-shaped teeth, eighth nerve deafness, and interstitial keratitis.
   b. rhagades, interstitial keratitis, and hepatosplenomeglay.
   c. pseudoretinitis pigmentosa, interstitial keratitis, and peg-shaped teeth.
   d. pseudoretinitis pigmentosa, eighth nerve deafness, and interstitial keratitis.
   e. interstitial keratitis, cataract, and pseudoretinitis pigmentosa.

34. Match each of the clinical characteristics listed in the left column with the appropriate agent (more than one agent may be assigned to each of the characteristics).

   a. frequently associated with a mild serous conjunctivitis developing within 24 hours of birth.
   b. typically associated with a hyperacute purulent conjunctivitis within 2 days of birth.
   c. generally associated with a follicular conjunctivitis developing 5 to 14 days following birth.
   d. if untreated, may progress to otitis media and pneumonitis.
   e. if untreated, may progress to corneal ulceration and endophthalmitis.
   f. if left untreated, may progress to meningitis.
   g. diagnosis may be made by Gram's stain alone.
   h. diagnosis may be made by Giemsa stain alone.
   i. requires intravenous penicillin for adequate treatment.
   j. may be treated with oral antibiotics.
   k. may be treated topically in an otherwise healthy infant.

   1. herpes simplex virus.
   2. chlamydiae, subtypes d through k.
   3. Neisseria gonorrhoeae.
   4. Credé prophylaxis.

35. Which of the following are considered common etiologic agents for conjunctivitis in children?

   1. *Streptococcus pneumoniae.*
   2. *Hemophilus influenzae.*
   3. *Staphylococcus aureus.*
   4. *Streptococcus pyogenes.*

   a. 1, 2, and 3.
   b. 1 and 3.
   c. 2 and 4.
   d. 4 only.
   e. 1, 2, 3, and 4.

36. Which of the following viral infections may be associated with a pronounced keratitis?

      1. herpes simplex.
      2. adenovirus type 8.
      3. herpes zoster.
      4. adenovirus type 3.

    a. 1, 2, and 3.
    b. 1 and 3.
    c. 2 and 4.
    d. 4 only.
    e. 1, 2, 3, and 4.

37. T or F -- The syndrome of infectious mononucleosis is rarely accompanied by a conjunctivitis.

38. Which of the following concerning Parinaud's oculoglandular syndrome is/are true?

      1. Common etiologic agents include the cat-scratch fever organism, rickettsiae, *Treponema pallidum*, and mycobacterial species.
      2. Clinically, follicles are prominent with a moderate discharge.
      3. Historical features may include contact with animals.
      4. Histopathology reveals follicles and granulomas.

    a. 1, 2, and 3.
    b. 1 and 3.
    c. 2 and 4.
    d. 4 only.
    e. 1, 2, 3, and 4.

39. The agent most commonly responsible for preseptal cellulitis in children is:

    a. *S. aureus.*
    b. *Pseudomonas aeruginosa.*
    c. *S. pyogenes.*
    d. *H. influenzae.*
    e. *Proteus mirabilis.*

40. The agent most frequently associated with orbital cellulitis following bacterial conjunctivitis is:

    a. *S. aureus.*
    b. *P. aeruginosa.*
    c. *S. pyogenes.*
    d. *H. influenzae.*
    e. *P. mirabilis.*

41. The focus of primary infection in most cases of orbital cellulitis is:

    a. maxillary sinus.
    b. ethmoid sinus.
    c. frontal sinus.
    d. orbital foreign body.
    e. meningitis with cavernous sinusitis.

42. Sudden deterioration in ocular motility without a dramatic increase in proptosis suggests which complication of orbital cellulitis?

    a. panophthalmitis.
    b. meningitis.
    c. central retinal artery occlusion.
    d. cavernous sinus thrombosis.
    e. subperiosteal abscess.

43. Which of the following concerning vernal conjunctivitis is/are true?

    1. It is primarily a disease of the first two decades of life.
    2. It affects girls more frequently than boys.
    3. Prominent symptoms include photophobia and itching.
    4. The palpebral form of the disease is typically more severe inferiorly.

    a. 1, 2, and 3.
    b. 1 and 3.
    c. 2 and 4.
    d. 4 only.
    e. 1, 2, 3, and 4.

44. Features distinguishing vernal conjunctivitis from trachoma include:

    1. true follicles with germinal centers in vernal disease.
    2. eosinophils in trachoma.
    3. limbal nodules in vernal disease.
    4. prominent subconjunctival scarring in trachoma.

    a. 1, 2, and 3.
    b. 1 and 3.
    c. 2 and 4.
    d. 4 only.
    e. 1, 2, 3, and 4.

45. T or F -- The limbal nodules of vernal keratoconjunctivitis are actually follicles.

46. T or F -- Horner-Trantas dots and Herbert's pits are histopathologically indistinguishable.

47. T or F -- The presence of superior corneal pannus favors the diagnosis of trachoma over vernal conjunctivitis.

48. Corneal manifestations of vernal disease may include:

   1. superficial punctate keratitis.
   2. superior corneal pannus.
   3. transverse oval sterile ulceration in the superior cornea.
   4. deep stromal vascularization.

   a. 1, 2, and 3.
   b. 1 and 3.
   c. 2 and 4.
   d. 4 only.
   e. 1, 2, 3, and 4.

49. T or F -- The shield ulcers of vernal keratoconjunctivitis are primarily due to mechanical abrasion by tarsal papillae.

50. Which of the following concerning Stevens-Johnson syndrome is/are true?

   1. This is a disorder restricted to childhood.
   2. Postinfectious, postvaccine, and drug-induced autoimmune disorders have all been implicated.
   3. The associated vasculitis leads to a vesicular rash and mucous membrane lesions.
   4. Clinical findings include fever, pharyngitis, and headache.

   a. 1, 2, and 3.
   b. 1 and 3.
   c. 2 and 4.
   d. 4 only.
   e. 1, 2, 3, and 4.

51. Along with a fever of greater than 5 days' duration, which of the following are diagnostic criteria for Kawasaki disease?

   1. bilateral conjunctival injection.
   2. mucous membrane injection with fissures.
   3. strawberry tongue.
   4. desquamating rash of the palms and/or soles.

   a. 1, 2, and 3.
   b. 1 and 3.
   c. 2 and 4.
   d. 4 only.
   e. 1, 2, 3, and 4.

52. Systemic mortality due to Kawasaki's disease is most frequently due to:

    a. stroke.
    b. respiratory failure.
    c. myocardial infarction.
    d. acute renal failure.
    e. acute adrenal insufficiency.

53. Which one of the following concerning the anatomy of the nasolacrimal system is false?

    a. The canaliculi normally run vertically for 1 or 2 mm before running medially toward the nasolacrimal sac.
    b. The medial palpebral ligament straddles the lower one-third of the nasolacrimal sac.
    c. The nasolacrimal canal extends downward, posteriorly, and laterally through the lateral nasal wall.
    d. The lining of the canaliculi is a stratified squamous epithelium, while that of the nasolacrimal sac and canal is a bilayered columnar epithelium.
    e. The medial portion of the eyelid is more susceptible to tearing injuries due to absence of the tarsal plate.

54. Which one of the following concerning congenital impatency of nasolacrimal system is false?

    a. It may mimic a medial canthal hemangioma.
    b. Acute dacryocystitis is uncommon.
    c. The defect in canalization is within the intraosseous portion of the nasolacrimal duct.
    d. Common symptoms include epiphora and mucus discharge.
    e. If canalization has not spontaneously occurred by the age of 12 to 15 months, it is unlikely to do so.

55. T or F -- Initial probing with irrigation of an impatent nasolacrimal system is successful 90% of the time.

56. T or F -- The neural crest migrates in toward the anterior portion of the optic cup in several waves, forming the entire cornea.

57. T or F -- In megalocornea, the cornea is normal except for its excessive diameter.

58. T or F -- Keratoglobus is frequently associated with the Marfan's syndrome.

59. Failure of proper migration and differentiation of neural crest cells may lead to all of the following disorders except:

a. internal ulcer of von Hippel.
b. Scheie's syndrome.
c. Peters' anomaly.
d. Rieger's syndrome.
e. posterior embryotoxon.

60. Features that serve to distinguish congenital hereditary endothelial dystrophy (CHED) from congenital glaucoma include:

    1. intraocular pressure.
    2. epithelial edema.
    3. corneal diameter.
    4. corneal thickness.

a. 1, 2, and 3.
b. 1 and 3.
c. 2 and 4.
d. 4 only.
e. 1, 2, 3, and 4.

61. Features that serve to differentiate congenital hereditary endothelial dystrophy (CHED) from congenital hereditary stromal dystrophy (CHSD) include:

    1. intraocular pressure (IOP).
    2. epithelial edema.
    3. corneal diameter.
    4. corneal thickness.

a. 1, 2, and 3.
b. 1 and 3.
c. 2 and 4.
d. 4 only.
e. 1, 2, 3, and 4.

62. Match the causes of congenital neonatal corneal clouding with their tendency to be unilateral or bilateral.

a. sclerocornea.
b. forceps injury.
c. mucopolysaccharidoses.
d. anterior segment dysgenesis (Peters' anomaly).
e. congenital hereditary endothelial dystrophy.
f. congenital hereditary stromal dystrophy.
g. corneal dermoids.
h. congenital glaucoma.

1. unilateral.
2. bilateral.
3. either.

63. T or F -- The crystalline deposits seen in the cornea in infantile cystinosis are found nowhere else in the eye.

64. Corneal ulceration and scarring seen in familial dysautonomia (Riley-Day syndrome) is secondary to:

        1. impaired epithelial-stromal adherence.
        2. impaired corneal sensation.
        3. impaired humoral immune responses.
        4. decreased tearing.

    a. 1, 2, and 3.
    b. 1 and 3.
    c. 2 and 4.
    d. 4 only.
    e. 1, 2, 3, and 4.

65. Which of the following concerning the epidemiology of infantile glaucoma is/are true?

        1. Most cases are bilateral.
        2. Subsequent offspring of parents with an affected child have approximately a 5% chance of manifesting the condition.
        3. A patient with infantile glaucoma has approximately a 5% chance of having a child similarly affected.
        4. The incidence of primary open-angle glaucoma in grandparents of an affected patient is elevated.

    a. 1, 2, and 3.
    b. 1 and 3.
    c. 2 and 4.
    d. 4 only.
    e. 1, 2, 3, and 4.

66. T or F -- The basic pathophysiologic mechanism in all cases of infantile glaucoma involves an imperforate membrane covering the angle.

67. Symptoms and/or signs of infantile glaucoma include:

        1. tearing.
        2. enlargement of corneal diameter.
        3. loss of corneal clarity.
        4. photophobia.

    a. 1, 2, and 3.
    b. 1 and 3.
    c. 2 and 4.
    d. 4 only.
    e. 1, 2, 3, and 4.

68. T or F -- Acute ruptures in Descemet's membrane associated with infantile glaucoma are typically vertical, while those associated with birth trauma are typically horizontal.

69. T or F -- Corneal clouding or tearing is more likely to be the presenting symptom with glaucoma whose onset is before the age of 3 months, whereas corneal enlargement will probably the presenting finding in older infants.

70. T or F -- Like optic nerve cupping, an afferent pupillary defect carries little prognostic significance in infantile glaucoma.

71. Recognized methods for long-term management of infantile glaucoma include:

    1. trabeculotomy.
    2. trabeculectomy.
    3. goniotomy.
    4. oral carbonic anhydrase inhibitors.

    a. 1, 2, and 3.
    b. 1 and 3.
    c. 2 and 4.
    d. 4 only.
    e. 1, 2, 3, and 4.

72. Which of the following are considered negative prognostic factors in infantile glaucoma?

    1. presence of an afferent pupillary defect.
    2. corneal diameter greater than 14 mm at the time of diagnosis.
    3. onset at less than 3 months of age.
    4. optic nerve cupping.

    a. 1, 2, and 3.
    b. 1 and 3.
    c. 2 and 4.
    d. 4 only.
    e. 1, 2, 3, and 4.

73. Systemic evaluation of the neonate with glaucoma should include:

    1. serum galactose levels.
    2. serum antirubella IgG levels.
    3. serum phytanic acid levels.
    4. urinalysis for proteinuria and aminoaciduria.

    a. 1, 2, and 3.
    b. 1 and 3.
    c. 2 and 4.
    d. 4 only.
    e. 1, 2, 3, and 4.

74. Which of the following agents used in general anesthesia tend to lower intraocular pressure (IOP)?

    1. halothane.
    2. ketamine.
    3. thiopental.
    4. succinycholine.

  a. 1, 2, and 3.
  b. 1 and 3.
  c. 2 and 4.
  d. 4 only.
  e. 1, 2, 3, and 4.

75. T or F -- The upper end of normal IOP for infants and children is felt to be the same as that for adults--22 mm Hg.

76. Which of the following concerning simple ectopia lentis is/are true?

    1. The dominant variety is more common than the recessive variety.
    2. The recessive variety is bilateral, while the dominant variety is unilateral.
    3. The recessive variety may be accompanied by a displaced and abnormally shaped pupil.
    4. All dominant forms of the disorder develop by age 20 years.

  a. 1, 2, and 3.
  b. 1 and 3.
  c. 2 and 4.
  d. 4 only.
  e. 1, 2, 3, and 4.

77. Which of the following concerning Marfan's syndrome is/are true?

    1. The majority of cases are sporadic.
    2. The majority of patients with the full syndrome develop ectopia lentis.
    3. The average refraction on patients with the syndrome reveals moderate hyperopia.
    4. Systemic treatment of the condition may include propranolol and antibiotic prophylaxis before dental procedures.

  a. 1, 2, and 3.
  b. 1 and 3.
  c. 2 and 4.
  d. 4 only.
  e. 1, 2, 3, and 4.

78. Which of the following concerning homocystinuria is/are true?

1. This disorder is inherited on an autosomal dominant basis.
2. The majority of patients will develop ectopia lentis.
3. Systemic mortality is due to a coagulopathy with clotting deficiency and bleeding diatheses.
4. The primary defect leading to lens dislocation is a structural deficiency in the zonules.

a. 1, 2, and 3.
b. 1 and 3.
c. 2 and 4.
d. 4 only.
e. 1, 2, 3, and 4.

79. Ectopia lentis associated with mental retardation may be seen in which of the following disorders:

1. Sturge-Weber syndrome.
2. Hyperlysinemia.
3. Down's syndrome.
4. Weill-Marchesani syndrome.

a. 1, 2, and 3.
b. 1 and 3.
c. 2 and 4.
d. 4 only.
e. 1, 2, 3, and 4.

80. Which of the following types of congenital cataract do not require systemic laboratory evaluation?

1. bilateral cataract with no family history.
2. monocular cataract with no family history.
3. cataract associated with retinal pigment epithelial abnormalities.
4. posterior lenticonus.

a. 1, 2, and 3.
b. 1 and 3.
c. 2 and 4.
d. 4 only.
e. 1, 2, 3, and 4.

81. In which of the following maternal-fetal infections is congenital cataract virtually unheard of ?

a. toxoplasmosis.
b. rubella.
c. cytomegalic inclusion disease.
d. herpes simplex.
e. syphilis.

82. Which of the following congenital cataract scenarios mandates the most urgent surgical intervention?

    a. monocular anterior polar cataract.
    b. binocular posterior lenticonus.
    c. monocular lamellar cataract.
    d. monocular nuclear cataract.
    e. binocular nuclear cataract.

83. Which one of the following statements regarding necessary alterations in surgical strategy for pediatric cataract extraction (relative to adults) is false?

    a. Intracapsular surgery is generally avoided in younger patients due to more prominent hyaloidocapsular attachments.
    b. Extracapsular nuclear expression is generally avoided because of the small, relatively soft nucleus of the juvenile cataract.
    c. Pediatric cataracts are usually soft and can be aspirated entirely.
    d. Primary posterior capsulectomy is generally not undertaken due to more prominent hyaloidocapsular attachments in the young eye.
    e. One or more peripheral iridectomies are generally indicated due to the higher risk of exaggerated inflammation and secondary pupillary block.

84. The systemic evaluation of a patient with bilateral congenital cataracts might include which of the following?

    1. bilateral audiograms.
    2. serum calcium level.
    3. urinalysis.
    4. karyotyping.

    a. 1, 2, and 3.
    b. 1 and 3.
    c. 2 and 4.
    d. 4 only.
    e. 1, 2, 3, and 4.

85. Match each of the systemic disorders listed in the left-hand column with its most likely manifestations.

a. Fabry's disease.
b. homocystinuria.
c. Refsum's disease.
d. Wilson's disease.
e. Lowe's syndrome.
f. Alport's syndrome.
g. myotonic dystrophy.
h. incontinentia pigmenti.
i. ichthyosis.
j. Hallermann-Streiff syndrome.

1. hematuria and hearing loss.
2. flaking dermopathy and enlarged corneal nerves.
3. conjunctival and retinal telangiectasis.
4. ectopia lentis, tall stature, and mental retardation.
5. frontal bossing, baldness, and testicular atrophy.
6. alopecia and bird-like facies.
7. progressive tapetoretinal degeneration and hearing loss.
8. peripheral retinal neovascularization.
9. hepatic failure, dementia, and peripheral pigmentation of Descemet's membrane.
10. aminoaciduria, hypotonia, and renal rickets.

86. Which of the following concerning juvenile rheumatoid arthritis (JRA) is/are true?

1. It is the most common etiology of anterior uveitis in the pediatric population.
2. Although it may have onset at any age, it is extraordinarily rare under the age of 2 years.
3. To conclude that uveitis is associated with JRA, there must be an antecedent history of joint symptoms.
4. The uveitis of JRA is nearly always entirely anterior.

a. 1, 2, and 3.
b. 1 and 3.
c. 2 and 4.
d. 4 only.
e. 1, 2, 3, and 4.

87. Which of the following concerning the five subtypes of JRA is/are true?

    1. With the exception of the pauciarticular, late-onset type (HLA-B27 positive), all of the subtypes of JRA are considerably more common in girls.
    2. The group at highest risk of developing anterior uveitis is the pauciarticular early-onset group with rheumatoid factor (RF) negative and antinuclear antibody (ANA) negative.
    3. Iridocyclitis is frequently seen as part of the syndrome of systemic JRA (Still's disease).
    4. The joints involved in patients with iridocyclitis are typically the large joints (knee, ankle, elbow).

  a. 1, 2, and 3.
  b. 1 and 3.
  c. 2 and 4.
  d. 4 only.
  e. 1, 2, 3, and 4.

88. Which of the following regarding the clinical manifestations of JRA is/are true?

    1. The findings of chronic uveitis may be discovered incidentally.
    2. Visual loss due to amblyopia is rarely a problem.
    3. Surgery for band keratopathy made be indicated for photophobia and discomfort, as well as for visual loss.
    4. Cataract surgery with intraocular lens (IOL) implantation may be indicated in cases of visually significant cataract.

  a. 1, 2, and 3.
  b. 1 and 3.
  c. 2 and 4.
  d. 4 only.
  e. 1, 2, 3, and 4.

89. Other etiologies of uveitis and joint complaints in children that must be considered in the differential diagnosis of JRA include:

    1. inflammatory bowel disease.
    2. sarcoidosis.
    3. Lyme disease.
    4. herpes simplex infection.

  a. 1, 2, and 3.
  b. 1 and 3.
  c. 2 and 4.
  d. 4 only.
  e. 1, 2, 3, and 4.

90. Which one of the following concerning the pediatric uveitis associated with herpes zoster virus (HZV) is false?

   a. Typically, the uveitis develops during convalescence from acute varicella infection.
   b. The uveitis in (reactivated) zoster ophthalmicus may have both anterior and posterior components.
   c. Reactivation disease may also be accompanied by a keratitis, either epithelial or stromal.
   d. In the setting of immunosuppression, reactivation disease should be treated with systemic as well as topical corticosteroids.
   e. Those at risk for reactivation disease include patients with acute leukemia and who are post-renal transplant.

91. T or F -- Pediatric uveitis due to herpes simplex virus (HSV) infection is usually accompanied by keratitis.

92. T or F -- Over 50% of uveitis in the pediatric population has a posterior component.

93. The most common etiology of posterior uveitis in the pediatric population is:

   a. toxocariasis.
   b. toxoplasmosis.
   c. syphilis.
   d. sarcoidosis.
   e. idiopathic.

94. Tissues in which the Toxoplasma parasite survives the best include:

   1. hepatic cells.
   2. cerebral neurons.
   3. red blood cells.
   4. ganglion cells.

   a. 1, 2, and 3.
   b. 1 and 3.
   c. 2 and 4.
   d. 4 only.
   e. 1, 2, 3, and 4.

95. Manifestations of acquired systemic toxoplasmosis include all the following except:

   a. acute arthritis.
   b. rash.
   c. meningoencephalitis.
   d. influenza-like syndrome.
   e. retinitis.

96. T or F -- Recurrent toxoplasmosis frequently presents as a granulomatous anterior uveitis.

97. Which one of the following concerning ocular histoplasmosis is false?

    a. Symptoms consistent with histoplasmosis include a flu-like syndrome and malaise.
    b. There is a geographic, but not a seasonal, predilection for the development of systemic or ocular histoplasmosis.
    c. The vitritis that may accompany the ocular infection may lead to decreased visual acuity.
    d. The initial infection consists of a choroidal granuloma.
    e. Although skin testing may support the diagnosis, it may lead to worsening of the macular disease.

98. Which of the following concerning toxocariasis is/are true?

    1. The infectious cycle in humans generally starts with the consumption of fecally-contaminated soil.
    2. The condition may present as a peripheral granuloma in an otherwise quiet eye.
    3. There may be an associated peripheral eosinophilia.
    4. The associated uveitis is due to a hypersensitivity reaction to living organism.

    a. 1, 2, and 3.
    b. 1 and 3.
    c. 2 and 4.
    d. 4 only.
    e. 1, 2, 3, and 4.

99. Which of the following concerning idiopathic pars planitis is/are true?

    1. It may have a mild course, with floaters as the only symptom.
    2. Peripheral retinal periphlebitis is frequently associated.
    3. Infectious etiologies are usually not found.
    4. It is usually unilateral.

    a. 1, 2, and 3.
    b. 1 and 3.
    c. 2 and 4.
    d. 4 only.
    e. 1, 2, 3, and 4.

100. Findings in a patient with known JRA and uveitis that should prompt an increase in topical steroid administration include:

        1. worsening cataract.
        2. flare.
        3. band keratopathy.
        4. aqueous cells.

    a. 1, 2, and 3.
    b. 1 and 3.
    c. 2 and 4.
    d. 4 only.
    e. 1, 2, 3, and 4.

101. Which one of the following concerning persistent hyperplastic primary vitreous (PHPV) is false?

    a. Mittendorf's dots and Bergmeister's papillae may be considered mild variants of the disorder.
    b. In severe cases, fibrovascular overgrowth within the primary vitreous may invade the lens substance itself.
    c. A common complication is glaucoma, either secondary to vitreous hemorrhage or secondary angle closure.
    d. The presence of dense leukocoria in an eye that is abnormally small suggests the diagnosis of retinoblastoma rather than PHPV.
    e. The condition is typically unilateral.

102. The incidence of retinopathy of prematurity (ROP) of any stage in premature children weighing less than 1250 gm at birth is approximately:

    a. 5%.
    b. 25%.
    c. 50%.
    d. 65%.
    e. 100%.

103. T or F -- The nasal retina is generally completely vascularized by the sixth gestational month, while the temporal retina is not completely vascularized until the eighth gestational month.

104. T or F -- The timing of the onset of various stages of ROP suggest that postdelivery age rather than postconceptional age is the critical factor.

105. Which of the following concerning risks factors for the development of ROP is/are true?

   1. Gestational age at birth is inversely proportional to the probability of development of ROP.
   2. Incidence and severity of ROP increases directly with average arterial oxygenation.
   3. Blacks may tend to develop less severe forms of the disorder.
   4. Necrotizing enterocolitis (NEC) is an independent risk factor for development of ROP.

   a. 1, 2, and 3.
   b. 1 and 3.
   c. 2 and 4.
   d. 4 only.
   e. 1, 2, 3, and 4.

106. T or F -- Zone I is considered to be a circular area with diameter 30 degrees centered around the optic nerve.

107. The Cryo-ROP study established that cryotherapy will reduce the incidence of unfavorable outcomes (posterior retinal detachment, fixed macular folds, or retrolental fibroplasia) in eyes with which of the following criteria?

   1. stage III disease or worse.
   2. "plus" disease.
   3. involvement of at least five contiguous or eight interrupted clock hours.
   4. disease involving only zone 1 or zone 2.

   a. 1, 2, and 3.
   b. 1 and 3.
   c. 2 and 4.
   d. 4 only.
   e. 1, 2, 3, and 4.

108. Sequelae of ROP may include:

   1. angle-closure glaucoma.
   2. cataract.
   3. pseudoexotropia.
   4. pseudoesotropia.

   a. 1, 2, and 3.
   b. 1 and 3.
   c. 2 and 4.
   d. 4 only.
   e. 1, 2, 3, and 4.

109. Which of the following concerning screening protocols for premature infants is/are true?

    1. Only infants of birth weight less than 1500 gm require screening.
    2. Initial examination should take place 4 to 6 weeks after birth or at 30 weeks' gestational age, whichever is later.
    3. In patients with mild or no ROP, examinations may be conducted every 2 weeks.
    4. In patients with threshold ROP, cryotherapy should be delivered within 72 hours.

    a. 1, 2, and 3.
    b. 1 and 3.
    c. 2 and 4.
    d. 4 only.
    e. 1, 2, 3, and 4.

110. Which one of the following concerning Coats' disease is false?

    a. True Coats' disease is a disorder of childhood, more often affecting boys.
    b. The condition is more commonly bilateral than unilateral.
    c. Diagnosis of Coats' disease may not be made in the setting of subretinal exudate without obvious abnormal retinal vessels.
    d. Full treatment involves obliteration of the abnormal vessels and subsequent treatment of associated retinal detachment.
    e. In up to one-half of untreated cases, the condition may be nonprogressive.

111. T or F -- Juvenile cataracts associated with type I diabetes mellitus generally develop independent of the level of blood sugar control.

112. Children of diabetic mothers are at increased risk for the development of:

    a. Coats' disease.
    b. pigmentary glaucoma.
    c. aniridia.
    d. optic nerve hypoplasia.
    e. pseudotumor cerebri.

113. The most common fundus finding in a patient with acute leukemic oculopathy is:

    a. choroidal infiltration (creamy elevated subretinal patches).
    b. nerve fiber layer hemorrhages.
    c. cotton-wool spots.
    d. Roth's spots.
    e. optic disc edema.

114. T or F -- A patient with known acute leukemia who presents with disc edema and loss of vision should be evaluated for radiotherapy within the next 2 weeks.

115. T or F -- Patients with leukemic optic neuropathy may be more sensitive to radiation neuropathy than other patients.

116. Other ocular manifestations common in leukemic oculopathy include:

> 1. uveitic glaucoma.
> 2. spontaneous hyphemas.
> 3. iris heterochromia.
> 4. cataract.

a. 1, 2, and 3.
b. 1 and 3.
c. 2 and 4.
d. 4 only.
e. 1, 2, 3, and 4.

117. Which of the following concerning the gangliosidoses is/are true:

> 1. The most common is GM^2, type I (Tay-Sachs disease).
> 2. Inheritance is generally on an X-linked recessive basis.
> 3. Prominent cherry-red spots are typically seen in Tay-Sachs and Sandhoff's diseases.
> 4. Patients generally succumb to neurologic deterioration in their late teens or early twenties.

a. 1, 2, and 3.
b. 1 and 3.
c. 2 and 4.
d. 4 only.
e. 1, 2, 3, and 4.

118. Which one of the following concerning the oculorenal syndromes is false?

a. Lowe's syndrome is inherited on an X-linked recessive basis.
b. Female carriers of Lowe's syndrome may be detected by punctate cortical opacities of the lens.
c. The most common ocular disorder in Lowe's syndrome is glaucoma.
d. The most common ocular finding in Alport's syndrome is anterior lenticonus and/or anterior polar cataract.
e. Unlike Alport's syndrome, Senior-Loken syndrome features a progressive retinal degeneration with profound visual symptoms.

119. Ocular findings consistent with renal failure from any etiology include:

       1. exudative retinal detachment.
       2. calcium crystals in the conjunctiva.
       3. macular edema.
       4. diffuse arteriolar attenuation.

    a. 1, 2, and 3.
    b. 1 and 3.
    c. 2 and 4.
    d. 4 only.
    e. 1, 2, 3, and 4.

120. T or F -- In albinism, more ganglion cell fibers decussate at the chiasm than in normal visual pathways.

121. T or F -- The tyrosinase-negative type of albinism generally has more severe clinical findings than the tyrosinase-positive type.

122. T or F -- The vitreous is normal in juvenile retinoschisis.

123. Reliable methods of distinguishing juvenile retinoschisis from Goldmann-Favre dystrophy include:

       1. macular examination.
       2. electro-oculography (EOG).
       3. electroretinogram (ERG).
       4. careful family history.

    a. 1, 2, and 3.
    b. 1 and 3.
    c. 2 and 4.
    d. 4 only.
    e. 1, 2, 3, and 4.

124. Fundus findings that may be seen in association with tapetoretinal degeneration include:

       1. cystoid macular edema.
       2. vitreous cells.
       3. posterior subcapsular cataract.
       4. subretinal exudation.

    a. 1, 2, and 3.
    b. 1 and 3.
    c. 2 and 4.
    d. 4 only.
    e. 1, 2, 3, and 4.

125. T or F -- Most cases of sector retinitis pigmentosa ultimately progress to macular involvement with a poor visual prognosis.

126. The most common underlying disorder in a patient with a "bull's-eye" maculopathy is:

    a. Stargardt's disease.
    b. cone dystrophy.
    c. chloroquine retinopathy.
    d. hydroxychloroquine retinopathy.
    e. Best's disease.

127. Which one of the following regarding the various forms of congenital stationary night blindness (CSNB) is false?

    a. Retinitis punctata albescens is associated with dots deep in the retina.
    b. Fundus albipunctatus reveals normalization of the scotopic ERG after prolonged dark adaptation (after 3-12 hours).
    c. One recessive form is frequently associated with high myopia.
    d. One variety may have a normal scotopic a-wave with no apparent b-wave.
    e. Oguchi's displays the Mizuo phenomenon--a golden sheen of the retina returning to normal after several hours of dark adaption.

128. T or F -- Visual acuity, though usually better in blue cone monochromatism than rod monochromatism, is not reliable for distinguishing between the two.

129. Clinical findings associated with Leber's congenital amaurosis include:

        1. oculodigital sign.
        2. keratoconus.
        3. high hyperopia.
        4. sensorineural hearing loss.

    a. 1, 2, and 3.
    b. 1 and 3.
    c. 2 and 4.
    d. 4 only.
    e. 1, 2, 3, and 4.

130. T or F -- In most cases designated as Stargardt's disease, the presenting symptom is night blindness.

131. T or F -- Visual function in the pattern dystrophies of the retinal pigment epithelium (RPE) is usually good.

132. All of the following are features of Aicardi syndrome except:

   a. X-linked recessive inheritance.
   b. agenesis of the corpus callosum.
   c. infantile spasms.
   d. lacunar chorioretinal degeneration.
   e. severe mental retardation.

133. T or F -- Morning glory disc anomaly is generally an incidental finding with little functional significance.

134. T or F -- Colobomata involving the optic nerve may be associated with nonrhegmatogenous retinal detachment.

135. T or F -- Medullation of optic nerve fibers generally begins at the optic chiasm and is completed by the end of the first month of life.

136. T or F -- Myelinated nerve fibers are more common in boys than girls.

137. Findings consistent with the tilted disc syndrome include:

   1. prominence of the superior portion of the disc.
   2. an inferior or inferonasal scleral crescent.
   3. situs inversus.
   4. binasal field defects.

   a. 1, 2, and 3.
   b. 1 and 3.
   c. 2 and 4.
   d. 4 only.
   e. 1, 2, 3, and 4.

138. Which of the following concerning optic nerve hypoplasia is/are true?

   1. The condition may be unilateral or bilateral.
   2. Visual acuity may vary from normal to no light perception.
   3. A classic sign is the double ring sign.
   4. The association of optic nerve hypoplasia, absence of the septum pellucidum, midline central nervous system (CNS) anomalies, and hypothalamic-pitutary abnormalities is stronger for unilateral than for bilateral optic nerve hypoplasia.

   a. 1, 2, and 3.
   b. 1 and 3.
   c. 2 and 4.
   d. 4 only.
   e. 1, 2, 3, and 4.

139. The most common location for optic disc pits is:

    a. superonasal.
    b. superotemporal.
    c. inferotemporal.
    d. inferonasal.
    e. central.

140. Aids in distinguishing pseudopapilledema with buried drusen from true papilledema include:

                1. red free photographs.
                2. CT scanning.
                3. visual fields.
                4. ultrasonography.

    a. 1, 2, and 3.
    b. 1 and 3.
    c. 2 and 4.
    d. 4 only.
    e. 1, 2, 3, and 4.

141. T or F -- The prognosis for visual recovery is better for the optic neuritis associated with Devic's disease than for idiopathic optic neuritis.

142. Which one of the following concerning histiocytosis X is false?

    a. These disorders reflect abnormal proliferation of dendritic histiocytes.
    b. Radiographically, these tumors produce osteosclerosis.
    c. Conventional radiography will frequently disclose a greater number of bony lesions than are apparent clinically.
    d. The classic triad in Hand-Schüller-Christian disease is diabetes insipidus, lytic skull lesions, and proptosis.
    e. Patients with Letterer-Siwe disease are frequently very ill.

143. Options for the treatment of the histiocytoses include:

                1. curettage.
                2. intralesion steroid injections.
                3. low-dose radiation.
                4. systemic steroid therapy.

    a. 1, 2, and 3.
    b. 1 and 3.
    c. 2 and 4.
    d. 4 only.
    e. 1, 2, 3, and 4.

144. Prognosis for the histiocytoses is unfavorable for children with:

        1. age of onset less than 2 years.
        2. multiple lesions of the skull.
        3. hepatic or bone marrow involvement.
        4. bilateral proptosis.

    a. 1, 2, and 3.
    b. 1 and 3.
    c. 2 and 4.
    d. 4 only.
    e. 1, 2, 3, and 4.

145. Which one of the following concerning the fibro-osseous disorders of the orbit is false?

    a. The distinction between fibrous dysplasia and ossifying fibroma is generally made radiologically.
    b. Fibrous dysplasia may be either sclerotic or lytic radiologically.
    c. Generally, fibrous dysplasia stabilizes after skeletal maturity is attained.
    d. The polyostotic variety of fibrous dysplasia may be accompanied by sexual precocity and hyperpigmented skin macules.
    e. The most significant visual implication of fibro-osseous orbital lesions is optic nerve compression.

146. Which one of the following concerning capillary hemangiomas is false?

    a. Systemic interferon may lead to involution.
    b. They are more common in girls than in boys.
    c. They characteristically blanch with pressure.
    d. Phlebolith formation is common.
    e. Indications for treatment include occlusion amblyopia and/or significant astigmatism.

147. T or F -- The pathology of the nevus flammeus (port-wine stain) is consistent with cavernous dilation of dermal blood vessels and cellular proliferation.

148. Which of the following concerning lymphangiomas is/are true?

        1. They are primarily a disorder of the pediatric age range.
        2. Superficial lesions may have a bluish or violaceous hue.
        3. Classic presenting symptoms include proptosis with crying and following upper respiratory infections, and spontaneous ecchymosis.
        4. Surgical intervention is indicated early in the course of the disorder in order to remove the tumor while it is small.

    a. 1, 2, and 3.
    b. 1 and 3.
    c. 2 and 4.
    d. 4 only.
    e. 1, 2, 3, and 4.

149. Which lesions may be associated with proptosis with Valsalva maneuver or crying?

        1. orbital lymphangioma.
        2. capillary hemangioma.
        3. orbital varix.
        4. orbital cavernous hemangioma.

  a. 1, 2, and 3.
  b. 1 and 3.
  c. 2 and 4.
  d. 4 only.
  e. 1, 2, 3, and 4.

150. Which of the following concerning the epidemiology of rhabdomyosarcoma is/are true:

        1. It is one of the most common soft-tissue malignancies in children.
        2. It is the most common solid malignant tumor of the orbit in children.
        3. A common presentation is an orbital cellulitis-like picture.
        4. The average age at diagnosis is 7 years.

  a. 1, 2, and 3.
  b. 1 and 3.
  c. 2 and 4.
  d. 4 only.
  e. 1, 2, 3, and 4.

151. T or F -- Any child with unexplained acquired ptosis should have radiographic imaging of the orbit to rule out rhabdomyosarcoma.

152. Which of the following regarding the histopathology of rhabdomyosarcoma is/are true?

        1. The embryonal type is the most common.
        2. The embryonal type has the best prognosis.
        3. The alveolar type has the worst prognosis.
        4. The differentiated (pleomorphic) type is the second most common.

  a. 1, 2, and 3.
  b. 1 and 3.
  c. 2 and 4.
  d. 4 only.
  e. 1, 2, 3, and 4.

153. The proper intervention for newly diagnosed rhabdomyosarcoma is:

  a. exenteration.
  b. radiotherapy.
  c. chemotherapy.
  d. a, b, and c.
  e. b and c.

154. Which of the following concerning the neurilemmoma (schwannoma) is/are true?

    1. The majority of patients with neurofibromatosis will develop at least one.
    2. The lesion can be exquisitely tender or painful.
    3. Malignant degeneration is common.
    4. There are two classic histopathologic patterns.

    a. 1, 2, and 3.
    b. 1 and 3.
    c. 2 and 4.
    d. 4 only.
    e. 1, 2, 3, and 4.

155. Which of the following concerning neurofibroma is/are true?

    1. The nodular neurofibroma is the most specific for neurofibromatosis.
    2. Like schwannomas, neurofibromas grow in close relation to peripheral nerves.
    3. Neurofibromas are generally osteosclerotic.
    4. The association of neurofibroma with congenital glaucoma is strongest with lesions of the upper eyelid.

    a. 1, 2, and 3.
    b. 1 and 3.
    c. 2 and 4.
    d. 4 only.
    e. 1, 2, 3, and 4.

156. Which of the following features might be used to differentiate between neurofibroma and neurilemmoma?

    1. the presence of axons and perineural cells in the neurofibroma.
    2. the presence of Schwann cells in the neurilemmoma.
    3. the presence of a true capsule around a neurilemmoma.
    4. positive S-100 staining for neurofibroma.

    a. 1, 2, and 3.
    b. 1 and 3.
    c. 2 and 4.
    d. 4 only.
    e. 1, 2, 3, and 4.

157. Which of the following concerning optic nerve glioma is/are true?

    1. The age range with the highest incidence is 2 to 6 years.
    2. Two commons means of presentation include visual loss and proptosis.
    3. The classic radiographic appearance of the lesion on CT scanning is a fusiform enlargement of the optic nerve.
    4. A syndrome strikingly similar to spasmus nutans may be seen in gliomas involving the hypothalmus or optic chiasm.

    a. 1, 2, and 3.
    b. 1 and 3.
    c. 2 and 4.
    d. 4 only.
    e. 1, 2, 3, and 4.

158. Which of the following regarding the treatment of optic nerve gliomas is/are true?

    1. Biopsy findings are important in guiding appropriate therapy.
    2. Extent of spread is important in guiding appropriate therapy.
    3. Tumors arising from the optic nerve have a poorer prognosis than those arising from the optic chiasm.
    4 Increased intracranial pressure and involvement of contiguous CNS structures confer a poorer prognosis.

    a. 1, 2, and 3.
    b. 1 and 3.
    c. 2 and 4.
    d. 4 only.
    e. 1, 2, 3, and 4.

159. T or F -- Meningiomas are more likely to appear osteolytic than osteoblastic on radiographic studies.

160. Which of the following regarding the epidemiology of neuroblastoma is/are true?

    1. In some pediatric series, the incidence is greater than that of rhabdomyosarcoma.
    2. The second most common site of origin is the retroperitoneal sympathetic chain.
    3. The site of origin is the adrenal gland in at least one-half of cases.
    4. This tumor presents as metastases in over one-half of cases.

    a. 1, 2, and 3.
    b. 1 and 3.
    c. 2 and 4.
    d. 4 only.
    e. 1, 2, 3, and 4.

161. Common presentations for neuroblastoma metastatic to the orbit include:

    1. rapidly developing proptosis.
    2. spontaneous ecchymoses.
    3. orbital cellulitis.
    4. enophthalmos.

    a. 1, 2, and 3.
    b. 1 and 3.
    c. 2 and 4.
    d. 4 only.
    e. 1, 2, 3, and 4.

162. All of the following are features of the histopathology of metastatic neuroblastoma except:

    a. sheets of indistinct round cells with scanty cytoplasm.
    b. copious mitotic figures.
    c. areas of tumor necrosis.
    d. Homer Wright rosettes.
    e. bony invasion.

163. Which of the following are considered ominous prognostic factors for metastatic neuroblastoma?

    1. liver metastases.
    2. age less than 1 year old.
    3. bone marrow metastases.
    4. bone metastases.

    a. 1, 2, and 3.
    b. 1 and 3.
    c. 2 and 4.
    d. 4 only.
    e. 1, 2, 3, and 4.

164. The paraneoplastic syndrome most commonly associated with metastatic neuroblastoma is:

    a. photoreceptor degeneration.
    b. optic neuropathy.
    c. opsoclonus.
    d. facial myokymia.
    e. cerebellar degeneration.

165. Which of the following concerning Ewing's sarcoma is/are true?

   1. Like neuroblastoma, this tumor may present with an orbital cellulitis-like picture.
   2. Invasion of the globe is common.
   3. The age at onset is older than for neuroblastoma.
   4. Unlike neuroblastoma, there is no role for radiotherapy.

   a. 1, 2, and 3.
   b. 1 and 3.
   c. 2 and 4.
   d. 4 only.
   e. 1, 2, 3, and 4.

166. The histopathologic "starry sky" (histiocytes scattered amidst a monotonous background of lymphocytes) is the classic appearance of:

   a. chloroma.
   b. Burkitt's lymphoma.
   c. Wilms' tumor.
   d. metastatic neuroblastoma.
   e. Ewing's sarcoma.

167. Which one of the following concerning ocular adnexal dermoid cysts is false?

   a. They are choristomatous arrests of epithelial tissue.
   b. The most common location is the superonasal orbital rim.
   c. Generally, they do not enlarge after the first year of life.
   d. Rupture may lead to an orbital cellulitis-like picture.
   e. Radiography of orbital lesions generally demonstrates bony excavation.

168. Which of the following may be considered features that distinguish pediatric orbital pseudotumor from that seen in adults?

   1. More frequent involvement of the lacrimal gland in children.
   2. More frequent constitutional symptoms such as headache, fever, vomiting, and lethargy in children.
   3. Greater resistance to steroid therapy in adults.
   4. Peripheral eosinophilia in children.

   a. 1, 2, and 3.
   b. 1 and 3.
   c. 2 and 4.
   d. 4 only.
   e. 1, 2, 3, and 4.

169. The epibulbar lesion most commonly seen in children under the age of 15 years is:

   a. dermoid.
   b. pyogenic granuloma.
   c. dermolipoma.
   d. nevus.
   e. epithelial inclusion cyst.

170. Findings consistent with the Goldenhar-Gorlin syndrome include:

   1. vertebral anomalies.
   2. eyelid colobomas.
   3. limbal dermoids.
   4. aniridia.

   a. 1, 2, and 3.
   b. 1 and 3.
   c. 2 and 4.
   d. 4 only.
   e. 1, 2, 3, and 4.

171. T or F -- Other than those seen in Goldenhar's syndrome, limbal dermoids are rarely associated with other abnormalities.

172. T or F -- Limbal dermoids are generally more difficult to excise completely than dermolipomas.

173. Which of the following concerning the incidence of retinoblastoma is/are true?

   1. The most frequent age at diagnosis is 18 months.
   2. Ninety percent of cases are diagnosed by the age of 3 years.
   3. Almost 95% of newly diagnosed cases will have no family history of retinoblastoma.
   4. The most reliable clue to the presence of a new germ-line mutation is unilateral involvement.

   a. 1, 2, and 3.
   b. 1 and 3.
   c. 2 and 4.
   d. 4 only.
   e. 1, 2, 3, and 4.

174. T or F -- Germ-line mutations leading to retinoblastoma are inherited on an autosomal dominant basis with 100% penetrance.

175. Which of the following regarding the genetics of inherited retinoblastoma is/are true?

       1. The locus is on the long arm of chromosome 13 (13q).
       2. The gene product of interest induces malignant transformation if produced in sufficient concentration.
       3. The chromosomal defect is expressed on an autosomal recessive basis.
       4. The effects of the retinoblastoma gene are expressed only within the eye.

    a. 1, 2, and 3.
    b. 1 and 3.
    c. 2 and 4.
    d. 4 only.
    e. 1, 2, 3, and 4.

176. A couple gives birth to a child who, at the age of 9 months, is diagnosed with bilateral retinoblastoma. There is no previous family history of the disorder. Which one of the following statements regarding this situation is incorrect?

    a. The child most likely carries one abnormal copy of chromosome 13 in each of his cells.
    b. The chance of this child having an affected brother or sister is approximately 6%.
    c. Either the mother or the father must carry an abnormal copy of chromosome 13 in their germ cells.
    d. The child's life expectancy is less than normal.
    e. Chromosomal analysis on the parents and affected child could elucidate the origin of the genetic defect.

177. Two years later, the same couple gives birth to another child who, at the age of 15 months, is diagnosed with bilateral retinoblastoma. When the parents inquire about the probability of their next child developing retinoblastoma, they should be told that the probability is approximately:

    a. less than 1%.
    b. 6%.
    c. 25%.
    d. 40%.
    e. 80%.

178. The probability of a patient who survives bilateral retinoblastoma giving birth to a child with retinoblastoma is:

    a. less than 1%.
    b. 6%.
    c. 25%.
    d. 40%.
    e. 80%.

179. Patients who have received radiation therapy for bilateral retinoblastoma are at increased risk for the development of:

    1. osteogenic sarcoma of the long bones.
    2. osteogenic sarcoma of the orbital bones.
    3. malignant melanoma of the eyelids.
    4. leiomyosarcomas of the eye or orbit.

    a. 1, 2, and 3.
    b. 1 and 3.
    c. 2 and 4.
    d. 4 only.
    e. 1, 2, 3, and 4.

180. T or F -- The prognosis for survival in patients who develop a second malignancy after treatment for retinoblastoma is poor.

181. Which of the following is the least common presentation for retinoblastoma?

    a. decreased vision.
    b. strabismus.
    c. orbital cellulitis.
    d. incidental finding.
    e. leukocoria.

182. Which of the following is the most common presentation for retinoblastoma?

    a. decreased vision.
    b. strabismus.
    c. orbital cellulitis.
    d. incidental finding.
    e. leukocoria.

183. Clinical features that are particularly helpful in the diagnosis of retinoblastoma include:

    1. spontaneous hyphema.
    2. ophthalmoscopically evident calcification.
    3. heterochromia iridis.
    4. vitreous seeding.

    a. 1, 2, and 3.
    b. 1 and 3.
    c. 2 and 4.
    d. 4 only.
    e. 1, 2, 3, and 4.

184. T or F -- Retinoblastoma that grows into the vitreous in a mushroom or spherical shape is termed exophytic.

185. Match the name of the histopathologic feature listed in the right-hand column with the light microscopic characteristics listed in the left-hand column.

a. a cluster of nearly mature-appearing photoreceptor elements.

b. a ring of nuclei surrounding parallel arranged fibrils with a central clear lumen.

c. a ring of nuclei and cell processes surrounding a blood vessel.

d. a ring of nuclei surrounding a mass of haphazardly arranged cell processes with no central lumen.

1. Flexner-Wintersteiner rosettes.
2. Homer Wright rosettes.
3. pseudorosettes.
4. fleurettes.

186. The blood vessels in a retinoblastoma may absorb released nucleic acids from the necrotic cells and take on what appearance microscopically?

a. eosinophilia.
b. basophilia.
c. fibrinoid necrosis.
d. xanthomatization.
e. congophilia.

187. T or F -- An interesting light microscopic characteristic of retinoblastoma is zonal necrosis of tumor surrounding blood vessels.

188. T or F -- The genetic implications of retinoma (retinocytoma) are identical to those of retinoblastoma.

189. Which of the following is the most common site of retinoblastoma spread outside the eye?

a. skull bones.
b. liver.
c. lymph nodes.
d. central nervous system (CNS).
e. distal bones.

190. T or F - Case reports of pineal gland neoplasms associated with retinoblastoma probably represent central nervous system metastasis.

191. Which of the following might be considered part of a workup for a patient with suspected retinoblastoma?

> 1. aqueous humor paracentesis.
> 2. CT scanning.
> 3. serum levels of carcinoembryonic antigen (CEA).
> 4. cranial magnetic resonance imaging (MRI).

a. 1, 2, and 3.
b. 1 and 3.
c. 2 and 4.
d. 4 only.
e. 1, 2, 3, and 4.

192. Metastatic workup for a patient with established retinoblastoma should include:

> 1. bone marrow biopsy.
> 2. bone scan.
> 3. lumbar puncture.
> 4. liver-spleen scan.

a. 1, 2, and 3.
b. 1 and 3.
c. 2 and 4.
d. 4 only.
e. 1, 2, 3, and 4.

193. Which one of the following regarding the treatment of retinoblastoma is false?

a. For large tumors, treatment generally includes enucleation.
b. In advanced or metastatic cases, chemotherapy is used.
c. Photocoagulation may be used for small, obviously localized tumors.
d. Cryotherapy is avoided because it typically leads to dissemination of viable tumor cells within the eye.
e. Cobalt plaque therapy has been used in eyes that have incompletely responded to external beam irradiation.

194. Match each of the fundus tumors of childhood with its systemic disorder.

a. capillary hemangioma of the retina.
b. astrocytic hamartoma of the optic nerve.
c. astrocytic hamartoma of the retina.
d. diffuse choroidal hemangioma.
e. peripheral acquired hemangioma of the retina.

1. neurofibromatosis.
2. Sturge-Weber syndrome.
3. von Hippel-Lindau disease.
4. none of the above.
5. no systemic association.

195. The typical color of a juvenile xanthogranuloma (JXG) is:

   a. black.
   b. pearly.
   c. orange.
   d. blue.
   e. salmon.

196. T or F -- The most common location of extraocular JXG is skeletal muscle.

197. T or F -- The skin lesions of JXG are generally left untreated, while iris lesions generally mandate intervention.

198. Which one of the following regarding medulloepithelioma (diktyoma) is false?

   a. The cell of origin is probably nonpigmented cilary epithelium.
   b. Like hemangiopericytoma, tumors with benign histopathologic features hide a significant metastatic potential.
   c. A teratoid variant exists that may contain cartilage, muscle, or neural tissue.
   d. Leukocoria may be the presenting finding.
   e. Enucleation before transscleral extension is frequently curative.

199. A 17-year-old girl undergoes dilated funduscopic examination after being fitted for contact lenses. A creamy orange, geographic placoid elevation deep to the retina is noted to extend superotemporally from the disc margin. There is subretinal fluid in the inferior periphery. Ultrasound reveals a very highly reflective thickening of choroid in the same region. Computed tomography reveals calcification. The most likely diagnosis is:

   a. amelanotic melanoma.
   b. choroidal hemangioma.
   c. choroidal osteoma.
   d. choroidal metastasis from an ovarian primary.
   e. regressed retinoblastoma.

200. Which of the following neoplastic disorders may involve intraocular structures?

   1. leukemia.
   2. rhabdomyosarcoma.
   3. Letter-Siwe syndrome.
   4. neuroblastoma.

   a. 1, 2, and 3.
   b. 1 and 3.
   c. 2 and 4.
   d. 4 only.
   e. 1, 2, 3, and 4.

201. T or F -- If indicated, prophylactic irradiation following the diagnosis of acute leukemia in childhood should involve both of the eyes.

202. Which of the following are found in greater than 90% of adolescents or adults with neurofibromatosis?

        1. café au lait spots.
        2. neurofibromas.
        3. Lisch nodules.
        4. gliomas.

a. 1, 2, and 3.
b. 1 and 3.
c. 2 and 4.
d. 4 only.
e. 1, 2, 3, and 4.

203. Each of the following is seen in increased frequency in patients with neurofibromatosis except:

a. malignant melanoma of the uveal tract.
b. Wilms' tumor.
c. rhabdomyosarcoma.
d. choroidal osteoma.
e. schwannomas.

204. T or F -- The light microscopic findings of Lisch nodules are indistinguishable from those of iris nevi.

205. T or F -- The optic nerve gliomas associated with neurofibromatosis generally have a poorer prognosis than isolated lesions.

206. Match the diagnostic criteria listed in the left column with the type of neurofibromatosis listed in the right column.

a. plexiform neurofibroma.
b. intertriginous freckling.
c. bilateral acoustic neuromas.
d. unilateral optic glioma.
e. first-degree relative with the same disorder plus two neurofibromas, meningiomas, gliomas, or schwannomas.
f. two or more Lisch nodules.
g. posterior subcapsular cataract.
h. sphenoidal dysplasia.

1. neurofibromatosis type 1.
2. neurofibromatosis type 2.
3. both.
4. neither.

207. Seizures, mental retardation, and facial angiofibroma form the classic triad for:

    a. neurofibromatosis.
    b. tuberous sclerosis.
    c. von Hippel-Lindau disease.
    d. ataxia-telangiectasia.
    e. Sturge-Weber syndrome.

208. T or F -- Adenoma sebaceum always presents by the end of puberty and may be confused with acne vulgaris.

209. T or F -- The complete Sturge-Weber syndrome includes facial hemangioma, ipsilateral glaucoma, and ipsilateral epilepsy.

210. T or F -- The classic fundus finding in a patient with Sturge-Weber syndrome is the focal choroidal hemangioma.

211. T or F -- The glaucoma seen ipsilateral to facial hemangioma in Sturge-Weber syndrome is due entirely to elevated episcleral venous pressure (EVP).

212. What percentage of patients with capillary hemangiomas of the retina will develop hemangioblastomas of the cerebellum?

    a. 5%.
    b. 20%.
    c. 50%.
    d. 75%.
    e. 100%.

213. T or F -- Like Sturge-Weber syndrome, iris neovascularization may complicate the course of retinal angiomatosis.

214. T or F -- The Wyburn-Mason syndrome is always unilateral.

215. Places to look for the vascular changes associated with ataxia-telangiectasia include:

    1. retroauricular skin.
    2. conjunctivae.
    3. popliteal fossae.
    4. malar skin.

    a. 1, 2, and 3.
    b. 1 and 3.
    c. 2 and 4.
    d. 4 only.
    e. 1, 2, 3, and 4.

216. Which of the following immune deviations is associated with ataxia-telangiectasia?

       1. hypogammaglobulinemia.
       2. thymus hypoplasia.
       3. monoclonal gammopathies.
       4. IgA deficiency.

  a. 1, 2, and 3.
  b. 1 and 3.
  c. 2 and 4.
  d. 4 only.
  e. 1, 2, 3, and 4.

217. T or F -- The life expectancy of patients with ataxia-telangiectasia is normal.

218. Which of the following disorders is inherited on an autosomal recessive basis?

  a. neurofibromatosis.
  b. tuberous sclerosis.
  c. Sturge-Weber syndrome.
  d. von Hippel-Lindau disease.
  e. ataxia-telangiectasia.

219. Which of the following disorders has no clear inheritance pattern?

  a. neurofibromatosis.
  b. tuberous sclerosis.
  c. Sturge-Weber syndrome.
  d. von Hippel-Lindau disease.
  e. ataxia-telangiectasia.

220. Potential ocular manifestations of the craniosynostoses include:

       1. papilledema.
       2. exposure keratitis.
       3. tortuous retinal vasculature.
       4. optic nerve hypoplasia.

  a. 1, 2, and 3.
  b. 1 and 3.
  c. 2 and 4.
  d. 4 only.
  e. 1, 2, 3, and 4.

221. The strabismus most frequently associated with the craniosynostoses is:

a. double elevator palsy.
b. Duane's syndrome.
c. V-pattern exotropia.
d. A-pattern esotropia.
e. infantile esotropia.

222. T or F -- In a patient with strabismus associated with craniosynostosis, it is best to correct the strabismus as early as possible to enhance binocular function.

223. Features of the Pierre Robin syndrome include:

1. cleft palate.
2. glossoptosis.
3. micrognathia.
4. bird face.

a. 1, 2, and 3.
b. 1 and 3.
c. 2 and 4.
d. 4 only.
e. 1, 2, 3, and 4.

224. Lower lid colobomas, pronounced antimongoloid slant (downward displacement of the lateral canthus), and orbital rim defects are typical of:

a. Hallermann-Streiff syndrome.
b. Treacher Collins syndrome.
c. Goldenhar's syndrome.
d. Waardenburg's syndrome.
e. Pierre Robin syndrome.

225. T or F -- The difference between primary telecanthus and secondary telecanthus is the presence of true hypertelorism in the former.

226. Ocular findings in the fetal alcohol syndrome include all of the following except:

a. a blepharophimosis-like picture.
b. hypertelorism.
c. anterior segment dysgeneses.
d. tortuous retinal vessels.
e. optic nerve hypoplasia.

227. In which of the following inborn errors of metabolism are corneal findings seen?

        1. MPS I-H (Hurler's syndrome).
        2. MPS III (Sanfilippo's syndrome).
        3. Fabry's disease.
        4. Tay-Sachs disease.

    a. 1, 2, and 3.
    b. 1 and 3.
    c. 2 and 4.
    d. 4 only.
    e. 1, 2, 3, and 4.

228. The pupillary light reflex can be shown to develop at approximately what age?

    a. 20 weeks' gestation.
    b. 30 weeks' gestation.
    c. 40 weeks' gestation.
    d. 4 weeks postnatally (44 weeks postconception).
    e. 8 weeks postnatally (48 weeks postconception).

229. Signs of poor vision in a 1-month-old infant might include:

        1. paradoxic pupillary response to light.
        2. oculodigital sign.
        3. fixation only on extremely bright lights.
        4. skew deviation.

    a. 1, 2, and 3.
    b. 1 and 3.
    c. 2 and 4.
    d. 4 only.
    e. 1, 2, 3, and 4.

230. An infant boy is born with a disorder not previously seen in his family, except for an older sister. Five other siblings are not affected. This is most consistent with what type of inheritance?

    a. autosomal dominant.
    b. autosomal recessive.
    c. X-linked dominant.
    d. X-linked recessive.
    e. mitochondrial.

231. Disorders to be considered in a neonate with very poor vision and a normal ocular examination include:

        1. Lowe's syndrome.
        2. achromatopsia.
        3. optic nerve hypoplasia.
        4. Leber's congential amaurosis.

    a. 1, 2, and 3.
    b. 1 and 3.
    c. 2 and 4.
    d. 4 only.
    e. 1, 2, 3, and 4.

232. Which of the following tests will always be normal in severe unilateral optic nerve hypoplasia?

    a. visual acuity test.
    b. swinging flashlight test.
    c. electroretinography.
    d. visual evoked responses.
    e. fluorescein angiography.

233. Ocular disorders associated with optic nerve hypoplasia include:

        1. albinism.
        2. aniridia.
        3. coloboma.
        4. Duane's syndrome.

    a. 1, 2, and 3.
    b. 1 and 3.
    c. 2 and 4.
    d. 4 only.
    e. 1, 2, 3, and 4.

234. T or F -- If a child's nystagmus has a rotary component, congenital nystagmus may be eliminated from the differential diagnosis.

235. Which of the following disorders should be considered in the differential diagnosis of congenital nystagmus associated with photophobia?

               1. oculocutaneous albinism.
               2. Leber's congenital amaurosis.
               3. achromatopsia.
               4. cystinosis.

a. 1, 2, and 3.
b. 1 and 3.
c. 2 and 4.
d. 4 only.
e. 1, 2, 3, and 4.

Answers

1.   c.   Axial length increases most rapidly over the first 4 years of life and more slowly thereafter until age 10 to 12 years.

2.   c.   The lens is proportionately the largest part of the infant eye.

3.   True.   Corneal diameters greater than 13 mm are termed megalocornea.

4.   d.

5.   False.   The optic nerve is generally myelinated to the lamina cribrosa 4 to 6 months <u>before</u> foveal maturation.

6.   a.   Acuity estimates are highest with VEP. OKN and PLT are fairly close. OKN is more cumbersome and difficult to quantify accurately than PLT.

7.   False.   VEP documents 20/20 acuity by age 6 to 8 months. PLT cannot document 20/20 until 24 to 30 months.

8.   False.   The globe obscured by the fused lids is typically disorganized.

9.   a.   The <u>upper</u> lids are more frequently involved. Other features include limbal dermoids, branchial cleft abnormalities and vertebral anomalies.

10.   False.   The <u>lower</u> lids are more frequently involved by congenital ectropion and congenital entropion.

11.   True.

12.   False.   There are <u>four</u> varieties of epicanthus:

                1. palpebralis (simple) -- broader <u>above</u>
                2. inversus -- broader <u>below</u>
                3. tarsalis -- equally broad above and below
                4. supraciliaris -- origin from <u>eyebrow</u>

13.   False.   Hypertelorism implies an abnormally wide distance between medial <u>orbital</u> walls. Telecanthus is an abnormally wide distance between medial <u>canthi</u>. Telecanthus may be isolated (primary) or secondary to hypertelorism!

14.   c.   Epicanthus <u>inversus</u> and telecanthus are the other components of this tetrad. Ectropion or euryblepharon is seen in some cases, as well.

15.   b.   Seventy percent of pregnant women are seronegative. Placental transfer of organism is common in the newly infected mother; however, many infected infants will <u>not</u> have systemic manifestations.

16.   True.

17. a.   Microphthalmos and cataracts are rare. Focal chorioretinal lesions are common. Diffuse retinopathy is not seen.

18. c.   IgG against toxoplasma found in the infant's serum is probably <u>maternal</u> and may reflect <u>old</u> maternal infection. IgM, on the other hand, does <u>not</u> cross the placenta and probably represents a response to fetal infection. CT evidence is very strong.

19. e.   Pyrimethamine (Daraprim) and sulfadiazine are antimicrobial agents effective against <u>Toxoplasma</u>. Prednisone reduces inflammatory tissue destruction. Pyrimethamine blocks synthesis of folinic acid, so it must be given as well. Note that folinic acid is synthesized from dietary folic acid, so folic acid administration is not sufficient!

20. d.   The later in the course of the pregnancy a mother is infected, the lower is the chance of fetal infection, and if infection occurs, the lower the likelihood of symptomatic defects. Infection early in pregancy leads to a <u>high</u> rate of abnormalities. Thanks to vaccinations (MMR), most mothers in developed countries are seropositive (protected).

21. c.   Many cases of "oculoauditory syndrome" are due to rubella.

22. c.   While children with congenital rubella syndrome may develop either cataract <u>or</u> glaucoma, their coincidence in an infant is rare.

23. e.   Virus in lens material can lead to rebound uveitis after cataract extraction.

24. d.   Excessive rebound uveitis is due to live virus retained within residual lens cortex.

25. c.   Approximately 2% of human infants are infected. Most cases are silent.

26. c.

27. False.   Most neonatal herpes is contracted at the time of delivery due to passage through an infected birth canal.

28. True.

29. False.   Most cases of congenital herpes declare themselves with vesicular dermatitis, keratoconjunctivitis, pneumonitis, or meningoencephalitis.

30. False.   A posterior inflammatory component is far more common in congenital disease, with severe retinitis and vitritis. This is unusual in acquired disease but may be the cause of some cases of acute retinal necrosis.

31. a.   Herpes simplex is generally transmitted at the time of birth as the child passes through an infected birth canal.

32. a.   Microphthalmia is an unusual manifestation of congenital syphilis.

33. a.   Rhagades, linear scars around the mouth, are characteristic of congenital lues, but not a part of Hutchinson's triad.

34. a. 4. The time of onset of neonatal conjunctivitides after birth is important. Silver
    b. 3. nitrate prophylaxis (medicamentosa) tends to present earliest, followed by
    c. 1, 2. gonococcus, herpes simplex, and chlamydiae. Gonorrhea must be treated with
    d. 2. intravenous antibiotics, while inclusion conjunctivitis may be eradicated with oral
    e. 3. antibiotics. Intravenous acyclovir is now used for all forms of neonatal herpes
    f. 1. simplex virus infections. Mild topical antibiotics, or no treatment at all, is sufficient
    g. 3. for chemical conjunctivitis.
    h. 2.
    i. 3.
    j. 2.
    k. 4.

35. a. *S. pyogenes* is an infrequent cause. *S. aureus*, *S. pneumococcus*, and *H. influenzae*
    are far more common.

36. a. Pharyngoconjunctival fever generally spares the cornea, although subepithelial
    infiltrates or superficial punctate keratitis may rarely be seen.

Both EKC + PCF are caused by Adenovirus type 3.

37. False. A self-limited conjunctivitis is very common but frequently obscured by other, more
    prominent symptoms and signs.

38. e. The inflammation in Parinaud's syndrome is always granulomatous.

39. a. The most common cause is minor skin trauma.

40. d.

41. b. Ethmoid sinusitis is the leading risk factor for the development of orbital cellulitis.

42. d. Cavernous sinus inflammation causes cranial nerve dysfunction without proptosis,
    leading to a sudden worsening of ocular motility without other changes in the
    examination.

43. b. Boys are more frequently involved than girls, and the upper tarsal conjunctiva is more
    commonly and more severely involved than the lower.

44. d. True follicles are rare in vernal disease, while eosinophils are numerous. Both
    conditions may have prominent limbal nodules (limbal papillae and Horner-Trantas
    dots in vernal, limbal follicles in trachoma). Trachoma scars extensively, while vernal
    rarely does.

45. False. The limbal lesions in vernal keratoconjunctivitis are more papilliform, since they have
    a central vascular core. When a central pit full of degenerated eosinophils forms, the
    term <u>Horner-Trantas dot</u> is applied.

46. False. Horner-Trantas dots are clumps of degenerated eosinophils, while Herbert's pits are
    depressed, necrotic follicles at the limbus.

47. True. Many experts have maintained that corneal vernal disease rarely, if ever, leads to
    vascularization of the cornea. Superficial vascularization is far more common with
    trachoma, but it has been reported to occur in severe vernal keratoconjunctivitis, as
    well.

48. a. Deep corneal vascularization is unlikely in vernal disease. So-called shield ulcers -- large oval, central epithelial defects--are classic corneal manifestations of the disease.

49. False. Debridement of giant palpebral papillae has been tried therapeutically, in an attempt to speed reepithelialization of shield ulcers. Typically, this fails, indicating that some factor other than mechanical irritation is at play. Some experts have suggested that inflammatory factors released by diseased conjunctiva may be responsible.

50. c. Stevens-Johnson syndrome can affect patients of all age and typically causes target-shaped macular, rather than vesicular, dermatitis. The mucous membrane lesions are vesicular.

51. e. Other diagnostic criteria include injected pharynx, edema of upper or lower extremities, nonspecific rash, and lymphadenopathy. Fever plus four of the other criteria must be present to make the diagnosis.

52. c. The vasculitis may involve the coronary arteries and lead to coronary artery aneurysm or occlusion.

53. b. The medial canthal tendon straddles the <u>superior</u> one-third of the nasolacrimal sac. Thus distention of the sac due to obstruction presents as a mass <u>below</u> the tendon.

54. c. Dacryocele, or congenital mucocele of the nasolacrimal sac, typically has a bluish-red hue, similar to a hemangioma, and results from chronic obstructive tear stasis. Recurrent conjunctivitis is far more common than dacryocystitis. Obstruction is nearly always at the inferior extreme of the nasolacrimal duct--the valve of Hasner (within the inferior nasal meatus). If it persists beyond 1 year of age, surgical intervention is generally required.

55. True. Failure is generally followed by a repeat probing and irrigation. If this fails a second time, then Silastic intubation is tried. If this also fails, then dacryocystorhinostomy is the next step.

56. False. The corneal endothelium and stroma are neural crest-derived, but the epithelium is derived from surface ectoderm!

57. True. If horizontal diameters exceed 13 mm with no other detectable abnormalities, then the term <u>megalocornea</u> may be applied.

58. False. Keratoconus is associated with Marfan's syndrome. Keratoglobus is associated with Ehlers-Danlos syndrome.

59. b. Scheie's syndrome, or MPS I-S, is a mucopolysaccharidosis, an inborn error of metabolism. Each of the other disorders is a "neurocristopathy."

60. b. CHED occurs secondary to a defect of the corneal endothelium and Descemet's membrane. Although the corneal edema may resemble that seen in congenital glaucoma, there is no elevated intraocular pressure or increased corneal diameter.

61. c. In CHSD, the cloudy stroma is of normal thickness, and the epithelium is normal. In CHED, there is epithelial edema and a thickened stroma. In both conditions, IOP is usually normal.

62. a. 3.
      b. 1.
      c. 2.
      d. 3.
      e. 2.
      f. 2.
      g. 1.
      h. 3.

63. False.   Cystine crystals may be found in the cornea, conjunctiva, and uvea.

64. c.   Corneal ulceration and scarring in familial dysautonomia (Riley-Day syndrome) is secondary to decreased or absent corneal sensation and decreased lacrimation.

65. a.   Approximately two-thirds of the cases of infantile glaucoma are bilateral, and approximately two-thirds are boys. An affected parent has about a 5% chance of having a child with infantile glaucoma, and the next subsequent sibling has approximately a 5% chance of being affected. The incidence of open-angle glaucoma in grandparents is no different from age-matched controls.

66. False.   There is controversy regarding the basic pathophysiologic mechanism underlying the cause of infantile glaucoma. Many anomalies in and around the chamber angle have been described. Barkan's theory involves the presence of an imperforate membrane covering the angle. This is probably only true in certain cases.

67. e.

68. False.   Ruptures in Descemet's membrane associated with infantile glaucoma are usually horizontal, and those associated with birth trauma are usually vertical.

69. True.   This is probably true because younger infants spend most of the day with their eyes closed, making corneal enlargement difficult to detect.

70. False.   While optic nerve cupping in infants may be reversible, the presence of an afferent pupillary defect carries a poor visual prognosis.

71. a.   Medication is used only for preoperative control of intraocular pressure in children. Definitive management consists of surgery.

72. a.   Optic cupping is reversible in children. Afferent pupillary defects generally indicate irreversible optic nerve damage.

73. d.   Rubella IgM titers might be of value in a neonate, but IgG titers are not diagnostic, since they are of <u>maternal</u> origin during the first 3 to 6 months of life. Glaucoma is not a feature of galactosemia or Refsum's disease. Lowe's syndrome must be considered.

74. b.   Ketamine and succinylcholine elevate IOP. Ketamine only does so at high doses. Succinylcholine does so by triggering undirected extraocular muscle contractions (fasciculations).

75. False.   Unlike adults, pressures in children over 20 mm Hg are suspicious for glaucoma.

76. b. All inherited forms are typically bilateral, but recessive forms may be asymmetric. Dominant varieties may not present until the third, fourth, fifth, or sixth decades.

77. c. Autosomal dominant patterns are most frequently reported, but 15% have no family history. Aortic valvular insufficiency and aneurysm may be life-threatening and should be treated with cardiac depressants and/or surgery. Mitral valve prolapse may also be found. Myopia, high astigmatism, or frank keratoconus is seen in association with ectopia lentis in many cases.

78. c. Homocystinuria is an elastosis and leads to hypercoagulability with thrombotic vascular occlusions. The elastosis also causes defective zonular function and ectopia lentis in 90% of patients. It is inherited on an autosomal recessive basis.

79. c. Mentation is typically normal in Sturge-Weber syndrome, while ectopia lentis is unusual in Down's syndrome (except after trauma).

80. c. Bilaterality makes a systemic condition more likely. Monocular cataracts rarely herald significant systemic derangements. Anterior lenticonus may be part of Lowe's syndrome, but isolated posterior lenticonus is usually isolated. Pigmentary retinopathy raises the possibility of congenital infections.

81. d. Congenital cataract formation secondary to a materal herpes simplex virus infection would be extremely unusual, since infection is typically acquired at birth.

82. d. Monocular visual deprivation, most likely with nuclear cataract, is the most "amblyogenic." Every visually significant infantile cataract should be operated on as soon as it is feasible.

83. d. Because of the high incidence of capsular opacification, many surgeons advocate primary posterior capsulotomy (at the time of cataract extraction).

84. e. A complete systemic evaluation of a patient with bilateral congenital cataracts should rule out congenital rubella infection, hypocalcemia, Lowe's syndrome, and trisomies.

85. a. 3.   f. 1.
    b. 4.   g. 5.
    c. 7.   h. 8.
    d. 9.   i. 2.
    e. 10. j. 6.

86. e. There is a pediatric uveitis identical to JRA with no previous history of joint disease, but this is generally considered as a separate disorder.

87. d. Pauciarticular, early-onset patients are most likely to develop uveitis, but they are generally ANA positive, RF negative. Uveitis is rare in Still's disease, which is more common in boys.

88. b. The symptoms of chronic uveitis in JRA may be minimal. As a result, routine examinations should be frequent to avoid amblyopia from undetected sequelae (cataract, keratopathy). Placement of an IOL is absolutely contraindicated following cataract surgery in these patients because of the aggressive postoperative inflammation aggravated by an IOL.

89. a.

90. d.   In immunocompromised patients, a high risk of systemic spread with severe complications exists and may be more likely if systemic steroids are used. Topical steroids may be used in immunocompromised patients.

91. True.   Although keratitis is not universal in patients with HSV uveitis, it is usually present in affected children.

92. True.

93. b.   Up to 50% of pediatric patients with posterior uveitis have ocular toxoplasmosis.

94. c.   The brain and retina (a part of the brain) are the sites where toxoplasma organisms survive best.

95. a.   Acute arthritis is not a typical finding in acquired systemic toxoplasmosis.

96. True.   The anterior flare-up may occur without obvious reactivation of retinal disease.

97. c.   In ocular histoplasmosis, there is no vitreous inflammation.

98. a.   The infectious cycle generally starts with a child consuming sand or dirt contaminated by the feces of a house pet that ingested the organism (dogs more often than cats). A peripheral granuloma with overlying vitreous opacification and chronic uveitis are typical findings in toxocarosis. The uveitis may die down and leave a quiescent peripheral granuloma. The inflammation in the eye often flares after the larva dies, and corticosteroids are the drug of choice in the treatment of this condition.

99. a.   Pars planitis is bilateral in about 75% of cases. Lyme disease or syphilis may be the underlying cause, but the work-up is usually negative.

100. d.   The number of aqueous cells in the anterior chamber, and not the amount of flare, should be the basis for treatment with topical steroids. Topical steroid may worsen cataract and will not reverse band keratopathy.

101. d.   PHPV occurs frequently in small eyes, while retinoblastoma rarely occurs in association with microphthalmia.

102. d.   Studies of the natural history of ROP show that 65% of premature infants with birth weight less than 1250 gm will develop some stage of the disease.

103. False. Vascularization of the nasal retina is complete by (approximately) the eighth gestational month. The temporal retina is completely vascularized 1 to 2 months later.

104. False. The risk of ROP does not correlate with the postdelivery age but with gestational age (postconception age).

105. b.   Although increased oxygen tension has been implicated in the pathogensis of ROP, the correlation with disease severity is not direct. Athough NEC shares similar risk factors with ROP (low birth weight), no known pathologic connection exists between the two conditions.

106. False.   Zone 1 is a circle of <u>radius</u> 30 degrees (twice the distance from optic disc to macula) centered on the optic disc. Zone 2 extends to the nasal ora and the temporal equator (radius 60 degrees). Zone 3 is the remaining crescent-shaped region anterior to zone 2 in the temporal retina.

107. e.   All of these criteria together define subjects shown to benefit from cryotherapy.

108. e.   All of these complications can occur from ROP. Pseudostrabismus results from a change in angle kappa due to macular ectopia from peripheral cicatrization. Pseudoexotropia is more common than pseudoesotropia.

109. e.   No reports of ROP developing before 30 weeks of gestational age have been made, so screening before that time is not performed. The risk of ROP in babies greater than 1500 gm is very low, so screening is not required. Examinations should be done every 2 weeks unless stage 3 prethreshold ROP is found, in which case examinations should be done at least weekly.

110. b.   Coats' disease is more commonly unilateral than bilateral. Abnormal vessels must be present, either by direct examination or fluorescein angiography, to make the diagnosis of Coats' disease.

111. False.   The incidence of juvenile cataracts appears to be higher in patients with poorly controlled diabetes.

112. d.   Optic nerve hypoplasia, particularly segmental, is more common in children of mothers with diabetes. Central vision is usually good, but sector or altitudinal field defects are frequently present.

113. b.   Flame-shaped nerve fiber hemorrhages are the one most common funduscopic finding. White-centered hemorrhages (Roth's spots), cotton-wool spots, optic disc swelling, and perivascular infiltration may also be seen but are less common. Choroidal infiltration is usually not ophthalmoscopically apparent.

114. False.   Permanent loss of central acuity may occur rapidly with leukemic involvement of the optic nerve. Radiation therapy should be undertaken (within 24-48 hours) on an emergent basis is such cases.

115. True.   The administration of chemotherapeutic agents to patients with leukemia makes the optic nerve more susceptible to radiation optic neuropathy than other eyes. Radiation dosage may need to be adjusted accordingly.

116. e.   Glaucoma may occur due to posterior synechiae formation with increased relative pupillary block or pupillary seclusion, from tumor cells clogging the trabecular meshwork or from spontaneous hyphema. Cataract may occur secondary to inflammation or radiation therapy.

117. b.   All of the gangliosidoses are autosomal recessive diseases. Most patients die in their first decade.

118. c.   The most common ocular disorder associated with Lowe's syndrome is a characteristic small, thick, opaque cataract.

119. a.   Diffuse arteriolar attenuation is not a characteristic finding in renal failure, although it may occur if there is severe associated hypertension.

120. False.   It is felt that <u>fewer</u> ganglion cells decussate at the chiasm than in normal subjects.

121. True.   Albino patients with the tyrosinase-negative variety usually have severe photophobia and nystagmus. Visual acuity is usually less than 20/200. As the name implies, tyrosinase-negative albinos have no tyrosinase enzyme in their hair shafts or skin.

122. False.   Extensive vitreous syneresis, vitreous veils, and strands are common features of X-linked juvenile retinoschisis.

123. c.   The EOG is abnormal in Goldmann-Favre disease and normal in X-linked juvenile retinoschisis. Goldmann-Favre disease is autosomal recessive. Both diseases have abnormal ERGs. In mild forms of juvenile retinoschisis, the scotopic b-wave is lost, with preservation of the a-wave. In severe cases, the ERG is extinguished, as it is in most cases of Goldmann-Favre. Both diseases are characterized by foveal and peripheral retinoschisis, as well as retinal pigment epithelial disturbances, although the latter are more severe in Goldmann-Favre.

124. e.   Some forms of tapetoretinal degeneration can have prominent subretinal exudation and mimic Coats' disease.

125. False.   Although electrophysiologic testing may show diffuse retinal involvement in sector retinitis pigmentosa, the condition rarely progresses, and the prognosis is good. This is reflected in normal b-wave implicit times.

126. b.   Cone dystrophy is the most common bull's-eye maculopathy.

127. a.   Retinitis punctata albescens is <u>not</u> a form of CSNB but is progressive (albeit more slowly than typical retinitis pigmentosa).

128. True.   With complete rod monochromatism, acuity is typically 20/200. With blue cone monochromatism, acuities are 20/40 to 20/200.

129. e.   The oculodigital sign refers to a tendency to gouge the eyes with a finger or fist. It is felt that afflicted patients do this to provide entopic stimulation of the neurosensory retina. Five to 10% of patients with Leber's congenital amaurosis have associated hearing loss.

130. False.   The presenting symptom is usually decreased central visual acuity.

131. True.   Central vision is usually preserved in the pattern dystrophies.

132. a.   Aicardi syndrome is limited to females because it is X-linked <u>dominant</u>. It is lethal in male infants or fetuses.

133. False.   Most cases of morning glory disc have poor vision. The condition is usually unilateral and may be associated with cranial vault abnormalities. It is more common in girls.

134. True.   Nonrhegmatogenous retinal detachments occur with optic nerve pits, primarily involving the macula.

135. False. Myelination of the optic nerve begins at the lateral geniculate ganglion, not at the optic chiasm. Myelination of the nerve is completed within a month of birth. Some studies claim it is complete to the lamina cribrosa by 1 month before birth; others claim 1 month after.

136. True. This condition occurs bilaterally in 20% of cases.

137. a. The visual field defects usually correspond to the area of fundus ectasia (inferior or inferonasal) and are consequently in the upper temporal field. They often cross the midline, unlike chiasmal defects.

138. a. DeMorsier's syndrome (septo-optic dysplasia) is far more common in bilateral optic nerve hypoplasia. Most authorities feel that neuro-imaging should be conducted in both unilateral and bilateral optic nerve hypoplasia.

139. c. Optic nerve pits are usually in the inferotemporal quadrant or central part of the disc.

140. c. Both CT scanning and ultrasonography will reveal the presence of disc drusen, if calcified. Red free photographs are of no value. However, disc drusen do autofluoresce on fluorescein angiography. To elicit this, fluorescein barrier filters must be used with no injection. The visual fields of chronic papilledema and disc drusen may appear similar and are of less value.

141. False. Devic's disease, or neuromyelitis optica, is considered by most experts as an entity separate from multiple sclerosis. It is characterized by acute optic neuritis (usually bilateral) and transverse myelitis. Visual prognosis is much poorer for this optic neuritis than for typical optic neuritis.

142. b. The tumors produce osteolysis, not osteosclerosis.

143. e. Depending on the extent of the disease, any or all of these treatments may be useful.

144. b. Children of age less than 2 years with multifocal disease (especially compromise of liver, lung, or hematopoiesis) have a poor prognosis.

145. a. The distinction between fibrous dysplasia and ossifying fibroma is generally made histologically. If osteoblasts are present, then the lesion is called an ossifying fibroma; if absent, the term fibrous dysplasia is applied.

146. d. Blood stagnation and phleboliths are characteristic of cavernous, not capillary, hemangiomas.

147. False. The pathology reveals dilated capillaries without the endothelial cell proliferation characterizing capillary hemangioma. This accounts for their flat clinical appearance.

148. a. Surgery is not prudent unless absolutely necessary, as these tumors are difficult to remove completely and have a propensity to hemorrhage.

149. a.

150. e. Wilm's tumor, neuroblastoma, and rhabdomyosarcoma are the three most common solid pediatric maligancies. Leukemia is the most common of all pediatric malignancies.

151. True. An unexplained mass in the lids or acquired ptosis in a child should prompt radio-imaging to rule out rhabdomyosarcoma.

152. b. Differentiated rhabdomyosarcoma in the least common type but has the best prognosis.

153. e. Exenteration is reserved for treatment failures and recurrences.

154. c. A minority of patients with neurofibromatosis (1.5%) will develop a schwannoma. It rarely undergoes malignant degeneration. The two classic histologic appearances are Antoni A (regular arrangement of eosinophilic spindle cells with palisading nuclei) and Antoni B (haphazardly arranged stellate cells in a myxomatous matrix). Perineural spread and compression account for pain.

155. d. Plexiform neurofibroma is most specific for neurofibromatosis. Unlike schwannomas, neurofibromas grow independent of peripheral nerves. In addition, they are generally osteolytic.

156. b. Schwann cells (neural crest derivatives) may be seen in both neurilemmomas and neurofibromas. Positive staining for S-100 is characteristic of any cell derived from the neural crest. Thus, this will also be seen in both lesions.

157. e. Pathologically, these are pilocytic astrocytomas of the juvenile type.

158. c. Optic gliomas are usually benign in children. If the tumor is located within the orbit, observation may be appropriate. On the other hand, if the tumor is posterior (chiasm, optic tract), radiation therapy may be appropriate to avoid hydrocephalus and damage to contiguous CNS structures.

159. False. Radiographically, meningiomas produce hyperplastic bony changes (although bone destruction can be seen).

160. a. The tumor presents with metastases in about one-third of patients.

161. a. Enophthalmos is characteristically seen with metastatic scirrhous carcinoma of the breast in adult women.

162. d. Homer Wright rosettes are usually not seen in orbital metastases, being limited to the better differentiated primary tumor.

163. c. Even with metastastes to the liver, bone marrow, and spleen, survival may be as high as 84%. Bone metastasis is a poor prognostic factor. Age at onset is the most powerful predictor of survival.

164. c. Opsoclonus ("dancing eyes") is the paraneoplastic syndrome most commonly associated with metastatic neuroblastoma.

165. b. Ewing's sarcoma is a primary intramedullary malignancy of bone, and periocular metastasis usually presents with proptosis, hemorrhage, and inflammation from tumor necrosis. It occurs in 10 to 25 year olds, older than the population with neuroblastoma. Usually there is no globe involvement, and treatment is principally chemotherapy, although radiation to remote sites has been used with some success.

166. b.

Answers

167. b.   The most common location is the superotemporal orbital rim, in association with the zygomatic-frontal suture line.

168. c.   In children, one-third of pseudotumor is bilateral but is rarely associated with systemic disease. One-half of patients have headache, abdominal pain, or lethargy. In addition, peripheral blood and local tissue eosinophilia are more common in children.

169. d.   One study of 302 epibulbar lesions removed from children less than 15 years old reported the following frequencies:

CHORISTOMAS 33% → Dermoid 19%
                    Dermolipom - 10%

nevus - 29%
dermoid- 19%
epithelial inclusion cyst - 11%
dermolipoma - 10%
pyogenic granuloma - 6%

170. a.   Goldenhar-Gorlin syndrome features limbal and conjunctival dermoids with upper lid colobomas, preauricular appendages, aural fistulas, and vertebral deformities. It is a syndromic abnormality of branchial arch development.

171. False.   Approximately 30% of epibulbar dermoids have associated systemic and ocular findings.

172. False.   Dermolipomas are often closely associated with extraocular muscles or lacrimal gland, and complete surgical excision is difficult.

173. a.   Retinoblastoma occurs in approximately 1 in 20,000 births. Only 6% have positive family history. The familial tumors appear to be inherited in an autosomal dominant pattern with 80% penetrance. Genetic counseling is complex, but bilateral retinoblastoma probably represents a genetic mutation.

174. False.   As in question 113, the inheritance pattern appears to be autosomal dominant with 80 to 90% penetrance. Thus, the offspring of a patient with bilateral retinoblastoma has approximately a 40% chance of developing a tumor (80% of 50%).

175. b.   The locus of the responsible gene is located on 13q14, and the defect must occur on both chromosomes 13 (recessive), consistent with Knudson's hypothesis. The absence of the growth regulatory gene results in the expression of the retinoblastoma. The retinoblastoma gene is likely expressed in other tissues as well. In particular, the pineal gland tumors accompanying some bilateral retinoblastoma are felt to be primary tumor and not metastasis. Musculoskeletal and integumentary systems are at increased risk of malignancy.

176. c.   With no family history and healthy parents, this child probably suffered a germ-line mutation of chromosome 13. His parents' copies are probably normal. Again, genetic counseling is complex, but the following generalizations serve as guidelines:

1. Healthy parents with one affected child have a 6% chance of producing more affected children.
2. If two or more siblings are affected, this implies a chromosomal defect in one parent. Thus, each additional child has a 40% chance of inheriting the tumor.
3. A parent with bilateral retinoblastoma has a 50% chance of transmitting the affected chromosome to his/her children. With 80% penetrance, 40% of offspring will be affected phenotypically.

177. d.   See answer 176.

178. d.   See answer 176.

179. e.   Patients who are postradiation therapy for retinoblastoma are susceptible to many malignancies, including all of the listed tumors but most notably osteogenic sarcoma.

180. True.   Life expectancy is markedly diminished.

181. c.   Although the presenting symptoms and signs depend on the extent of the tumor, the frequency of some of the presenting signs and symptoms are summarized below, with leukocoria and strabismus presenting the majority of the presentations:

leukocoria - 60%
strabismus - 22%
decreased vision - 5%
incidental finding - 4%
orbital cellulitis - 2%

182. e.

183. c.   Two diagnostic features of retinoblastoma are chalky white deposits on the tumor (which represent calcifications) and multiple clumps of tumor cells floating in the vitreous (vitreous seeding).

184. False.   Growth into the vitreous is termed endophytic. Growth outward from the retina through sclera is exophytic.

185. a. 4.   Note that Flexner-Wintersteiner rosettes are more specific for retinoblastoma
      b. 1.   than Homer Wright rosettes.
      c. 3.
      d. 2.

186. b.   Given the acidic nature of nuclei acids, they will be basophilic.

187. False.   The rapid tumor growth exceeds the blood supply. Necrosis occurs with preservation of cells around blood vessels.

188. True.   Although the course of retinoma is benign, the fellow eye may show a retinoblastoma, and the genetic implications are identical.

189. d.   Direct spread into the optic nerve and CNS is most common. Bone metastasis is seen in over one-half of metastatic cases. Lymph node metastases are second most common.

190. False.   This relationship is common enough to be labeled "trilateral" retinoblastoma and likely represents a primary malignancy of the pineal gland.

191. e.   CT scanning and ultrasonography are standard, since they can demonstrate otherwise undetectable calcifications. MRI is helpful in determining the extent of tumor spread. Serum levels of CEA may be elevated in large tumors. Paracentesis is not a typical part of the work-up but may be used in difficult cases to show an elevated level of lactate dehydrogenase in aqueous humor (relative to serum levels).

192. a.

193. d.   Cryotherapy is as effective as photocoagulation for small tumors difficult to manage with photocoagulation.

194. a. 3.   Capillary hemangioma of the retina may be accompanied by intracranial
     b. 1.   hemangioblastomas and other systemic tumors in von Hippel-Lindau disease.
     c. 1.   Glial tumors of the retina and and optic disc such as astrocytic hamartoma of the
     d. 2.   optic disc and retina are seen with tuberous sclerosis but may also be associated
     e. 5.   with neurofibromatosis. Diffuse choroidal hemangioma can be associated with Sturge-Weber syndrome.

195. c.   The combination of high lipid content (yellow) and vascularity (red) leads to the color of these benign growths. They can also be yellow-brown, especially when located on the iris.

196. False.   Skin lesions are more common than those in skeletal muscle.

197. True.   The risk of spontaneous hyphema from iris lesions is high enough to prompt treatment.

198. b.   The only medulloepitheliomas associated with significant metastic risk are those that extend into the orbit.

199. c.   This is a classic description of a choroidal osteoma. These tumors are composed of mature bone; they commonly become yellow-white by the late teenage years (secondary to overlying RPE atrophy).

200. b.   Both of these neoplasms can involve the choroid. The other two are primarily extraocular/orbital neoplasms.

201. True.   The highly vascular uveal tissues are common sites for leukemic infiltration.

202. a.   Gliomas and other CNS neoplasms (aside from neurofibromas) are found in less than 10% of patients with this disorder.

203. d.   Cutaneous melanoma does not appear to be more frequent.

204. True.   Lisch nodules, like nevi, are composed of groups of benign, nevus-type melanocytes.

205. False.   These gliomas are more "hamartomatous" and less neoplastic than isolated glioma.

206. a. 1.   e. 3.
     b. 1.   f. 1.
     c. 2.   g. 2.
     d. 1.   h. 1.

207. b.   Adenoma sebaceum consists microscopically of an angiofibroma.

208. True.

209. False.   The seizures are contralateral (secondary to the presence of leptomeningeal hemangioma overlying the ipsilateral cerebral convexity).

210. False.   <u>Diffuse</u> choroidal hemangioma is classic, leading to the so-called tomato - catsup fundus. Focal choroidal hemangioma is also seen in this disorder but is more frequently isolated.

211. False.   This is a leading candidate for the etiology, but it has not been shown to be the sole cause (or even a definitive primary cause). Some patients have less elevated EVP with an angle anomaly. Rubeosis may occur later in the disease course, as well.

212. b.

213. True.   In Sturge-Weber syndrome, the retina overlying a diffuse hemangioma may develop serous detachment or ischemia and provoke neovascularization. In retinal angiomatosis, the cause tends to be serous detachment of the retina secondary to leakage at the capillary hemangioma.

214. True.

215. e.

216. c.

217. False.   Patients with ataxia-telangiectasia tend to die from recurrent respiratory infections or leukemia/lymphoma before reaching middle age.

218. e.   The others are autosomal dominant, except for Sturge-Weber syndrome which is sporadic.   *WYBURN MASON Has No Hereditary inheritance either!*

219. c.   See answer 218.

220. a.   Optic nerve atrophy -- from chronically high intracranial pressure or abnormalities of the optic canal -- has been described, but hypoplasia is not a common finding.

221. c.

222. False.   Abnormalities in the development and origins of the extraocular muscles make correction of the strabismus very difficult; furthermore, should reconstructive surgery for the orbits be necessary, as is often the case, any good results obtained from muscle surgery would almost certainly be ruined.

223. a.   The findings of this deformity/anomaly are present in a number of specific syndromes.

224. b.

225. False.   Primary telecanthus is an increased distance between the medial canthi that is the result of soft-tissue abnormality alone; secondary telecanthus is, as the name implies, caused by an underlying process such as hypertelorism (in which the medial walls of the bony orbits are actually further apart).

226. b.   Primary telecanthus may be seen, but not hypertelorism (See #225).

227. b.   Marked corneal clouding is seen with Hurler's syndrome, and a spiral or whorl pattern (cornea verticillata) is associated with Fabry's disease.

228. b.

229. a.   Skew deviation may occur without reason for alarm during the early perinatal period. The other signs are of great concern.

230. b.   The disorder could not be dominant, or at least one of the parents would have had it. X-linked recessive is unlikely, because the children's father would have had to have the phenotype for the daughter to inherit it (she would need two affected X chromosomes). Some previous history, in the maternal lineage, would be necessary to support a mitochondrial mode of inheritance; also, one would expect more affected siblings.

231. c.   Achromatopsia, with few or no functioning cones, and Leber's congenital amaurosis, with few or no functioning photoreceptors, cause severe visual compromise. While it may be subtle, hypoplastic optic nerves usually appear small on examination. Lowe's syndrome should feature an abnormal examination (cataracts or glaucoma).

232. c.   The photoreceptors should not be affected, and the ERG will be normal.

233. e.

234. False.   A rotary component is a common finding in congenital nystagmus.

235. b.   Nystagmus is prominent in Leber's congenital amaurosis, but photophobia would be extremely unusual. Photophobia is prominent in cystinosis, but unless there are other complicating features, nystagmus would not be expected.

References

1. Richard, James. "Section 6: Pediatric Ophthalmology and Strabismus." in F.M. Wilson (ed.). Basic and Clinical Science Course. San Francisco: American Academy of Ophthalmology, 1991-1992.

2. Taylor, David (ed.). Pediatric Ophthalmology. Boston: Blackwell Scientific Publications, 1990.

6: Orbit and Oculoplastic Surgery

1. T or F -- The medial walls of each orbit are parallel.

2. T or F -- The lateral walls of each orbit are parallel.

3. T or F -- The widest dimension of the orbit is at the anterior orbital rim.

4. T or F -- The volume of the average human orbit is approximately 2 tablespoons (30 cc).

5. Match the combinations of bones listed in the left-hand column with the wall of the orbit to which they contribute listed in the right-hand column.

   a. zygomatic, greater wing of sphenoid.   1. orbital roof.
   b. maxillary, palatine, and zygomatic.   2. lateral orbital wall.
   c. frontal, lesser wing of sphenoid.   3. medial orbital wall.
   d. ethmoid, lacrimal, sphenoid, and maxillary.   4. orbital floor.

6. Match the orbital structures listed in the left-hand column with the orbital wall that contains them listed in the right-hand column.

   a. infraorbital groove.   1. orbital roof.
   b. lacrimal gland fossa, trochlea.   2. lateral orbital wall.
   c. lacrimal sac fossa.   3. medial orbital wall.
   d. orbital tubercle of Whitnall.   4. orbital floor.

7. The globe is least protected by the orbit, and thus most vulnerable to trauma:

   a. superiorly.
   b. laterally.
   c. inferiorly.
   d. medially.
   e. the globe is equally protected on all four sides.

8. The strongest orbital wall is the:

   a. roof.
   b. medial wall.
   c. floor.
   d. lateral wall.
   e. all four walls are equally strong.

9. The weakest orbital wall is the:

   a. roof.
   b. medial wall.
   c. floor.
   d. lateral wall.
   e. all four walls are equally strong.

10. Within which orbital bone are the optic foramen and canal contained?

    a. frontal.
    b. ethmoid.
    c. lesser wing of sphenoid.
    d. greater wing of sphenoid.
    e. palatine.

11. Match the structures listed in the left-hand column with their appropriate portals of entry or exit from the intracranial space.

    a. cranial nerve VI.
    b. cranial nerve III.
    c. potential route for spread of infectious sinusitis.
    d. ophthalmic artery.
    e. cranial nerve V-3.
    f. cranial nerve IV.
    g. superior ophthalmic vein.
    h. cranial nerve II.
    i. sympathetic nerve fibers to the iris dilator muscle.
    j. infraorbital nerve.
    k. cranial nerve V-2.
    l. sympathetic nerve fibers to ocular and orbital blood vessels.
    m. internal carotid artery.

    1. optic canal.
    2. foramen ovale.
    3. inferior orbital fissure.
    4. foramen lacerum.
    5. ethmoidal foramina.
    6. superior orbital fissure.
    7. foramen rotundum.

12. Which of the following terminal branches of the ophthalmic artery anastomose with branches of the external carotid system?

> 1. the supraorbital artery.
> 2. the lacrimal artery.
> 3. the dorsonasal artery.
> 4. the angular artery.

    a. 1, 2, and 3.
    b. 1 and 3.
    c. 2 and 4.
    d. 4 only.
    e. 1, 2, 3, and 4.

13. Match the descriptions listed in the left-hand column with the appropriate orbital soft tissues listed in the right-hand column.

    a. travel(s) within fat compartments with radiating branches.
    b. fibrous origin of the extraocular muscles.
    c. travel(s) in orbital septa in a complex of rings.
    d. continuous with the orbital septum anteriorly and dura posteriorly.
    e. splits lacrimal gland into two lobes.
    f. acts as suspensory ligament of the globe.
    g. three layers, thinnest posteriorly and thickest anteriorly.

    1. orbital arteries.
    2. annulus of Zinn.
    3. Lockwood's ligament.
    4. optic nerve sheath.
    5. periorbita.
    6. orbital veins.
    7. levator aponeurosis.

14. Which sinus system aerates first?

    a. frontal.
    b. ethmoid.
    c. sphenoid.
    d. maxillary.
    e. pyriform.

15. For each of the sinus systems listed on the left, select the nasal area into which it drains, listed on the right.

    a. sphenoid sinus.
    b. frontal sinus.
    c. anterior ethmoid air cells.
    d. posterior ethmoid air cells.
    e. maxillary sinus.
    f. nasolacrimal duct.

    1. sphenoethmoidal recess.
    2. superior meatus.
    3. middle meatus.
    4. inferior meatus.

16. Which of the following orbital disorders are marked by prominent pain?

> 1. orbital pseudotumor.
> 2. thyroid ophthalmopathy.
> 3. malignant mixed tumor of the lacrimal gland.
> 4. optic nerve sheath meningioma.

    a. 1, 2, and 3.
    b. 1 and 3.
    c. 2 and 4.
    d. 4 only.
    e. 1, 2, 3, and 4.

17. Which one of the following disorders typically produces downward and lateral displacement of the globe?

    a. thyroid ophthalmopathy.
    b. malignant mixed tumor of the lacrimal gland.
    c. frontal sinus mucocele.
    d. squamous cell carcinoma of the maxillary sinus.
    e. optic nerve sheath meningioma.

18. All of the following disorders typically present with a rapid onset except:

    a. orbital cellulitis.
    b. rhabdomyosarcoma.
    c. benign mixed tumor of the lacrimal gland.
    d. bacterial dacryoadenitis.
    e. ruptured dermoid cyst.

19. T of F -- Hypertelorism and exorbitism are synonymous.

20. The upper limit of normal for exophthalmometry in white men is:

    a. 16 mm.
    b. 20 mm.
    c. 22 mm.
    d. 25 mm.
    e. 28 mm.

21. The upper limit of normal for exophthalmometry in black men is:

    a. 16 mm.
    b. 20 mm.
    c. 22 mm.
    d. 25 mm.
    e. 28 mm.

22. The most frequent cause of bilateral proptosis in adults is:

    a. lymphoma.
    b. cavernous hemangioma.
    c. carotid-cavernous fistula.
    d. thyroid ophthalmopathy.
    e. sphenoid wing meningioma.

23. The most common cause of unilateral proptosis in adults is:

    a. lymphoma.
    b. cavernous hemangioma.
    c. carotid-cavernous fistula.
    d. thyroid ophthalmopathy.
    e. sphenoid wing meningioma.

24. The most common cause of unilateral proptosis in children is:

    a. acute leukemia.
    b. orbital cellulitis.
    c. orbital pseudotumor.
    d. thyroid ophthalmopathy.
    e. rhabdomyosarcoma.

25. T or F -- Unlike children, enlargement of orbital dimensions in an adult implies a chronic process.

26. Match the anatomic structures listed in the left column with the conventional radiography technique that best images them.

    a. optic foramena.   1. Caldwell's projection.
    b. orbital floors.   2. Waters' projection.
    c. orbital rims.   3. lateral projection.
    d. orbital roofs.   4. oblique projection.
    e. medial orbital wall.
    f. sella turcica.

27. T or F -- One disadvantage of computed tomography (CT) compared to conventional tomography is its higher radiation dosage.

28. The optimal sound wave frequency for ocular and orbital ultrasound is:

    a. 10 hertz (Hz).
    b. 10 kilohertz (kHz).
    c. 10 megahertz (MHz).
    d. 20 kHz.
    e. 20 MHz.

29. T or F -- Resolution of ultrasound images increases with stimulus frequency.

30. T or F -- Ultrasound depth penetration increases with stimulus frequency.

31. Which method of echography provides the greatest amount of dynamic information, particularly for vascular structures?

   a. standardized echography.
   b. A-scan echography.
   c. B-scan echography.
   d. Doppler echography.
   e. immersion echography.

32. Orbital echography reveals a rounded extraconal lesion with well-defined, smooth borders and very low internal reflectivity. Which one of the following is the most likely tissue diagnosis?

   a. orbital neurofibroma.
   b. sinus mucocele with orbital extension.
   c. orbital lymphangioma.
   d. carcinoma metastatic to the orbit.
   e. orbital pseudotumor.

33. A 34-year-old woman presents with explosive proptosis, chemosis, photophobia, and pain with exquisite tenderness. There is global limitation of ocular motility and enlargement of the lacrimal gland clinically. There is no discharge, fever, or leukocytosis. Orbital ultrasound may have characteristics including:

   1. regular, smooth, rounded borders.
   2. poor internal sound transmission (high reflectivity).
   3. prominent vascular pulsation.
   4. enlargement of extraocular muscles.

   a. 1, 2, and 3.
   b. 1 and 3.
   c. 2 and 4.
   d. 4 only.
   e. 1, 2, 3, and 4.

34. State-of-the-art computed tomography (CT) scans permit a spatial resolution of:

   a. 1 mm^3.
   b. 5 mm^3.
   c. 1 cm^3.
   d. 5 cm^3.
   e. 10 cm^3.

35. Which of the following features should be requested to maximize information gained from orbital CT scanning?

        1. thin slices (1-2 mm cuts).
        2. intrathecal metrizamide injection.
        3. coronal sections.
        4. 1.5 tesla magnet.

    a. 1, 2, and 3.
    b. 1 and 3.
    c. 2 and 4.
    d. 4 only.
    e. 1, 2, 3, and 4.

36. Which of the following features are necessary for generation of magnetic resonance images (MRI)?

        1. high-power magnetic field.
        2. atomic nuclei with electrical dipoles.
        3. radiofrequency energy pulses.
        4. presence of water or calcium.

    a. 1, 2, and 3.
    b. 1 and 3.
    c. 2 and 4.
    d. 4 only.
    e. 1, 2, 3, and 4.

37. T or F -- The magnetic field strength used to generate an MRI approaches that of the earth's magnetic field.

38. Which one of the following statements regarding the physics of MRI scanning is false?

    a. Nuclear dipoles are aligned with each other via a strong external magnetic field.
    b. The direction of nuclear dipole alignment is acutely altered by application of a radiofrequency pulse, either 90 degrees or 180 degrees away from original alignment.
    c. The times required for the return of dipole alignment with the external magnetic field--relaxation times--determine the scan's appearance.
    d. Substances with long T1 times (longitudinal relaxation time) appear bright on T1-weighted images.
    e. Substances with long T2 times (transverse relaxation time) appear bright on T2-weighted scans.

39. T or F -- Vitreous appears bright on T1-weighted images.

40. T or F -- Orbital fat appears bright on T1-weighted images.

41. Compared to MRI, which of the following may be considered advantages of CT scanning?

    1. better definition of bony tissues.
    2. better definition of soft tissues.
    3. ability to detect metallic foreign bodies.
    4. better definition of chiasmal pathology.

    a. 1, 2, and 3.
    b. 1 and 3.
    c. 2 and 4.
    d. 4 only.
    e. 1, 2, 3, and 4.

42. Relative to CT imaging, MRI has which of the following advantages?

    1. greater patient comfort.
    2. lower cost and greater accessibility.
    3. less motion artifact.
    4. wider selection of scanning planes.

    a. 1, 2, and 3.
    b. 1 and 3.
    c. 2 and 4.
    d. 4 only.
    e. 1, 2, 3, and 4.

43. Match the blood tests listed in the left column with the conditions for which they are most likely to be positive or helpful (items in the right column may be used more than once).

a. angiotensin converting enzyme (ACE).	1. Wegener's granulomatosis.
b. antinuclear antibody (ANA).	2. sarcoidosis.
c. perinuclear antineutrophil cytoplasmic antibodies (p-ANCA).	3. Sjögren's syndrome.
d. cytoplasmic antineutrophil cytoplasmic antibody (c-ANCA).	4. systemic lupus erythematosus.
e. anti-SS-A and B antibodies.	5. metastatic neuroblastoma.
f. carcinoembryonic antigen (CEA).	6. Graves' disease.
g. lysozyme.	7. polyarteritis nodosa.
h. sensitive thyroid stimulating hormone (TSH).	8. metastatic carcinoma.
i. vanillylmandelic acid.	
j. hepatitis B antigen.	

44. T or F -- Anophthalmos is more common than microphthalmos.

45. T or F -- Normal orbital development is dependent on the presence of a grossly normal globe during childhood.

46. Craniofacial cleft syndromes that affect the orbit, eyelids, or eye include:

> 1. Treacher Collins syndrome.
> 2. Apert's syndrome.
> 3. Goldenhar's syndrome.
> 4. Crouzon's disease.

   a. 1, 2, and 3.
   b. 1 and 3.
   c. 2 and 4.
   d. 4 only.
   e. 1, 2, 3, and 4.

47. The most common location for an orbital meningocele is the:

   a. medial canthus.
   b. infraorbital notch.
   c. lateral canthus.
   d. supraorbital notch.
   e. lacrimal gland fossa.

48. The most common orbital or eyelid finding in the craniosynostosis syndromes is:

   a. blepharophimosis.
   b. ptosis.
   c. hypertelorism.
   d. ankyloblepharon.
   e. large orbit with apparent enophthalmos.

49. Features serving to differentiate preseptal cellulitis from orbital cellulitis include:

> 1. pain with eye movement.
> 2. diplopia with limitation in ductions.
> 3. sharply demarcated border of erythematous skin at the orbital margin.
> 4. marked warmth and tenderness of periorbital tissues.

   a. 1, 2, and 3.
   b. 1 and 3.
   c. 2 and 4.
   d. 4 only.
   e. 1, 2, 3, and 4.

50. T or F -- In adults, preseptal cellulitis may rapidly spread to involve the orbits with bacteremia and meningitis.

51. The organisms most frequently implicated in preseptal cellulitis in adults are:

   a. *Staphylococcus* species.
   b. *Streptococcus* species.
   c. *Hemophilus* species.
   d. *Pseudomonas* species.
   e. *Bacillus* species.

52. The most common risk factor for the development of preseptal cellulitis is:

   a. recent dental surgery.
   b. recent upper respiratory infection.
   c. recent orbital fracture.
   d. recent skin trauma.
   e. sinusitis.

53. Drugs of choice in the treatment of typical preseptal cellulitis include:

   1. Trimethoprim/sulfamethoxazole (Bactrim).
   2. Dicloxacillin.
   3. Tetracycline.
   4. Cephalexin.

   a. 1, 2, and 3.
   b. 1 and 3.
   c. 2 and 4.
   d. 4 only.
   e. 1, 2, 3, and 4.

54. The agent most likely to cause a severe preseptal cellulitis leading to secondary orbital cellulitis and central nervous system infection in infants and toddlers is:

   a. *Staphylococcus aureus.*
   b. *Streptococcus pneumoniae.*
   c. *Hemophilus influenzae.*
   d. *Streptococcus pyogenes.*
   e. *Neisseria meningitidis.*

55. The most common historical risk factor for the development of orbital cellulitis is:

   a. recent upper respiratory infection.
   b. ethmoid sinusitis.
   c. recent dental extraction.
   d. preseptal cellulitis.
   e. recent orbital fracture.

56. Decreased visual acuity in the setting of suspected orbital cellulitis must be evaluated with which of the following tests?

        1. MRI scanning.
        2. swinging flashlight test.
        3. fluorescein angiography.
        4. CT scanning.

    a. 1, 2, and 3.
    b. 1 and 3.
    c. 2 and 4.
    d. 4 only.
    e. 1, 2, 3, and 4.

57. A patient with suspected orbital cellulitis suddenly worsens with a virtually frozen globe, despite an inapparent increase in proptosis. Corneal sensation is likewise diminished. The most likely explanation for these events is:

    a. orbital apex syndrome.
    b. orbital compartment syndrome.
    c. meningitis secondary to orbital cellulitis.
    d. panophthalmitis secondary to orbital cellulitis.
    e. cavernous sinus thrombosis.

58. Tests that are important for distinguishing infectious orbital cellulitis from inflammatory orbital pseudotumor include:

        1. oral temperature.
        2. orbital CT scan.
        3. complete blood count with differential.
        4. sedimentation rate.

    a. 1, 2, and 3.
    b. 1 and 3.
    c. 2 and 4.
    d. 4 only.
    e. 1, 2, 3, and 4.

59. A 19-year-old patient presents to the ophthalmologist with redness of his left eye. The skin of the upper and lower left eyelids is red and inflamed. There is a small eschar on the left upper lid medially. Visual acuity is normal. The patient is orthotropic in primary gaze, and ductions appear full bilaterally. On far right gaze, the patient develops a small exotropia. The deviation is slightly more noticeable when he fixes with his left eye. Hertel exophthalmometry reads 16 mm OD and 18 mm OS. There is no orbital tenderness, but he describes a slight discomfort with right gaze. Oral temperature is 99.2°F. White blood count is 9100 with a normal differential. The examination finding that most strongly argues against the diagnosis of simple preseptal cellulitis is:

a. exophthalmometry.
b. ocular motility findings.
c. external examination findings (erythema, warmth).
d. oral temperature.
e. white blood cell count.

60. The patient in question 59 undergoes CT scanning, which reveals a dense left ethmoid sinusitis with irregular densities of the orbital fat on the left. The patient is hospitalized and started on intravenous antibiotics. Appropriate antibiotic choices for these findings include:

1. nafcillin.
2. cefuroxime.
3. chloramphenicol.
4. cefazolin.

a. 1, 2, and 3.
b. 1 and 3.
c. 2 and 4.
d. 4 only.
e. 1, 2, 3, and 4.

61. Following admission, the clinical status of the patient in questions 59 and 60 slightly deteriorates over the initial 12 hours. This is followed by a 24- to 36-hour period of modest improvement. After 2 days, however, 3 mm of proptosis persists, and there is still pain with attempted adduction OS. These findings suggest the possibility of:

a. cavernous sinus thrombosis.
b. spread of infection to adjacent sinuses.
c. inappropriate choice of antibiotic.
d. subperiosteal abscess.
e. meningitis.

62. What test must be performed to evaluate the findings described in question 61?

a. orbital ultrasound.
b. ocular ultrasound.
c. cerebral angiography.
d. lumbar puncture.
e. orbital CT scanning.

63. The diagnostic maneuver of choice in question 62 is performed and confirms suspicions. What therapeutic step must now be undertaken?

    a. surgical drainage.
    b. intrathecal antibiotics.
    c. pars plana vitrectomy with intraocular antibiotics.
    d. use of broader spectrum intravenous antibiotic agents.
    e. orbital decompression.

64. T or F -- The phakomatoses are generalized disorders featuring multiple hamartomas-- disordered growths containing tissue elements not normally found at the site of involvement.

65. Which one of the following regarding dermoid and epidermoid cysts is false?

    a. They share a common pathophysiology.
    b. The key distinguishing feature between the two is the nature of the wall of the cystic cavity.
    c. In children, nearly all of these lesions are anterior to the orbital septum.
    d. In adults, nearly all of these lesions are anterior to the orbital septum.
    e. Dermoid cysts may induce bony erosion on radiography.

66. Features shared by dermoid cysts and lipodermoids include:

                    1. typical location.
                    2. general surgical strategies.
                    3. gross pathology.
                    4. cellular constituents on histopathology.

    a. 1, 2, and 3.
    b. 1 and 3.
    c. 2 and 4.
    d. 4 only.
    e. 1, 2, 3, and 4.

67. T or F -- The definition of an orbital teratoma is a lesion containing all three germinal cell layers.

68. T or F -- Orbital teratomas may simulate malignancy but rarely, if ever, metastasize.

69. Greater that 90% of periocular capillary hemangiomas become manifest by:

    a. 4 to 8 weeks of life.
    b. 6 to 8 months of age.
    c. 12 to 18 months of age.
    d. 24 to 30 months of age.
    e. 3 to 4 years of age.

70. Most capillary hemangiomas reach their peak size at approximately what age?

    a. 2 to 3 months.
    b. 6 to 12 months.
    c. 12 to 24 months.
    d. 3 to 5 years.
    e. 5 to 7 years.

71. Potentially important complications of capillary hemangiomas in childhood are:

                1. occlusion amblyopia.
                2. proptosis with exposure.
                3. significant astigmatism.
                4. ocular invasion.

    a. 1, 2, and 3.
    b. 1 and 3.
    c. 2 and 4.
    d. 4 only.
    e. 1, 2, 3, and 4.

72. The "nevus flammeus," which may be confused for a capillary hemangioma, is seen as a part of what systemic disorder?

    a. neurofibromatosis.
    b. Treacher Collins syndrome.
    c. von Hippel's disease.
    d. Sturge-Weber syndrome.
    e. Goldenhar's syndrome.

73. The key clinical feature distinguishing between nevus flammmeus and capillary hemangioma is:

    a. extent of skin thickening.
    b. lesion color.
    c. area of skin affected.
    d. presence of absence of blanching with pressure.
    e. pulsations.

74. T or F -- It is rare for an eyelid hemangioma in a child to be associated with hemangiomas in other organ systems.

75. Indications for treatment of eyelid capillary hemangiomas in childhood include:

                    1. significant astigmatism.
                    2. significant cosmetic deformity.
                    3. significant occlusion.
                    4. lack of initial resolution by age 2 years.

   a. 1, 2, and 3.
   b. 1 and 3.
   c. 2 and 4.
   d. 4 only.
   e. 1, 2, 3, and 4.

76. The least likely complication of treatment of eyelid capillary hemangiomas is:

   a. cataract.
   b. soft-tissue atrophy.
   c. endophthalmitis.
   d. rebound growth upon cessation of therapy.
   e. future malignancy in the treated area.

77. Key features differentiating cavernous hemangioma and capillary hemangioma include:

                    1. age of affected patients.
                    2. volume of blood flow through each.
                    3. size of blood-filled spaces on micropathology.
                    4. tendency to metastasize.

   a. 1, 2, and 3.
   b. 1 and 3.
   c. 2 and 4.
   d. 4 only.
   e. 1, 2, 3, and 4.

78. T or F -- Orbital lymphangiomas are believed to develop from abnormal sequestrations of lymphatic channels from the remainder of the orbital lymphatic system.

79. Which of the following regarding the histopathology of orbital lymphangioma is/are true?

    1. Unlike capillary hemangioma, the cystic spaces are large.
    2. Lymphoid tissue, even follicles, may be found within the substance of the tumor.
    3. Loculated areas of old hemorrhage, "chocolate cysts," may be found.
    4. There is generally a well-defined fibrous capsule surrounding the tumor.

    a. 1, 2, and 3.
    b. 1 and 3.
    c. 2 and 4.
    d. 4 only.
    e. 1, 2, 3, and 4.

80. Which of the following regarding the surgical therapy of orbital lymphangioma is/are true?

    1. Careful dissection will generally lead to complete tumor excision.
    2. Significant cosmetic deformity and recurrent orbital hemorrhage are the most common indications for surgical therapy.
    3. Recurrence is rare.
    4. Carbon dioxide laser or orbital decompression techniques may be helpful in the surgical therapy of this tumor.

    a. 1, 2, and 3.
    b. 1 and 3.
    c. 2 and 4.
    d. 4 only.
    e. 1, 2, 3, and 4.

81. Which of the following orbital tumors is least likely to present as a "masquerade syndrome"?

    a. optic nerve glioma.
    b. orbital dermoid cyst.
    c. rhabdomyosarcoma.
    d. acute leukemic orbital infiltration.
    e. metastatic neuroblastoma.

82. Which one of the following clinical findings at presentation is inconsistent with the diagnosis of optic nerve glioma?

    a. insidious onset.
    b. afferent pupillary defect.
    c. pain.
    d. axial proptosis.
    e. unilaterality.

83. Which one of the following radiographic features is considered "pathognomonic" for optic nerve glioma?

    a. adjacent bony erosion.
    b. "kinking" of the optic nerve.
    c. multiple cystic cavities within the optic nerve.
    d. "tram-track" enlargement of the optic nerve.
    e. traction on posterior globe with "tenting."

84. The study of choice for defining the presence or extent of intracranial involvement with optic nerve glioma is:

    a. polytomography.
    b. ultrasonography.
    c. CT scanning.
    d. MRI scanning.
    e. carotid angiography.

85. T or F -- Incisional biopsy of suspected optic nerve glioma may be easily misinterpreted as optic nerve meningioma.

86. Modalities that may be of use in the treatment of optic nerve glioma include:

    1. observation.
    2. radiotherapy.
    3. surgical resection.
    4. chemotherapy.

    a. 1, 2, and 3.
    b. 1 and 3.
    c. 2 and 4.
    d. 4 only.
    e. 1, 2, 3, and 4.

87. Indications for therapeutic intervention for optic nerve glioma include:

    1. presence of afferent pupillary defect.
    2. rapidly progressive tumor growth.
    3. proptosis.
    4. involvement of intracranial optic nerve with field loss in the contralateral eye.

    a. 1, 2, and 3.
    b. 1 and 3.
    c. 2 and 4.
    d. 4 only.
    e. 1, 2, 3, and 4.

88. A patient with known neurofibromatosis presents with pulsating proptosis of long duration. CT scan of the orbit will most likely reveal:

   a. orbital neurofibroma.
   b. cavernous hemangioma.
   c. abnormality of the sphenoid bone.
   d. optic nerve glioma.
   e. carotid-cavernous fistula.

89. A 7-year-old boy presents with a 3-day history of progressive proptosis, injection, and pain of the left eye. He is systemically well with normal temperature. White blood cell count is normal, and emergent orbital CT scanning reveals superonasal orbital infiltration with bony erosion. The diagnosis that must be excluded at this point is:

   a. bacterial orbital cellulitis.
   b. optic nerve glioma.
   c. frontal sinus mucocele.
   d. rhabdomyosarcoma.
   e. orbital neurofibroma.

90. Which one of the following regarding a biopsy of orbital rhabdomyosarcoma is false?

   a. Care must be taken to prevent local seeding or distant dissemination with tumor cells.
   b. Electron microscopic studies are frequently necessary to secure the diagnosis.
   c. In cases of high suspicion, lumbar puncture and bone marrow biopsy should be performed at the time of biopsy.
   d. The embryonal pattern is the most common pathologic variant.
   e. The most malignant variant, alveolar rhabdomyosarcoma, occurs most frequently in the superior orbit.

91. Match the clinical characteristics listed in the left column with the histologic patterns listed in the right column.

   a. best prognosis.
   b. most differentiated (most likely to see cross-striations on light microscopy).
   c. more commonly occurs in inferior orbit.
   d. most common pattern seen in children.
   e. worst prognosis.
   f. least common of the primary orbital varieties.
   g. orbital involvement reflects secondary invasion from sinuses or conjunctiva.

   1. alveolar.
   2. botryoid.
   3. embryonal.
   4. pleomorphic.

92. T or F -- The cell of origin for most rhabdomyosarcomas is the myocyte of extraocular muscle.

93. T or F -- Like adults, metastases in children more frequently involve the eye (uvea) than the orbit.

94. Fungal species likely to lead to a necrotizing orbital cellulitis include:

        1. Candida.
        2. Aspergillus.
        3. Fusarium.
        4. Mucor.

    a. 1, 2, and 3.
    b. 1 and 3.
    c. 2 and 4.
    d. 4 only.
    e. 1, 2, 3, and 4.

95. T or F -- Both mucormycosis and aspergillosis of the orbit occur only in patients with immune dysfunction (e.g., diabetics).

96. A 33-year-old patient with type I diabetes mellitus presents with a 2-week history of gradually progressive proptosis, redness, and irritation OS. Visual acuities are 20/20 OD and 20/100 OS. There is an afferent pupillary defect on the left, along with 4 mm of proptosis and moderate conjunctival injection. Ductions are normal on the right and globally reduced on the left. CT scanning reveals left ethmoid and maxillary sinusitis with evidence of orbital involvement. The next step in the proper evaluation of this patient is:

    a. complete blood count.
    b. blood glucose.
    c. careful ENT evaluation.
    d. oral temperature.
    e. orbital MRI scan.

97. Which of the following orbital or adnexal tumors affect women significantly more frequently than men?

        1. cavernous hemangioma.
        2. sebaceous cell carcinoma.
        3. meningioma.
        4. fibrous histiocytoma.

    a. 1, 2, and 3.
    b. 1 and 3.
    c. 2 and 4.
    d. 4 only.
    e. 1, 2, 3, and 4.

98. A patient presents to the ophthalmologist with a history of gradually progressive prominence of the left eye. There are no visual complaints, although the patient notes a mild throbbing pain intermittently on the left side of his head. Visual acuities are normal and symmetric, and there is 4 mm of axial proptosis on the left. There is no lid retraction evident in primary gaze. There is questionable lid lag on downgaze. The eye examination is otherwise normal, including no evidence of inflammation. The historical feature most convincingly arguing against the diagnosis of Graves' ophthalmopathy is:

a. male sex.
b. unilateral involvement.
c. throbbing sensation.
d. full eye movements.
e. no lid retraction.

99. Arrange the extraocular muscles listed below in order of decreasing frequency of involvement with Graves' ophthalmopathy (1 being the most frequently involved and 4 being the least frequently involved).

a. superior rectus.   1.
b. lateral rectus.   2.
c. inferior rectus.   3.
d. medial rectus.   4.

100. Surveillance of the patient with Graves' ophthalmopathy must include:

        1. visual acuity testing.
        2. visual field testing.
        3. color vision testing.
        4. fluorescein angiography.

a. 1, 2, and 3.
b. 1 and 3.
c. 2 and 4.
d. 4 only.
e. 1, 2, 3, and 4.

101. T or F -- If laboratory evidence of a dysthyroid state fails to develop within 10 years of the diagnosis of Graves' ophthalmopathy, the ophthalmic diagnosis should be questioned seriously.

102. Surgical procedures that may be indicated during the active, inflammatory phase of Graves' ophthalmopathy include:

    1. strabismus surgery.
    2. lateral tarsorrhaphy.
    3. recession of the levator aponeurosis.
    4. orbital decompression.

    a. 1, 2, and 3.
    b. 1 and 3.
    c. 2 and 4.
    d. 4 only.
    e. 1, 2, 3, and 4.

103. A 45-year-old woman presents with mild bilateral proptosis and lid retraction. There is no previous history of thyroid disease, and the patient denies any periocular pain. The one blood test that is most likely to be of value in this circumstance is:

    a. total thyroxine (T 4) levels.
    b. free T 4 levels.
    c. total triiodothyronine (T 3) levels.
    d. thyroid hormone index (total T 4 and thyroid binding globulin levels).
    e. sensitive thyroid-simulating hormone levels (TSH)--immunometric assay.

104. T or F -- The pathologic changes seen in extraocular muscle involvement with Graves' ophthalmopathy reflect primary inflammatory destruction of muscle cells.

105. T or F -- The histopathologic changes evident in extraocular muscle specimens from patients with Graves' ophthalmopathy may also be seen in the lacrimal glands.

106. Which one of the following signs is considered classic for CT scanning in Graves' ophthalmopathy?

    a. nodular muscle enlargement.
    b. solitary muscle enlargement.
    c. "kinking" of extraocular muscles.
    d. fusiform muscle enlargement with sparing of tendons.
    e. enhancement of posterior sclera with intravenous contrast injection.

107. A patient with brittle type I diabetes and labile hypertension presents with obvious Graves' ophthalmopathy. There is an afferent pupillary defect, decreased visual acuity, and an abnormal visual field, all on the right side. The patient is markedly hyperthyroid, and general anesthesia is felt to be risky as the patient is on the brink of thyroid storm. The patient's blood sugar is running in the mid 200s, and renal function studies are normal. Which of the following interventions might be appropriate for control of vision-threatening ophthalmopathy?

> 1. orbital radiation.
> 2. oral corticosteroids.
> 3. oral cyclosporine.
> 4. lateral tarsorrhaphy.

a. 1, 2, and 3.
b. 1 and 3.
c. 2 and 4.
d. 4 only.
e. 1, 2, 3, and 4.

108. Before undertaking surgical correction of strabismus in Graves' ophthalmopathy, the angle of deviation should be stable for what period of time?

a. 1 month.
b. 3 months.
c. 6 months.
d. 1 year.
e. 2 years.

109. A patient with a known history of hyperthyroidism presents with bilateral proptosis, unilateral decreased vision with associated afferent pupillary defect, dyschromatopsia, and visual field defects. There is associated vertical strabismus and severe lid retraction with cosmetic significance bilaterally. The corneas are normal bilaterally. Arrange the surgical procedures listed below in their proper chronologic order (1 being the first procedure to be performed and 3 being the final procedure to be performed).

a. vertical rectus muscle recession with adjustable sutures.   1.
b. orbital decompression.   2.
c. levator recessions with interposition spacer grafts.   3.

110. Manifestations of idiopathic orbital inflammation (pseudotumor) include all of the following except:

a. dacryoadenitis.
b. peripheral ulcerative keratitis.
c. extraocular myositis.
d. periscleritis.
e. optic perineuritis.

111. Clinical findings that are more likely in pediatric orbital pseudotumor than in the adult variety of the disease include all of the following except:

a. bilateral involvement.
b. systemic symptoms and signs (malaise, fever, vomiting).
c. minimal periocular pain.
d. peripheral eosinophilia.
e. cells in cerebrospinal fluid.

112. Which of the following are features of sclerosing orbital pseudotumor?

1. insidious onset.
2. more frequently steroid-resistant than other variants.
3. may be misdiagnosed as an orbital neoplasm.
4. pain is a less prominent complaint.

a. 1, 2, and 3.
b. 1 and 3.
c. 2 and 4.
d. 4 only.
e. 1, 2, 3, and 4.

113. A patient with presumed inflammatory orbital pseudotumor is treated with oral prednisone, 60 mg, daily for 2 weeks. No improvement in clinical findings is seen. The next therapeutic step should be:

a. doubling of oral prednisone dosage.
b. induction with intravenous methylprednisolone.
c. orbital irradiation.
d. oral cyclophosphamide (Cytoxan).
e. orbital biopsy.

114. Which of the following regarding the biopsy findings of orbital pseudotumor is/are true?

1. Compared to orbital lymphoma, the lesions are relatively hypocellular.
2. A microscopic specimen of involved extraocular muscle could be indistinguishable from that of Graves' ophthalmopathy.
3. The presence of many eosinophils in an adult's biopsy suggest the presence of an underlying systemic vasculitis.
4. The presence of neutrophils makes the diagnosis of pseudotumor unlikely.

a. 1, 2, and 3.
b. 1 and 3.
c. 2 and 4.
d. 4 only.
e. 1, 2, 3, and 4.

115. CT findings that differentiate orbital pseudotumor from Graves' ophthalmopathy include:

       1. enlargement of multiple extraocular muscles.
       2. enlargement of extraocular muscle tendons.
       3. unilateral involvement.
       4. enhancement of posterior sclera with intravenous contrast injection.

    a. 1, 2, and 3.
    b. 1 and 3.
    c. 2 and 4.
    d. 4 only.
    e. 1, 2, 3, and 4.

116. All of the following disorders may be associated with a clinical presentation indistinguishable from typical inflammatory orbital pseudotumor except:

    a. systemic lupus erythematosus (SLE).
    b. polyarteritis nodosa.
    c. Wegener's granulomatosis.
    d. sarcoidosis.
    e. Churg-Strauss syndrome.

117. For which of the following disorders is bilateral, painless enlargement of the lacrimal glands considered a typical presentation?

       1. Sjögren's syndrome.
       2. sarcoidosis.
       3. inflammatory orbital pseudotumor.
       4. benign lymphoepithelial lesions.

    a. 1, 2, and 3.
    b. 1 and 3.
    c. 2 and 4.
    d. 4 only.
    e. 1, 2, 3, and 4.

118. Which of the following regarding cavernous hemangioma of the orbit is/are true?

       1. Women are more frequently affected than men.
       2. It is the most common etiology of neoplastic unilateral proptosis in adults.
       3. A-scan ultrasonography reveals high internal reflectivity.
       4. There is generally an associated bruit.

    a. 1, 2, and 3.
    b. 1 and 3.
    c. 2 and 4.
    d. 4 only.
    e. 1, 2, 3, and 4.

119. T or F -- Hemangiopericytomas are more likely to limit ocular motility than cavernous hemangiomas.

120. T or F -- The most important prognostic indicator for systemic mortality from orbital hemangiopericytoma is cellular morphology on biopsy.

121. A 28-year-old man presents to an ophthalmologist 1 week after motor vehicle accident with resultant blunt head trauma. He is complaining of irritation and redness of the left eye. Visual acuity is normal bilaterally. There is marked conjunctival injection of the left eye, with prominence of the superficial and deep vessels all the way to the limbus. There is 5 mm of proptosis on the involved side. Slit-lamp examination is normal. Intraocular pressures are 16 mm Hg OD and 25 mm Hg OS. Funduscopic examination is normal on the right but reveals dilated, tortuous retinal veins on the left. On careful questioning, the patient reports hearing a rushing noise intermittently. Auscultation of the left orbit reveals a faint bruit. "Arterialization" of his orbit is due to a disturbance in the:

    a. intraorbital central retinal artery.
    b. intracranial ophthalmic artery.
    c. intracravernous internal carotid artery.
    d. cervical common carotid artery.
    e. branches of the middle meningeal artery.

122. A 73-year-old woman presents to the ophthalmologist complaining of mild redness and irritation of her left eye for approximately 2 months. She denies any head trauma. Visual acuity is normal bilaterally. There is 3 mm of proptosis on the left with mild to moderate vascular congestion of the conjunctiva consisting of prominent deep and superficial vessels all the way to the limbus. Slit-lamp examination is normal. Intraocular pressures are 16 mm Hg OD and 25 mm Hg OS. Funduscopic examination reveals mildly dilated retinal venules bilaterally. The patient denies hearing any abnormal sounds, and there is no audible bruit over either orbit. "Arterialization" of her orbit is due to a disturbance in the:

    a. intraorbital central retinal artery.
    b. intracranial ophthalmic artery.
    c. intracavernous internal carotid artery.
    d. cervical common carotid artery.
    e. branches of the middle meningeal artery.

123. T or F -- The clinical finding considered classic for orbital varices is an audible bruit with corkscrewing of conjunctival vessels.

124. T or F -- Most orbital meningiomas arise outside the orbit and invade secondarily.

125. T or F -- The growth patterns of meningiomas associated with neurofibromatosis are indistinguishable from isolated tumors.

126. Which of the following regarding the radiographic evaluation of meningioma is/are true?

> 1. Associated bony changes may be either osteolytic or osteoblastic.
> 2. Angiography generally reveals a highly vascularized tumor ("tumor blush").
> 3. CT scanning is the modality of choice in the initial evaluation of a patient with optic nerve meningioma.
> 4. MRI scanning is particularly useful for evaluating suspected intracranial extension.

    a. 1, 2, and 3.
    b. 1 and 3.
    c. 2 and 4.
    d. 4 only.
    e. 1, 2, 3, and 4.

127. T or F -- Excisional biopsy of optic nerve meningioma is possible with preservation of vision.

128. Indications for the removal of orbital meningioma include:

> 1. severe loss of vision.
> 2. progressive tumor growth in a child.
> 3. evidence of intracranial extension.
> 4. afferent pupillary defect.

    a. 1, 2, and 3.
    b. 1 and 3.
    c. 2 and 4.
    d. 4 only.
    e. 1, 2, 3, and 4.

129. T or F -- Anterior visual pathway gliomas in adults are particularly malignant, but only when associated with neurofibromatosis.

130. In the general ophthalmologist's practice, what percentage of lacrimal gland lesions will be inflammatory or lymphoid?

    a. 10%.
    b. 20%.
    c. 40%.
    d. 50%.
    e. greater than 75%.

131. The most common neoplasm of the lacrimal gland is the:

    a. adenoid cystic carcinoma.
    b. malignant mixed tumor.
    c. benign mixed tumor.
    d. adenocarcinoma.
    e. mucoepidermoid carcinoma.

132. Which historical features are considered essential in the clinical evaluation of lacrimal gland lesions?

    1. presence or absence of double vision.
    2. presence or absence of pain.
    3. presence or absence of dry eye symptoms.
    4. duration of symptoms.

    a. 1, 2, and 3.
    b. 1 and 3.
    c. 2 and 4.
    d. 4 only.
    e. 1, 2, 3, and 4.

133. Which radiographic features of CT scanning are considered essential in the evaluation of lacrimal gland lesions?

    1. degree of enhancement with intravenous contrast injection.
    2. soft-tissue outlines of glandular enlargement.
    3. presence or absence of glandular calcification.
    4. presence or absence of adjacent bony change.

    a. 1, 2, and 3.
    b. 1 and 3.
    c. 2 and 4.
    d. 4 only.
    e. 1, 2, 3, and 4.

134. Match the clinical characteristics listed in the left-hand column with the type of lacrimal gland lesion (the choices in the right hand column may be used more than once).

a. pain.
b. adjacent osteolysis.
c. "pancake" enlargement of lacrimal gland.
d. symptoms present for greater than 1 year.
e. globular enlargement of the lacrimal gland.
f. adjacent bony molding (pressure-induced bony change).
g. symptoms present for less than 1 year.
h. enlargement of lacrimal gland anterior to the orbital rim on CT scanning.
i. normal adjacent bone on CT scanning.

1. lymphoid.
2. inflammatory.
3. benign neoplasm.
4. malignant neoplasm.
5. 1 and 2.
6. 3 and 4.
7. 2 and 4.
8. 1, 2, and 4.

135. A 30-year-old man presents with a 2-year history of gradually progressive proptosis of the right eye. There is no associated pain or inflammation. CT scanning reveals globular enlargement of the lacrimal gland with no extension anterior to the orbital rim. Adjacent bone is normal. Which one of the following regarding this clinical situation is false?

a. The most likely diagnosis is more frequently encountered in men.
b. Initial approach to the patient should include an incisional biopsy.
c. Any surgical intervention must be undertaken with very careful dissection.
d. Definitive treatment will necessitate lateral orbitotomy.
e. Histopathology may reveal areas of cartilage.

136. The most common malignant neoplasm of the the lacrimal gland is the:

a. pleomorphic adenoma.
b. malignant mixed tumor.
c. adenoid cystic carcinoma.
d. mucoepidermoid carcinoma.
e. adenocarcinoma.

137. T or F -- Adenoid cystic carcinoma of the lacrimal gland is frequently painful due to extreme reactive inflammation and orbital swelling.

138. Which of the following regarding fibrous dysplasia is/are true?

1. Orbital involvement in a girl under the age of 10 years is associated with a high probability of precocious puberty.
2. The hallmark of the histopathology is aggregation of lamellar bone.
3. The treatment of choice is high-dose radiotherapy.
4. The most frequent visual sequelae are related to optic nerve compression.

a. 1, 2, and 3.
b. 1 and 3.
c. 2 and 4.
d. 4 only.
e. 1, 2, 3, and 4.

139. Which one of the following histiocytic disorders is most likely to involve orbital bone?

a. Letterer-Siwe disease.
b. Hand-Schüller-Christian disease.
c. eosinophilic granuloma.
d. juvenile xanthogranuloma.
e. sinus histiocytosis.

140. T or F -- The therapy for eosinophilic granuloma is identical to that for the disseminated histiocytoses.

141. The most common mesenchymal tumor of the orbit in humans is:

a. ossifying fibroma.
b. fibrous dysplasia.
c. hemangiopericytoma.
d. fibrous histiocytoma.
e. osteogenic sarcoma.

142. T or F -- Fibrous histiocytoma may behave in a locally aggressive fashion but rarely if ever metastasizes.

143. T or F -- Clinical and/or radiographic features frequently allow differentiation between reactive lymphoid hyperplasia and orbital lymphoma.

144. The systemic evaluation of a patient with biopsy-proven orbital lymphoma generally includes all of the following except:

    a. bone scan.
    b. bone marrow biopsy.
    c. liver and spleen scan.
    d. lumbar puncture.
    e. serum immunoelectrophoresis.

145. Features that support the histopathologic diagnosis of "reactive" lymphoid hyperplasia over ocular adnexal lymphoma include all of the following except:

    a. high degree of cellular heterogeneity.
    b. low degree of cellular atypia.
    c. low degree of endothelial cell proliferation.
    d. numerous reactive germinal centers.
    e. preponderance of T-lymphocytes.

146. Key features supporting the diagnosis of lymphoproliferative lesions over idiopathic inflammatory orbital syndrome (pseudotumor) include:

    1. absence of significant fibrous stroma.
    2. polyclonal lymphocyte expansion.
    3. hypercellularity.
    4. cellular heterogeneity (lymphocytes plus plasma cells, eosinophils, neutrophils).

    a. 1, 2, and 3.
    b. 1 and 3.
    c. 2 and 4.
    d. 4 only.
    e. 1, 2, 3, and 4.

147. Exceptions to the rule of thumb that all orbital tumors are dark on T1-weighted MRI scans include:

    1. retrobulbar hemorrhage of at least 24 hours.
    2. melanoma.
    3. mucocele.
    4. meningioma.

    a. 1, 2, and 3.
    b. 1 and 3.
    c. 2 and 4.
    d. 4 only.
    e. 1, 2, 3, and 4.

148. T or F--The most common site of origin for tumors that secondarily invade the orbit is the cranial cavity.

149. The most common sinus lesion that invades the orbit is the:

    a. osteoma.
    b. mucocele.
    c. mucoepidermoid carcinoma.
    d. squamous cell carcinoma.
    e. inverted papilloma.

150. The most common site of a primary tumor metastatic to the orbit in women is:

    a. breast.
    b. lung.
    c. ovary.
    d. colon.
    e. uterine.

151. The most common site of a primary tumor metastatic to the orbit in men is:

    a. colon.
    b. lung.
    c. carcinoid.
    d. prostatic.
    e. cutaneous melanoma.

152. Match the radiographic characteristics listed in the left-hand column with the type of facial fractures listed in the right-hand column.

    a. craniofacial dysjunction.   1. Le Fort I.
    b. low transverse maxillary fracture.   2. Le Fort II.
    c. orbital floor, medial wall, lateral wall   3. Le Fort III.
       fractures.
    d. pyramidal maxillary fracture.
    e. no orbital bony involvement.
    f. medial orbital floor fractures.

153. Classic features of a "tripod" fracture include all of the following except:

    a. downward displacement of the lateral canthus.
    b. infraorbital hypesthesia.
    c. trismus.
    d. deficit of upgaze.
    e. temporal subconjunctival hemorrhage.

154. A sensitive finding in direct naso-orbital-ethmoid fracture is:

   a. subconjunctival hemorrhage.
   b. epistaxis.
   c. telecanthus.
   d. hypoglobus.
   e. infraorbital hypesthesia.

155. T or F -- Indirect orbital floor fractures are frequently associated with inferior orbital rim fractures.

156. Which of the following findings in orbital floor fractures are exacerbated by the presence of a coincident medial orbital wall fracture?

               1. infraorbital hypesthesia.
               2. enophthalmos.
               3. vertical diplopia.
               4. subcutaneous emphysema.

   a. 1, 2, and 3.
   b. 1 and 3.
   c. 2 and 4.
   d. 4 only.
   e. 1, 2, 3, and 4.

157. All of the following findings are consistent with an inferior orbital wall fracture and entrapment except:

   a. infraorbital hypesthesia.
   b. enophthalmos.
   c. subcutaneous emphysema.
   d. limitation in ocular motility in all fields of gaze.
   e. hypoglobus.

158. T or F -- The diagnostic study of choice in probable orbital floor fracture is the Waters view (conventional radiograms).

159. T or F -- Forced duction testing is generally helpful in the acute setting to determine if ocular motility limitations are due to entrapment or muscle dysfunction.

160. T or F -- If exophthalmometry performed at the time of orbital floor fracture does not reveal enophthalmos, it is unlikely to develop subsequently.

161. T or F -- Most diplopia associated with orbital contusion disappears within 7 to 14 days following injury.

162. Which of the following are considered indications for surgical repair of orbital floor fractures?

       1. disabling diplopia present 7 to 10 days after the original injury.
       2. large fracture on acute CT scan.
       3. enophthalmos greater than 2 mm.
       4. infraorbital hypesthesia.

    a. 1, 2, and 3.
    b. 1 and 3.
    c. 2 and 4.
    d. 4 only.
    e. 1, 2, 3, and 4.

163. T or F -- Larger, complex, comminuted floor fractures are more likely to lead to entrapment than small, posterior floor fractures.

164. The optimal time for surgical repair of orbital floor fractures is generally considered to be:

    a. within 24 hours of injury.
    b. 1 to 3 days following injury.
    c. 3 to 7 days following injury.
    d. 7 to 14 days following injury.
    e. 4 to 6 weeks following injury.

165. Which of the following are considered indications for removal of an intraorbital foreign body?

       1. vegetable foreign body.
       2. any lead foreign body.
       3. anterior, easily approachable foreign bodies.
       4. orbital apex location with good vision.

    a. 1, 2, and 3.
    b. 1 and 3.
    c. 2 and 4.
    d. 4 only.
    e. 1, 2, 3, and 4.

166. A patient presents to an ophthalmology emergency room after being struck over the left eye with a baseball bat. Examination reveals a 24-year-old man in acute distress. Visual acuity is 20/20 OD and light perception OS. There is an obvious left afferent pupillary defect. There is taut ecchymosis of the left upper and lower lid, with 3 mm of proptosis on the left. With the left lids tensely pried apart, ductions are normal OD and barely detectable OS. There is hemorrhagic chemosis 360 degrees OS and a microhyphema. Funduscopic examination is normal with the exception of obvious arterial pulsations. Intraocular pressue is 75 mm Hg. The next step to be taken is emergent:

    a. CT scanning.
    b. intravenous methylprednisolone.
    c. exploration of the globe.
    d. lateral canthotomy and cantholysis.
    e. intravenous acetazolamide and mannitol.

167. A patient presents to an ophthalmology emergency room after tumbling off a bicycle and striking his head on the pavement. Examination reveals a 24-year-old man in mild discomfort holding his head. There is a 5-mm abrasion on the left temple. Visual acuity is 20/20 OD and light perception OS. There is an obvious left afferent pupillary defect. There is no periorbital edema, and extraocular movements are full. The slit-lamp examination, fundus examination, and intraocular pressures are normal. Confrontation visual fields are full OD. The next step to be taken is emergent:

    a. CT scanning.
    b. oral prednisone.
    c. exploration of the globe.
    d. lateral canthotomy and cantholysis.
    e. intravenous acetazolamide and mannitol.

168. T or F -- The distinction between direct and indirect optic nerve trauma is the involvement of a foreign body in the former.

169. A CT scan performed on the bicyclist described in question 167 is entirely normal. The next appropriate step to be taken in this situation is emergent:

    a. intravenous methylprednisolone.
    b. exploration of the globe.
    c. lateral canthotomy and cantholysis.
    d. intravenous acetazolamide and mannitol.
    e. optic nerve sheath decompression.

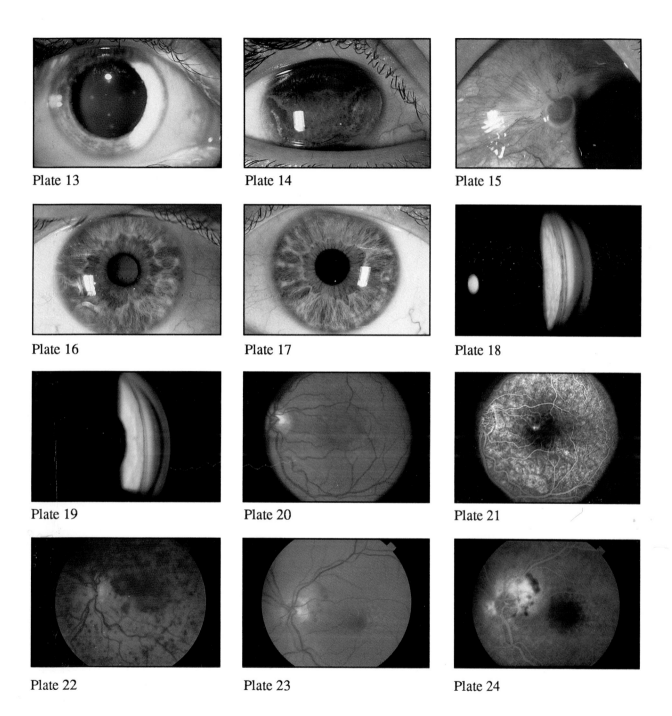

Plate 13

Plate 14

Plate 15

Plate 16

Plate 17

Plate 18

Plate 19

Plate 20

Plate 21

Plate 22

Plate 23

Plate 24

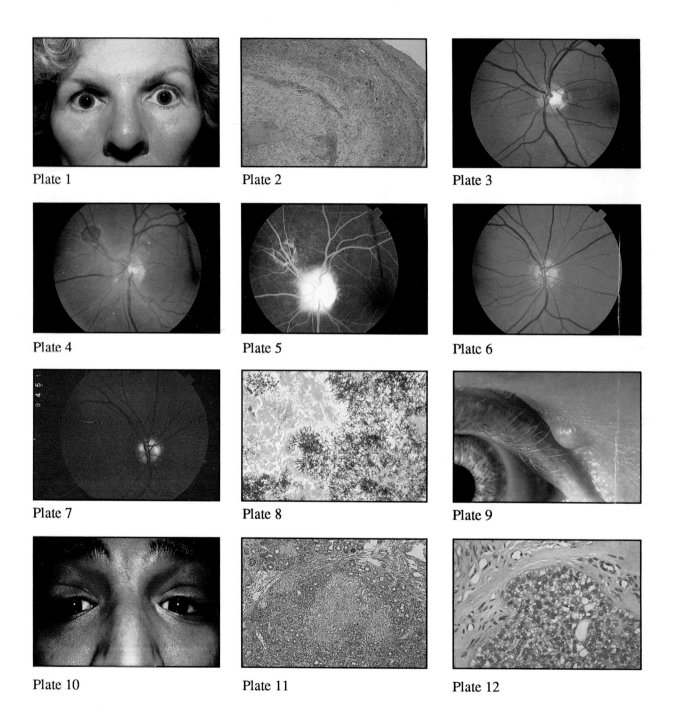

Plate 1

Plate 2

Plate 3

Plate 4

Plate 5

Platc 6

Plate 7

Plate 8

Plate 9

Plate 10

Plate 11

Plate 12

170. For which of the following clinical situations is enucleation, rather than evisceration, preferred?

        1. suspected intraocular malignancy.
        2. painful blind eye.
        3. blind eye following significant penetrating trauma.
        4. cosmetically unacceptable phthisical eye.

    a. 1, 2, and 3.
    b. 1 and 3.
    c. 2 and 4.
    d. 4 only.
    e. 1, 2, 3, and 4.

171. The most common postoperative complication of enucleation is:

    a. superior sulcus deformity.
    b. socket contracture.
    c. enophthalmos.
    d. exophthalmos.
    e. extrusion of implant.

172. Which of the following features increase the risk of extrusion of orbital implants?

        1. implant too large for the orbit.
        2. comformer too large for the fornix.
        3. exposed synthetic integrated implants.
        4. orbital tissue infection.

    a. 1, 2, and 3.
    b. 1 and 3.
    c. 2 and 4.
    d. 4 only.
    e. 1, 2, 3, and 4.

173. T or F -- The primary advantage of evisceration over enucleation is the statically lower probability of sympathetic ophthalmia.

174. T or F -- The procedure of choice in severe socket contracture following enucleation involves the use of buccal mucosa grafts.

175. T or F -- The difference between subtotal and total exenteration is preservation of periorbita and eyelids in the former.

176. T or F -- The difference between total and extended exenterations is preservation of bony orbital walls in the former.

177. Which one of the following statements regarding the orbicularis oculi muscle is false?

    a. The orbital portion is primarily involved in forceful eyelid closure (winking and spasm).
    b. The palpebral portion is primarily involved in involuntary closure (blinking).
    c. The superficial medial head of the pretarsal portion of the muscle (Horner's tensor muscle) is critical to adequate lacrimal drainage.
    d. The lateral terminations of the pretarsal portion of the muscle constitute the lateral canthal tendon.
    e. The lateral terminations of the preseptal portion of the muscle constitute the lateral palpebral raphe.

178. Which of the following regarding the orbital septum is/are true?

    1. The septum arises both superiorly and inferiorly from the periosteum of the orbital rim.
    2. An intact, healthy orbital septum provides a relative barrier to intraorbital spread of subcutaneous infection.
    3. When fat is encountered intraoperatively, it implies retroseptal penetration.
    4. The orbital septum normally fuses with the levator aponeurosis in the upper lid in the same position as it does with the capsulopalpebral fascia in the lower lid.

    a. 1, 2, and 3.
    b. 1 and 3.
    c. 2 and 4.
    d. 4 only.
    e. 1, 2, 3, and 4.

179. Which of the following regarding Whitnall's ligament (superior suspensory ligament of the globe) is/are true?

    1. It is a condensation or extension of the sheath of the levator muscle.
    2. It acts as an important fulcrum for appropriate function of the levator muscle.
    3. It runs from the trochlea medially to the lateral orbital wall laterally.
    4. Standard ptosis surgery includes transection of Whitnall's ligament.

    a. 1, 2, and 3.
    b. 1 and 3.
    c. 2 and 4.
    d. 4 only.
    e. 1, 2, 3, and 4.

180. Which one of the following regarding the levator palpebrae superioris is false?

    a. The muscular portion is longer than the aponeurotic portion.
    b. It originates in close proximity to the superior rectus origin, just above the annulus of Zinn.
    c. Its superficial portion inserts into the orbicularis muscle and subcutaneous tissues.
    d. Its deeper portion inserts into the superior border of the tarsus.
    e. It runs from the posterior lacrimal crest medially to the lateral orbital tubercle laterally.

181. T or F -- Müller's muscle (superior tarsal muscle) generally accounts for approximately 4 mm of palpebral fissure height.

182. T or F -- The superior and inferior tarsal muscles both insert into the peripheral border of their respective tarsi.

183. Which of the following regarding the lower eyelid retractors is/are true?

    1. The lower eyelid analog of the levator aponeurosis is the capsulopalpebral fascia.
    2. The capsulopalpebral fascia arises from the common sheaths of the inferior oblique and inferior rectus muscles.
    3. Both the capsulopalpebral fascia and the inferior tarsal muscle insert into the inferior conjunctival fornix.
    4. The orbital septum inserts into the capsulopalpebral fascia 3 to 4 mm inferior to the inferior tarsal margin.

    a. 1, 2, and 3.
    b. 1 and 3.
    c. 2 and 4.
    d. 4 only.
    e. 1, 2, 3, and 4.

184. T or F -- The superior peripheral palpebral arterial arcade lies in a plane between the levator aponeurosis and Müller's muscle.

185. T or F -- The accessory lacrimal glands of Krause are found in the conjunctival fornix, while the glands of Wolfring are found at the tarsal border in the subconjunctival space.

186. T or F -- The anterior insertion of the medial canthal tendon is more important than the posterior insertion for maintenance of normal medial canthal appearance and function.

187. T or F -- "Antimongoloid" slant of the palpebral fissure occurs when the lateral canthus is greater than 3 mm higher than the medial canthus.

188. The structure that gives rise to the gray line of the eyelid margin is/are:

a. meibomian glands.
b. Moll's glands.
c. tarsal border.
d. the mucocutaneous junction.
e. the marginal strip of pretarsal orbicularis muscle.

189. The normal horizontal extent of the human palpebral fissure is approximately:

a. 20 mm.
b. 25 mm.
c. 30 mm.
d. 35 mm.
e. 40 mm.

190. T or F -- The palpebral arterial arcades provide numerous anastomotic connections between internal and external carotid circulations.

191. Arrange in order, from superficial (1) to deep (7), the structures listed below as encountered through an eyelid incision in the upper eyelid crease.

a. levator aponeurosis.	1.
b. skin.	2.
c. conjunctiva.	3.
d. Müller's muscle.	4.
e. orbicularis oculi.	5.
f. orbital fat.	6.
g. orbital septum.	7.

192. Which of the following are considered defining features of the blepharophimosis syndrome?

1. ptosis.
2. epicanthus tarsalis.
3. telecanthus.
4. lower lid ectropion.

a. 1, 2, and 3.
b. 1 and 3.
c. 2 and 4.
d. 4 only.
e. 1, 2, 3, and 4.

193. T or F -- The blepharophimosis syndrome is generally inherited on an autosomal dominant basis.

194. The systemic disorder most commonly associated with the blepharophimosis syndrome is:

   a. hypospadias.
   b. dry, redundant skin.
   c. primary amenorrhea.
   d. diabetes mellitus.
   e. coarctation of the aorta.

195. Match the anatomic definitions listed in the left-hand column with the correct terms listed in the right-hand column.

   a. fold of skin over the medial canthus, broader in the upper lid.
   b. pretarsal muscle and skin riding above the lid margin with vertical eyelashes.
   c. fold of skin over the medial canthus, broader over the lower lid.
   d. horizontal widening of palpebral fissure associated with antimongoloid slant and loss of contact between the lid and globe.
   e. partial or complete fusion of eyelids laterally by webs of skin.
   f. fold of skin over the medial canthus that is equally broad in both the upper and lower eyelids.

   1. euryblepharon.
   2. ankyloblepharon.
   3. epicanthus tarsalis.
   4. epicanthus palpebralis.
   5. epicanthus inversus.
   6. epiblepharon.

196. T or F -- Congenital coloboma of the upper eyelid is generally isolated, while that of the lower lid is more commonly associated with other facial abnormalities.

197. T or F -- In cryptophthalmos, the eye underlying the lid defect is generally normal.

198. Disadvantages of intralesion steroid treatment of chalazia relative to incision and curettage include:

   1. higher incidence of infection.
   2. potential depigmentation of overlying skin.
   3. steroid-induced glaucoma.
   4. lower success rate.

   a. 1, 2, and 3.
   b. 1 and 3.
   c. 2 and 4.
   d. 4 only.
   e. 1, 2, 3, and 4.

199. The most likely outcome following inadvertent suturing of the orbital septum into subcutaneous tissues while repairing a partial-thickness eyelid laceration is:

a. ectropion.
b. entropion.
c. kink of the lid margin.
d. lid retraction in downgaze.
e. ptosis.

200. The most reliable sign that the orbital septum has been involved in a partial-thickness lid laceration is:

a. ptosis.
b. orbital fat herniation.
c. entropion.
d. ectropion.
e. lid retraction in downgaze.

201. T or F -- In medial canthal tendon (MCT) avulsion, the critical maneuver in reestablishing cosmetic and anatomic integrity is reattachment of the anterior limb of the medial canthal tendon.

202. T or F -- Transnasal wiring or titanium plate fixation of the medial canthal tendon (MCT) is indicated in the presence of posterior medial canthal tendon avulsion and naso-orbital-ethmoid fracture.

203. Which of the following donor sites are considered acceptable for free skin grafts in the setting of lid lacerations with tissue loss?

1. retroauricular skin.
2. contralateral upper eyelid.
3. supraclavicular space.
4. buttock skin.

a. 1, 2, and 3.
b. 1 and 3.
c. 2 and 4.
d. 4 only.
e. 1, 2, 3, and 4.

204. To allow maximal spontaneous return of function before surgical repair, it is generally wise to observe traumatic ptosis in an adult for what period of time?

a. 4 weeks.
b. 2 months.
c. 3 months.
d. 6 months.
e. 12 months.

205. T or F -- Involutional ectropion is more common in the upper eyelid than in the lower eyelid.

206. Which of the following factors are important to evaluate before planning therapy for involutional ectropion?

    1. position of the inferior punctum.
    2. stability of the lower limb of the medial canthal tendon.
    3. stability of the lateral canthal tendon.
    4. presence or absence of contracture of the orbicularis muscle.

    a. 1, 2, and 3.
    b. 1 and 3.
    c. 2 and 4.
    d. 4 only.
    e. 1, 2, 3, and 4.

207. An acceptable temporizing measure for paralytic ectropion and severe corneal exposure associated with typical Bell's palsy might be:

    a. pentagonal wedge resection of the lower eyelid.
    b. temporary lateral tarsorrhaphy.
    c. frontalis brow suspension.
    d. punctal electrocautery.
    e. inferior retractor recession with full-thickness skin grafting of the lower lid.

208. T or F -- Adequate repair of severe cicatricial ectropion can be accomplished with scar relaxation techniques combined with horizontal tightening procedures.

209. T or F -- Involutional entropion is more commonly seen in the upper lid.

210. T or F -- The "snapback" test is useful in the evaluation of a patient with presumed involutional entropion.

211. T or F -- Digital pressure along the inferior border of the inferior tarsus will temporarily correct involutional entropion but not cicatricial entropion.

212. Which of the following is true regarding cryotherapy for trichiasis?

> 1. The treatment is probably more effective than electrolysis.
> 2. It employs a freeze-thaw-freeze technique.
> 3. Local anesthesia is required to minimize pain.
> 4. The only complication associated with the treatment is failure to eliminate trichiasis completely.

   a. 1, 2, and 3.
   b. 1 and 3.
   c. 2 and 4.
   d. 4 only.
   e. 1, 2, 3, and 4.

213. Critical components in the evaluation of corneal protection mechanisms prior to ptosis surgery include all of the following except:

   a. assessment of lagophthalmos.
   b. measurement of the margin-reflex distance.
   c. assessment of Bell's phenomenon.
   d. Schirmer's testing.
   e. assessment of corneal sensation.

214. The primary abnormality seen in simple congenital ptosis is in the:

   a. levator muscle.
   b. levator aponeurosis.
   c. levator innervation.
   d. third nerve nucleus.
   e. supranuclear control of lid function.

215. T or F -- In acquired myogenic ptosis, the amount of ptosis generally correlates well with the degree of residual levator function.

216. The primary abnormality seen in ptosis after cataract surgery is in the:

   a. levator muscle.
   b. levator aponeurosis.
   c. levator innervation.
   d. third nerve nucleus.
   e. supranuclear control of lid function.

217. T or F -- In aponeurotic ptosis, the amount of ptosis generally correlates well with the degree of residual levator function.

218. T or F -- The ptosis of myasthenia gravis almost always responds well to systemic anticholinesterase medication.

219. The ptosis associated with Marcus Gunn syndrome is due to aberrant connections between the levator muscle and which cranial nerve?

a. V.
b. VII.
c. IX.
d. X.
e. XII.

220. The procedure of choice for moderate unilateral acquired ptosis associated with good levator function and a normal upper eyelid crease should be:

a. Müller's muscle resection.
b. levator muscle resection.
c. reinsertion of levator aponeurosis.
d. bilateral frontalis suspension.
e. unilateral frontalis suspension.

221. The procedure of choice in a child with asymmetric but bilateral, moderate to severe congenital ptosis would be:

a. Müller's muscle resection.
b. levator muscle resection.
c. reinsertion of levator aponeurosis.
d. bilateral frontalis suspension.
e. unilateral frontalis suspension.

222. The procedure of choice in a patient with ptosis following cataract surgery (good levator function and a high or effaced upper eyelid crease) would be:

a. Müller's muscle resection.
b. levator muscle resection.
c. reinsertion of levator aponeurosis.
d. bilateral frontalis suspension.
e. unilateral frontalis.

223. T or F -- Unlike thyroid eye disease, the lid retraction of Collier's sign features greater retraction of the lateral lid than the medial lid.

224. T or F -- A subset of patients with congenital ptosis will also have impaired ipsilateral upgaze but no other signs of third nerve palsy.

225. All of the following are included in the differential diagnosis of eyelid retraction except:

    a. thyroid eye disease.
    b. cirrhosis.
    c. resection of superior rectus muscle.
    d. dorsal midbrain compression.
    e. myasthenia gravis.

226. T or F -- In the management of lid abnormalities and thyroid eye disease, inferior lid retraction is generally more easily and successfully repaired than superior lid retraction.

227. Which one of the following papillomatous lesions of the eyelid is considered premalignant?

    a. verruca vulgaris.
    b. seborrheic keratosis.
    c. actinic keratosis.
    d. nevus verruca.
    e. acanthosis nigricans.

228. Which of following papillomatous lesions of the eyelid may be associated with underlying systemic malignancy?

    a. verruca vulgaris.
    b. seborrheic keratosis.
    c. actinic keratosis.
    d. nevus verruca.
    e. acanthosis nigricans.

229. Which of the following eyelid lesions are typically slightly elevated with a central ulcerated area or crater?

    1. molluscum contagiosum.
    2. basal cell carcinoma.
    3. keratoacanthoma.
    4. verruca vulgaris.

    a. 1, 2, and 3.
    b. 1 and 3.
    c. 2 and 4.
    d. 4 only.
    e. 1, 2, 3, and 4.

230. Which of the following regarding basal cell carcinoma of the eyelid is/are true?

    1. It is the most common eyelid malignancy.
    2. It may be clinically indistinguishable from sebaceous cell carcinoma of the eyelid.
    3. The morpheaform pattern has the worst prognosis.
    4. It more frequently involves the lower eyelid than the upper eyelid.

    a. 1, 2, and 3.
    b. 1 and 3.
    c. 2 and 4.
    d. 4 only.
    e. 1, 2, 3, and 4.

231. Which one of the following regarding the treatment of basal cell carcinoma of the eyelid is false?

    a. Five-year mortality for all cases of ocular basal cell carcinoma approaches 3%.
    b. Complete surgical excision is the treatment of choice in virtually all cases.
    c. Following Mohs' resection of basal cell carcinoma, spontaneous granulation generally leads to the optimal cosmetic outcome.
    d. Cryotherapy of adnexal lesions may be considered in patients who are extremely poor candidates for surgery.
    e. Extirpation of medial canthal lesions may require resection of the lacrimal drainage system and/or subtotal exenteration.

232. T or F -- The clinical course of squamous cell carcinoma of the ocular adnexa is generally more indolent than that of basal cell carcinoma.

233. Which one of the following regarding sebaceous cell carcinoma is false?

    a. The primary focus may be either eyelid or caruncle.
    b. Recognition is often delayed due to misdiagnosis as innocent eyelid inflammation.
    c. Shave biopsy techniques are inadequate.
    d. As for basal cell carcinoma, the Mohs' surgical techniques offer optimal cosmetic outcome and long-term survival.
    e. The hallmarks of the histopathology of the condition include skip areas and pagetoid intraepithelial spread of malignancy.

234. Which one of the following regarding malignant melanoma of eyelid skin is false?

    a. The incidence of this neoplasm is increasing.
    b. The most common form, superficial spreading melanoma, has no direct relation to sun exposure.
    c. Nodular melanoma has the worst prognosis.
    d. The factor of greatest prognostic significant is depth of invasion.
    e. Like conjunctival melanosis, eyelid melanoma may be controlled with cryotherapy.

235. T or F -- In general, eyelid marginal defects of 25% or less may be repaired by direct closure, while larger defects require grafting or advancement techniques.

236. Which of the following may serve to distinguish dermatochalasis from blepharochalasis?

     1. age of onset.
     2. history of recurrent eyelid swelling.
     3. herniation of the orbital lobe of the lacrimal gland.
     4. coincident presence of true ptosis.

    a. 1, 2, and 3.
    b. 1 and 3.
    c. 2 and 4.
    d. 4 only.
    e. 1, 2, 3, and 4.

237. The most significant complication of blepharoplasty is:

    a. overcorrection.
    b. undercorrection.
    c. diplopia.
    d. orbital hemorrhage.
    e. cellulitis.

238. All of the following favor the diagnosis of benign essential blepharospasm over hemifacial spasm except:

    a. no involvement of lower facial muscles along with orbicularis muscle.
    b. bilateral involvement.
    c. absence of abnormal movements during sleep.
    d. synchronous contractures of involved muscles.
    e. lack of response to neurosurgical decompression of the facial nerve.

239. Which of the following regarding the treatment of essential blepharospasm is/are true?

     1. Botulinum injections offer effective but temporary relief.
     2. Stripping of orbicularis muscle fibers is a surgical alternative to botulinum injections.
     3. Treatment of essential blepharospasm may exacerbate coexistent dry eye syndrome.
     4. Facial nerve avulsion is a surgical modality preferable to orbicularis myectomy.

    a. 1, 2, and 3.
    b. 1 and 3.
    c. 2 and 4.
    d. 4 only.
    e. 1, 2, 3, and 4.

240. Which of the following regarding the secretory apparatus of the lacrimal system is/are true?

1. The lacrimal gland is split into two lobes by the check ligament of lateral rectus muscle.
2. Surgical removal of the orbital portion of the lacrimal gland with preservation of the palpebral portion will result in normal reflex tear secretion.
3. Surgical removal of the palpebral portion of the lacrimal gland with preservation of the orbital portion will result in preserved reflex tear secretion.
4. Efferent fibers to the lacrimal gland originate in the superior salivatory nucleus of the mid-pons.

a. 1, 2, and 3.
b. 1 and 3.
c. 2 and 4.
d. 4 only.
e. 1, 2, 3, and 4.

241. Which one of the following ganglia serves as the home for cell bodies providing postganglionic innervation of the lacrimal gland?

a. geniculate.
b. superior cervical.
c. ciliary.
d. pterygopalatine.
e. gasserian.

242. T or F -- The accessory lacrimal glands of Krause and Wolfring are responsible for basal tear secretion.

243. The average distance from lacrimal punctum to nasolacrimal sac is:

a. 2 mm.
b. 8 mm.
c. 10 mm.
d. 30 mm.
e. highly variable.

244. The average distance from lacrimal punctum to inferior nasal meatus is:

a. 2 mm.
b. 8 mm.
c. 10 mm.
d. 30 mm.
e. 50 mm.

245. T or F -- The flap of soft tissue that prevents reflex of nasal secretions into the nasolacrimal duct system is called the valve of Rosenmüller.

246. T or F -- The sites of obstruction in congenital and acquired nasolacrimal obstruction are identical.

247. Which one of the following functional tests of lacrimal drainage is most likely to yield a "false positive" result?

    a. primary dye test (Jones I test).
    b. secondary dye test (Jones II test).
    c. Schirmer's test.
    d. dye disappearance test.
    e. lacrimal scintigraphy.

248. Which one of the following functional tests of lacrimal drainage allows identification of a failure of the lacrimal pump mechanism?

    a. primary dye test (Jones I test).
    b. secondary dye test (Jones II test).
    c. Schirmer's test.
    d. dye disappearance test.
    e. lacrimal scintigraphy.

249. T or F -- As with congenital impatency of nasolacrimal system, probing of the nasolacrimal duct in acquired impatency may have long-lasting therapeutic benefit.

250. Diagnostic evaluation in the patient complaining of tearing whose functional tests are normal might include:

                1. examination of tear film.
                2. tear breakup-time testing (TBUT).
                3. complete Schirmer's testing.
                4. corneal sensation testing.

    a. 1, 2, and 3.
    b. 1 and 3.
    c. 2 and 4.
    d. 4 only.
    e. 1, 2, 3, and 4.

251. T or F -- Both superior and inferior canalicular systems must be patent for normal tear drainage.

252. Common causes of canalicular obstruction include all of the following except:

    a. congenital.
    b. trauma.
    c. phospholine iodide.
    d. Actinomyces infection.
    e. idoxuridine use.

253. A 65-year-old man is noted to have a chronic mucoid discharge coming from a mildly inflamed right lower punctum. Pressure on the right inferior canaliculus causes reflux of whitish-yellow granular and mucoid debris. A sample is obtained and sent for Gram's, Giemsa, and Gomori-methenamine silver stains, the last of which is shown in color plate 8. Treatment should consist of:

    1. warm compresses.
    2. topical penicillin.
    3. curettage of the canaliculus.
    4. dacryocystorhinostomy (DCR).

    a. 1, 2, and 3.
    b. 1 and 3.
    c. 2 and 4.
    d. 4 only.
    e. 1, 2, 3, and 4.

254. Intubation of the canalicular system following lacerating trauma is recommended for approximately what length of time?

    a. 1 to 2 weeks.
    b. 2 to 4 weeks.
    c. 4 to 6 weeks.
    d. 8 to 12 weeks.
    e. 3 to 6 months.

255. The most important predisposing factor for acute dacryocystitis is:

    a. chronic blepharitis.
    b. acute bacterial conjunctivitis.
    c. tear stasis of any etiology.
    d. ethmoid sinusitis.
    e. dry eye.

256. The initial management of acute dacryocystitis should include which of the following:

    1. irrigation and probing of the affected system.
    2. warm compresses.
    3. emergent dacryocystorhinostomy.
    4. oral antibiotics.

    a. 1, 2, and 3.
    b. 1 and 3.
    c. 2 and 4.
    d. 4 only.
    e. 1, 2, 3, and 4.

257. Acute, lancinating pain in the medial canthal region with minimal noninflamed enlargement of the lacrimal sac is most subjective of:

a. acute dacryocystitis.
b. chronic dacryocystitis.
c. impacted dacryolith.
d. <u>Actinomyces</u> canaliculitis.
e. Wegener's granulomatosis of the lacrimal sac.

258. T or F -- The most common malignant tumor of the lacrimal sac is adenocarcinoma.

259. T or F -- Congenital swelling of the medial canthus above the medial canthal tendon, in the absence of any active inflammation, probably represents congenital dacryocele.

260. Which of the following regarding congenital obstruction of the nasolacrimal system is/are true?

1. Approximately one third are bilateral.
2. If spontaneous resolution has not occurred by age 9 to 12 months, it is unlikely to occur.
3. Successful surgical management with probing alone becomes significantly less likely after the age of 1 year.
4. General anesthesia is generally necessary after the age of 6 months.

a. 1, 2, and 3.
b. 1 and 3.
c. 2 and 4.
d. 4 only.
e. 1, 2, 3, and 4.

261. T or F -- Following unsuccessful probings of a congenitally impatent nasolacrimal system, the next appropriate step is dacryocystorhinostomy.

262. The most common site of organic obstruction in acquired nasolacrimal obstruction is:

a. punctum.
b. canaliculus.
c. valve of Rosenmüller.
d. intraosseus nasolacrimal duct.
e. valve of Hasner.

263. Which of the following constitute indications for dacryocystorhinostomy?

      1. recurrent acute dacryocystitis.
      2. chronic discharge or symptomatic epiphora with a positive secondary dye test (organic obstruction).
      3. persistent epiphora in a child after probing and Silastic intubation of a congenitally impatent system.
      4. chronic discharge or symptomatic epiphora with a negative secondary dye test (functional obstruction).

    a. 1, 2, and 3.
    b. 1 and 3.
    c. 2 and 4.
    d. 4 only.
    e. 1, 2, 3, and 4.

264. T or F -- In probing the nasolacrimal system of an infant with congenital stenosis, it is better to start with the superior canaliculus.

265. The surgical approach of choice in a patient complaining of epiphora with severe canalicular trauma and scarring is:

    a. dacryocystorhinostomy (DCR).
    b. canaliculo-DCR.
    c. conjunctivo-DCR.
    d. Silastic intubation of the nasolacrimal system.
    e. marsupialization of the canalicular system.

266. A 27-year-old man presents with multiple nodules on all four eyelids, the largest of which is depicted in color plate 9. The lesions vary in size, but all appear similar, having a central crater. There is mild follicular conjunctivitis in both eyes. Which of the following regarding this patient's findings is/are true?

      1. The lesions are neoplastic.
      2. The patient's sexual and drug abuse histories should be taken.
      3. Actinic exposure plays a role in pathogenesis.
      4. Biopsy may reveal huge intracytoplasmic inclusions.

    a. 1, 2, and 3.
    b. 1 and 3.
    c. 2 and 4.
    d. 4 only.
    e. 1, 2, 3, and 4.

267. A 29-year-old black man presents for evaluation of "swollen eyes," which developed over 2 to 3 months. His external appearance is shown in color plate 10. With traction on the upper lid and the patient looking down, there is obvious prolapse of the palpebral lobe of the lacrimal gland, associated with conjunctival injection. There is no pain or tenderness. A biopsy of the lacrimal gland is shown in color plate 11. Which of the following is/are true?

1. The disorder may be associated with systemic metastatic calcification.
2. Total exenteration of the orbit should be undertaken immediately.
3. Plain radiograms of the chest should be obtained.
4. The patient is likely to have anti-SS antibodies in serum.

a. 1, 2, and 3.
b. 1 and 3.
c. 2 and 4.
d. 4 only.
e. 1, 2, 3, and 4.

Answers

1. True.

2. False. Each lateral orbital wall diverges at an angle of approximately 45 degrees from the midline.

3. False. The orbit is pear-shaped. Its widest dimension is a several millimeters <u>inside</u> the anterior rim.

4. True. The average human orbit has a volume of approximately 30 cc.

5. a. 2.
    b. 4.
    c. 1.
    d. 3.

6. a. 4.
    b. 1.
    c. 3.
    d. 2.

7. b. Blunt orbital trauma from the temporal side is most dangerous to the globe because it is most exposed laterally. (Of course, there is <u>no</u> orbital protection anteriorly!)

8. d.

9. b. The anterior portion of the medial wall is also known as the lamina papyracea, or paper-thin layer.

10. c. Blunt cranial trauma is often transmitted to the sphenoid, with secondary indirect traumatic optic neuropathy as a consequence.

11. a. 6.   h. 1.
    b. 6.   i. 6.
    c. 5.   j. 3.
    d. 1.   k. 7.
    e. 2.   l. 1.
    f. 6.   m. 4.

12. a. These anastomoses may prove critical in the setting of high-grade carotid stenosis. (The angular artery is the terminal branch of the facial artery, a branch of the external carotid system.)

13. a. 1.
    b. 2.
    c. 6.
    d. 5.
    e. 7.
    f. 3.
    g. 4.

14. b.

15. a. 1.
    b. 3.
    c. 3.
    d. 2.
    e. 3.
    f. 4.

16. b.   If pain is present, Graves' disease is almost certainly <u>not</u> the cause of the orbitopathy.

17. c.   The proptosis of Graves' disease is variable but usually axial (as is the case with meningioma). Lacrimal gland malignancies may produce proptosis, which is typically down and inward. Sinus tumors push the eye up.

18. c.   The history of proptosis due to pleomorphic adenoma is characteristically greater than 6 to 12 months.

19. False.   In hypertelorism, the medial orbital walls are separated excessively. In exorbitism, the lateral walls <u>diverge</u> excessively (greater than 90 degrees).

20. c.

21. d.

22. d.

23. d.

24. b.

25. True.   Children's orbits are more plastic, so disorders with a <u>short</u> duration can cause orbital enlargement. This is not the case in adults.

26. a. 4.
    b. 2.
    c. 1.
    d. 2.
    e. 1.
    f. 3.

27. False.   While CT does use greater radiation than plain films, it involves less than plain film tomography, which requires multiple exposures.

28. c.   Higher frequencies give better resolution. Lower frequencies give better penetration.

29. True.   See answer 28.

30. False.   See answer 28.

31. d.

32. b.   Neurofibromas will have high reflectivity. Lymphangioma will have irregular borders. Metastatic cancer and pseudotumor will have irregular borders and high reflectivity.

33. c.   Idiopathic orbital inflammation (pseudotumor) is the likely diagnosis.

34. a.   This represents considerable improvement over first-generation scanners, whose resolution was frequently no greater than 5 mm^3.

35. b.   Orbital studies are incomplete without coronal sections. Thin slices enhance sensitivity. Intrathecal metrizamide is rarely used since the advent of magnetic resonance imaging scanning (MRI), which is enhanced with powerful 1.5 tesla magnets.

36. a.   MRI scans are generated by exposing dipolar molecules to a radio frequency pulse after alignment with a powerful external magnetic field. Calcium is bright on standard x-rays but dark (hypointense) and poorly imaged with MRI.

37. False.   The magnet field used for MRI is several orders of magnitude <u>greater</u> than the earth's.

38. d.   Long T1 times render a substance hypointense (dark) on MRI scans.

39. False.   Vitreous appears <u>dark</u> on T1-weighted (long T1) and bright on T2-weighted (long T2) images.

40. True.   Orbital fat behaves <u>opposite</u> to vitreous. To determine the type of MRI image, look for which is brighter. If the fat is brighter, it is a T1-weighted image. If the vitreous is brighter, it is a T2-weighted image.

41. b.   CT is better for calcified structures. MRI is superior for soft tissues and intracranial evaluation. MRI is contraindicated in the setting of possible metallic foreign body, since it may be dislodged by the magnet (if the foreign body is ferromagnetic).

42. d.   MRI offers simultaneously available axial, coronal, and sagittal images. It takes longer to generate, increasing motion artifact. The "box" that patients must lie in may be "claustrophobogenic." MRI is at least twice as expensive and less accessible than CT scanning. This may not be true for long!

43. a. 2.   f. 8.
    b. 4, 3.   g. 2.
    c. 7.   h. 6.
    d. 1.   i. 5.
    e. 3.   j. 7.

44. False.   Anophthalmos is very rare.

45. True.   Enucleation in early childhood can lead to underdevelopment of the involved orbit. This is aggravated by irradiation.

46. b.   Apert's syndrome and Crouzon's disease are synostoses, not cleft syndromes.

47. a.   A bluish bulge <u>above</u> the medial canthal tendon is typically a meningocele, while one <u>below</u> is typically a dacryocele.

48. c. The orbits of patients with craniosynostoses are usually <u>small,</u> with resultant proptosis and exposure.

49. a. Both forms of inflammation will feature superficial erythema (rubor) and warmth (calor).

50. False. An intact orbital septum is an important, but not inviolable, barrier to infectious spread. Inappropriate treatment increases the risk. Rapid central spread of preseptal infection may be seen in infants and toddlers.

51. a. *Streptococcus* species are a close second.

52. d.

53. c. Dicloxacillin offers some advantage against beta-lactamase-producing organisms. Cephalexin (Keflex) is less expensive, yet still efficacious.

54. c. Intravenous antibiotics are indicated for *H. influenzae* cellulitis in children.

55. b. The other options listed are also risk factors, but ethmoid sinusitis is the most common.

56. c. Decreased vision suggests an acute orbital apex syndrome, requiring prompt decompression.

57. e. This is one of the most dreaded complications of orbital cellulitis, with a significant increase in systemic morbidity and mortality.

58. a. Patients with orbital cellulitis are typically febrile. For pseudotumor, this is uncommon except in children. A leukocytosis with "left-shift" is also more common in cellulitis. The sedimentation rate may be elevated in either condition, and in both, CT may show a nonspecific retrobulbar infiltrate but may have signs specific to one of the two disorders (e.g., muscle enlargement, subperiosteal abscess).

59. b. Two mm of discrepancy on exophthalmometry is the upper limit of normal. The external findings are consistent with either preseptal or orbital cellulitis. The "fever" is low grade and nonspecific. Strabismus indicates possible orbital inflammation.

60. a. First-generation cephalosporins are generally not sufficient for covering *H. influenzae* or anaerobes. Second-generation agents are preferred. Beta-lactamase-resistant penicillins, combined with the appropriate cephalosporin or chloramphenicol, are routinely used.

61. d. Failure to dramatically improve after 48 to 72 hours of antibiotic can indicate a subperiosteal abscess. Relapse after switching to oral antibiotics may also be a sign. Inappropriate choice of antibiotic should <u>not</u> be associated with modest improvement.

62. e.

63. a. Antibiotic penetration into abscesses is notoriously poor. "Pus must pass."

64. False. The phakomatoses <u>are</u> hamartomatous disorders. However, hamartomas are nests of abnormal tissue growth involving <u>normally native</u> tissue types. (Hamartoma--abnormal tissue in a normal place; choristoma--normal tissue in an abnormal place.)

65. d.   Both types are ectopic epithelial rests created by aberrant "pinching off" in utero. The variety that is silent until adulthood is generally intraorbital (retroseptal).

66. d.   Dermolipomas are more frequently on the bulbar surface and are generally solid (rather than cystic). Surgical excision is much more difficult due to unsuspected extension and periocular infiltration.

67. False.   More than one of the three germinative layers (ectoderm, mesoderm, and edoderm) must be present to label a lesion a teratoma, but all three need not be.

68. True.   They are frequently quite large at birth and thus simulate malignancy.

69. b.   Greater than half are obvious by 1 to 2 months of age.

70. b.   These tumors generally spontaneously regress, starting in the second year of life.

71. b.   These are two of the three primary indications for intervention. The third is significant cosmetic deformity.

72. d.   The nevus flammeus (port-wine stain) is a cavernous hemangioma of the dermis. Some pathology textbooks also refer to the lesion as a dermal telangiectasia.

73. d.   Capillary hemangiomata will blanch with pressure, while the nevus flammeus does not. There is considerable overlap between the other features listed.

74. False.   Many affected children have a systemic angiogenic disorder including pulmonary, soft-tissue, and/or skin lesions.

75. a.   Spontaneous involution continues over 4 to 7 years.

76. c.   Systemic and/or intralesional steroids may be associated with typical side effects (glaucoma and cataract), as well as rebound growth after cessation of therapy (steroid dependence). Steroid injections typically do cause soft-tissue atrophy and hypopigmentation. Radiation, rarely used except in the most severe cases, carries the most ominous risks, including future malignancy.

77. b.   Neither capillary nor cavernous hemagioma have high blood flow, and neither metastasize. Cavernous hemangioma are rarely seen in youth. As the name of each implies, the blood-filled spaces are tiny in the capillary hemangiomata and large in the cavernous variety.

78. False.   The orbit has no native lymphatic system. The origin of orbital lymphangioma is unclear.

79. a.   The lack of a well-defined capsule makes complete surgical excision very difficult. The growth pattern is infiltrative.

80. c.   Surgical strategies are frequently limited to "debulking" by any safe means possible, since complete excision is usually not possible.

81. a.   Each of the others may present and be treated as orbital cellulitis. Metastatic neuroblastoma may also simulate trauma, presenting with spontaneous periocular ecchymosis.

82. c.   Each of the others is considered typical. Pain is quite unusual.

83. b.   Tram-tracking is considered classic for meningioma.

84. d.   MRI has been a major advance in the management of patients with optic nerve tumors.

85. True.   The tumor may induce a secondary meningothelial hyperplastic response misinterpreted as meningioma.

86. e.   The management of optic nerve glioma in children is a subject of much discussion and honest disagreement among the experts. Any of the options may be correct in a given situation, and the ultimate choice must be individualized to the patient's circumstances (e.g., vision, size of tumor, extent of centripetal spread, age).

87. c.   Most experts agree that intracranial spread (or a high likelihood of such), rapid growth simulating a malignant variety, and loss of functional vision constitute indications for intervention.

88. c.   Dysplasia or aplasia of the sphenoid bone creates large posterior orbital defects. This leads to pulsating exophthalmos, as brain tissue herniates outward.

89. d.   Orbital pseudotumor should not cause bony erosion. Mucocele, glioma, and neurofibromas are rarely so inflammatory. Rhabdomyosarcoma responds well to treatment and should be promptly diagnosed.

90. e.   All the statements are true, except that alveolar rhabomyosarcoma has a predilection for the inferior orbit. The embryonal variant is more common superonasally. Metastatic workup includes lumbar puncture and bone marrow biopsy, best done under anesthesia.

91. a. 4.   e. 1.
     b. 4.   f. 4.
     c. 1.   g. 2.
     d. 3.

92. False. The tumor does not arise from malignant transformation of extraocular muscle. The cell of origin is probably a mesodermal anlage (remnant) within orbital connective tissue.

93. False. Most periocular metastases in children are orbital, unlike in adults. The most common is neuroblastoma.

94. c.

95. False. Mucormycosis is generally seen only in the immunocompromised (chemotherapy, post-transplant, diabetics). Aspergillosis is probably more common in this population, as well, but it may be seen in otherwise healthy individuals.

96. c.   Orbital phycomycosis generally results from invasion by necrotizing fungal sinusitis. Black eschar in the nasal cavity is virtually diagnostic, but is a late finding. (Its absence does not exclude the diagnosis.)

97. a.   Fibrous histiocytoma is slightly more common in men. The others are more common in women, by a ratio of at least 1.5:1.

98. c.   If pain is present, Graves' disease is highly unlikely.

99. 1. c.
     2. d.
     3. a.
     4. b.

100. a.   Decreasing acuity, relative afferent pupillary defect, impairment of color vision, and evidence of scotomata may all be indicative of optic nerve compression. Maculopathy is uncommon in Graves' disease.

101. False. Thyroid-related orbitopathy can occur despite a persistently euthyroid state (as indicated by clinical and laboratory findings).

102. c.   Acute corneal decompensation and evidence of optic nerve compression are indications for immediate surgical intervention. Strabismus surgery should be delayed until the inflammation is quiescent and the examination has stabilized. Levator aponeurosis recession may yield unpredictable results in the setting of active inflammation.

103. e.   This is the most sensitive way to detect hyperthyroidism; feedback regulation can lead to a reliably detectable decrease in TSH, even when fluctuating levels of T4 and T3 may not be indicative.

104. False. The atrophy of myofibrils is felt to be secondary to compression by surrounding edema. The latter occurs with deposition of glycosaminoglycans in the presence of inflammatory cell and fibroblast infiltration. Primary destruction of myocytes does not seem to occur.

105. True.   Fibrosis tends to be less severe, leading to partial loss of the normal glandular tissue.

106. d.   The enlargement generally features smooth contours. Although sometimes only a single muscle is enlarged, this should be considered an atypical finding. Posterior scleral enhancement is more suggestive of orbital inflammatory syndrome/pseudotumor or posterior scleritis.

107. b.   Corticosteroids would be relatively contraindicated in light of the patient's diabetes. Tarsorrhaphy, though safe, would do nothing for the optic nerve compromise.

108. c.   This allows adequate time for stability of the condition to be established, allowing for a more predictable outcome.

109. 1. b.   Optic nerve decompression gets the highest priority, as does
     2. a.   tarsorrhaphy for corneal exposure. Strabismus surgery should be
     3. c.   performed before lid surgery because the former can cause changes in resting lid position.

110. b.   Changes in corneal sensation may occur, but frank ulceration -- especially peripherally--is unusual.

111. c.   Orbital pseudotumor is generally quite painful for both children and adults.

112. e.   The lack of pain as a prominent symptom contributes to the insidious progress of this condition and the possibility of misdiagnosis as a neoplasm. Its tendency to be diagnosed at a later stage, when fibrosis has already occurred, may contribute to the diminished response to steroids(relative to other forms of the disease).

113. b. A dosage of 60 mg of prednisone is at the lower end of the usual range. Further attempt should be made to bring about a response with stronger steroid therapy before subjecting the patient to the risks of biopsy. (Dramatic worsening of the patient's condition might provoke earlier biopsy, however.)

114. a. The inflammatory infiltrate is polymorphous and may include neutrophils. Graves' myositis may look identical.

115. c. Unlike Graves' ophthalmopathy, pseudotumor can and commonly does involve the muscle tendons as well as their insertions, along with posterior Tenon's fascia.

116. d. Sarcoidosis is generally not associated with pain and usually spares orbital soft tissues.

117. c. Sjögren's syndrome typically would present with keratoconjunctivitis sicca and/or a dry mouth, usually along with symptoms of (or a diagnosis of) a collagen-vascular disease like rheumatoid arthritis. Furthermore, the lacrimal glands are usually small. Orbital pseudotumor is usually painful.

118. a. These lesions generally do not have the high arterial blood flow usually associated with bruits. Their composition--densely packed vascular channels--leads to a high internal reflectively on ultrasound.

119. True. Hemangiopericytomas tend to be more rapidly expansile and aggressive tumors, increasing the likelihood of adversely affecting ocular motility.

120. False. Benign-appearing tumors of this type may turn out to be invasive and eventually spread metastatically. Some that appear quite malignant, with poor differentiation and many mitotic figures, may remain relatively quiescent!

121. c. This would be a classic presentation of an internal carotid-cavernous sinus fistula, often resulting from the shearing effect of rapid acceleration/deceleration trauma on the relatively fixed/immobile artery passing through the sinus.

122. e. This is, in contrast to the previous question, a classic presentation of a cavernous sinus wall-dural shunt, featuring lower arterial flow and a more insidious onset.

123. False. Varices are venous structures that usually would not have sufficient blood flow to produce an audible bruit. The classic presentation is proptosis with the Valsalva maneuver.

124. True. Most are of intracranial origin; however, with the widespread use of computed tomography, it has become apparent that primary optic nerve sheath meningiomas are much more common than was once thought--many being asymptomatic lesions found incidentally.

125. False. In neurofibromatosis, the growth pattern tends to be paraxial (diffusely along the nerve sheath) rather than focal.

126. e. Although it could be argued that MRI may better delineate the tumor initially, bony changes--particularly those that are subtle--will be better seen with CT. Gadolinium-enhanced MRI is particularly valuable for detecting intracranial spread.

127. False. The fragile pial vessels supplying the optic nerve are easily disrupted by any attempt to remove the tumor.

128. a.   As these tumors are usually histologically benign--despite being locally destructive--
            they can often be observed for years without risking the loss of vision that would
            accompany excision. When vision has become too poor to counterbalance the risk
            of tumor spread (if such is occurring), or if tumor growth is becoming potentially
            life-threatening, surgical intervention is indicated. Pediatric meningiomas are more
            aggressive than adult tumors and are removed earlier.

129. False. Although optic nerve gliomas presenting in adulthood do tend to be particularly
            malignant, this applies to isolated tumors (not associated with neurofibromatosis).
            The latter generally (in adults and children) have a better prognosis.

130. e.   In contrast, orbit specialists probably see 50% epithelial neoplasms and 50%
            inflammatory/lymphoid lesions.

131. c.   Adenoid cystic carcinoma is the most common malignant neoplasm of this location.

132. c.   Pain is more typical of <u>acute</u> inflammatory, infectious, or malignant lesions.
            Duration of symptoms is helpful in separating slowly progressive (benign) lesions,
            such as the benign mixed tumor, from more acute conditions, such as malignant
            neoplasm or inflammation. Radiologic findings are the third critical feature in the
            evaluation. Osteolysis strongly favors a malignant lesion.

133. c.   Soft-tissue contour analysis can help differentiate between lymphoid tumors
            (elongated smooth masses-- "pancakes") from parenchymal tumors (globular
            masses). Adenoid cystic carcinomas usually produce bony destruction. Benign
            mixed cell tumors often cause concave pressure changes in the adjacent bone.
            Lymphoid and inflammatory lesions rarely cause bony changes.

134. a. 7.
     b. 4.
     c. 5.
     d. 3.
     e. 6.
     f. 3
     g. 8.
     h. 5.
     i. 5.

135. b.   The most likely diagnosis is that of benign mixed cell tumor.   The male-female ratio
            is 3:2. The tumor should be approached through a lateral orbitotomy with careful
            excision to avoid rupture of the tumor's pseudocapsule. Incisional or incomplete
            biopsy techniques can lead to infiltrative tumor recurrence and, occasionally,
            malignant transformation.

136. c.   Mucoepidermoid carcinoma is distinctly uncommon.

137. False. Although adenoid cystic carcinomas may cause severe pain, it is usually due to
            perineural invasion and bony destruction.

138. d.   Fibrous dysplasia may be monostotic (affect only one bone) or polyostotic. The
            polyostotic variety may present with precocious puberty and dermal hyperpigmented
            macules. This disorder, Albright's syndrome, <u>rarely</u> involves the orbit. Orbital
            disease is nearly always monostotic and rarely associated with precocious puberty,
            regardless of age. Surgical curettage or excision is usually undertaken.

139. c.   Eosinophilic granuloma frequently involves the orbital bones. The classic triad of Hand-Schüller-Christian disease consists of proptosis, lytic skull lesions, and diabetes insipidus. Orbital involvement is rare in Letterer-Siwe disease.

140. False.   Chemotherapy (vincristine or vinblastine) is required for patients with disseminated disease. In contrast, the lesions of eosinophilic granuloma may (1) be observed for spontaneous regression, (2) be excised, or (3) receive radiotherapy (if advanced).

141. d.

142. False.   Ten percent have metastatic potential. Another 16% are termed "locally aggressive" but not frankly malignant.

143. False.   It is impossible to differentiate clinically or radiologically between benign reactive lymphoid hyperplasia and orbital lymphoma. Biopsy with light microscopy, immunochemical staining, and electron microscopy is necessary to distinguish between them.

144. d.   The central nervous system (CNS) is not routinely surveyed in patients with orbital lymphoma. This is in distinction to patients with intraocular lymphoma. When CNS involvement is suspected, CT or MRI is the starting point.

145. c.   Benign reactive hyperplasia tends to produce a high degree of endothelial cell proliferation, with numerous germinal centers. T-cells predominate in a mixture of acute and chronic cells. In some borderline lesions, atypical cells may be seen. These may be thought of as "atypical reactive lymphoid hyperplasia."

146. b.   Both orbital inflammatory syndrome and lymphoproliferation are composed of polyclonal lymphocytes (although lymphoma contains a monoclonal subpopulation). Cellular heterogenity is a feature of both orbital inflammatory syndrome and reactive lymphoid hyperplasia. The key features separating the two are (1) prominent fibrovascular stroma and (2) hypocellularity, both seen in pseudotumor and not in lymphoid activation.

147. a.   The three orbital deposits that are hyperintense on T1 weighted images are:

1. blood
2. melanin
3. mucous

148. False.   The nose and paranasal sinuses are more frequently the focus of tumors that secondarily invade the orbit.

149. b.   The most common sinus neoplasm to invade the orbit is squamous cell carcinoma.

150. a.   Typically, the orbital metastasis occurs months to years after diagnosis and treatment of the primary tumor. A classic (but uncommon) presentation is progressive enophthalmos due to scirrhous breast carcinoma, which contracts and scars, drawing the eye inward.

151. b.   An orbital metastasis is more likely to be the mode of presentation for bronchogenic carcinoma than for a breast primary.

152. a. 3.
    b. 1.
    c. 3.
    d. 2.
    e. 1.
    f. 2.

153. d. The tripod complex is produced by three distinct fractures along suture lines--zygomaticofrontal, zygomaticomaxillary, and the zygomatic arch. Ocular motility may or may not be normal in pure tripod fractures, but upgaze should be spared. Repair is indicated when there is marked cosmetic deformity or potential mandibular instability.

154. c. Telecanthus is definded as an abnormally large distance between medial canthi, regardless of intraorbital distance.

155. False. The qualifier "indirect" implies that forces other than direct contact with a blunt object led to orbital wall fracture (for instance, suddenly increasing intraorbital pressure). This type is rarely associated with orbital rim fracture, which is seen more frequently as a component of direct orbital wall fractures.

156. c. Subcutaneous emphysema is usually produced by medial or inferior orbital wall fractures into the ethmoid or maxillary sinuses. The addition of volume to the orbit also aggravates enophthalmos.

157. d. Orbital floor fractures usually produce vertical limitations of gaze. Global motility deficits generally indicate blunt trauma with muscle and/or nerve contusion.

158. False. CT of the orbit with coronal and sagittal views gives better definition of the soft tissue and bony structures than plain films. MRI has no role, since bone is dark.

159. False. With severe muscle contusion, edema, or hemorrhage, forced ductions may be falsely positive or impossible to interpret. They are more fruitful if performed 5 to 10 days after injury.

160. False. Enopthalmos often develops after the swelling subsides from an initially exophthalmic orbit.

161. True. Most diplopia is due to reversible muscle contusion.

162. a. Infraorbital hypesthesia may or may not resolve on its own. Whether it is affected by orbital surgery is controversial. Its functional impact is minimal.

163. False. Large, complex anterior fractures lead to marked inferior orbital herniation without entrapment. This causes hypoglobus and enopthalmos. Small, posterior fractures can cause significant entrapment as a crowded muscle belly is forced or pinched into the defect. In these cases, enophthalmos is minimal.

164. d. This time period provides a chance for orbital swelling and "contusion diplopia" to resolve and yet is early enough to avoid problems with scarring of a significant floor fracture.

165. b.   Vegetable foreign bodies carry a high risk of infection. Lead can cause a granulomatous reaction, but if far posterior should be left in place. Orbital apex foreign bodies are hazardous to remove and should be pursued only if there is convincing evidence of direct optic nerve compromise (decreased vision, afferent pupillary defect, dyschromatopsia).

166. d.   When ocular or optic disc perfusion is severely compromised by an orbital compartment syndrome, immediate canthotomy with <u>cantholysis</u> should be performed to decompress the orbit.

167. a.   In cases where the ocular examination suggests optic nerve trauma (afferent pupillary defect, poor vision), neuro-imaging is indicated to rule out direct optic nerve injury (e.g., optic canal fracture).

168. False.   In direct optic nerve trauma, something physically impinges on the optic nerve, but it need not be a foreign body (e.g., bone fragments). In indirect trauma, nothing can be found to have directly struck the nerve.

169. a.   Since no obvious lesion can be identified on the CT scan, the optic nerve injury is most likely indirect. Emergent high-dose intravenous methylprednisolone is indicated to reduce swelling associated with the injury. Optic canal decompression should also be considered.

170. b.   Each of these constitute indications for enucleations. However, evisceration provides better cosmesis and is technically easier to perform. The advantages of enucleation are preservation of ocular pathology for microscopic review and lower risk of sympathetic ophthalmia. A cosmetically unacceptable phthisical eye may be covered with a prosthetic shell.

171. a.   This complication results from inadequate volume replacement when the eye is removed from the orbit.

172. e.   All of these factors increase the likelihood of orbital implant extrusion. (A conformer that is too large will place stress on the soft-tissue closure).

173. False.   Theoretically, the chance of sympathetic ophthalmia is greater with evisceration than enucleation (see answer 170).

174. True.   Buccal mucosal grafting is ideal for the treatment of socket contracture. Care must be taken to avoid damaging the duct from the parotid gland when harvesting the graft.

175. True.

176. True.

177. c.   The <u>deep</u> head of the pretarsal muscle (Horner's tensor tarsi) is a localized bundle of pretarsal orbicularis that is critical to adequate tear drainage.

178. a.   In the lower eyelid, the orbital septum fuses with the capsulopalpebral fascia at or immediately below the inferior tarsal border. In the upper eyelid of whites, the septum fuses with the levator aponeurois about 3 mm above the superior tarsal border.

179. a.   Whitnall's ligament should not be confused with the horns of the levator aponeurosis, which <u>are</u> structures to be cut during ptosis surgery.

180. d.   The deeper or posterior portion inserts onto the anterior surface of the lower half of the tarsus, not to its superior border. Müller's muscle inserts into the superior border of the tarsus.

181. False.   Müller's muscle accounts for about 2 mm of vertical palpebral fissure height.

182. True.

183. a.   The orbital septum fuses with the capsulopalpebral fascia at or immediately below the inferior tarsal border.

184. True.   This arcade is found immediately above the superior tarsal border in the plane between the levator aponeurosis and Müller's muscle.

185. True.   These accessory lacrimal glands are responsible for basal lacrimal secretion; in contrast, the lacrimal gland is responsible for reflex tear secretion.

186. False.   The posterior portion of the medial canthal tendon inserts into the posterior lacrimal crest and is highly important in maintaining normal medial canthal appearance and function.

187. False.   The normal "mongoloid" slant of the palpebral fissure occurs because of the higher insertion of the lateral canthal tendon (3 mm higher than the medial canthal tendon). "Antimongoloid" slant occurs when the lateral tendon inserts lower than the medial.

188. e.   This strip is also known as the muscle of Riolan.

189. c.   The normal adult palpebral fissure is 30 mm horizontally and 8 to 11 mm vertically.

190. True.   The internal carotid artery provides blood by route of the ophthalmic artery and its branches, while the external carotid artery provides blood by route of the angular and temporal arteries of the face.

191. 1. b.
     2. e.
     3. g.
     4. f.
     5. a.
     6. d.
     7. c.

192. b.   Blepharophimosis syndrome (congenital eyelid syndrome) is characterized by telecanthus, epicanthus inversus, severe ptosis, and blepharophimosis. Ectropion is a variable feature.

193. True.

194. c.   This is the only known association with blepharophimosis.

195. a. 3.
    b. 6.
    c. 5.
    d. 1.
    e. 2.
    f. 4.

196. True.

197. False.   Severe ocular defects are usually hidden by the fused lids.

198. c.

199. d.

200. b.   Orbital fat is "sandwiched" between orbital septum (superficial) and levator aponeurosis (deep).

201. False.   The posterior limb of the tendon must be reattached to posterior lacrimal crest, or the lid contour will ride away from the globe surface.

202. True.   Adequate MCT fixation requires a firm base. A high nasal fracture precludes this without a plate or contralateral (transnasal) fixation.

203. a.   Hairless skin of similar pigmentation must be chosen. Buttock skin has hair!

204. d.

205. False.   It is far more common in the lower eyelid.

206. e.

207. b.

208. False.   Skin grafting must be included for success.

209. False.   Entropion of any etiology is more common in the lower lid.

210. True.   This is a simple test of skin elasticity.

211. True.   In cicatricial entropion, vertical foreshortening is present, rather than the redundancy of involutional entropion.

212. a.   Lid notching, scarring, hypopigmentation, and edema may be seen after lash cryoepilation.

213. b.   Margin-reflex distance is a measure of ptosis severity and has nothing to do with corneal protection mechanisms.

214. a.   Congenital myogenic ptosis, in isolation, is a muscular dystrophy (maldevelopment) typically affecting only the levator-superior rectus complex (see answer 224).

215. True.

216. b.   Aponeurotic dehiscence has been blamed on anesthetic injections, lid specula, and bridle sutures. The exact cause is not clear.

217. False.   The muscle is spared, so despite severe ptosis, levator function is usually good.

218. False.   Actually, the ptosis is often medication resistant.

219. a.   Levator innervation is derived from the trigeminal supply (V) to the pterygoids and masseters!

220. b.   Müllers' resections only offer 1 to 3 mm of improvement. Aponeurosis surgery is indicated for a blunted or high eyelid crease. Frontalis suspension is bilateral surgery for severe bilateral ptosis.

221. d.   See answer 220.

222. c.   See answer 220.

223. False.   The converse is true: Lateral lid retraction is greater than medial in Graves' disease.

224. True.   A combined levator-superior rectus dystrophy is cited as the cause.

225. c.   Recession of the superior rectus muscle may cause lid retraction. Resection will lead to ptosis.

226. False.   Both may be difficult, but lower lid retraction is more challenging. Its repair may necessitate spacer grafts (e.g., auricular cartilage, hard palate).

227. c.   Acanthosis nigricans is associated with internal malignancy but not transformation. Actinic keratosis is related to UV exposure and may develop into squamous cell carcinoma.

228. e.   See answer 227.

229. a.   Verruca are typically papilliform without central excavation.

230. e.   The fibrosing, or morpheaform, pattern extends in thin, fingerlike projections, which escape excision or radiation.

231. c.   Mohs' surgeons may permit healing by secondary intention (granulation), but most prefer early (delayed primary) closure via flaps or grafts.

232. False.   Squamous cell carcinoma is less common but clinically more aggressive.

233. d.   There may be multicentric foci of tumor with skip areas, and negative margins do not necessarily imply complete excision of the tumor. Hence, Mohs' surgery should not be undertaken. Wide surgical margins should be used, with map biopsies taken over the entire ocular surface.

234. e.   Cryotheraphy selectively destroys melanocytes but is insufficient for cutaneous melanoma and should be considered a palliative treatment.

235. True.

236. a.   Blepharochalasis is a rare idiopathic disorder leading to inflammatory edema of the eyelids. It is familial, and younger patients, especially females, are affected. The repeated episodes of edema may cause ptosis and herniation of the orbital lobe of the lacrimal gland. Dermatochalasis is redundant preseptal skin due to aging. True ptosis (involutional) may be present in either disorder.

237. d.   Injury to orbital fat pads, vessels, or orbicularis may result in retrobulbar hemorrhage that dissects into the posterior orbit and compresses the optic nerve.

238. d.   Hemifacial spasm is rarely bilateral and is usually due to vascular compression of the seventh cranial nerve at the brainstem and can result in synchronous contractions of the entire side of the face. Along with partial complex seizures and myoclonic epilepsy, essential blepharospasm is effaced by sleep.

239. a.   Any treatment for belpharospasm is designed to decrease eyelid closure. Thus, dry eye will be aggravated. Facial nerve ablation suffers from recurrence rates as high as 30% and is associated with complications such as paralysis of the entire face. Orbicularis myectomy is usually preferred to facial nerve avulsion. Botulinim injection is the initial treatment of choice.

240. d.   The lateral horn of the levator aponeurosis divides the lacrimal gland. Removal of the orbital lacrimal gland removes the efferent input and interferes with reflex tearing, whereas removal of the palpebral lobe damages the ducts from the orbital portion, which run through the palprebral lobe. This impairs reflex tearing as well.

241. d.

242. True.

243. c.   It is 2 mm down (ampulla), then 8 mm across (canaliculus).

244. d.   The sac plus duct add another 20 to 25 mm, for 30 mm total from punctum to inferior meatus.

245. False.   The valve of Hasner provides this protection. The valve of Rosenmüller prevents tear reflux from lacrimal sac to canaliculi.

246. False.   In congenital obstruction, the blockage is at the valve of Hasner. In acquired cases, the blockage is within the intraosseous nasolacrimal duct.

247. a.   Jones I test consists of placing 2% fluorescein in the conjunctival fornices and attempting to recover fluorescein with a swab at the inferior meatus. Unfortunately, one-third of normal patients will have abnormal results with this test.

248. b.   Jones II test is performed after dye disappearance test or after Jones I indicates blockage. The fornix is irrigated, and the lacrimal sac cannulated and irrigated. If dye is recovered in the inferior meatus, then incomplete blockage of the nasolacrimal duct, patent upper system, and functioning lacrimal pump is indicated. However, if only clear fluid is recovered, then a nonfunctioning lacrimal pump or blocked upper system is indicated.

249. False.   Probing of acquired obstructions rarely yields permanent patency.

250. a.   If no functional or organic obstruction is discovered, then hyperlacrimation probably accounts for tearing. The evaluation of the tear film and lacrimal secretory function should be performed. Abnormal tear film precipitates or mucus may be discovered, and TBUT less than 10 seconds indicates poor function of the inner mucinous layer of the tear. Schirmer's testing provides information on reflex and basal secretion of lacrimal gland.

251. False.   A single functioning punctum and canaliculus is usually sufficient.

252. a.   Congenital obstructions usually occur at the valve of Hasner. Canalicular impatency is rare in infants.

253. a.   The Gomori-methenamine silver (GMS) stain shows slender branching organisms reminiscent of fungus. Bacteria known to resemble fungus in routine stains include Nocardia and Actinomyces. The former is distinguished by acid-fast positivity, while the latter by its dependency on vitamin K in culture media. Fungal canaliculitis is relatively uncommon compared to Actinomyces infections. Appropriate treatment generally consists of canalicular clean-out combined with topical penicillin. DCR may ultimately be required, but less invasive maneuvers should be attempted first.

254. e.   The longer, the better!

255. c.   Strictures, narrow or long ducts, and nasal and sinus inflammatory disease may cause tear stasis and lead to acute dacryocystitis.

256. c.   Again, less invasive maneuvers should be tried first. Probing and irrigation offer little here.

257. c.   This is the ocular equivalent of a kidney stone!

258. False.   The most common malignant tumor of the lacrimal sac is squamous cell carcinoma.

259. False.   Dacryocele is usually below the medial canthal tendon. Encephalocele is usually above the medial canthal tendon.

260. e.

261. False.   The next appropriate step is Silastic intubation. DCR follows if this is unsuccessful.

262. d.   See answer 240.

263. a.   A negative secondary dye test indicates poor lacrimal pump function; DCR would not be helpful.

264. True.   The superior canaliculus possesses more maneuverable angles and hence is easier to probe. Furthermore, there is less functional significance if a false passage is created.

265. c.   Complete bypass of the canalicular system is required, and conjunctivo-DCR with placement of a Jones tube is the only choice to provide this bypass.

266. c.   Eyelid nodules with central craters generate the following first-order differential diagnosis: (1) basal cell carcinoma (BCC), (2) keratoacanthoma, and (3) molluscum contagiosum. Only molluscum would be expected to present with multiple distinct nodules (in the basal cell nevus syndrome, BCC might present multiply). While healthy individuals can certainly develop molluscum, multiple large lesions suggest an underlying immune deficiency. The pathognomonic finding on light microscopy is the presence of huge eosinophilic intracytoplasmic inclusions.

267. b.   This young black man has bilateral painless enlargement of the lacrimal glands. Biopsy is consistent with the most likely etiology--sarcoidosis. Hypercalcemia due to enhanced vitamin D activity may lead to metastatic calcification. Chest x-ray may indicate pulmonary disease (hilar adenopathy); treatment is usually reserved for pulmonary symptoms or compromised pulmonary function tests. Anti-SS antibodies are typical of Sjögren's syndrome (autoimune lymphocytic dacryoadenitis) and are rarely seen in sarcoidosis. Furthermore, lacrimal gland enlargement is relatively uncommon with Sjögren's syndrome. Certainly, orbital exenteration for this bilateral immunologic disorder is not indicated.

References

1. Katowitz, J. A. "Section 7: Orbit, Eyelids, and Lacrimal System." in F.M. Wilson (ed.). Basic and Clinical Science Course. San Francisco: American Academy of Ophthalmology, 1991-1992.

2. Hornblass, Albert (ed.). Oculoplastic, Orbital, and Reconstructive Surgery. Baltimore: Williams and Wilkins, 1990.

7: Cornea and External Disease

1. The cardinal signs of inflammation include all of the following except:

   a. redness.
   b. irreversible architectural disruption.
   c. tenderness or pain.
   d. loss of function.
   e. warmth.

2. T or F -- The key difference between a toxic agent and an immune agent is that cellular damage by the former is independent of previous exposure.

3. T or F -- Macrophages and polymorphonuclear leukocytes (PMNs) incite similar degrees of local tissue damage in acute inflammatory reactions.

4. Which of the following markers of ocular inflammation are relatively nonspecific in the determination of etiology?

   1. conjunctival papillae.
   2. conjunctival follicles.
   3. chemosis
   4. giant conjunctival papillae.

   a. 1, 2, and 3.
   b. 1 and 3.
   c. 2 and 4.
   d. 4 only.
   e. 1, 2, 3, and 4.

5. Conjunctival papillae can be seen in inflammation of the:

   1. conjunctival fornices.
   2. tarsal conjunctiva.
   3. bulbar conjunctiva.
   4. limbal conjunctiva.

   a. 1, 2, and 3.
   b. 1 and 3.
   c. 2 and 4.
   d. 4 only.
   e. 1, 2, 3, and 4.

6. A conjunctival inflammatory response characterized by multiple polygonal nodules with central fibrovascular cores is consistent with a:

   a. follicular response.
   b. papillary response.
   c. phlyctenular response.
   d. giant papillary response.
   e. ligneous response.

7. Connective tissue septa in the subepithelial space are responsible for the development of which inflammatory morphology?

   a. papillae.
   b. follicles.
   c. phlyctenules.
   d. Herbert's pits.
   e. giant papillae.

8. The least reliable location of a conjunctival papillary response for etiologic interpretation is the:

   a. inferior fornix.
   b. superior fornix.
   c. superior edge of superior tarsus.
   d. inferior edge of superior tarsus.
   e. limbus.

9. T or F -- The definition of a giant papilla is a papilla greater than 5 mm in diameter.

10. The differential diagnosis of a true giant papillary conjunctivitis (GPC) includes all of the following except:

    a. contact lens-related conjunctivitis.
    b. trachoma.
    c. atopic keratoconjunctivitis.
    d. ocular prosthesis-related conjunctivitis.
    e. vernal keratoconjunctivitis.

11. Clumps of calcific degeneration and eosinophils at the limbus are termed:

    a. Herbert's pits.
    b. von Arlt's line.
    c. Fuchs' spots.
    d. Horner-Trantas dots.
    e. Cogan's patches.

12. Rounded, depressed regions of necrotic limbal follicles are termed:

    a. Herbert's pits.
    b. von Arlt's line.
    c. Fuchs' spots.
    d. Horner-Trantas dots.
    e. Cogan's patches.

13. T or F -- The various forms of giant papillary conjunctivitis (GPC) are indistinguishable clinically.

14. T or F -- With adequate treatment, the clinical symptoms of contact lens-related GPC generally remit before the papillae disappear.

15. Mild contact lens-related GPC may be differentiated from an infectious follicular conjunctivitis by:

    1. the presence of itching in the former.
    2. the presence of mucous and serous discharge in the latter.
    3. injection of bulbar conjunctiva in the latter.
    4. findings in the inferior conjunctival fornix of the latter.

    a. 1, 2, and 3.
    b. 1 and 3.
    c. 2 and 4.
    d. 4 only.
    e. 1, 2, 3, and 4.

16. Rounded, gelatinous-appearing lesions of the conjunctiva with vessels at the periphery, but never within the nodular substance, are called:

    a. follicles.
    b. papillae.
    c. phlyctenules.
    d. giant papillae.
    e. pseudomembranes.

17. Follicular conjunctivitides are typically more severe inferiorly than superiorly, except for:

    a. adult inclusion conjunctivitis.
    b. epidemic keratoconjunctivitis.
    c. Parinaud's syndrome.
    d. trachoma.
    e. medicamentosa.

18. By definition, a conjunctivitis may be termed "chronic" if it lasts longer than:

    a. 2 weeks.
    b. 4 weeks.
    c. 6 weeks.
    d. 8 weeks.
    e. 12 weeks.

19. The differential diagnosis for acute follicular conjunctivitis includes all of the following except:

    a. epidemic keratoconjunctivitis (EKC).
    b. herpes simplex keratoconjunctivitis.
    c. medicamentosa.
    d. trachoma.
    e. adult inclusion conjunctivitis.

20. The differential diagnosis for chronic follicular conjunctivitis includes all of the following except:

    a. EKC.
    b. medicamentosa.
    c. Parinud's oculoglandular syndrome.
    d. benign folliculosis.
    e. trachoma.

21. Infectious etiologies of pseudomembranous or membranous conjunctivitis include all of the following except:

    a. gonococcus.
    b. herpes simplex.
    c. adult inclusion conjunctivitis.
    d. diphtheria.
    e. *Candida.*

22. Immunologic etiologies of a pseudomembranous or membranous conjunctivitis include all of the following except:

    a. ocular cicatricial pemphigoid (OCP).
    b. vernal keratoconjunctivitis.
    c. ligneous keratoconjunctivitis.
    d. Stevens-Johnson syndrome.
    e. atopic keratoconjunctivitis.

23. T or F -- Microcystic corneal epithelial edema consists of fluid in the intracellular space, due to cellular hypoxia.

24. T or F -- Pathophysiologic factors critical for the development of a filamentary keratopathy include corneal stromal thickening and increased mucus production.

25. Entities to be considered in the differential diagnosis of a filamentary keratitis include all of the following except:

    a. ptosis.
    b. neurotrophic keratopathy.
    c. recurrent erosion syndrome.
    d. OCP.
    e. medicamentosa.

26. Superficial opacification of the cornea in a horizontal fashion between the eyelid margins is best referred to as:

    a. superficial punctate keratitis.
    b. micropannus.
    c. band keratopathy.
    d. gross corneal pannus.
    e. interstitial keratitis.

27. Cellular infiltrates that characterize corneal stromal inflammation can be derived from:

    a. limbal vasculature.
    b. aqueous humor.
    c. tears.
    d. a and c.
    e. a, b, and c.

28. The predominant cell forms seen in nongranulomatous keratic precipitates (KPs) are:

                    1. lymphocytes.
                    2. epithelioid cells.
                    3. PMNs.
                    4. macrophages.

    a. 1, 2, and 3.
    b. 1 and 3.
    c. 2 and 4.
    d. 4 only.
    e. 1, 2, 3, and 4.

29. The predominant cell forms seen in "mutton-fat" KP are :

                    1. lymphocytes.
                    2. epithelioid cells.
                    3. PMNs.
                    4. macrophages.

    a. 1, 2, and 3.
    b. 1 and 3.
    c. 2 and 4.
    d. 4 only.
    e. 1, 2, 3, and 4.

30. Match the gram-positive organisms listed in the right-hand column with staining, culture, and clinical characteristics listed in the left-hand column (note that each organism may be used more than once).

a. grow in pairs of lancet-shaped cocci with alpha hemolysis.
b. bacterium that resembles filamentous fungi and is vitamin K dependent.
c. a slender, curved rod with pseudohyphae or beading.
d. cocci in chains or rarely clusters; the most resistant gram-positive coccus.
e. pleomorphic bacilli resembling Chinese letters.
f. cocci in clusters, producing coagulase.
g. bacilli found in soil and vegetation.
h. organism most commonly responsible for traumatic endophthalmitis.
i. cocci in clusters; do not produce coagulase.
j. organism frequently associated with chronic recurrent canaliculitis.
k. alpha-hemolytic cocci associated with crystalline keratopathy.
l. frequently associated with chronic recurrent dacryocystitis in patients with nasolacrimal stenosis.
m. an acid-fast filamentous bacterium confused with fungus; associated with multifocal abscesses.
n. organism most frequently associated with hypersensitivity marginal keratitis.

1. *Staphylococcus aureus.*
2. *Staphylococcus epidermidis.*
3. *Streptococcus viridans.*
4. *Streptococcus pneumoniae.*
5. *Streptococcus faecalis.*
6. *Corynebacterium.*
7. *Proprionibacterium acnes.*
8. *Bacillus cereus.*
9. *Actinomyces.*
10. *Nocardia.*

31. Match the gram negative organisms listed in the right-hand column with staining, culture, and clinical characteristics listed in the left-hand column.

a. gram-negative rod growing in gray-blue colonies with a sweet grape aroma.
b. dumbbell or boxcar-shaped diplobacilli, always end-to-end.
c. associated with central nervous system (CNS) infections in adolescents and young adults.
d. associated with hyperacute purulent conjunctivitis in neonates and adults.
e. associated with a fulminant sclerokeratitis.
f. may grow as satellites of *S. aureus* on blood agar.
g. gram-negative rod requiring 5% carbon dioxide, fermenting glucose only.
h. pleomorphic rod requiring hemin and nicotinamide-adenine dinucleotide (NAD), associated with otitis and meningitis, and potentially fatal septicemia in children.
i. commonly associated with angular blepharitis and corneal ulcer in alcoholics.
j. common etiology of bleb-associated endophthalmitis.
k. enterobacterium that overgrows culture plate quickly.

1. *Pseudomonas aeruginosa.*
2. *Neisseria gonorrhoeae.*
3. *Neisseria meningitidis.*
4. *Hemophilus influenzae.*
5. *Moraxella.*
6. *Proteus.*

32. A corneal ulcer recalcitrant to routine treatment is rescraped for special staining and cultures. Gram's stain shows moderate diphtheroids. Which special stain is most likely to be of value in determining the actual diagnosis?

a. Ziehl-Neelsen stain.
b. Warthin-Starry stain.
c. Methenamine silver stain.
d. Giemsa stain.
e. Periodic acid-Schiff (PAS) stain.

33. Which culture media should be used in addition to routine broth to isolate the organism suspected in the previous question?

1. blood agar.
2. Sabouraud's medium.
3. Löwenstein-Jensen medium.
4. blood agar with *S. aureus* colonies.

a. 1, 2, and 3.
b. 1 and 3.
c. 2 and 4.
d. 4 only.
e. 1, 2, 3, and 4.

34. Antibiotics useful in the topical treatment of mycobacterial keratitis include:

    1. kanamycin.
    2. rifampin.
    3. amikacin.
    4. vancomycin.

    a. 1, 2, and 3.
    b. 1 and 3.
    c. 2 and 4.
    d. 4 only.
    e. 1, 2, 3, and 4.

35. T or F -- To localize treponemes from infected tissues or secretions, the preparations must be fresh.

36. T or F -- The *Treponema pallidum* immobilization (TPI) test is as sensitive and specific as the FTA-Abs test.

37. T or F -- The fluorescent treponemal antibody absorption (FTA-ABS) test is as sensitive and specific as the microhemagglutination of treponema pallidum test (MHA-TP).

38. A case of secondary acquired syphilis is adequately treated with parenteral penicillin. Which of the following blood tests would be expected to normalize?

    1. VDRL (Venereal Disease Research Laboratory).
    2. MHA-TP.
    3. Rapid plasma reagin (RPR).
    4. FTA-ABS.

    a. 1, 2, and 3.
    b. 1 and 3.
    c. 2 and 4.
    d. 4 only.
    e. 1, 2, 3, and 4.

39. T or F -- As culture methods have improved, these have become more reliable than serology in the diagnosis of Lyme disease.

40. The most common agent involved in mycotic ocular infections in the northern half of the United States is:

    a. Alternaria.
    b. Aspergillus.
    c. Fusarium.
    d. Penicillium.
    e. Candida.

41. The most common agent involved in mycotic ocular infections in the southern half of the United States is:

    a. Alternaria.
    b. Aspergillus.
    c. Fusarium.
    d. Penicillium.
    e. Candida.

42. The most basic difference between Candida and Fusarium is:

    a. Fusarium is a mold, and Candida is dimorphic.
    b. Fusarium is dimorphic, and Candida is a mold.
    c. Fusarium is a mold, and Candida is a yeast.
    d. Fusarium is a yeast, and Candida is a mold.
    e. Fusarium as a yeast has pseudohyphae, while Candida has true hyphae.

43. The most basic difference between Fusarium and Mucor is:

    a. Fusarium is a mold, and Mucor is dimorphic.
    b. Fusarium is dimorphic, and Mucor is a mold.
    c. Fusarium is a mold, and Mucor is a yeast.
    d. Fusarium is a yeast, and Mucor is a mold.
    e. Fusarium has septate hyphae, while Mucor has nonseptate hyphae.

44. The most common ocular manifestation of cryptococcal infection is:

    a. membranous conjunctivitis.
    b. orbital cellulitis.
    c. lid abscesses.
    d. endogenous endophthalmitis.
    e. ulcerative keratitis.

45. T or F -- Dimorphic fungi are frequently encountered in mycotic keratitis.

46. Factors that increase the difficulty of laboratory identification of fungal pathogens include all of the following except:

    a. inclusion of cycloheximide in various media.
    b. fastidiousness of the fungal agents.
    c. discarding of plates before full identification of fungal species.
    d. discarding of plates before full exploration of fungal sensitivities.
    e. confusion of pathogenic fungal species as contaminants.

47. Which of the following regarding the epidemiology of herpes simplex virus (HSV) infections in man is/are true:

    1. Type I typically causes recurrent perioral cold sores.
    2. Ocular herpes infections are split evenly between types I and II.
    3. Type II typically causes genital disease.
    4. Acute and convalescent antibody titers are helpful in the diagnosis of acute and recurrent disease.

    a. 1, 2, and 3.
    b. 1 and 3.
    c. 2 and 4.
    d. 4 only.
    e. 1, 2, 3, and 4.

48. T or F -- Intranuclear inclusion bodies of HSV epithelial infection are best highlighted with Papanicolaou (Pap) smear.

49. T or F -- The multinucleated giant cells seen in epithelial HSV infection are best seen with Giemsa stain.

50. T or F -- The herpes zoster virus (HZV) produces the same inclusion bodies and giant cells as HSV.

51. Which of the following Epstein-Barr virus (EBV) antibodies peak in serum level within the first 6 to 12 weeks of infection?

    1. Viral capsid antigen IgM (VCA-IgM).
    2. VCA-IgG.
    3. Early antigen-diffuse (EA-D).
    4. Epstein-Barr nuclear antigen (EBNA).

    a. 1, 2, and 3.
    b. 1 and 3.
    c. 2 and 4.
    d. 4 only.
    e. 1, 2, 3, and 4.

52. Which of the following EBV antibodies are detectable in serum for life following infection?

    1. VCA-IgM.
    2. VCA-IgG.
    3. EA-D.
    4. EBNA.

    a. 1, 2, and 3.
    b. 1 and 3.
    c. 2 and 4.
    d. 4 only.
    e. 1, 2, 3, and 4.

Cornea and External Disease

53. Match the clinical manifestations listed in the left-hand column with each's viral etiology.

   a. pustular rash of the eyelids and conjunctiva after vaccination.
   b. leads to follicular conjunctivitis in poultry handlers.
   c. causes severe membranous conjunctivitis and punctate keratitis.
   d. a nonspecific conjunctivitis and benign punctate keratitis universally accompanies the exanthem.
   e. may be associated with a secondary toxic follicular conjunctivitis, particularly inferiorly.

   1. adenovirus.
   2. molluscum contagiousum.
   3. vaccinia.
   4. rubeola.
   5. Newcastle disease.

54. Biologic features of chlamydiae that render them closer to bacterial than viral life forms include all of the following except:

   a. nucleic acid content.
   b. mechanism of replication.
   c. cell wall properties.
   d. full complement of organelles.
   e. response to certain antimicrobial agents.

55. T or F -- Accurate diagnosis of ocular chlamydial infection relies on recovery and culture of live organism.

56. Acceptable alternatives for adequate treatment of ocular chlamydial infection include:

   1. erythromycin orally for 1 week.
   2. rifampin orally for 3 weeks.
   3. erythromycin ointment for 3 weeks.
   4. tetracycline orally for 3 weeks.

   a. 1, 2, and 3.
   b. 1 and 3.
   c. 2 and 4.
   d. 4 only.
   e. 1, 2, 3, and 4.

57. Chlamydial serotypes associated with trachoma in humans include:

  1. A.
  2. E.
  3. C.
  4. L.

   a. 1, 2, and 3.
   b. 1 and 3.
   c. 2 and 4.
   d. 4 only.
   e. 1, 2, 3, and 4.

58. Which one of the following regarding *Acanthamoeba* and its ocular manifestations is false?

   a. The organism, particularly in its cyst form, is very hearty.
   b. Culture technique generally involves non-nutrient agar overlaid with *Escherichia coli*.
   c. Diagnostic yield from conjunctival fornix culture is high (75%).
   d. Calcofluor white is the stain of choice and requires fluorescence microscopy.
   e. The organism may induce an optic neuritis.

59. Match the clinical characteristics listed in the left-hand column with the roundworms listed in the right-hand column.

   a. generally contracted by ingestion of fecally contaminated soil or raw vegetables.
   b. generally contracted by ingestion of raw pork..
   c. generally spread by the black fly vector, breeding in rivers.
   d. most common site of infection is extraocular muscle and orbit tissues.
   e. most common site of infection is intraretinal.
   f. most common sites of infection are intraocular tissues, either anterior or posterior.
   g. may rarely be associated with systemic roundworm infection (visceral larva migrans).
   h. may manifest as pain with eye movement or subconjunctival hemorrhage only.
   i. a leading cause of blindness worldwide due to sclerosing keratitis.
   j. serum antibody titers helpful in diagnosis.
   k. treated with suramin or ivermectin.
   l. treated with steroids and diethylcarbamazine.
   m. treated with thiabendazole.

   1. *Onchocerca volvulus*.
   2. *Trichinella spiralis*.
   3. *Toxocara*.

60. Which one of the following regarding louse infections of the eye is false?

    a. *Pediculus capitis* and *Phthirus pubis* are the only organisms that infect the periocular structures.
    b. Ocular irritation is due to injection of toxic louse saliva into lid tissue.
    c. Sexual contact is felt to be the significant mode of transmission.
    d. The same organisms that infect eyelashes infect pubic hairs.
    e. Eradication of organisms depends on suffocation, either by bland ointments or paralytic medications such as eserine.

61. Which of the following regarding arachnid infections of the eye is/are true?

    1. The most common genus involved is *Demodex*.
    2. These organisms are normal commensals.
    3. The classic slit-lamp sign is sleeving of eyelash bases.
    4. Antiparisitic therapy rests on suffocation of the organisms with bland ointments or paralytic medications (eserine).

    a. 1, 2, and 3.
    b. 1 and 3.
    c. 2 and 4.
    d. 4 only.
    e. 1, 2, 3, and 4.

62. Members of the normal flora of human conjunctiva include all of the following except:

    a. *S. epidermidis*.
    b. Diphtheroids.
    c. *S. viridans*.
    d. *B. cereus*.
    e. *S. aureus*.

63. T or F -- In an adult inclusion conjunctivitis, the likelihood of finding cytoplasmic or intranuclear inclusions is high.

64. T or F -- In neonatal inclusion conjunctivitis, the likelihood of finding cytoplasmic or intranuclear inclusions is high.

65. Match the special equipment needed for corneal scraping listed in the left-hand column with the proper organisms listed in the right-hand column (note that there may be more than one correct answer for each item in the left-hand column).

    a. thioglycolate broth.
    b. Giemsa stain.
    c. blood agar with *S. aureus* cultures.
    d. Sabouraud's agar.
    e. Ziehl-Neelsen stain.
    f. Calcofluor white smear.
    g. Löwenstein-Jensen agar.
    h. non-nutrient agar with *E. coli* overgrowth.
    i. Gomori-methenamine silver stain.

    1. *H. influenzae*.
    2. anaerobic organisms.
    3. filamentous fungi.
    4. *Mycobacteria*.
    5. *Acanthamoeba*.
    6. *Chlamydia*.
    7. *Nocardia*.

66. The method of choice for documenting intracytoplasmic inclusion bodies is:

    a. thioglycolate broth.
    b. Giemsa stain.
    c. blood agar with *S. aureus* cultures.
    d. Sabouraud's agar.
    e. Ziehl-Neelsen stain.

67. Which of the following agents has in vivo activity against herpes simplex virus?

    1. idoxuridine (IDU).
    2. vidarabine (Vira-A).
    3. trifluridine (Viroptic).
    4. acyclovir.

    a. 1, 2, and 3.
    b. 1 and 3.
    c. 2 and 4.
    d. 4 only.
    e. 1, 2, 3, and 4.

68. Which of the following antivirals has in vivo activity against herpes zoster virus?

    1. idoxuridine (IDU).
    2. vidarabine (Vira-A).
    3. trifluridine (Viroptic).
    4. acyclovir.

    a. 1, 2, and 3.
    b. 1 and 3.
    c. 2 and 4.
    d. 4 only.
    e. 1, 2, 3, and 4.

69. Which of the following antivirals has an ophthalmic ointment preparation?

    1. idoxuridine.
    2. trifluridine.
    3. vidarabine.
    4. acyclovir.

    a. 1, 2, and 3.
    b. 1 and 3.
    c. 2 and 4.
    d. 4 only.
    e. 1, 2, 3, and 4.

70. Which of the following antivirals blocks viral replication by interference with DNA synthesis?

                    1. idoxuridine.
                    2. trifluridine.
                    3. vidarabine.
                    4. acyclovir.

   a. 1, 2, and 3.
   b. 1 and 3.
   c. 2 and 4.
   d. 4 only.
   e. 1, 2, 3, and 4.

71. T or F -- Hypersensitivity to one antiviral does not imply hypersensitivity to all antivirals.

72. T or F -- Resistance to one antiviral does not imply resistance to all antivirals.

73. Which of the following antivirals has a mechanism of action specific for herpes viruses, with scarely no effect on host cells?

                    1. idoxuridine (IDU).
                    2. trifluridine (Viroptic).
                    3. vidarabine (Vira-A).
                    4. acyclovir.

   a. 1, 2, and 3.
   b. 1 and 3.
   c. 2 and 4.
   d. 4 only.
   e. 1, 2, 3, and 4.

74. T or F -- The drug of choice in the treatment of an indolent, steroid-resistant, infectious herpetic ulcer is vidarabine.

75. Arrange the antivirals listed below in order of descending topical toxicity (1 being the most toxic and 4 being the least toxic).

   a. idoxuridine.   1.
   b. acyclovir.   2.
   c. trifluridine.   3.
   d. vidarabine.   4.

76. All of the following have been described as signs of antiviral toxicity except:

   a. punctate epithelial keratopathy.
   b. follicular conjunctivitis.
   c. anterior uveitis.
   d. indolent corneal ulceration.
   e. preauricular lymphadenopathy.

77. The drug of choice for presumed filamentous keratomycosis is:

   a. topical amphotericin.
   b. oral ketoconazole.
   c. topical clotrimazole.
   d. topical natamycin.
   e. topical flucytosine.

78. Which one of the following regarding the polyene class of antifungal agents is false?

   a. They are classified by the number of double bonds present.
   b. Amphotericin has the greatest topical activity against filamentous fungi.
   c. The corneal epithelium is a significant barrier to penetration of natamycin.
   d. Acceptable intraocular concentrations of polyene antifungals can only be achieved with direct intravitreal injection.
   e. Topical amphotericin must be stored in dark glass or opaque containers.

79. Which one of the following antifungal agents is most likely to encounter fungal resistance?

   a. natamycin.
   b. flucytosine.
   c. amphotericin.
   d. miconazole.
   e. thimerosal.

80. The drug of choice for Aspergillus keratitis is:

   a. clotrimazole.
   b. flucytosine.
   c. natamycin.
   d. amphotericin.
   e. tolnaftate.

81. Which of the following organ systems is most likely to be the target of toxicity from the polyene class of antifungal agents?

   a. central nervous system.
   b. cardiovascular.
   c. renal.
   d. hematopoietic.
   e. hepatic.

82. Which of the following organ systems is most likely to be the target of the imidazole class of antifungal agents?

 a. central nervous system.
 b. cardiovascular.
 c. renal.
 d. hematopoietic.
 e. hepatic.

83. Which of the following antifungal agents are in the same class?

 1. flucytosine.
 2. natamycin.
 3. miconazole.
 4. amphotericin.

 a. 1, 2, and 3.
 b. 1 and 3.
 c. 2 and 4.
 d. 4 only.
 e. 1, 2, 3, and 4.

84. Which of the following antifungal agents are in the same class?

 1. ketoconazole.
 2. miconazole.
 3. clotrimazole.
 4. nystatin.

 a. 1, 2, and 3.
 b. 1 and 3.
 c. 2 and 4.
 d. 4 only.
 e. 1, 2, 3, and 4.

85. Agents recognized to be useful in the medical therapy of Acanthamoeba keratitis include:

 1. propamidine (Brolene).
 2. clotrimazole.
 3. neomycin.
 4. pentamidine.

 a. 1, 2, and 3.
 b. 1 and 3.
 c. 2 and 4.
 d. 4 only.
 e. 1, 2, 3, and 4.

86. The cellular element generally responsible for inflammatory corneal damage is the:

    a. macrophage.
    b. lymphocyte.
    c. polymorphonuclear leukocycte (PMN).
    d. T-lymphocyte.
    e. eosinophil.

87. Arrange the various glucocorticoid agents listed in the left-hand column in order of decreasing systemic potency (1 being the most potent and 5 being the least potent).

    a. methylprednisolone.   1.
    b. hydrocortisone.   2.
    c. cortisone.   3.
    d. prednisone.   4.
    e. dexamethasone.   5.

88. T or F -- Phosphate preparations of topical steroids are generally more soluble in water than acetate preparations and may be dispensed in solution rather than suspension.

89. The topical steroid preparation with the greatest anti-inflammatory activity within the cornea is:

    a. prednisolone phosphate 1.0% (Inflamase Forte).
    b. dexamethasone phosphate 1.0% ointment (Decadron).
    c. prednisolone acetate 1.0% (Pred Forte).
    d. dexamethasone alcohol 0.1% suspension (Maxidex).
    e. fluorometholone alcohol 0.1% suspension (FML).

90. The ocular corticosteroid that is least likely to induce intraocular pressure (IOP) elevation is:

    a. prednisolone phosphate.
    b. prednisolone acetate.
    c. dexamethasone alcohol.
    d. fluorometholone.
    e. medrysone.

91. T or F -- Topical corticosteroid treatment can lead to reactivation of HSV keratitis in a quiet eye with a history of previous herpetic disease.

92. Topical corticosteroids should probably be withheld in any eye with:

      1. active dendritic epithelial keratitis.
      2. disciform keratitis.
      3. presumed fungal keratitis.
      4. pseudodendritic epithelial keratitis.

  a. 1, 2, and 3.
  b. 1 and 3.
  c. 2 and 4.
  d. 4 only.
  e. 1, 2, 3, and 4.

93. Etiologies recognized in the pathogenesis of conjunctival papilloma include:

      1. immunologic.
      2. neoplastic.
      3. toxic.
      4. infectious.

  a. 1, 2, and 3.
  b. 1 and 3.
  c. 2 and 4.
  d. 4 only.
  e. 1, 2, 3, and 4.

94. Assign the distinguishing features listed in the left column with the type of papillomas listed in the right column.

  a. usually seen in older adults.
  b. usually seen in children or adolescents.
  c. rarely bilateral.
  d. occasionally bilateral.
  e. rarely multiple.
  f. occasionally multiple.
  g. usually on palpebral conjunctiva.
  h. generally on bulbar conjunctiva.
  i. incomplete excision generally associated with solitary recurrence.
  j. incomplete excision associated with multiple recurrences.
  k. may be associated with fulminant conjunctivitis.
  l. rarely associated with conjunctivitis.
  m. may spontaneously improve.
  n. rarely spontaneously improves.

  1. neoplastic papilloma.
  2. viral papilloma.
  3. both.
  4. neither.

95. A patient presents 6 hours after receiving a prescription for topical pencillin for a suspected bacterial blepharoconjunctivitis. The patient complains of itching and tearing, and an examination documents severe chemosis and mild hyperemia. The most likely diagnosis is:

    a. antibiotic resistance.
    b. toxic follicular conjunctivitis.
    c. toxic papillary conjunctivitis.
    d. anaphylactoid reaction.
    e. contact allergic reaction.

96. A patient presents approximately 6 days after daily use of Polysporin ointment following cataract surgery. The patient describes a gradual onset of scaling and itching of the skin and increasing redness of the eye. The hypersensitivity pattern most likely at play is:

    a. Type I.
    b. Type II.
    c. Type III.
    d. Type IV.
    e. Type V.

97. Which type of hypersensitivity conjunctivitis takes the longest to develop?

    a. toxic follicular conjunctivitis.
    b. toxic papillary conjunctivitis.
    c. contact dermatitis with conjunctivitis.
    d. anaphylactoid reaction.
    e. no clear time pattern can be assigned to any of the reactions.

98. T or F -- Most patients who develop contact lens-induced papillary conjunctivitis develop giant papillae.

99. Presenting symptoms compatible with the diagnosis of contact lens-induced papillary conjunctivitis include:

                1. itching.
                2. mucoid discharge.
                3. conjunctival injection.
                4. preauricular lymphadenopathy.

    a. 1, 2, and 3.
    b. 1 and 3.
    c. 2 and 4.
    d. 4 only.
    e. 1, 2, 3, and 4.

100. T or F -- The incidence of GPC is greatest with soft contact lenses (SCL) and least with polymethylmethacrylate (PMMA) lenses.

101. Manipulations in the contact lens regimen that are helpful in the control of contact lens-induced papillary conjunctivitis include:

  1. change of contact lens brand or style.
  2. change to heat sterilization methods.
  3. use of topical mast cell inhibitors.
  4. decreasing the frequency of enzyme treatments.

  a. 1, 2, and 3.
  b. 1 and 3.
  c. 2 and 4.
  d. 4 only.
  e. 1, 2, 3, and 4.

102. The classic clinical sign of staphylococcal blepharoconjunctivitis is:

  a. inferior follicular conjunctivitis.
  b. scurf.
  c. limbal papillae.
  d. collarettes.
  e. sleeving of lashes.

103. Symptoms consistent with staphylococcal blepharoconjunctivitis include which of the following:

  1. red eyes.
  2. epiphora.
  3. photophobia.
  4. no symptoms.

  a. 1, 2, and 3.
  b. 1 and 3.
  c. 2 and 4.
  d. 4 only.
  e. 1, 2, 3, and 4.

104. T or F -- Culture techniques offer nothing diagnostically or therapeutically in staphylococcal blepharoconjunctivitis.

105. Which of the following, when combined with lid hygiene, is not an appropriate treatment regimen for staphylococcal blepharoconjunctivitis?

  a. bacitracin ointment plus prednisolone 1/8% twice a day.
  b. warm compresses twice a day.
  c. warm compresses followed by bacitracin twice a day.
  d. prednisolone 1/8% twice a day.
  e. warm compresses followed by bacitracin ointment and prednisolone 1/8% twice a day.

106. Which of the following may be direct manifestations of ocular infection?

  1. hordeolum.
  2. chalazion.
  3. meibomitis.
  4. phlyctenulosis.

  a. 1, 2, and 3.
  b. 1 and 3.
  c. 2 and 4.
  d. 4 only.
  e. 1, 2, 3, and 4.

107. The two organisms most frequently involved in phlyctenulosis are:

  a. *Coccidioides immitis* and *M. tuberculosis*.
  b. *Coccidioides* and *Staphylococcus*.
  c. *Chlamydia trachomatis* and *Staphylococcus*.
  d. *Mycobacterium tuberculosis* and *Staphylococcus*.
  e. *Coccidioides* and *Candida*.

108. Phlyctenules are a manifestation of what type hypersensitivity?

  a. Type I.
  b. Type II.
  c. Type III.
  d. Type IV.
  e. Type V.

109. Bacterial conjunctivitides in a healthy host are self-limited with the exception(s) of:

  1. *N. gonorrhoeae*.
  2. *Hemophilus* species.
  3. *N. meningitidis*.
  4. *Staphylococcus*.

  a. 1, 2, and 3.
  b. 1 and 3.
  c. 2 and 4.
  d. 4 only.
  e. 1, 2, 3, and 4.

110. The most common cause of hyperacute purulent conjunctivitis is:

  a. *Hemophilus aegyptius*.
  b. *N. meningitidis*.
  c. *S. pneumoniae*.
  d. *N. gonorrhoeae*.
  e. *H. influenzae*.

111. The only bacterial conjunctivitis that routinely leads to preauricular lymphadenopathy is:

    a. *H. aegyptius*.
    b. *N. meningitidis*.
    c. *S. pneumoniae*.
    d. *N. gonorrhoeae*.
    e. *H. influenzae*.

112. The treatment of choice in culture-proven gonococcal conjunctivitis is:

    a. topical pencillin G QID for 14 days.
    b. topical pencillin G QID with doxycycline 100 mg orally BID for 1 week.
    c. topical pencillin G QID and topical tetracycline QID for 1 week.
    d. ceftriaxone one gm I.M. daily for 5 days.
    e. ceftriaxone one gm I.M. daily for 5 days and doxycycline orally BID for 3 weeks.

113. A pearly eyelid nodule with a central crater and associated inferior follicular conjunctivitis is the classic picture for:

    a. phlyctenulosis.
    b. staphylococcal blepharoconjunctivitis.
    c. phthiriasis.
    d. primary herpes simplex dermatitis.
    e. molluscum contagiosum.

114. Classic epidemic keratoconjunctivitis (EKC) is typically caused by:

    a. enterovirus type 70.
    b. adenovirus types 3 and 7.
    c. Newcastle virus.
    d. adenovirus types 8 and 19.
    e. coxsackievirus A24.

115. T or F -- Late cicatrization excludes the diagnosis of EKC.

116. The most important element in the management of a patient with EKC is:

    a. topical bacitracin ointment.
    b. topical trifluridine drops.
    c. warm compresses.
    d. topical prednisolone.
    e. fastidious hygiene.

117. T or F -- The key feature distinguishing acute hemorrhagic conjunctivitis from EKC is the presence of subconjunctival hemorrhage in the former.

118. Which one of the following regarding trachoma is false?

    a. Serotypes A through C are responsible.
    b. Blinding complications of the infection are due to the pronounced hypersensitivity responses to *Chlamydia*.
    c. In the MacCallan classification, stages I and II feature follicles with no scarring, while stages III and IV have pronounced subepithelial fibrosis.
    d. The World Health Organization has a simplified grading system based on the presence or absence of follicles, intense inflammation, scarring, trichiasis, or corneal opacification.
    e. Treatment with antibiotics should be prolonged and may require retreatment with multiple agents due to resistance.

119. Which one of the following regarding inclusion conjunctivitis is false?

    a. Except for transmission in swimming pools, the adult form is venereally transmitted.
    b. Unlike trachoma, adult inclusion conjunctivitis affects the inferior conjunctiva more than the superior conjunctiva.
    c. Unlike EKC, inclusion conjunctivitis is never membranous.
    d. Unlike EKC, associated keratitis may be localized to the superior one-third of the cornea.
    e. Unlike EKC, corneal neovascularization can be seen.

120. Successful long-term management of adult inclusion conjunctivitis includes:

    a. recurrent topical tetracycline.
    b. recurrent oral tetracycline therapy.
    c. chronic daily use of a mild topical steroid preparation.
    d. conjunctival transplantation.
    e. examination with treatment, if necessary, of personal contacts.

121. Important differences between neonatal inclusion conjunctivitis and adult inclusion conjunctivitis include all of the following except:

    a. more prominent follicular response in neonates.
    b. more discharge in neonates.
    c. pseudomembranes or membranes in neonates.
    d. more prominent cytoplasmic inclusion bodies in neonates.
    e. better response to topical therapy in neonates.

122. T or F -- Because of its response to topical therapy, neonatal inclusion conjunctivitis can be treated by this route alone.

123. The spectrum of atopic ocular disease includes all of the following except:

    a. seasonal allergic conjunctivitis.
    b. phlyctenulosis.
    c. atopic keratoconjunctivitis.
    d. giant papillary conjunctivitis.
    e. vernal keratoconjunctivitis.

124. Which of the following disorders is most likely to respond quickly to topical antihistamine therapy?

    a. season allergic conjunctivitis.
    b. phlyctenulosis.
    c. atopic keratoconjunctivitis.
    d. giant papillary conjunctivitis.
    e. vernal keratoconjunctivitis.

125. For which disorder is chronic use of systemic antihistamine most important?

    a. season allergic conjunctivitis.
    b. phlyctenulosis.
    c. atopic keratoconjunctivitis.
    d. giant papillary conjunctivitis.
    e. vernal keratoconjunctivitis.

126. Clinical features distinguishing seasonal allergic conjunctivitis from vernal keratoconjunctivitis include:

    1. prominent itching.
    2. response to topical antihistamine.
    3. seasonal occurrence.
    4. the presence of giant papillae.

    a. 1, 2, and 3.
    b. 1 and 3.
    c. 2 and 4.
    d. 4 only.
    e. 1, 2, 3, and 4.

127. Which of the following regarding limbal vernal keratoconjunctivitis is/are true?

    1. It is more common in blacks than palpebral vernal conjunctivitis.
    2. This variety is more commonly associated with shield corneal ulcer than the palpebral form.
    3. Collections of cellular debris and eosinophils may accumulate at the surface of limbal papillae.
    4. Long-term management is centered around daily corticosteroid use.

    a. 1, 2, and 3.
    b. 1 and 3.
    c. 2 and 4.
    d. 4 only.
    e. 1, 2, 3, and 4.

128. Features distinguishing atopic keratoconjunctivitis from vernal keratoconjunctivitis include:

        1. age range of typically affected patient.
        2. seasonal variations of incidence.
        3. presence of extensive conjunctival and corneal scarring.
        4. presence of eosinophils in conjunctival scrapings.

a. 1, 2, and 3.
b. 1 and 3.
c. 2 and 4.
d. 4 only.
e. 1, 2, 3, and 4.

129. To secure the diagnosis of atopic keratoconjunctivitis, it is critical to inquire about a previous or active history of:

a. asthma.
b. sinusitis.
c. vesicular rash consistent with HSV.
d. eczema.
e. aspirin hypersensitivity.

130. Clinical findings consistent with a diagnosis of Reiter's syndrome include all of the following except:

a. keratoderma blenorrhagicum.
b. severe retinal vasculitis.
c. nonerosive oligoarthritis.
d. papillary conjunctivitis with corneal neovascularization.
e. acute nongranulomatous iridocyclitis.

131. An obese 35-year-old man presents to an ophthalmologist complaining of increasing redness and irritation of his left eye, progressive over the previous 4 to 6 months. Examination discloses mildly edematous and erythematous left eyelids with mild conjunctival injection and scant mucus discharge. The conjunctival findings are much more prominent superiorly. The right eye appears normal. With this patient, the critical historical feature to inquire about is:

a. use of over-the-counter eye medications.
b. any history of previous sexually transmitted diseases.
c. which side of his body he generally chooses to sleep on.
d. any previous history of allergic disorders.
e. any previous history of arthritic disorders.

132. T or F -- One feature that characterizes infectious marginal keratitis is tendency for centripetal spread.

133. The two leading causes of corneal blindness in the United States are:

    a. trachoma and trauma.
    b. trachoma and herpes simplex.
    c. trauma and herpes simplex.
    d. trachoma and onchocerciasis.
    e. trauma and onchocerciasis.

134. T or F -- The most common means of developing a type 1 HSV genital infection is by orogenital sexual activity.

135. T or F -- The most common means of developing a type 2 HSV ocular infection is by orogenital sexual activity.

136. Latent type 1 HSV (responsible for recurrent orofacial infection) generally resides in the:

    a. oculomotor nucleus.
    b. gasserian ganglion.
    c. geniculate ganglion.
    d. sphenopalatine ganglion.
    e. superior cervical ganglion.

137. Clinical features differentiating primary from recurrent HSV infection include:

    1. prominent follicular membranous conjunctivitis.
    2. preauricular lymphadenopathy.
    3. duration and size of corneal dendrites.
    4. vesicular blepharitis.

    a. 1, 2, and 3.
    b. 1 and 3.
    c. 2 and 4.
    d. 4 only.
    e. 1, 2, 3, and 4.

138. T or F -- Decreased corneal sensation is a sensitive and specific sign of recurrent herpetic keratitis.

139. Which of the following regarding the treatment of recurrent herpetic epithelial keratitis is/are true?

    1. Debridement of active dendrites may be of value.
    2. No improvement in epithelial disease after 7 to 10 days of therapy indicates resistance to the selected medication.
    3. Oral acyclovir may play a role in the treatment of recurrent epithelial HSV keratitis.
    4. Topical steroids in low doses are recommended to minimize corneal scarring.

    a. 1, 2, and 3.
    b. 1 and 3.
    c. 2 and 4.
    d. 4 onlly.
    e. 1, 2, 3, and 4.

140. Potential outcomes of overtreatment with topical antivirals for HSV keratitis include:

    1. sterile corneal ulceration.
    2. pseudodendrites.
    3. punctate keratitis with photophobia.
    4. bacterial superinfection.

    a. 1, 2, and 3.
    b. 1 and 3.
    c. 2 and 4.
    d. 4 only.
    e. 1, 2, 3, and 4.

141. Two weeks after initial diagnosis and topical therapy of HSV epithelial keratitis, a patient returns with a 4 mm, oval, central epithelial defect with smooth rolled edges. Factors that may be important in the pathogenesis of this finding include:

    1. underlying stromal inflammation.
    2. overuse of prescribed topical antivirals.
    3. impaired corneal sensation.
    4. active intraepithelial virus replication.

    a. 1, 2, and 3.
    b. 1 and 3.
    c. 2 and 4.
    d. 4 only.
    e. 1, 2, 3, and 4.

142. T or F -- The descriptor "disciform" is specific for autoimmune keratitis due to HSV infection.

143. Which of the following is/are seen as part of the spectrum of HSV disciform keratitis?

> 1. Descemet's folds.
> 2. mild anterior uveitis with scattered KP.
> 3. glaucoma.
> 4. peripheral anterior synechiae.

a. 1, 2, and 3.
b. 1 and 3.
c. 2 and 4.
d. 4 only.
e. 1, 2, 3, and 4.

144. A circular, superficial distribution of neutrophils around an area of corneal edema or inflammation is called:

a. Wessely ring.
b. disciform keratitis.
c. corneal abscess.
d. metaherpetic ulcer.
e. ring ulcer.

145. The differential diagnosis of the lesion described in question 144 includes all of the following except:

a. HSV.
b. Reiter's syndrome.
c. Acanthamoeba keratitis.
d. Anesthetic keratopathy.
e. Behçet's disease.

146. T or F -- Topical steroids play a role in the management of all cases of disciform keratitis.

147. T or F -- Herpetic interstitial keratitis (IK) is generally more aggressive than disciform keratitis.

148. Which of the following are justifications for the use of oral acyclovir in the management of herpes simplex ocular infection?

 1. primary infection.
 2. concomitant chronic oral steroid therapy for a nonrelated disorder.
 3. recalcitrant epithelial or stromal keratitis.
 4. systemic immune deficiency.

 a. 1, 2, and 3.
 b. 1 and 3.
 c. 2 and 4.
 d. 4 only.
 e. 1, 2, 3, and 4.

149. T or F -- Cutaneous vesicles at the side of the tip of the nose (Hutchinson's sign) indicate a high probability of ocular involvement by HSV.

150. T or F -- All cases of herpes zoster ophthalmicus (HZO) represent reactivation of latent trigeminal ganglion infection.

151. T or F -- The dermatitis associated with herpes zoster reactivation is generally more protracted than the ocular inflammation.

152. Medications useful in the control of postherpetic neuralgia include:

 1. cimetidine orally for the first 7 days of active dermatitis.
 2. oral tricyclic antidepressant.
 3. acyclovir.
 4. prednisone orally, started 7 to 10 days after eruption of active dermatitis.

 a. 1, 2, and 3.
 b. 1 and 3.
 c. 2 and 4.
 d. 4 only.
 e. 1, 2, 3, and 4.

153. All of the following features of corneal dendrites favor the diagnosis of herpes zoster ophthalmicus except:

 a. a large, frequently branching dendrite.
 b. a dendrite with overlying plaque of epithelial cells.
 c. a dendrite with no terminal bulb.
 d. coarse, ropy dendrites with blunt ends.
 e. a dendrite with dull fluorescein and no rose-bengal staining.

154. Which of the following are systemic risk factors for the development of bacterial keratitis?

1. drug abuse.
2. aging.
3. vitamin deficiency.
4. diabetes mellitus.

a. 1, 2, and 3.
b. 1 and 3.
c. 2 and 4.
d. 4 only.
e. 1, 2, 3, and 4.

155. Local factors that may increase the risk for bacterial keratitis include:

1. dry eye syndrome.
2. impaired corneal sensation.
3. recurrent erosions.
4. chronic topical steroid therapy.

a. 1, 2, and 3.
b. 1 and 3.
c. 2 and 4.
d. 4 only.
e. 1, 2, 3, and 4.

156. T or F -- Compared to gram-negative organisms, gram-positive organisms tend to produce focal infiltrates.

157. T or F -- Compared to gram-positive organisms, gram-negative organisms are more likely to produce fulminant liquefactive corneal necrosis.

158. Which of the following constitute independent risk factors for the development of *Acanthamoeba* keratitis?

1. diabetes mellitus.
2. frequent use of hot tubs.
3. previous history of a corneal transplant.
4. contact lens use.

a. 1, 2, and 3.
b. 1 and 3.
c. 2 and 4.
d. 4 only.
e. 1, 2, 3, and 4.

159. Which of the following features of contact lens use constitutes the greatest risk for the development of *Acanthamoeba* keratitis?

   a. homemade saline storage solutions.
   b. use of solutions containing thimerosal.
   c. heat sterilization techniques.
   d. chemical sterilization techniques.
   e. insufficient enzyme treatments.

160. Which clinical feature is nearly universal in *Acanthamoeba* keratitis?

   a. tearing.
   b. pseudoptosis.
   c. severe pain.
   d. ring infiltrate.
   e. hypopyon.

161. Which of the following may be considered independent risk factors for the development of fungal keratitis?

   1. prolonged use of topical corticosteroids.
   2. prolonged use of broad-spectrum topical antibiotics.
   3. corneal trauma.
   4. previous history of herpetic keratitis.

   a. 1, 2, and 3.
   b. 1 and 3.
   c. 2 and 4.
   d. 4 only.
   e. 1, 2, 3, and 4.

162. Leading causes of interstitial keratitis (IK) in the United States include all of the following except:

   a. sarcoidosis.
   b. lepromatous leprosy.
   c. Cogan's syndrome.
   d. herpes zoster virus.
   e. syphilis.

163. T or F -- Interstitial keratitis is more frequently seen as a complication of congenital syphilis than acquired syphilis.

164. T or F -- Compared to congenital syphilis, tuberculous interstitial keratitis is more frequently unilateral and sectoral.

165. Cogan's syndrome is frequently associated with which systemic disorder?

   a. polyarteritis nodosa.
   b. Wegener's granulomatosis.
   c. rheumatoid arthritis.
   d. adenocarcinoma, usually bronchogenic.
   e. systemic lupus erythematosus.

166. Which one of the following regarding Thygeson's superficial punctate keratitis is false?

   a. There may be an HLA association.
   b. The presenting symptom is typically photophobia or tearing.
   c. There is usually an associated follicular conjunctivitis.
   d. The corneal deposits may resemble those of EKC.
   e. Topical steroids have been used for symptomatic relief but may prolong the natural history of the disorder.

167. There is a probable association of superior limbic keratoconjunctivitis (SLK) with:

   a. valvular heart disease.
   b. thyroid disease.
   c. inflammatory bowel disease.
   d. systemic lupus erythematosus.
   e. bacillary dysentery.

168. Modalities helpful in long-term control of SLK include:

   1. topical silver nitrate.
   2. cauterization of bulbar conjunctiva.
   3. pressure patching or contact lenses.
   4. topical corticosteroids.

   a. 1, 2, and 3.
   b. 1 and 3.
   c. 2 and 4.
   d. 4 only.
   e. 1, 2, 3, and 4.

169. T or F -- The approach to SLK in a patient with a history of soft contact lenses use is identical to that for a patient with no such history.

170. Which class of chemicals constitutes the greatest threat for ocular injury?

   a. solvents.
   b. petroleum products.
   c. acid.
   d. alkali.
   e. detergents.

171. T or F -- The pathophysiology of alkali burns involves protein denaturation and precipitation of previously soluble tissue protein.

172. T or F -- The tissue damage due to acid burns tends to be self-limited by tissue buffering and barrier effects of the tissue damage itself.

173. T or F -- Glaucoma is more likely to be a long-term sequela of alkali burns than acid burns.

174. Clinical features to be observed at the initial evaluation of a chemical burn include:

   1. tear pH.
   2. extent of epithelial defects.
   3. extent of limbal ischemia.
   4. corneal clarity.

   a. 1, 2, and 3.
   b. 1 and 3.
   c. 2 and 4.
   d. 4 only.
   e. 1, 2, 3, and 4.

175. After thorough and copious irrigation of the conjunctival fornices, the next most important step in initial management of a patient with a chemical burn is:

   a. topical steroid agents.
   b. topical antibodic agents.
   c. debridement of any foreign bodies.
   d. topical ascorbate.
   e. topical citrate.

176. The primary goal in intermediate therapy of chemical burns is:

   a. normalization of intraocular pressure.
   b. reestablishment of limbal blood flow.
   c. control of intraocular inflammation.
   d. normalization of tear and conjunctival pH.
   e. reepithelization of the corneal surface.

177. T or F -- The best antibiotic prophylaxis following a chemical burn is a broad-spectrum antibiotic such as gentamicin.

178. T or F -- The optimal time for the administration of topical corticosteroids for dampening inflammation is 7 to 14 days following chemical injury.

179. T or F -- Long-term management following severe ocular chemical injury involves reestablishment of healthy epithelial surfaces with conjunctival and/or corneal transplants.

180. Which one of the following regarding episcleritis is false?

    a. Both nodular and diffuse forms have been described.
    b. The majority of cases are sectoral.
    c. The majority of cases will be recurrent.
    d. The condition may lead to scleritis if not promptly treated.
    e. Treatment consisting of topical steroids or nonsteroidal agents is generally ameliorative.

181. Features distinguishing episcleritis from scleritis include all of the following except:

    a. the presence of pain.
    b. the color of affected sclera.
    c. response to topical phenylephrine.
    d. the presence of episcleral versus scleral edema.
    e. association with systemic connective tissue disorders.

182. The most benign form of scleritis is:

    a. diffuse anterior scleritis.
    b. nodular anterior scleritis.
    c. necrotizing scleritis with inflammation.
    d. scleromalacia perforans.
    e. posterior scleritis.

183. The scleritis associated with the gravest systemic prognosis is:

    a. nodular diffuse anterior scleritis.
    b. nodular anterior scleritis.
    c. necrotizing scleritis with inflammation.
    d. scleromalacia perforans.
    e. posterior scleritis.

184. The scleritis most likely to be associated with rheumatoid arthritis is:

    a. diffuse anterior scleritis.
    b. nodular anterior scleritits.
    c. necrotizing scleritis with inflammation.
    d. scleromalacia perforans.
    e. posterior scleritis.

185. The scleritis most likely to present with proptosis and visual loss is:

    a. nodular diffuse anterior scleritis.
    b. nodular anterior scleritits.
    c. necrotizing scleritis with inflammation.
    d. scleromalacia perforans.
    e. posterior scleritis.

186. T or F -- Posterior uveitis (vitreous cells, papillitis, macular edema with exudates) is common in scleritis; anterior uveitis is rare.

187. T or F -- The pathophysiology of scleritis may also be manifest in the cornea as either a sclerosing or a lytic marginal keratitis.

188. Infectious scleritis may be seen due to all of the following except:

    a. Chlamydia.
    b. syphilis.
    c. tuberculosis.
    d. herpes zoster.
    e. leprosy.

189. Systemic disease associations for scleritis include:

                    1. rheumatoid arthritis.
                    2. Wegener's granulomatosis.
                    3. polyarteritis nodosa.
                    4. inflammatory bowel disease.

    a. 1, 2, and 3.
    b. 1 and 3.
    c. 2 and 4.
    d. 4 only.
    e. 1, 2, 3, and 4.

190. Agents helpful in the medical management of autoinflammatory sclerokeratitis include all of the following except:

    a. topical indomethacin.
    b. oral prednisone.
    c. subtenon's corticosteroid.
    d. cyclophosphamide.
    e. cyclosporine A.

191. The most common cause of acute, painful enlargement of the lacrimal gland is:

    a. sarcoidosis.
    b. Sjögren's syndrome.
    c. bacterial dacryoadenitis.
    d. leprosy.
    e. herpes zoster virus.

192. The most common cause of painless, bilateral enlargement of lacrimal glands is:

   a. sarcoidosis.
   b. Sjögren's syndrome.
   c. bacterial dacryoadenitis.
   d. leprosy.
   e. herpes zoster virus.

193. Mikulicz's syndrome refers to the combination of chronic dacryoadenitis with:

   a. rheumatoid arthritis.
   b. enlargement and inflammation of the parotid glands.
   c. keratoconjunctivitis sicca.
   d. systemic lupus erythematosus.
   e. dacryocele.

194. The treatment of choice for the most common cause of chronic canaliculitis is:

   a. topical tetracycline for 2 weeks.
   b. oral tetracycline for 3 weeks.
   c. surgical evacuation of the canaliculus.
   d. topical corticosteroids.
   e. oral acyclovir for 2 weeks.

195. Chronic asymptomatic dacryocystitis is most frequently caused by:

   a. *S. aureus.*
   b. *S. pneumoniae.*
   c. *S. epidermidis.*
   d. *H. influenzae.*
   e. *P. aeruginosa.*

196. A patient presents with a tender mass below the medial canthal tendon and mucopurulent discharge from the inferior canaliculus. One week of oral antibiotic treatment and warm compresses leads to an increase in size and fluctuance of the mass. The next step in treatment should be:

   a. increasing the frequency of warm compresses.
   b. change in antibiotic agents.
   c. increasing the frequency of dosage of the antibiotic agent.
   d. probing and irrigation of the nasolacrimal system.
   e. incision and drainage of the fluctuant mass.

197. A 2-month-old infant with unilateral epiphora OS is brought to the ophthalmologist by her parents. Gentle compression of the lacrimal sac produces reflux of mucus from the canaliculi, but only on the left. There is obviously increased tear flow on the left as well. The next step should probably be:

   a. warm compresses to the left eye.
   b. probing and irrigation of the nasolacrimal system on the left.
   c. reassurance with once daily antibiotic ointment and gentle medial canthal massage.
   d. incision and drainage of the lacrimal sac.
   e. oral antibiotics.

198. An 8-month-old infant with chronic epiphora and discharge OS is brought to the ophthalmologist by his parents. Gentle massage of the medial canthal area produces a reflux of mucus from the left canaliculi. The next step in management should be:

   a. warm compresses to the left eye.
   b. probing and irrigation of the nasolacrimal system on the left.
   c. reassurance with once daily antibiotic ointment and gentle medial canthal massage.
   d. incision and drainage of the lacrimal sac.
   e. oral antibiotics.

199. T or F -- Following unsuccessful probing of a congenitally impatent nasolacrimal system, the next therapuetic step should be dacryocystorhinostomy.

200. The epithelium of eyelid skin is:

   a. keratinizing stratified squamous.
   b. nonkeratinizing stratified squamous.
   c. keratinizing stratified columnar.
   d. nonkeratinizing stratified columnar.
   e. keratinizing pseudostratified.

201. Match the histologic features listed in the left-hand column with the various layers of the epidermis.

   a. flattened, elongated squamous cells with multiple keratohyaline granules.
   b. cuboid or columnar cells with large nuclei aligned in a single row above the basement membrane.
   c. multiple eosinophilic layers of protein with no cellular details visible.
   d. polygonal cells with numerous hair-like filamentous connections between cells.

   1. Basal cell layer.
   2. Prickle cell layer.
   3. Granular layer.
   4. Keratin layer.

202. Match the mechanics of secretion listed in the left-hand column with the gland listed in the right-hand column.

    a. secretion by simple exocytosis.
    b. secretion by release of entire cellular contents (disruption of cell).
    c. secretion by pinching or budding off of a portion of cellular cytoplasm.

    1. apocrine.
    2. eccrine.
    3. holocrine.

203. Match the eyelid glands listed in the left-hand column with the mode of secretion in the right-hand column.

    a. meibomian glands.
    b. glands of Zeis.
    c. Moll's glands.
    d. typical sweat glands.

    1. apocrine.
    2. eccrine.
    3. holocrine.

204. Features differentiating epibulbar epithelium from epidermal epithelium include:

    1. lack of rete ridges.
    2. lack of a granular layer.
    3. presence of goblet cells.
    4. lack of a prickle cell layer.

    a. 1, 2, and 3.
    b. 1 and 3.
    c. 2 and 4.
    d. 4 only.
    e. 1, 2, 3, and 4.

205. Features differentiating conjunctival from corneal epithelium include:

    1. lack of rete ridges.
    2. lack of granular cell layer.
    3. lack of a keratin layer.
    4. presence of goblet cells.

    a. 1, 2, and 3.
    b. 1 and 3.
    c. 2 and 4.
    d. 4 only.
    e. 1, 2, 3, and 4.

206. Match the epithelial growth features described in the left-hand column with the appropriate histopathologic terminology.

a. individual cellular enlargement, pleomorphism prominent nucleoli, hyperchromasia, and abnormal mitoses.
b. loss of maturational order and normal layering of the epithelium.
c. severe atypia and abnormal polarity.
d. full-thickness dysplasia.
e. invasion of epithelial basement membrane by dysplastic squamous epithelium.
f. keratinization and formation of skin-like features by mucosal epithelium.

1. squamous cell carcinoma.
2. atypia.
3. carcinoma in situ.
4. epidermidalization.
5. abnormal polarity.
6. anaplasia.

207. T or F -- A melanophage is a melanocyte that has differentiated into a phagocytic cell.

208. Which of the following are common features of conjunctival papillomas?

1. hyperkeratosis.
2. acanthosis.
3. parakeratosis.
4. anaplasia.

a. 1, 2, and 3.
b. 1 and 3.
c. 2 and 4.
d. 4 only.
e. 1, 2, 3, and 4.

209. Which of the following eyelid or conjunctival lesions may assume a papillomatous growth pattern?

1. seborrheic keratosis.
2. actinic keratosis.
3. verruca.
4. squamous cell carcinoma.

a. 1, 2, and 3.
b. 1 and 3.
c. 2 and 4.
d. 4 only.
e. 1, 2, 3, and 4.

Cornea and External Disease

210. A 33-year-old man presents to an ophthalmologist complaining of a "growth" on his eyelid. He maintains that the lesion developed over the preceding 4 weeks and is nontender. He produces a driver's license photo from 4 months earlier which shows normal eyelids. Examination discloses a 3.5-cm round elevated lesion of the right lower eyelid with a central depressed area and debris within. There is no pigmentation. The most likely diagnosis is:

    a. seborrheic keratosis.
    b. actinic keratosis.
    c. keratoacanthoma.
    d. basal cell carcinoma.
    e. squamous cell carcinoma.

211. T or F -- If diagnostic suspicion proves correct for the patient in question 210, biopsy may reveal severe dysplasia.

212. T or F -- If diagnostic suspicion proves correct for the patient question 210, biopsy may reveal significant inflammation.

213. T or F -- If the patient in questions 210 is not troubled by the cosmetic features, he may be reassured and instructed to follow-up in 3 to 6 months.

214. Which one of the following regarding seborrheic keratosis is false?

    a. It is a lesion most commonly seen in elderly people.
    b. There may be an inherited tendency for its development.
    c. Texturally, the lesion appears dry and scaly.
    d. Histopathologically, there is prominent dyskeratosis and hyperpigmentation in a papillary growth pattern.
    e. The lesion must be carefully distinguished from actinic keratosis.

215. The key differentiating feature between a dermoid cyst and an epidermoid cyst is:

    a. dermoid cysts contain keratin within the cyst cavity.
    b. dermoid cysts are solid.
    c. dermoid cysts contain sebum within the cyst cavity.
    d. dermoid cysts are morphologically identical, but follow trauma or surgery.
    e. dermoid cysts contain dermal appendages within the cyst wall.

216. T or F -- The lesions of molluscum contagiosum are similar to keratoacanthoma, except the former are generally more inflamed.

217. Features serving to differentiate between actinic keratosis and seborrheic keratosis include:

        1. hyperpigmentation.
        2. elastosis.
        3. chronic dermal inflammation.
        4. epithelial atypia.

    a. 1, 2, and 3.
    b. 1 and 3.
    c. 2 and 4.
    d. 4 only.
    e. 1, 2, 3, and 4.

218. Which of the following growth patterns of basal cell carcinoma carries the worst prognosis?

    a. fibrosing.
    b. cystic.
    c. adenoid.
    d. adenocystic.
    e. nodular.

219. Which one of the following regarding basal cell carcinoma is true?

    a. Growth is usually is explosively rapid.
    b. In 25%, the conjunctiva is primarily involved with secondary skin involvement.
    c. The upper eyelid is affected more frequently than the lower eyelid.
    d. Nuclei at the periphery of tumor cell nests retain polarity with palisading.
    e. There are usually numerous mitotic figures per high power field.

220. Which location of basal cell carcinoma carries the poorest prognosis?

    a. medial lower lid.
    b. lateral lower lid.
    c. lateral canthus.
    d. upper lid.
    e. medial canthus.

221. Basal cell carcinoma causes the most significant systemic morbidity and mortality via:

    a. hematogenous metastasis to the brain.
    b. local invasion of skull and central nervous system.
    c. lymphatic metastasis.
    d. hematogenous metastasis to the lung.
    e. hematogenous metastasis to liver.

222. Which one of the following regarding squamous cell carcinoma of the eyelid is false?

    a. It is less common than basal cell carcinoma.
    b. Chronic actinic exposure plays a role in its development.
    c. The upper eyelid is more frequently involved than the lower eyelid.
    d. Metastatic potential is greater than for basal cell carcinoma.
    e. Growth pattern is usually rapid.

223. A 68-year-old woman complains to her ophthalmologist that her stye just won't go away, despite 3 months of warm compresses and two surgical drainages. She undergoes full-thickness biopsy of her lower lid; a light microscopic section is shown in color plate 12. Which of the following are true regarding her situation?

    1. The disorder typically affects middle-aged or elderly people.
    2. Prompt drainage of the initial chalazion would have been curative.
    3. Grossly, the lesion may have an orange-yellow hue.
    4. Mohs' micrographic techniques can be curative at this stage.

    a. 1, 2, and 3.
    b. 1 and 3.
    c. 2 and 4.
    d. 4 only.
    e. 1, 2, 3, and 4.

224. The biopsy specimen from the patient in the preceding question should also have undergone which one of the following histopathologic techniques?

    a. electron microscopy.
    b. cell surface marker studies.
    c. cellular adhesion studies.
    d. frozen section processing.
    e. serial section techniques.

225. All of the following features can be seen in sebaceous cell carcinoma except:

    a. epithelial xanthomatization.
    b. peripheral palisading of tumor cell nuclei.
    c. intraepithelial tumor cells.
    d. multifocal tumor cell nests.
    e. intraepithelial inflammatory cells.

226. Potential sites of origin of sebaceous cell carcinoma include:

       1. the glands of Zeis.
       2. the glands of the caruncle.
       3. the meibomian glands.
       4. Moll's glands.

    a. 1, 2, and 3.
    b. 2 and 4.
    c. 1 and 3.
    d. 4 only.
    e. 1, 2, 3, and 4.

227. Adnexal tumors of hair follicle origin include all of the following except:

    a. syringoma.
    b. trichoepithelioma.
    c. trichilemmoma.
    d. pilomatrixoma.
    e. trichofolliculoma.

228. Which of the following tumors is most likely to calcify?

    a. syringoma.
    b. trichoepithelioma.
    c. trichilemmoma.
    d. pilomatrixoma.
    e. trichofolliculoma.

229. T or F -- The difference between ephelis and lentigo is an increased number of melanocytes in the latter.

230. T or F -- The difference between nevi and lentigo is modification of the melanocyte population in nevi.

231. Which one of the following regarding nevi is false?

    a. Pigmentation and growth generally increase around the onset of puberty.
    b. With time, nevi tend to advance superficially, toward the surface epithelium.
    c. Junctional activity carries the greatest potential for malignant transformation.
    d. Subepithelial or dermal activity carries the least potential for malignant transformation.
    e. Nevi may be considered hamartomatous abnormalities.

232. Match the cellular features listed in the left-hand column with the appropriate type of nevus in the right-hand column.

   a. diffuse congenital deep dermal nevus of the periocular skin.
   b. nests of nevus cells in the basal epithelial layer.
   c. deeply located dermal nevus present at birth with very little elevation.
   d. compound nevus of childhood with bizarre cellular components but no malignant potential.
   e. deep dermal nevus present at birth with many dendritic nevus cells.

   1. junctional nevus.
   2. spindle cell nevus.
   3. blue nevus.
   4. cellular blue nevus.
   5. nevus of Ota.

233. Each of the following lesions is related to chronic sun exposure except:

   a. squamous cell carcinoma of the eyelid.
   b. lentigo maligna.
   c. sebaceous cell carcinoma.
   d. basal cell carcinoma.
   e. malignant melanoma.

234. The textural term most frequently applied to the consistency of a plexiform neurofibroma of the upper eyelid is:

   a. micropebbly.
   b. "bag of marbles."
   c. gravelly.
   d. "bag of worms."
   e. corduroy.

235. Which one of the following regarding Kaposi's sarcoma is false?

   a. It may be considered the malignant counterpart of a pyogenic granuloma.
   b. The disorder is endemic in Central Africa.
   c. In the setting of normal immune regulation, the disease typically affects the lower extremities of older men.
   d. Radiation plays no role in the management of ocular Kaposi's sarcoma.
   e. The disorder is generally more aggressive and lethal in the immunocompromised individual.

236. A stye or external hordeolum must arise from:

        1. Glands of Zeis.
        2. eccrine sweat glands.
        3. hair follicles.
        4. meibomian glands.

    a. 1, 2, and 3.
    b. 1 and 3.
    c. 2 and 4.
    d. 4 only.
    e. 1, 2, 3, and 4.

237. T or F -- All styes (external hordeola) are infectious.

238. Features critical in the definition of chalazion include:

        1. no history of pain.
        2. involvement of sebaceous glands.
        3. insidious onset.
        4. granulomatous inflammation.

    a. 1, 2, and 3.
    b. 1 and 3.
    c. 2 and 4.
    d. 4 only.
    e. 1, 2, 3, and 4.

239. Potential etiologies for multiple discrete eyelid nodules include all of the following except:

    a. juvenile xanthogranuloma.
    b. Hand-Schüller-Christian disease.
    c. xanthelasma.
    d. lipoid proteinosis.
    e. syringoma.

240. T or F -- The key difference between epibulbar and adnexal dermoid tumors is the presence of all three cell lines (ectoderm, mesoderm, and endoderm) in epibulbar dermoids.

241. A 32-year-old man from North Carolina presents to an ophthalmologist for routine examination. The ophthalmologist notes bilateral bulbar leukoplakia at the nasal and temporal limbus. On further questioning, the patient reports that these lesions have been present for many years and that several of his siblings have similar findings. Examination of which of the following is most likely to confirm the probable diagnosis:

a. medication history.
b. history of sunlight exposure.
c. intertriginous areas of the patient's body.
d. the patient's mouth.
e. the patient's fundus.

242. Epithelial neoplasms of the conjunctiva and cornea bear striking pathologic similarities to neoplasms of the:

a. stomach.
b. ovary.
c. cervix.
d. urinary bladder.
e. colon.

243. Match the terms for conjunctival and/or corneal intraepithelial neoplasia listed in the left-hand column with the histopathologic findings listed in the right-hand column.

a. mild dysplasia.
b. moderate dysplasia.
c. severe dysplasia.
d. carcinoma in situ.
e. microinvasive carcinoma.
f. squamous cell carcinoma.

1. atypia and loss of polarity involving the basal two-thirds of the epithelium.
2. full-thickness atypia and loss of polarity with limited areas of basement membrane invasion.
3. atypia and loss of polarity involving the basal one-third of the epithelium.
4. full-thickness atypia and loss of polarity with no remaining normal underlying architecture.
5. full-thickness atypia and loss of polarity of the epithelium, limited by intact basement membrane.

244. The most common location of origin for corneal intraepithelial neoplasia is:

a. the inferior fornix.
b. the superior fornix.
c. the limbus.
d. the bulbar conjunctiva.
e. the palpebral conjunctiva.

245. The key structure preventing local invasion of squamous cell carcinoma of the cornea is:

    a. epithelial basement membrane.
    b. Bowman's zone.
    c. corneal stroma.
    d. Descemet's membrane.
    e. endothelium.

246. Which one of the following regarding conjunctival nevi is false?

    a. Because of the absence of a dermal layer, conjunctival nevi are of the junctional variety only.
    b. Conjunctival nevi are frequently cystic.
    c. Due to sudden enlargement, mucus secretion within nevi can lead to the false impression of malignant transformation.
    d. Conjunctival nevi are more frequently amelanotic or lightly pigmented than skin nevi.
    e. Malignant transformation to melanoma is rare.

247. Which of the following statements regarding congenital melanosis oculi is accurate?

    a. Ocular melanocytosis is more common in blacks and Orientals, in whom malignant transformation is more common.
    b. Ocular melanocytosis is more common in whites, but malignant transformation to melanoma is more common in blacks and Orientals.
    c. Oculodermal melanocytosis is more common in Orientals and blacks, in whom malignant transformation is more common.
    d. Oculodermal melanocytosis is more common in blacks and Orientals, but malignant transformation is more common in whites.
    e. Oculodermal melanocytosis is equally common among whites, blacks, and Orientals.

248. Which of the following regarding primary acquired melanosis of the conjunctiva is/are true?

    1. The pigmented lesions represent proliferation of intraepithelial melanocytes.
    2. It is primarily a disorder of the middle-aged and elderly.
    3. The most troublesome sign (indicating potential malignant transformation) is nodular thickening.
    4. The most frequently involved region is the palpebral conjunctiva.

    a. 1, 2, and 3.
    b. 1 and 3.
    c. 2 and 4.
    d. 4 only.
    e. 1, 2, 3, and 4.

249. T or F -- Biopsy of acquired melanosis of the conjunctiva should be undertaken only when absolutely necessary, and always excisionally, to avoid seeding and spread of tumor.

250. T or F -- The most important adjunctive therapy to excisional biopsy of conjunctival melanoma is radiotherapy.

251. Features suggestive of benign reactive lymphoid hyperplasia rather than conjunctival lymphoma include:

    1. presence of prominent vascularity.
    2. heterogeneous cell population (neutrophils, eosinophils, plasma cells, and numerous lymphocytes).
    3. presence of numerous follicles.
    4. nodular, fleshy appearance on bulbar conjunctiva.

    a. 1, 2, and 3.
    b. 1 and 3.
    c. 2 and 4.
    d. 4 only.
    e. 1, 2, 3, and 4.

252. T or F -- The vast majority of conjunctival lymphomas are derived from T-lymphocytes.

253. T or F -- The best indicator of conjunctival lymphoma (rather than a reactive lesion) is light microscopic evidence of cellular atypia.

254. Which one of the following regarding abnormalities of corneal size is false?

    a. Megalocornea is defined as a cornea whose horizontal diameter is greater than 13 mm.
    b. The majority of megalocornea is bilateral and seen in men.
    c. Megalocornea may be associated with systemic abnormalities like Down's syndrome, Marfan's syndrome, or Alport's syndrome.
    d. Microcornea is often transmitted familially.
    e. In isolated microcornea, the eye is generally myopic.

255. The anterior segment dysgeneses reflect developmental abnormalities related to what cell line?

    a. surface ectoderm.
    b. neuroectoderm.
    c. neural crest.
    d. mesoderm.
    e. endoderm.

256. Schwalbe's ring represents the normal:

    a. peripheral termination of corneal epithelium.
    b. peripheral border between corneal and trabecular endothelium.
    c. peripheral border between nonpigmented and pigmented trabecular meshwork.
    d. peripheral termination of Bowman's zone.
    e. anterior insertion point of ciliary muscle.

257. An abnormally prominent Schwalbe's line is referred to as:

a. posterior embryotoxon.
b. Rieger's anomaly.
c. Peters' anomaly.
d. Axenfeld's anomaly.
e. internal ulcer of von Hippel.

258. A patient presents with unilateral glaucoma. Gonioscopy reveals an anteriorly displaced, prominent Schwalbe's line with attached iris processes. The angle is otherwise open. This clinical picture is most correctly referred to as:

a. posterior embryotoxon.
b. Axenfeld's anomaly.
c. Rieger's anomaly.
d. Axenfeld's syndrome.
e. Rieger's syndrome.

259. The brother of the patient described in question 258 is examined and also found to have elevated intraocular pressure. Gonioscopy on this patient reveals similar findings to the initial patient, but with additional findings of iris stromal hypoplasia and polycoria. There are no other obvious systemic abnormalities noted. This patients clinical condition would be most correctly termed:

a. posterior embryotoxon.
b. Axenfeld's anomaly.
c. Rieger's anomaly.
d. Axenfeld's syndrome.
e. Rieger's syndrome.

260. All cases of Peters' anomaly share which of the following features?

1. polycoria.
2. central absence of Descemet's membrane and endothelium.
3. cataract or ectopia lentis.
4. corneal leukoma.

a. 1, 2, and 3.
b. 1 and 3.
c. 2 and 4.
d. 4 only.
e. 1, 2, 3, and 4.

261. T or F -- Like Rieger's syndrome and anomaly, over half of patients with Peter's anomaly have glaucoma and are bilaterally affected.

262. Which of the following regarding corneal birth trauma is/are true?

    1. There are no means of distinguishing the findings from those of congenital glaucoma.
    2. The presenting finding is typically corneal haziness (stromal edema), in the first postnatal week.
    3. If corneal edema clears, there are no visual consequences and no permanent physical findings.
    4. Corneal stromal edema may recur later in life.

    a. 1, 2, and 3.
    b. 1 and 3.
    c. 2 and 4.
    d. 4 only.
    e. 1, 2, 3, and 4.

263. Which one of the following regarding pingueculae is false?

    a. The agent most frequently implicated in the pathogenesis is ultraviolet light.
    b. Histologically, accumulation of abnormal elastin material can be observed.
    c. The nasal limbus is more frequently involved than the temporal limbus.
    d. The lesions may calcify or become chronically inflamed.
    e. Surgical excision is generally not pursued unless there are cosmetic or comfort issues.

264. Which of the following regarding pterygia is/are true?

    1. Epidemiologically and histologically, pterygia are clearly extensions of pingueculae.
    2. Corneal invasion is limited in depth by the epithelial basement membrane.
    3. Mild inflammation and iron lines at the leading edge are typically seen.
    4. Like pingueculae, surgical intervention is usually mandated for comfort.

    a. 1, 2, and 3.
    b. 1 and 3.
    c. 2 and 4.
    d. 4 only.
    e. 1, 2, 3, and 4.

265. Methods to diminish the recurrence rate of pterygia following excision include:

        1. conjunctival autotransplantation.
        2. beta-irradiation.
        3. topical mitomycin C.
        4. 5-fluorouracil.

    a. 1, 2, and 3.
    b. 1 and 3.
    c. 2 and 4.
    d. 4 only.
    e. 1, 2, 3, and 4

266. The stain of choice for suspected amyloid deposits of the external eye is:

    a. Hematoxylin and eosin (H & E).
    b. Congo red.
    c. Periodic acid-Schiff (PAS).
    d. alcian blue.
    e. mucicarmine.

267. A conjunctival deposit of amyloid is biopsied and stained with Congo red. As a polarizing filter between the illuminating light and the specimen is rotated 90 degrees, the amyloid deposits seem to change from cherry red to apple green. This phenomenon is known as:

    a. birefringence.
    b. autofluorescence.
    c. metachromasia.
    d. fruit-looping.
    e. dichroism.

268. The most common form of conjunctival amyloidosis is:

    a. primary localized.
    b. primary systemic.
    c. heredofamilial.
    d. secondary localized.
    e. secondary systemic.

269. The most common type of eyelid amyloidosis is:

    a. primary localized.
    b. primary systemic.
    c. heredofamilial.
    d. secondary localized.
    e. secondary systemic.

270. Corneal forms of amyloidosis inlcude all of the following except:

    a. limbal girdle of Vogt.
    b. primary gelatinous drop-like dystrophy.
    c. lattice dystrophy Type I.
    d. polymorphic amyloid degeneration.
    e. Meretoja's syndrome.

271. Which one of the following regarding corneal arcus is false?

    a. The deposits generally begin in the interpalpebral fissure and spread superiorly and inferiorly with time.
    b. Incidence approaches 100% in patients over the age of 80.
    c. There is an increased incidence of arcus in blacks.
    d. There is generally a lucent zone between the limbus and the peripheral edge of the arcus.
    e. Unilateral corneal arcus may be seen in the setting of contralateral high-grade carotid stenosis.

272. T or F -- Hassall-Henle bodies develop from a pathophysiologic mechanism identical to corneal guttae.

273. T or F -- Hassall-Henle warts are forerunners of corneal edema.

274. A 65-year-old woman is examined as part of a routine annual checkup. On retroillumination of the cornea, fleck-like deposits in the deep corneal stroma are detectable centrally. Visual acuity is normal, and there are no other are ocular findings. The most likely diagnosis is:

    a. Hassall-Henle warts.
    b. cornea guttae.
    c. cornea farinata.
    d. central cloudy dystrophy.
    e. Fuchs' dystrophy.

275. The most common etiology of calcific band keratopathy is:

    a. chronic ocular inflammation.
    b. systemic hypercalcemia.
    c. primary hereditary band keratopathy.
    d. renal failure.
    e. chronic mercurial exposure.

276. Clinically and histopathologically, the earliest calcium deposits in band keratopathy are located in the:

    a. horizontal peripheral cornea, Descemet's membrane.
    b. vertical peripheral cornea, Descemet's membrane.
    c. vertical peripheral cornea, Bowman's zone.
    d. horizontal peripheral cornea, Bowman's zone.
    e. central cornea, Descemet's membrane.

277. The two most commonly encountered chemical compositions of band keratopathy are:

    a. urate and amyloid.
    b. urate and cholesterol.
    c. cholesterol and calcium.
    d. urate and calcium.
    e. cholesterol and amyloid.

278. T or F -- The pathophysiologic mechanisms at work in spheroidal corneal degeneration (climatic droplet keratopathy) are the same as for pterygia and pingueculae.

279. Which of the following corneal degenerations are generally seen only in association with corneal neovascularization?

    1. Salzmann's nodular degeneration.
    2. Spheroidal degeneration.
    3. Coats' white ring.
    4. Lipid keratopathy.

    a. 1, 2, and 3.
    b. 1 and 3.
    c. 2 and 4.
    d. 4 only.
    e. 1, 2, 3, and 4.

280. A 63-year-old woman presents with a red, painful right eye. Examination discloses an ulcerative, circumferential marginal keratitis with a leading, undermined edge and early neovascularization. Which one of the following regarding the condition is false?

    a. There is dysregulation in both cellular and humoral immunity.
    b. A more mild, less painful variant may be seen in young black men.
    c. Medical management might include oral prednisone, cyclophosphamide or methotrexate.
    d. Surgical intervention might include conjunctival resection or lamellar keratoplasty.
    e. An evaluation for connective tissue disease is mandatory.

281. Match the clinical characteristics in the left-hand column with the correct form of marginal degeneration listed in the right-hand column.

a. red, inflamed eyes.
b. white, quiet eyes.
c. prominent lipid deposition.
d. undermined edge of corneal stroma.
e. generally begins superiorly.
f. may begin anywhere peripherally.
g. spontaneous perforation possible.
h. spontaneous perforation unlikely.
i. associated with systemic collagen vascular disease.
j. may lead to disabling against-the-rule astigmatism.
k. may respond to immunosuppressives.

1. Mooren's ulcer.
2. Terrien's marginal degeneration.
3. both.
4. neither.

282. Ulcerative marginal keratitis indistinguishable from Mooren's ulcer may develop in patients with:

1. acne rosacea.
2. relapsing polychondritis.
3. Wegener's granulomatosis.
4. polymyositis.

a. 1, 2, and 3.
b. 1 and 3.
c. 2 and 4.
d. 4 only.
e. 1, 2, 3, and 4.

283. T or F -- There is a high spontaneous perforation rate in senile furrow degeneration.

284. Match the clinical characteristics listed in the left column with the classifications of corneal disorders in the right column.

a. associated with previous or concurrent disorders, diseases, or aging.
b. generally associated with family history.
c. generally begins centrally.
d. generally begins peripherally.
e. bilaterally symmetric.
f. unilateral or asymmetric.
g. progressive over time.
h. may be stationary.
i. may cause decreased vision.
j. may involve deposition of material not normally found in the cornea.

1. dystrophies.
2. degenerations.
3. both.
4. neither.

285. T or F -- The most common classification for corneal dystrophies is by the biochemical nature of the corneal deposits.

286. The most common anterior corneal dystrophy is:

a. Meesman's dystrophy.
b. Map-dot-fingerprint dystrophy.
c. lattice dystrophy type 1.
d. central cloudy dystrophy.
e. Reis-Bückler's dystrophy.

287. Which one of the following regarding anterior membrane dystrophy is false?

a. Examination of family members may disclose a familial pattern.
b. A disorder indistinguishable from the inherited form may be seen secondary to chronic blepharoconjunctivitis.
c. Abnormalities in basement membrane production are manifested as map and fingerprint lines.
d. Dots represents calcification of epithelial debris.
e. Symptoms are generally related to defective epithelial adherence.

288. Treatment modalities useful in symptomatic anterior membrane dystrophy include all of the following except:

a. epithelial debridement.
b. copious lubrication.
c. hypertonic saline ointments.
d. stromal puncture.
e. penetrating keratoplasty.

289. A 28-year-old patient presents to an ophthalmologist complaining of irritation and episodic blurry vision bilaterally. Slit-lamp examination reveals too-numerous-to-count bubbles visible only on retroillumination, intraepithelially. These bubbles appear entirely transparent. A lamellar keratoplasty specimen should reveal:

a. areas of reduplicated basement membrane and trapped epithelial cells.
b. PAS staining of epithelially contained "peculiar substance."
c. focal areas of absence of basement membrane and fibrocellular invasion of Bowman's zone.
d. hyaline deposits in the anterior stroma.
e. congophilic deposits in the anterior and midstroma.

290. Recurrent erosions are prominent features of which corneal dystrophies?

        1. anterior membrane dystrophy.
        2. Meesman's dystrophy.
        3. Reis-Bückler's dystrophy.
        4. central cloudy dystrophy.

    a. 1, 2, and 3.
    b. 1 and 3.
    c. 2 and 4.
    d. 4 only.
    e. 1, 2, 3, and 4.

291. Which of the following corneal dystrophies is the most disabling visually?

    a. anterior membrane dystrophy.
    b. Reis-Bückler's dystrophy.
    c. Meesman's dystrophy.
    d. central cloudy dystrophy.
    e. pre-Descemet's dystrophy.

292. A 29-year-old woman undergoes a routine ophthalmic examination. Visual acuity is normal. Slit-lamp examination discloses numerous crumb-like deposits in the anterior corneal stroma, which are bilaterally symmetric, densest centrally. Intervening stroma is clear. Which one of the following is likely to be false?

    a. Careful history may elicit a history of recurrent corneal erosions.
    b. Examination of family members will disclose similar findings.
    c. Visual acuity generally remains normal throughout life.
    d. Histopathologic review will reveal hyaline deposits on the Masson trichrome stain.
    e. Histopathologic review may reveal congophilic deposits resembling amyloid.

293. A 38-year-old man presents to the ophthalmologist complaining of gradual diminution in vision bilaterally. Visual acuity is 20/100 OU. Slit-lamp examination reveals focal gray crumb-like deposits in the stroma, densest centrally but extending to the limbus. Intervening areas of stroma have an ill-defined haze. Which one of the following regarding this condition is likely to be false?

    a. The patient's siblings may be affected, but his offspring are unlikely to be.
    b. It is the stromal dystrophy most likely to be associated with recurrent erosions.
    c. It is the least common of the stromal dystrophies.
    d. A blood test may aid in the diagnosis.
    e. The stain of choice for the corneal biopsy specimen is alcian blue.

294. A 59-year-old woman presents to the ophthalmologist complaining of gradual loss of vision in each eye over the previous 5 years. Visual acuity is 20/80 OU. Slit-lamp examination reveals multiple crumb-like deposits in the anterior central stroma along with refractile, branching, linear stromal deposits centrally. The peripheral corneal is clear. Both eyes are symmetrically involved. Which one of the following statements is likely to be false?

   a. Each of the patient's children has a 50% chance of being affected with the same disorder.
   b. Recurrent erosions are more likely to develop in this disorder than any of the other related disorders.
   c. Recurrence in donor corneas following penetrating keratoplasty is more likely with this disorder than any other related disorder.
   d. The patient, on further questioning, will probably complain of a history of double vision or facial droop.
   e. With a polarizing filters on both side of the specimen, light microscopic evaluation of the patient's corneal button following keratoplasty will reveal birefringence of the abnormal deposits.

295. Which of the stromal dystrophies, like arcus and xanthelasma, may be associated with systemic hyperlipidemia?

   a. granular dystrophy.
   b. central crystalline dystrophy.
   c. fleck dystrophy.
   d. central cloudy dystrophy of Francois.
   e. posterior amorphous stromal dystrophy.

296. Which one of the stromal dystrophies may be associated with keratoconus, atopy, or pseudoxanthoma elasticum?

   a. granular dystrophy.
   b. central crystalline dystrophy.
   c. fleck dystrophy.
   d. central cloudy dystrophy of Francois.
   e. posterior amorphous stromal dystrophy.

297. Which one of the following stromal dystrophies is least likely to be associated with poor vision?

   a. granular dystrophy.
   b. lattice dystrophy.
   c. macular dystrophy.
   d. central cloudy dystrophy of Francois.
   e. congenital hereditary stromal dystrophy.

298. T or F -- Pathophysiologically, the deposits representing corneal guttae are similar to macular drusen.

299. Which one of the following regarding Fuch's endothelial dystrophy is false?

 a. At one end of the spectrum are corneal guttae; at the other are epithelial bullae.
 b. Symptoms usually consist of blurry vision and pain, worse in the evening.
 c. Typically, stromal edema develops before epithelial abnormalities are noted.
 d. Specular microscopy reveals larger, irregular cells (endothelial polymegathism) and decreased cell counts.
 e. Penetrating keratoplasty may need to be undertaken at the time of cataract surgery, even though corneal symptoms are minimal or nonexistent.

300. An infant is born with bilaterally thickened, hazy corneas with epithelial edema. Corneal diameters are normal. There is associated nystagmus. Which one of the following regarding this condition is false?

 a. Intraocular pressure (IOP) is likely to be elevated.
 b. Another variant of the disorder exists in which there is no nystagmus and the onset is later.
 c. Features distinguishing this disorder from congenital hereditary stromal dystrophy include corneal thickening and epithelial edema.
 d. Descemet's membrane may thickened but there are no guttae.
 e. This disorder reflects an abnormality in neural crest cell migration or differentiation.

301. A 28-year-old man presents claiming "someone said my eyes look funny." Visual acuity is normal bilaterally. Slit-lamp examination reveals multiple abnormalities on the posterior corneal surface, including groups of blister-like deposits, scalloped banding, and irregular map-like grayish deposits on the endothelium with focal stromal edema. These findings are bilateral, as is corectopia, with the pupil drawn temporally. Careful questioning fails to reveal any family history of eye disorders. Which one of the following regarding this condition is probably false?

 a. Careful examination of a sibling may reveal milder but similar findings.
 b. Intraocular pressure may be elevated.
 c. Gonioscopy may reveal anteriorly placed peripheral anterior synechiae.
 d. Histopathologic findings of the eye, if reviewed, would reveal an abnormally proliferative corneal endothelium with desmosomes and microvilli.
 e. The most likely diagnosis is iridocorneal endothelial syndrome (ICE).

302. If corneal transplantation were required on the eye of the patient in question 301, the pathology would be strikingly similar to that seen in:

 a. keratoconus.
 b. epithelial downgrowth.
 c. Fuchs' dystrophy.
 d. granular dystrophy.
 e. macular dystrophy.

303. The most common finding in the contralateral eye of a patient with unilateral keratoconus is:

  a. Vogt's striae.
  b. horizontal breaks in Descemet's membrane.
  c. fleck dystrophy.
  d. myopia with high astigmatism.
  e. Brushfield spots.

304. The time of greatest progression of keratoconus is during the:

  a. first decade.
  b. second decade.
  c. third decade.
  d. fourth decade.
  e. the condition is generally static.

305. Match the clinical findings of keratoconus listed in the left-hand column with the appropriate eponymic designation in the right-hand column.

  a. conical reflection of light from a temporal light source on the nasal cornea.
  b. pointed deviation of the lower eyelid in downgaze.
  c. iron deposition in basal epithelial cells at the inferior aspect of the cone.
  d. vertical oblique lines within the corneal stroma that disappear with digital pressure on the eye.

  1. Munson's sign.
  2. Vogt's striae.
  3. Rizzutti's sign.
  4. Fleischer's ring.

306. A patient with known keratoconus presents to the ophthalmologist with a sudden decrease in vision and tearing from the right eye. Which one of the following regarding this situation is probably false?

  a. The "tearing" represents spontaneous perforation and demands immediate surgery.
  b. The corneal findings at the slit lamp may slowly resolve with time.
  c. There may be considerable associated pain.
  d. Typically, the condition is painless.
  e. This process may accelerate scarring.

307. A patient presents to the ophthalmologist unhappy with his latest refraction. Examination discloses vision of 20/50 with each eye through his new pair of spectacles. This improves to 20/25+ with a pinhole over either lens. Keratometry reveals 45.5 D at 180 degrees and 53.5 D at 90 degrees in each eye. The next logical intervention should be:

  a. photorefractive keratectomy.
  b. toric soft contact lens fitting.
  c. rigid contact lens fitting.
  d. thermal keratoplasty.
  e. penetrating keratoplasty.

308. T or F -- Keratoglobus usually offers a better visual prognosis either with or without penetrating keratoplasty than keratoconus.

309. Contact lens fitting is usually most challenging for patients with:

    a. keratoconus.
    b. keratoglobus.
    c. pellucid marginal degeneration.
    d. posterior keratoconus.
    e. microcornea.

310. Match the anatomic and clinical characteristics listed in the left-hand column with the correct tear film layer in the right-hand column.

    a. the innermost layer (closest to the cornea).
    b. permits diffusion of oxygen and metabolites to the cornea readily.
    c. retards tear evaporation.
    d. constitutes the bulk of tear volume (greater than 90%).
    e. outermost layer (exposed to air).
    f. secreted by the conjunctiva.
    g. the middle layer.
    h. secreted by the glands of Krause and Wolfring.
    i. permits smooth, even distribution of tear film over corneal epithelium.
    j. secreted by meibomian glands.

    1. aqueous phase.
    2. lipid phase.
    3. mucus phase.

311. Which one of the following regarding tear deficiency states is false?

    a. Prominent symptoms include blurry vision and pain with blinking.
    b. Classic signs include ropy mucus discharge, corneal filaments, and punctate rose bengal staining in the exposure zone.
    c. Pathophysiologically, the problem is a loss of adequate tear volume.
    d. Patients may complain of epiphora.
    e. Tests to be considered in the evaluation of potential tear deficency include Schirmer's tests, rose bengal stain, and observation of tear breakup time.

312. T or F -- The purpose of topical anesthesia before Schirmer's testing is to reduce spontaneous blinking and prevent dislodging of the testing strips.

313. T or F -- Normal tear production during anesthetized Schirmer's test is 10 mm or more after 5 minutes.

314. Match the staining characterisitics in the left-hand column with the stains listed in the right-hand column.

a. adheres well to mucus.
b. stains mucus less vividly.
c. adheres firmly to exposed basement membrane.
d. adheres to dead or devitalized cells.
e. diffuses into intercellular epithelial spaces and stroma.
f. does not diffuse into intercellular spaces.
g. stain of choice for tear deficiency states.
h. stain of choice for epithelial defects.
i. stain of choice for herpes simplex epithelial keratitis.
j. requires dilution in aqueous solution for visualization.

1. rose bengal.
2. fluorescein.
3. both.
4. neither.

315. A patient presents with complaints typical for dry eye syndrome. Schirmer's testing with and without anesthesia is normal. A hypothesis of tear deficiency state due to inadequate tear lipid or mucus layer would be best confirmed by:

a. repeat Schirmer's testing.
b. tear breakup time testing.
c. tear osmolarity testing.
d. rose bengal staining.
e. tear lysozyme testing.

316. Which of the following historical features favor the diagnosis of a tear deficiency state?

1. symptoms worse in the morning.
2. symptoms aggravated by warm, dry conditions.
3. history of chalazia.
4. symptoms aggravated in windy conditions.

a. 1, 2, and 3.
b. 1 and 3.
c. 2 and 4.
d. 4 only.
e. 1, 2, 3, and 4.

317. Classic Sjögren's syndrome consists of keratoconjunctivitis sicca, xerostomia, and:

a. eczema.
b. arthritis.
c. Raynaud's phenomenon.
d. SS-A and SS-B autoantibodies.
e. Hashimoto's thyroiditis.

318. The critical difference between patients with primary and secondary Sjögren's syndrome is:

    a. the presence of autoantibodies in the primary group.
    b. the presence of autoantibodies in the secondary group.
    c. salivary gland involvement.
    d. HLA-Dw3 subtype in the primary group.
    e. association with systemic connective tissue disease in the secondary group.

319. Patients with primary Sjögren's syndrome are at increased risk for subsequent development of:

                1. autoimmune thyroiditis.
                2. Waldenström's macroglobulinemia.
                3. lymphoma.
                4. adenoid cystic carcinoma of the lacrimal gland.

    a. 1, 2, and 3.
    b. 1 and 3.
    c. 2 and 4.
    d. 4 only.
    e. 1, 2, 3, and 4.

320. A patient with established dry eye syndrome is suffering persistent discomfort and blurry vision despite hourly topical artificial tears. The next most appropriate intervention might be:

    a. warm compresses to both eyes twice a day.
    b. swimmers' goggles to be worn during the day.
    c. lateral tarsorrhaphy.
    d. a trial of temporary inferior punctal occlusion with collagen plugs.
    e. permanent thermal punctal occlusion for all four puncta.

321. Tear deficiency may play a pathophysiologic role in all of the following conditions except:

    a. corneal foreign body.
    b. ocular cicatricial pemphigoid (OCP).
    c. Bell's palsy.
    d. use of oral contraceptives.
    e. previous herpes zoster keratitis.

322. T or F -- The distribution of keratopathy seen in long-standing Bell's palsy is quite similar to that seen in primary Sjögren's syndrome.

323. T or F -- The distribution of keratopathy seen in long-standing neurotrophic keratitis is quite similar to that seen in primary Sjögren's syndrome.

324. A patient with a history of previous severe herpes zoster keratitis presents with Bell's palsy. Appropriate intervention at this point should include:

    a. hourly artificial tears.
    b. bandage contact lens.
    c. lateral tarsorrhaphy.
    d. conjunctival flap.
    e. oral acyclovir.

325. Which one of the following regarding rosacea is false?

    a. It is more common in fair-skinned races.
    b. Facial lesions include telangiectasis, papules, pustules, and comedones.
    c. Nasal skin thickening (rhinophyma) is a late sign.
    d. Mid-facial flushing may be enhanced with spicy food intake or hot beverages.
    e. Alcohol consumption can aggravate the disorder.

326. The most common ocular manifestation of rosacea is:

    a. chronic or recurrent meibomitis.
    b. marginal keratitis.
    c. episcleritis.
    d. peripheral keratitis.
    e. anterior uveitis.

327. T or F -- Tear deficiency state is more common in patients with rosacea than in patients with no evidence of the disorder.

328. Which of the following true regarding the pathology of acne rosacea is/are true?

    1. *Demodex* infestation may play an inciting or aggravating role.
    2. Biopsy of involved tissues frequently reveals granulomatous inflammation.
    3. There may be irreversible obliteration of meibomian glands.
    4. Type IV hypersensitivity may play a role in the pathogenesis.

    a. 1, 2, and 3.
    b. 1 and 3.
    c. 2 and 4.
    d. 4 only.
    e. 1, 2, 3, and 4.

329. A 42-year-old man of Irish descent presents to the ophthalmologist complaining that his eyes have been red for several months. Examination discloses multiple brow and cheek telangiectasias with small papillary rash at the tip of the nose. All four eyelids are thickened with telangiectasias crossing the lid margin. There is focal meibomian gland loss. Both eyes have moderate conjunctival injection, and the right eye has a marginal infiltrate under intact epithelium at the inferior temporal limbus. An effective treatment strategy might include all of the following except:

a. warm compresses to both eyes twice a day.
b. topical bacitracin ointment to the eyelids twice a day.
c. topical prednisolone 1.0% to the right eye every 2 to 4 hours.
d. topical metronidazole for the skin findings.
e. long-term oral doxycycline.

330. Which one of the following regarding erythema multiforme is false?

a. The distinction between minor and major variants is the involvement of mucous membranes in the latter.
b. The acute phase of the major type lasts longer than the minor type.
c. Inflammation is generally confined to the dermis or submucosal stroma.
d. Both major and minor varieties are self-limited and resolve uneventfully with proper supportive care.
e. The inflammation is primarily angiocentric.

331. The most commonly implicated inciting agent in erythema multiforme is:

a. recent use of pencillin.
b. recent herpes simplex infection.
c. recent mycoplasma infection.
d. recent use of sulfonamides.
e. recent use of anticonvulsants.

332. T or F -- Like the skin, the classic mucous membrane lesion of erythema multiforme resembles a target, or bull's-eye.

333. Which one of following regarding the acute care and long-term prognosis of erythema multiforme is false?

a. Mortality approaches 20% in severe cases.
b. The most frequent cause of death is secondary infection.
c. Systemic corticosteroids have substantially diminished mortality.
d. Aggressive ocular lubrication and lysis of symblepharons significantly reduce ultimate scarring.
e. The long-term ocular prognosis in toxic epidermal necrolysis is somewhat better than that of systemic erythema multiforme.

334. The mucous membrane most frequently involved in cicatricial pemphigoid is:

    a. oral.
    b. conjunctival.
    c. pharyngeal.
    d. esophageal.
    e. genitourinary.

335. T or F -- The pathophysiology of cicatricial pemphigoid (OCP) is identical of that of Stevens-Johnson syndrome (erythema multiforme major).

336. Which one of the following regarding the clinical features of OCP is false?

    a. The disorder is rarely seen in patients under the age of 30.
    b. Women are more commonly affected than men.
    c. The disease most typically presents as insidious, bilaterally asymmetric chronic conjunctivitis.
    d. Chronic use of topical ocular medications may induce a clinically identical picture.
    e. The most sensitive region of the eye to examine for early findings is the superior tarsus.

337. The classic histologic finding in OCP is:

    a. hypersensitivity angiitis in submucosal stroma.
    b. intraepithelial immunoglobulin and intraepithelial bullae.
    c. granulomatous destruction of epithelial basement membrane.
    d. complement and immunoglobulin bound to epithelial basement membrane.
    e. mast cells and eosinophils in the epithelium and subepithelial stroma.

338. T or F -- The initial drug of choice in all cases of OCP is dapsone.

339. Ocular findings consistent with vitamin A deficiency include:

    1. keratinization and bacterial superinfection of bulbar conjunctiva.
    2. tear deficiency state.
    3. deep white lesions of the peripheral retina.
    4. diffuse corneal necrosis with ulceration.

    a. 1, 2, and 3.
    b. 1 and 3.
    c. 2 and 4.
    d. 4 only.
    e. 1, 2, 3, and 4.

340. Bilateral corneal ulceration should be presumed to be due to vitamin A deficiency until proved otherwise in patients with:

    1. cystic fibrosis.
    2. history of gastric bypass surgery.
    3. cirrhosis.
    4. patients with a history of heavy smoking but normal nutrition.

a. 1, 2, and 3.
b. 1 and 3.
c. 2 and 4.
d. 4 only.
e. 1, 2, 3, and 4.

341. A 32-year-old woman presents to the ophthalmologist complaining of recurrent pain and tearing of her right eye over the previous 1 to 2 months. Closer questioning discloses that her symptoms are virtually always upon awakening and disappear after 2 or 3 hours. She denies any history of contact lens use. Which of the following statements is/are likely to be true?

    1. Careful questioning may reveal a history of corneal abrasion or trauma in the right eye.
    2. Careful examination of the right eye may disclose a focal abnormality in tear breakup.
    3. Careful examination of the left eye may reveal map or fingerprint abnormalities.
    4. This syndrome may be seen more frequently in patients with diabetes mellitus.

a. 1, 2, and 3.
b. 1 and 3.
c. 2 and 4.
d. 4 only.
e. 1, 2, 3, and 4.

342. Modalities accepted for treatment of the syndrome described in question 341 include all of the following except:

a. pressure patching.
b. copious lubricating ointments.
c. Five percent sodium chloride ointment at bedtime for 2 to 4 weeks.
d. bandage contact lens.
e. anterior stromal puncture with a 27-gauge needle.

343. Which one of the following regarding ligneous conjunctivitis is false?

a. This is primarily a disorder of childhood.
b. It is typically bilateral.
c. It typically presents as an acute membranous conjunctivitis.
d. Topical cyclosporine may be the most promising medical treatment.
e. Surgical resection of involved conjunctiva is the definitive treatment.

344. Which of the following concerning the mucopolysaccharidoses (MPS) is/are true?

   1. Lysosomal enzyme defects lead to accumulation of metabolites within keratocytes.
   2. The MPS least likely to demonstrate corneal clouding is type III (Sanfilippo's syndrome).
   3. Metabolites that accumulate include keratan sulfate, dermatan sulfate, and heparan sulfate.
   4. These disorders are all inherited on autosomal recessive bases.

   a. 1, 2, and 3.
   b. 1 and 3.
   c. 2 and 4.
   d. 4 only.
   e. 1, 2, 3, and 4.

345. The typical corneal finding in patient with Fabry's disease is:

   a. corneal clouding.
   b. anterior membrane dystrophy.
   c. vortex keratopathy.
   d. corneal guttae.
   e. corneal neovascularization.

346. A 26-year-old woman presents for a routine ophthalmic examination. Slit-lamp examination discloses a vortex keratopathy bilaterally with telangiectatic conjunctival vessels. Her mother and father are both healthy. Which one of the following is false?

   a. A careful drug history should be taken.
   b. The patient should be warned of potentially lethal renal failure.
   c. Other slit-lamp findings might include subtle posterior subcapsular cataract.
   d. Fundus findings might include telangiectatic retinal vessels.
   e. Half of the patient's brothers will be seriously affected by the same disorder.

347. A patient presents with photophobia and blurry vision. Examination discloses crystalline deposits throughout the entire stroma, densest peripherally. Findings important in determining the correct diagnosis include all of the following except:

   a. family history of eye findings.
   b. previous history of kidney transplant.
   c. history of peptic ulcer disease (PUD).
   d. presence of pigmentary retinopathy in each eye.
   e. serum immunoelectrophoresis.

348. The corneal findings in tyrosinemia most closely resemble those of:

   a. anterior membrane dystrophy.
   b. herpes simplex keratitis.
   c. Wilson's disease.
   d. chronic indomethacin usage.
   e. ochronosis.

349. Which one of the following regarding vortex keratopathy is false?

   a. Drugs associated with the finding include amiodarone, indomethacin, chloroquine, and chlorpromazine.
   b. The findings in drug-induced vortex keratopathy are identical to those of Fabry's disease.
   c. The pathophysiology of the deposits in drug-induced vortex keratopathy is identical to that of Fabry's disease.
   d. The drug-induced varieties are accompanied by a pigmentary retinopathy.
   e. Cessation of drug therapy will usually lead to resolution of vortex keratopathy.

350. A patient is sent to an ophthalmologist by a gastroenterologist to "rule out Wilson's disease." The key part of the ophthalmologist's examination should be:

   a. visual acuity measurement.
   b. slit-lamp examination.
   c. tonometry.
   d. gonioscopy.
   e. dilated funduscopy.

351. A Kayser-Fleischer ring may be seen in which of the following disorders?

   1. primary biliary cirrhosis.
   2. chronic active hepatitis.
   3. Wilson's disease.
   4. chalcosis.

   a. 1, 2, and 3.
   b. 1 and 3.
   c. 2 and 4.
   d. 4 only.
   e. 1, 2, 3, and 4.

352. Match the associated clinical findings listed in the left-hand column with the various disorders associated with enlarged corneal nerves listed in the right-hand column.

a. pigmentary retinopathy, hearing loss, mental retardation.
b. optic nerve glioma, multiple iris nevi.
c. sclerosing interstitial keratitis, anterior uveitis, and iris granulomas.
d. enlarged corneal diameter, horizontal breaks in Descemet's membrane, and dislocated lens.
e. scaly, tight skin.
f. hypertension, hypocalcemia, mucocutaneous neuromas.
g. myopic astigmatism, Munson's sign.
h. Hudson-Stahli line, cataract, Hassall-Henle warts.

1. old age.
2. neurofibromatosis, type I.
3. congenital glaucoma.
4. multiple endocrine neoplasia, type III.
5. keratoconus.
6. Hansen's disease.
7. Refsum's disease.
8. Ichthyosis.

353. The most accurate characterization of donor endothelial cell counts following penetrating keratoplasty is:

a. no significant change.
b. steady, progressive loss of endothelial cells forever.
c. slow, steady increase in endothelial cell count over 10 to 15 years.
d. rapid loss of endothelial cells over the first postoperative year, slow loss of endothelial cells over the next 10 to 15 years, with stable cell counts after 15 years.
e. slow, progressive loss of endothelial cells over 10 to 15 years with stabilization thereafter.

354. Currently, the most frequent indication for penetrating keratoplasty in the United States is:

a. keratoconus.
b. bullous keratopathy following cataract extraction.
c. Fuchs' dystrophy.
d. herpes simplex keratitis.
e. corneal stromal dystrophy.

355. Which of the following are considered favorable prognostic factors for penetrating keratoplasty?

1. relatively young age.
2. glaucoma.
3. large graft size (greater than 8.5 mm).
4. no previous history of graft rejection.

a. 1, 2, and 3.
b. 2 and 4.
c. 1 and 3.
d. 4 only.
e. 1, 2, 3, and 4.

356. Which of the following are considered unfavorable prognostic factors for penetrating keratoplasty?

       1. considerable stromal vascularization.
       2. tear deficiency state.
       3. active intraocular inflammation.
       4. corneal hypesthesia.

    a. 1, 2, and 3.
    b. 1 and 3.
    c. 2 and 4.
    d. 4 only.
    e. 1, 2, 3, and 4.

357. The primary cause of poor vision following penetrating keratoplasty for aphakic bullous keratopathy is:

    a. glaucoma.
    b. endophthalmitis.
    c. cystoid macular edema.
    d. graft rejection.
    e. retinal detachment.

358. Preoperative steps that are helpful in penetrating keratoplasty include:

       1. pilocarpine 1% preoperatively.
       2. Honan balloon placement prior to surgery.
       3. intravenous mannitol preoperatively.
       4. phospholine iodide, preoperatively.

    a. 1, 2, and 3.
    b. 1 and 3.
    c. 2 and 4.
    d. 4 only.
    e. 1, 2, 3, and 4.

359. T or F -- A scleral support ring (Flieringa ring) during penetrating keratoplasty is most helpful in eyes that are aphakic (or will become so during the procedure).

360. T or F -- The main advantage of small donor button size (7mm or less) is decreased astigmatism, while the main disadvantage is increased risk of rejection.

361. T or F -- The main advantage of oversizing the donor button (0.5 mm or more larger than the host bed) is to decrease the incidence of peripheral anterior synechiae and subsequent elevated intraocular pressure.

362. The condition in which same-size or smaller-than-host-bed donor buttons are often used is:

a. keratoconus.
b. Fuchs' dystrophy.
c. herpetic keratitis.
d. bullous keratopathy after cataract surgery.
e. corneal stromal dystrophies.

363. Which method of closure of penetrating keratoplasty causes the greatest amount of irregular astigmatism (prior to suture removal):

a. interrupted.
b. single running.
c. double running.
d. combined interrupted plus single running.
e. combined interrupted plus double running.

364. A patient returns for follow-up 8 weeks after penetrating keratoplasty. The central cornea is clear but too irregular to permit accurate keratometry. Vision is 20/400, pinholing to 20/30. What is the most reliable and effective method of visual rehabilitation?

a. random removal of sutures, one per week.
b. removal of sutures that appear tightest at the slit lamp.
c. use of keratoscope to guide suture removal.
d. removal of all sutures simultaneously.
e. contact lens refraction and correction.

365. T or F -- In penetrating keratoplasty (PK) for bullous keratopathy associated with anterior chamber intraocular lenses (ACIOL), the IOL should be removed in all cases.

366. T or F -- In the setting of severe corneal disease combined with cataract, the corneal transplantation should be performed initially, with cataract extraction performed later as a secondary procedure.

367. A 62-year-old woman presents complaining of slow loss of vision in each eye. She denies any previous ocular history. Visual acuities are 20/400 OD and 20/100 OS. Slit-lamp examination reveals corneal guttae OU with central stromal thickening more prominent on the right. The corneal epithelium is normal bilaterally. There is dense nuclear sclerosis on the right and moderate nuclear sclerosis on the left. The view of the fundus is consistent with the patients vision. The next appropriate step for visual rehabilitation in this patient might be:

a. extracapsular cataract extraction only (ECCE), OD.
b. ECCE with posterior chamber intraocular lens (PCIOL), OD.
c. penetrating keratoplasty alone (PK), OD.
d. PK with ECCE, OD.
e. PK, ECCE, PCIOL, OD.

368. A 65-year-old man presents to the ophthalmologist complaining of slow loss of vision in each eye. He denies any previous ocular history. Examination reveals visual acuities of 20/400 OD and 20/100 OS. Slit-lamp examination reveals severe corneal guttae bilaterally. The corneal epithelium and stroma are normal. There is dense nuclear sclerosis in the right eye and moderate nuclear sclerosis in the left eye. The next step for visual rehabilitation of this patient might be:

a. extracapsular cataract extraction only (ECCE), OD.
b. ECCE with posterior chamber intraocular lens (PCIOL), OD.
c. penetrating keratoplasty alone (PK), OD.
d. PK with ECCE, OD.
e. PK, ECCE, PCIOL, OD.

369. Mucous membrane grafting in anticipation of penetrating keratoplasty is most hazardous in patients with:

a. Stevens-Johnson syndrome.
b. ocular cicatricial pemphigoid (OCP).
c. trachoma.
d. keratoconjunctivitis sicca.
e. herpes zoster ophthalmicus.

370. Persistent epithelial defects of the donor cornea following PK are likely to be seen in all of the following except:

a. ocular cicatricial pemphigoid (OCP).
b. alkali burns.
c. keratoconus.
d. keratoconjunctivitis sicca.
e. herpes zoster ophthalmicus.

371. Recurrence of the original disease process has been reported following penetrating keratoplasty for each of the following conditions except:

a. lattice dystrophy.
b. herpes simplex keratitis.
c. Reis-Bückler dystrophy.
d. Fuchs' dystrophy.
e. macular dystrophy.

372. The most common postoperative complication seen after penetrating keratoplasty (PK) is:

a. infectious keratitis.
b. recurrence of the original disease process.
c. acute glaucoma.
d. high astigmatism.
e. wound leak.

373. A patient presents to the ophthalmologist 12 weeks following penetrating keratoplasty. Complaints consist of increasing redness and discomfort in the operated eye. Visual acuity is the same as the previous office visit 2 weeks earlier. Examination discloses a white, crystalline infiltrate at the donor/host interface between sutures. The infiltrate has indistinct borders, and the stroma appears thickened by it. There is overlying epithelial irregularity but no confluent epithelial defect. Gram's stain of a corneal scraping reveals gram-positive cocci in chains. Cultures on blood agar grow multiple colonies with alpha hemolysis. Which one of the following statements regarding this condition is false?

    a. The causative organism, as with cases originally described, is *S. viridans*.
    b. This infection is generally slowly progressive.
    c. This condition is generally quite responsive to topical antibiotics.
    d. Historical factors most significant in the development of the lesion include topical steroid use and keratoplasty.
    e. Other organisms reported to cause a similar condition include coagulase-negative *Staphylococcus* and *Candida* species.

374. A patient presents the day following penetrating keratoplasty for keratoconus. Examination discloses visual acuity of counting fingers at 1 foot. Slit-lamp examination shows diffuse corneal stromal edema with epithelial irregularity. Intraocular pressure is normal. Which of the following concerning this condition is/are true?

    1. By definition this constitutes primary graft failure.
    2. The probable cause of this condition is inadequate donor endothelium.
    3. A potential cause is inadvertent trauma to the donor button at the time of transplant.
    4. It may represent the earliest sign of immunologic graft rejection.

    a. 1, 2, and 3.
    b. 1 and 3.
    c. 2 and 4.
    d. 4 only.
    e. 1, 2, 3, and 4.

375. The most important mechanism for corneal allograft reaction is believed to be:

    a. Type I hypersensitivity.
    b. Type II hypersensitivity.
    c. Type III hypersensitivity.
    d. Type IV hypersensitivity.
    e. Type V hypersensitivity.

376. A patient presents to the ophthalmologist 1 week following his second penetrating keratoplasty in his right eye for herpes simplex keratitis. Visual acuity has dropped to hand motions. There is stromal edema of the inferior three-quarters of the donor button. The epithelium overlying this area is irregular. There are fine granular deposits on the endothelium along with a moderate anterior chamber reaction. The eye is aphakic (prior cataract surgery). Which one of the following concerning this situation is probably false?

    a. This is too early to represent corneal allograft rejection.
    b. Elevated intraocular pressure should be ruled out as a potential mechanism of corneal stromal edema.
    c. Vitreous-endothelial touch should ruled out as a potential cause of corneal edema.
    d. An important clue for determining the etiology of the findings is the absence of similar signs in the host bed.
    e. A linear array of KPs may have been observed along the endothelium earlier in the process.

377. Which one of the following regarding corneal allograft rejection is false?

    a. Epithelial rejection frequently manifests as subepithelial keratitis identical to EKC.
    b. Endothelial-stromal rejection is unlikely to develop in a first graft before 10 to 14 days postoperatively.
    c. Endothelial-stromal rejection may be incited by suture removal or intraocular laser procedures.
    d. Endothelial-stromal graft rejection should be treated as an emergency with intensive topical and systemic steroids.
    e. Epithelial rejection is generally more severe and damaging to the donor button than endothelial-stromal rejection.

378. The potential advantages of lamellar keratoplasty over penetrating keratoplasty include which of the following?

        1. Restrictions on donor material are not as stringent.
        2. The donor/host interface generally remains clearer.
        3. There is a lower incidence of allograft rejection.
        4. It is technically easier to perform.

    a. 1, 2, and 3.
    b. 1 and 3.
    c. 2 and 4.
    d. 4 only.
    e. 1, 2, 3, and 4.

379. Indications for lamellar keratoplasty include all of the following except:

    a. Reis-Bückler's dystrophy.
    b. a large corneal perforation in the bed of an infectious corneal ulcer.
    c. superficial traumatic corneal scars.
    d. lattice dystrophy.
    e. Terrien's marginal degeneration.

380. Which one of the following regarding tissue adhesive closure of corneal defects is false?

   a. Polymerization is rapid when the adhesive contacts free anions.
   b. All epithelium and necrotic tissue must be cleared from around the perforation to enhance adhesion.
   c. The bed to which the adhesive is to be attached must be dry at the time of treatment.
   d. Polymerization releases considerable amounts of heat (exothermic).
   e. Bandage contact lenses are generally needed following successful adhesive application.

381. Indications for conjunctival flap surgery include all of the following except:

   a. bullous keratopathy.
   b. chronic painful band keratopathy.
   c. neurotrophic ulceration.
   d. large perforation in the bed of an infectious corneal ulcer.
   e. severe surface disruption with pain following chemical alkali burn.

382. A 30-year-old woman presents complaining of episodic bilateral eye pain, worse on the left and associated with blurry vision. On further questioning, she relates a history of severe red eyes approximately 3 weeks ago, which have gradually improved as her current symptoms have developed. Best corrected acuity is 20/25 OD and 20/40 OS. External examination is unremarkable, and there is no lymphadenopathy. Slit-lamp examination reveals bilateral corneal findings, worse on the left, as shown in color plate 13. Which one of the following regarding her condition is false?

   a. Three weeks earlier, she may have had a membranous conjunctivitis.
   b. The corneal lesions represent active microbial replication.
   c. Topical steroids could provide significant symptomatic relief.
   d. Topical steroids could considerably increase the duration of the disease process.
   e. Similar corneal findings can be seen in the absence of antecendent red eye.

383. A 21-year-old patient presents with a history of chronically poor vision OD and slit-lamp findings shown in color plate 14. Which of the following laboratory tests is useful for initial evaluation?

   1. serum calcium levels.
   2. chest x-ray.
   3. FTA-Abs.
   4. complete HLA typing.

   a. 1, 2, and 3.
   b. 1 and 3.
   c. 2 and 4.
   d. 4 only.
   e. 1, 2, 3, and 4.

384. Three weeks after undergoing primary "bare-sclera" excision of a pterygium, a patient returns concerned about his eye (color plate 15). The surgeon should offer the patient:

   a. beta-irradiation to the surgical bed.
   b. mitomycin C drops immediately.
   c. assurance and frequent topical prednisolone.
   d. reoperation with conjunctival transplantation.
   e. wide excision with map biopsies and cryotherapy.

Answers

1.   b.   There are five cardinal features of inflammation: rubor (redness), calor (warmth), dolor (pain), tumor (swelling), and loss of function. Many forms of inflammation, for example, type I hypersensitivity, do not cause irreversible structural damage to involved tissues.

2.   True.   The final common pathway can be the same--inflammation-mediated tissue effects. An immune agent, by definition, can elicit an anamnestic response and cause inflammation.

3.   False.   PMNs are far more destructive. They are the "kamikaze" cells of inflammation. Macrophages are critical for the initiation of the afferent immune response, as well as "clean-up" duties.

4.   b.   Conjunctival papillae form whenever there is conjunctival swelling of any cause in certain areas. The tarsal and limbal conjunctiva are unique because their subepithelial substantia propria contains fibrous tissue septa that interconnect to form polygonal lobules with a central vascular bundle. Any inflammation in these regions will result in papillae. Papillae less than 1 mm in diameter are entirely nonspecific. When papillae are greater than 1 mm in diameter (giant papillae), they are more specific (see question 10). Conjunctival follicles represent focal lymphoid aggregates in the substantia propria. These are also more specific than papillae (see questions 19 and 20). Chemosis represents subepithelial edema and is nonspecific.

5.   c.   See answer 4.

6.   b.   This is essentially the morphologic definition of a conjunctival papilla.

7.   a.   See answer 4.

8.   c.   Most young people with healthy eyes will have small conjunctival papillae along the superior margin of the upper tarsus (remember that, when everted, this will be the <u>lower</u> edge of the tarsus).

9.   False.   The cutoff for giant papillae is 1 mm in diameter.

10.   b.   The four disorders associated with true giant papillae are vernal and atopic keratoconjunctivitis, and contact lens-related and prosthesis-related GPC. Trachoma has a more pronounced follicular response (although papillae may be seen as a non-specific sign).

11.   d.   Horner-Trantas dots are pathognomic for vernal keratoconjunctivitis. Herbert's pits are punched-out limbal lesions representing necrotic limbal follicles associated with trachoma. Von Arlt's line is linear subconjunctival scarring seen on the upper tarsus in "burned-out" trachoma. Fuchs' spots are areas of punched-out chorioretinal atrophy in the maculae of high myopes. Cogan's patches are focal areas of scleral compaction (dellen) anterior to horizontal rectus insertions in the elderly.

12.   a.   See answer 11.

13. False.   As a rule, the giant papillae in vernal are more solid-appearing, with sharper margins and greater elevation. In atopic keratoconjunctivitis, the giant papillae are less well defined, less elevated, and creamier in appearance.

14. True.   The papillae in contact lens-related GPC may last for several months or years after the symptoms are controlled.

15. d.   Itching and discharge may be seen in both contact lens-related GPC and viral conjunctivitis. Likewise, in both cases, the bulbar conjunctiva may be mildly to severely injected. In GPC, the inferior fornix is generally the least involved, while in viral conjunctivitis, it tends to be the most severely involved.

16. a.   See question 4.

17. d.   Trachoma is nearly always a disease of the superior conjunctiva. This is in stark contrast to inclusion conjunctivitis, another chlamydial disease, which is more severe inferiorly. Toxic follicular conjunctivitis secondary to medications and viral keratoconjunctivitis are also more severe inferiorly.

18. b.

19. d.   Trachoma generally presents insidiously. By the time the patient is seen by the ophthalmologist, there is usually a history of red eyes for several months (or of several recurrences).

20. a.   While the subepithelial keratitis may last for several months, the "red eye" (conjunctivitis) of EKC is nearly always gone after 3 to 4 weeks.

21. c.   Neonatal inclusion conjunctivitis may be pseudomembranous or membranous, but this is rare in adults. A pseudomembrane or membrane is a plaque of inflammatory debris--that is, mucus, fibrin, inflammatory cells, and/or hemorrhage--which can be stripped off of a mucosal surface. The distinction between a true and a pseudomembrane is that, when a true membrane is stripped, there is bleeding. This is because a true membrane is fused with and incorporated into the mucosal epithelium. Clinically, this distinction between a pseudomembrane and a true membrane may be a pseudo-distinction. That is, their appearances are similar and the differential diagnosis virtually identical.

22. e.   This is a feature that may help in differentiating between the two type I hypersensitivity causes of GPC. Atopic rarely comes with a (pseudo)membrane, while vernal may.

23. False.   Typical microcystic corneal epithelial edema is in the intercellular space and results from an imbalance between corneal turgescence (swelling due to intraocular pressure) and deturgescence (drying due to endothelial pumping). Intracellular epithelial edema does occur, as a result of epithelial hypoxia, but this appears different clinically--as a fine, frosted-glass appearance (Sattler's veil), generally associated with contact lens use.

24. False.   Two pathophysiologic factors are felt to be necessary for the development of corneal epithelial filaments--increased mucus production along with increased, deranged epithelial turnover. The filaments themselves are composed of mucus and desquamated epithelial cells.

25. d. It would be unusual for filaments to be seen in OCP, since mucus production is generally diminished in this disorder.

26. c. The depositions that form the horizontal band across the exposed portions of the cornea generally start peripherally and proceed centrally, but this is not invariable. The material that forms the deposit is most often calcium salts but may also be composed of urate salts.

27. e. For cells to enter the corneal stroma from the aqueous humor, there must be a breach in the endothelium.

28. b.

29. d. Note that "granulomatous" KPs may have a characteristic greasy, mutton-fat appearance without actually being granulomas themselves. Macrophages are responsible for the clinical appearance.

30. a. 4.   h. 2.
    b. 9.   i. 2.
    c. 7.   j. 9.
    d. 5.   k. 3.
    e. 6.   l. 4.
    f. 1.   m. 10.
    g. 8.   n. 2.

31. a. 1.   g. 2.
    b. 5.   h. 4.
    c. 3.   i. 5.
    d. 2.   j. 4.
    e. 1.   k. 6.
    f. 4.

32. a. On Gram's stain, mycobacteria may resemble corynebacteria--small pleomorphic gram-positive rods resembling Chinese letters. Acid-fast staining will highlight the mycobacteria, not diphtheroids.

33. b. Many mycobacteria will grow well on blood agar, but the Löwenstein-Jensen medium is designed for more fastidious mycobacteria.

34. a. The standard antimycobacterial agents for *Mycobacterium tuberculosis* are isoniazid, ethambutol, and rifampin. Aminoglycosides are also effective, particularly against some of the atypical mycobacteria.

35. True. Wet-field preparations, viewed with dark-field illumination, must be performed promptly.

36. False. The FTA-Abs is both more specific and more sensitive than TPI, and it is also easier to perform.

37. True. These two, FTA and MHA-TP, are the closest thing to a "gold standard" for syphilis testing.

38. b.   The VDRL and RPR tests reflect treponemal infection and revert to normal when treated. The value of these tests is primarily to monitor response to treatment, since they are less sensitive and specific. The FTA and MHA-TP offer greater sensitivity and specificity and do <u>not</u> normalize with treatment. They are lifelong markers of previous or active treponemal infection.

39. False.   The organism responsible for Lyme disease, *Borrelia burgdorferi*, is notoriously difficult to culture. Serology is not very sensitive but remains superior to culture techniques.

40. e.   Therapy of ocular mycosis is heavily dependent on geographic locale.

41. c.

42. c.   Fungi may be classified into three groups: (1) molds, or filamentous fungi (e.g., *Fusarium, Penicillium*), (2) yeasts (e.g., *Candida*), and (3) dimorphs (may exist as either mold or yeast, depending on environment).

43. e.   Filamentous fungi grow as rods (hyphae), which may or may not have internal divisions (septa).

44. d.   Cryptococcal keratitis is uncommon.

45. False.   Molds are most common, yeasts are second most common, and dimorphs (e.g., *Histoplasma, Coccidioides*) are rare.

46. b.   Fungi are typically hearty.

47. b.   Most periocular herpes infections are type I. Antibody titers may be helpful in primary disease, but not secondary (reactivation) cases.

48. True.   These are called Lipschütz bodies.

49. True.   This known as the Tzanck prep.

50. True.   Papanicalaou smears and Giemsa stains from the two viral infections may be indistinguishable.

51. a.   There are five anti-EBV antibodies: (1) VCA-IgG, (2) VCA-IgM, (3) EA-D, (4) EA-R (early antigen--restricted), and (5) EBNA (Epstein-Barr nuclear antigen). Only EBNA does not peak in the first 6 to 8 weeks of infection.

52. c.   VCA-IgG and EBNA provide lifelong evidence of EBV infection.

53. a. 3.
    b. 5.
    c. 1.
    d. 4.
    e. 2.

54. d.   Like bacteria (and unlike viruses), chlamydiae have both DNA and RNA, replicate via binary fission, have lipopolysaccharide cell walls, and respond to certain antibiotics. Unlike bacteria, chlamydiae do not possess all organelles and require a host cell for replication.

55. False.   Like Lyme disease, culture for chlamydial disorders is difficult. Detection of <u>antigen</u> in tissue scrapings using immunofluorescent techniques is the diagnostic standard.

56. c.   Treatment must consist of <u>oral</u> agents (erythromycin, tetracycline, or rifampin) for at least 21 days.

57. b.   Serotypes A, B, and C cause trachoma. Types D through K cause inclusion conjunctivitis, and LGV1 through 3 cause lymphogranuloma venereum.

58. c.   As with chlamydiae, culture of *Acanthamoeba* is difficult.

59. a. 3.   h. 2.
    b. 2.   i. 1.
    c. 1.   j. 3.
    d. 2.   k. 1.
    e. 3.   l. 3.
    f. 1.   m. 2.
    g. 3.

60. a.   Only *Phthiris pubis* (crab) has been associated with lash infestation. *Pediculus capitis* (head louse) resides only in the scalp. Therefore, ocular "pediculosis" is a misnomer (better term is "phthiriasis").

61. a.   Suffocation techniques helpful with phthiriasis are <u>not</u> effective for *Demodex* infestation.

62. d.

63. False.

64. True.   This is in distinction to adult forms of the disease.

65. a. 2.   Ziehl-Neelsen staining is a type of acid-fast stain.
    b. 3, 6.
    c. 1.
    d. 3.
    e. 4, 7.
    f. 3, 5.
    g. 4.
    h. 5.
    i. 3.

66. b.   This is useful for suspected chlamydial disease.

67. e.

68. d.   Topical acyclovir is available in Europe for HSV and HZV keratitis.

69. b. Idoxuridine and Vidarabine come in ointment preparations, which can be useful with children.

70. e. Idoxuridine and Vidarabine inhibit DNA synthesis by acting as false nucleic acids (analogs). Trifluridine inhibits thymidylate synthetase, a herpes-specific enzyme. Acyclovir, a guanosine analog, is activated only by thymidine kinase, another virus-specific enzyme. Both thymidylate synthetase and thymidine kinase are critical for herpetic DNA synthesis.

71. True.

72. True. Antivirals have different mechanisms of action, and resistance to one does not indicate resistance to all.

73. c. Acyclovir is activated byt viral thymidine kinase and is relatively nontoxic to mammalian cells. Trifluridine (Viroptic) inhibits another virus-specific enzyme, thymidylate synthetase. At high concentrations, it may act as a false nucleoside and affect human DNA synthesis, as well.

74. False. Trifluridine is more effective for herpetic ulcers.

75. 1. a.
    2. d.
    3. c.
    4. b.

76. c. The hypersensitivity reaction to idoxuridine is so strong that it may induce lymphadenopathy!

77. d.

78. b.

79. b. Flucytosine appears to have the most frequent viral resistance.

80. a.

81. c. Polyenes are insoluble in water and have systemic toxicity via binding to renal tubular cells and erythrocytes.

82. e. Thus, liver enzymes should be monitored during long-term ketoconazole therapy.

83. c. Natamycin and amphotericin are polyenes. Flucytosine is a pyrimidine, and miconazole is an imidazole.

84. a. Ketoconazole, miconazole, and clotrimazole are imidazoles. Nystatin is a polyene.

85. a. Although varied, treatment regimens for *Acanthamoeba* keratitis have included neomycin and propamidine. For resistant, aggressive cases topical imidazoles have also been used. Pentamidine's effect on *Acanthamoeba* keratitis is unknown at the present.

86. c. PMNs release hydrolytic enzymes that denature protein and cause tissue necrosis.

87. 1. e.
    2. a.
    3. d.
    4. b.
    5. c.

88. True. Suspensions must be shaken to be effective. Acetate preparations (suspensions) are more potent than phosphate preparations.

89. c. While drug levels in the cornea do not necessarily correlate with anti-inflammatory activity, studies involving rabbit corneas indicate that prednisolone acetate has the greatest anti-inflammatory activity.

90. e. Medrysone has poor anti-inflammatory activity but the lowest risk of IOP elevation.

91. False. Local steroids do not reactivate latent virus, but caution should be exercised, since intermittent shedding of the virus from the trigeminal ganglion (unrelated to steroid use) may coincide with steroid use and exacerbate subsequent disease.

92. b. In active dendritic epithelial keratitis, live virus proliferates but usually does not cause permanent ocular damage, and steroids are not indicated. Also, steroids can excerbate fungal keratitis and make its control more difficult.

93. c.

94. a. 1.   h. 1.
    b. 2.   i. 1.
    c. 1.   j. 2.
    d. 2.   k. 1.
    e. 1.   l. 2.
    f. 2.   m. 2.
    g. 2.   n. 1.

95. d. Anaphylactoid reaction is rapid in onset with itching, conjunctival erythema, and chemosis and is usually caused by penicillin, bacitracin, sulfacetamide, or anesthetics.

96. d. Allergic contact reactions (type IV) are slow and gradual in onset and characterized by itching with eczematoid dermatitis and conjunctival injection.

97. a. Toxic follicular conjunctivitis may take weeks, months, or even years to develop.

98. False. Small papillae (< 1 mm diameter) are far more common. True GPC is uncommon.

99. a. Preauricular lymphadnopathy usually indicates viral conjunctivitis.

100. True. The incidence of GPC is greatest with SCL, followed by rigid gas-permeable lenses, then PMMA lenses.

101. b. Contact lens-induced papillary conjunctivitis is felt to be secondary to immune system interactions with mucus or materials absorbed on the lens. Increased frequency of enzyme treatments may help. Heat sterilization "bakes" the irritating deposits onto the lens, so chemical methods (avoiding thimerosal) are preferred.

102. d. Collarettes indicate staphylococci; scurf indicates seborrhea. Sleeving of the lashes is a sign of *Demodex* infestation.

Answers

103. e.   Staphylococcal blepharoconjunctivitis may be asymptomatic or may present with red eyes and symptoms of ocular inflammation such as superficial punctate keratitis and subsequent epiphora and photophobia.

104. False.   Cultures may help direct the antibiotic regimen, since resistant *Staphylococcus* species are encountered in intractable cases.

105. d.   Steroids are usually used only in acute exercerbations and only with concurrent antibiotic therapy. During treatment, episodic intraocular pressure measurement and slit-lamp examination (for cataracts) are essential.

106. b.   A hordeolum may be an acute staphylococcal infection of the eyelid. Meibomitis can rarely result from bacterial infection. A chalazion and phlyctenulosis are secondary inflammatory disorders, not primary ocular infections.

107. d.   The most common cause of phlyctenulosis is *Staphylococcus*, followed by active or latent tuberculosis.

108. d.

109. a.   *Neisseria* species can invade intact corneal epithelium, causing keratitis and endophthalmitis. *H. influenzae* can cause orbital cellulitis or septicemia, in children.

110. d.   It is important to recognize and treat hyperacute purulent conjuctivits; untreated, it can rapidly progress to corneal ulceration and perforation.

111. d.   This is the only bacterial conjunctivitis that causes preauricular adenopathy.

112. e.   Doxycyline (or tetracycline) is added to treat potential chlamydial infection (sexually transmitted diseases tend to run together).

113. e.   Removal of the lesion is curative.

114. d.   Pharyngoconjunctival fever in caused by adenovirus types 3 and 7.

115. False.   Symblepharon formation is a possible sequela of adenoviral infection.

116. e.   Adenoviral conjunctivitis is highly contagious, and infection can be transferred by fomites several weeks after onset.

117. False.   Epidemic keratoconjunctivitis may produce a hemorrhagic or membranous conjunctivitis. Keratitis is not seen in acute hemorrhagic conjunctivitis caused by picornavirus.

118. b.   The complications of trachoma are due to scarring and cicatrization of the ocular surface.

119. c.   Inclusion conjunctivitis of the newborn may produce a pseudomembrane.

120. e.   Personal contacts must be examined and treated because of the venereal nature of the disease.

121. a.   The follicular response of inclusion conjunctivitis is rarely seen in the neonatal form.

122. False.   Although neonatal inclusion conjunctivitis usually responds to topical therapy, systemic erythromycin is recommended because of associated chlamydial infections, such as otitis media and pneumonitis.

123. b.   Phlyctenules are type IV-- delayed type hypersensitivity reactions. They are not seen in ocular atopic disease (type I).

124. a.   Seasonal allergic conjunctivitis is ideally treated with topical antihistamines.

125. c.   Topical antihistamines do not work well in atopic keratoconjunctivitis; systemic antihistamines are critical for its control.

126. c.   The key differentiating feature is the presence of giant papillae. Vernal is also less likely to respond to topical antihistamines.

127. b.   Long-term corticosteroid use should be avoided because of possible side effects. Topical cromolyn sodium is a useful adjunct for long-term management. Palpebral vernal is more commonly associated with shield ulcers.

128. a.   While conjunctival scraping in atopic disease usually reveals fewer eosinophils than in vernal keratoconjunctivitis, their mere presence is not a useful differentiating factor.

129. d.   By definition, atopic keratoconjunctivitis is an IgE-mediated process that occurs in patients who have atopic dermatitis (eczema).

130. b.   While posterior uveitis may occur in Reiter's syndrome, including cystoid macular edema, a severe retinal vasculitis is not a feature of this syndrome.

131. c.   This history is classic for the floppy eyelid syndrome. Spontaneous eyelid eversion occurs during sleep with minimal pillow (or bedsheet) contact. The condition is treated by mechanically protecting the involved eye (taping, shield). If these conservative measures fail, horizontal lid tightening procedures may be attempted.

132. True.   Noninfectious inflammatory marginal keratitis tends to remain peripheral.

133. c.   Trachoma is the most common cause of irreversible blindness in the world, but not in the United States.

134. True.   Genital herpes is usually type 2; however, type 1 herpes may affect the genitalia after orogenital sexual activity.

135. True.   Most ocular herpetic infections are caused by type 1 herpes; however, type 2 herpes may cause ocular infection following orogenital sexual activity.

136. b.   Type 2 herpes usually resides latently in spinal ganglia.

137. a.   Vesicular blepharitis may occur in either primary or recurrent HSV infection. Dendrites are fleeting in primary infection. Lymphadenopathy is rare in secondary disease.

138. False.   Decreased corneal sensation is sometimes difficult to detect and certainly not specific for herpetic infection.

139. b.   Topical antiviral medication may require up to 21 days to work. Topical steroids are contraindicated in active epithelial herpetic disease.

140. a.   Overtreatment with topical antivirals is common and should be avoided. Bacterial superinfection is not a complication of overtreatment.

141. a.   This ulcer is typical of a "metaherpetic" lesion and does not reflect epitheliitis. Corneal epithelial healing is impaired by decreased sensation, stromal inflammation, and antiviral toxicity.

142. False.   Disciform keratitis is a description only and may be seen with herpes zoster, mumps, or chemical injury. (See question 145).

143. a.   Peripheral anterior synechiae occur commonly following anterior uveitis due to HSV but are not usually seen with disciform keratitis.

144. a.   The phenomenon is identical to the immunoprecipate formed in the Ouchterlony gel.

145. b.   The differential diagnoses for disciform keratitis and Wessely rings are very similar. (See question 142).

146. False.   Herpetologists feel that either (1) the visual axis must be involved or (2) neovascularization must be progressing before steroids are indicated.

147. True.   Stromal necrosis can be devastating in IK.

148. e.

149. False.   Hutchinson's sign (vesicles at the tip of the nose) indicates a high probability of ocular involvement with herpes zoster virus.

150. False.   Reinfection has been reported to lead to typical HZO.

151. False.   Typically, the ophthalmologist is left handling ocular complications long after the rash is gone!

152. c.   Some experts feel that postherpetic neuralgia is less severe if the reactivation is treated promptly with acyclovir; others disagree. Prednisone is generally delayed until virus replication has ceased. Cimetidine is controversial but has fallen from favor.

153. a.   Herpes zoster "dendrites" (pseudodendrites) are typically smaller and less branching than their simplex counterparts.

154. e.   Drug abuse, particularly crack cocaine smoking, is associated with contamination and damage of corneal epithelium. Diabetes mellitus is associated with defective epithelial adherence, as is aging (which also comes with relative hypesthesia).

155. e.

156. True.

157. True.

158. c.   Contaminated water supplies, particularly hot tubs and homemade contact lens saline solution, are frequently implicated. Contact lens use alone is a risk factor.

159. a.   See answer 158.

160. c.   The organism classically causes a radial keratoneuritis with pain out of proportion to findings.

161. a.   Fortunately, herpetic keratitis does not appear to increase the risk of subsequent fungal keratitis.

162. b.   Leprosy is a cause of IK worldwide, but not in the United States.

163. True.

164. True.

165. a.   Patients are also at risk of aortitis with dissecting aneurysms.

166. c.   The conjunctiva is usually <u>normal</u> in Thygeson's disease.

167. b.   About one-half of patients with SLK have some form of thyroid disease. Treatment of the thyroid disorder, however, has little effect on the SLK.

168. a.   Most experts now agree that steroids are not effective therapy for SLK. Surgical resection of the superior bulbar conjunctiva is definitive.

169. False.   Discontinuation of contact lenses, at least temporarily, is therapeutic for contact lens-related SLK.

170. d.

171. False.   This protein-centered effect is typical of <u>acid</u> burns. Alkaline substances saponify cell membranes.

172. True.   This is in distinction to alkali burns, which propagate rapidly.

173. True.   This reflects greater intraocular penetration by alkaline substances.

174. e.   The ocular surface <u>must</u> be irrigated until pH is normal (6.8-7.2). Corneal epithelial loss, clarity, and limbal ischemia (whitening) are critical early prognostic factors.

175. c.   Retained foreign bodies represent a hazardous depot of alkaline material. These <u>must</u> be removed immediately upon detection.

176. e.   Epithelial continuity is essential for the prevention of infections, inflammation, and scarring. Unfortunately, severe chemical injuries retard healing.

177. False.   Avoiding drugs that are toxic to the epithelium (e.g., neomycin, tobramycin, gentamicin) is very important, as these agents are detrimental to the healing of the corneal epithelium.

178. False.   If corticosteroids are to be used, they should be restricted to the first 5 to 10 days. They are useful in reducing corneal and intraocular inflammation and helpful in combating the formation of symblepharons. However, corticosteroids may enhance collagenase-induced corneal melting, which often begins 1 to 2 weeks after the injury.

179. True.   Repair of cicatricial entropion and autologous conjunctival transplantion or mucous membrane grafts may be helpful in late therapy of severe chemical injury. Penetrating keratoplasty has increased success if the procedure is performed 1 to 2 years after the chemical injury.

180. d.   Episcleritis is a recurrent, transient, self-limited, and usually nonspecific disease of young adults. Simple episcleritis is sectoral in 70% and generalized in 30% of cases. Pingueculas may show a distinct form of episcleritis with local superficial inflammation similar to nodular episcleritis. Episcleritis rarely progresses to scleritis; however, episcleritis nearly always accompanies scleritis. Two-thirds of patients with episcleritis have recurrences, and the condition is usually self-limited without treatment. The condition can be treated with topical steroids and/or oral nonsteroidal agents.

181. a.   Generally, episcleritis causes minimal pain, whereas scleritis is moderately to severely painful. Episcleritis is usually of rapid onset as opposed to scleritis, which is usually gradual, over days. In scleritis, the scleral (deep episcleral) plexus is immobile and bluish-red in color; episcleritis appears salmon pink. Scleral vessels do not blanch with phenylephrine, as do those in episcleritis. Lastly, scleritis is frequently seen with systemic connective tissue disorders; this is not true of episcleritis.

182. a.   Diffuse anterior scleritis is the most benign form of scleritis and is associated with the least severe systemic conditions.

183. c.   Necrotizing scleritis with inflammation is the most destructive form of scleritis. Sixtyy percent of affected patients develop complications (in addition to scleral thinning), and 40% suffer visual loss. These patients often die within a few years, secondary to associated autoimmune disease.

184. d.   Patients with scleromalacia perforans (necrotizing scleritis without signs of inflammation) often have long-standing rheumatoid arthritis.

185. e.   Patients with posterior scleritis present with proptosis, pain, visual loss, and occasionally motility restrictions. Choroidal folds, papilledema, exudative retinal detachment, and even angle-closure glaucoma are possible. Histopathologically, posterior scleritis is a granulomatous process.

186. False.   Posterior uveitis occurs in virtually all patients with posterior scleritis and is not uncommon in anterior scleritis. Anterior uveitis occurs in about one-third of all patients with scleritis.

187. True.   Sclerokeratitis occurs when corneal changes develop in conjunction with scleritis. There are three forms: acute stromal keratitis, sclerosing keratitis, and marginal keratolysis (associated with collagenase production, seen in patients with autoimmune connective tissue disease).

188. a.　Scleritis can occur in association with various systemic infectious diseases, including leprosy, tuberculosis, herpes zoster, and syphilis. Metabolic diseases such as gout may also be associated with scleritis. Approximately one-half of patients with scleritis have an associated systemic disease.

189. e.　Scleritis is frequently associated with autoimmune connective tissue diseases such as systemic lupus erythematosus, rheumatoid arthritis, polyarteritis nodosa, or Wegener's granulomatosis. Inflammatory bowel disease has also been reported in conjunction with peripheral ulcerative keratitis.

190. c.　Subtenon injections of corticosteroids are relatively contraindicated, as these drugs may result in scleral thinning and increased potential for perforation.

191. c.　Acute dacryoadenitis is most often caused by ascending staphylococcal infection, often in patients who suffer from dehydration, and is associated with a purulent conjunctival discharge. Viral dacryoadenitis is frequently painless.

192. a.　Chronic dacryoadenitis is usually associated with systemic disease such as lymphoma, sarcoidosis, syphilis, or tuberculosis. Sarcoidosis is the most common cause of painless bilateral enlargement of the lacrimal gland.

193. b.　Chronic dacryoadenitis is sometimes accompanied by inflammation and swelling of the salivary glands which is referred to as Mikulicz's syndrome. Biopsy may be required for diagnosis.

194. c.　*Actinomyces israelii* is usually found with expression or curettage of the canaliculus. *A. israelii* is a gram positive, branching, filamentous bacterium. Canaliculitis occurs more frequently in females.

195. b.　Silent dacrocystitis is usually produced by *S. pneumoniae* and may present with no clinical symptoms other then occasional epiphora.

196. e.　A lacrimal sac abcess has formed and is not responsive to oral antibiotics. It must be drained.

197. c.　Congenital obstruction of the nasolacrimal system usually produces epiphora. The lumen of the nasolacrimal duct is blocked near the lower ostium (valve of Hasner) by epithelial debris or a mucosal membrane. The ostium will open spontaneously in 90% during the first 9 months of life. Gentle probing and irrigation of the nasolacrimal system are performed by 6 to 9 months of age, if the system does not open spontaneously. If probing is unsuccessful, silicone tube intubation should be considered.

198. b.　Because of the patient's age, probing and irrigation should be performed; few blocked ducts will open spontaneously after 9 months of age.

199. False.　If probing of a congenitally impatent nasolacrimal system is unsuccessful, silicone tube intubation should be considered and is 85% effective. Dacryocystorhinostomy should be delayed until age 3 for long-standing success.

200. a.

201. a. 3.   The epidermis is a keratinizing stratified squamous epithelium and is composed
    b. 1.   of five layers, from the bottom to top: basal cell layer (stratum germinativum),
    c. 4.   prickle cell layer, squamous layer, granular layer (stratum granulosum), and keratin
    d. 2.   layer (stratum corneum).

202. a. 2.   There are three accessory cutaneous structures: eccrine glands (i.e., sweat glands),
    b. 3.   apocrine glands (associated with hair follicles, i.e., Moll's glands) and holocrine
    c. 1.   glands (i.e. meibomian glands, sebaceous glands, and glands of Zeis).

203. a. 3.
    b. 3.
    c. 1.
    d. 2.

204. a.   Mucosal epithelia differ from epidermis in that they do not normally keratinize
           (absence of granular and keratin layer) and they do not have rete ridges. Mucosal
           epithelia also contain globlet cells.

205. d.   The conjunctiva, but not the cornea, contains many mucin-secreting goblet cells and
           accessory lacrimal glands. They are otherwise essentially identical epithelia.

206. a. 2.   Dysplasia is characterized by acanthosis (thickening of the prickle cell layer) with
    b. 5.   cellular atypia and loss of normal polarity. Anaplasia is dysplasia of such
    c. 6.   severity as to be obviously malignant. Epidermidalization can be found in benign
    d. 3.   or malignant tumors of squamous tissue.
    e. 1.
    f. 4.

207. False.   A melanophage is a macrophage that has engulfed melanin, not a melanocyte.

208. a.   These benign tumors demonstrate hyperkeratosis, parakeratosis, and
           epidermidalization in addition to lobular acanthosis surrounding vascular cores.
           Papillomas of the eyelid in young people are often caused by the human
           papillomavirus.

209. e.

210. c.   Keratoacanthoma is a benign and reactive tumor that develops rapidly over 4 to 8
           weeks. It is a large, elevated, and round cutaneous tumor that contains a central core
           of keratin. Although acanthosis, hyperkeratosis, and dyskeratosis may be extreme,
           dysplasia is absent. Inflammation is prominent, as keratoacanthoma is a type of
           pseudoepitheliomatous hyperplasia. This lesion is often mistaken for squamous
           carcinoma but spontaneously regresses. The other lesions listed in the question are
           primarily disorders of the elderly.

211. False.   Keratoacanthomas contain areas of acanthosis, hyperkeratosis, and dyskeratosis, but
           not dysplasia. They are not malignant or premalignant lesions, although their clinical
           presentation and behavior may raise this concern (pseudoepitheliomatous hyperplasia
           may simulate dysplasia microscopically).

212. True.

213. True.   Spontaneous regression is typical. It is, however, relatively easy to excise these
           lesions without recurrence.

214. c.   Seborrheic keratoses are usually verrucoid and "greasy" looking.

215. e.

216. False.   Keratocanthomas show more inflammation and are generally significantly larger. (Both are nodules with central craters.)

217. c.   Hyperpigmentation may be found in both lesions, as may inflammatory cells.

218. a.   This pattern features strands of tumor cells infiltrating out from the central, clinically apparent lesion. Thus, it is much more difficult to define the margins of the lesion. They are also less responsive to radiation therapy. The other forms listed tend to be more localized.

219. d.   This is a slowly growing tumor of the skin--conjunctival involvement being vanishingly rare--most commonly found on the lower lid.

220. e.   Tumors here tend to be more deeply invasive, and the involved structures are more difficult to free of tumor.

221. b.   Distant metastases of any kind are very rare for this tumor.

222. e.   These lesions tend to be slow growing.

223. b.   The histopathology indicates a sebaceous cell carcinoma of the eyelid, a disorder of later life. Only prompt recognition of the diagnostic possibility with prompt resection offers hope for complete cure. All too often, chalazia are repeatedly drained, with no pathologic review to exclude this critical diagnosis. Because of this tumor's tendency to produce "skip" lesions (discontinuous areas of diseased tissue), Mohs' techniques may leave residual tumor behind. Map biopsies are generally necessary.

224. d.   Frozen section techniques allow for preservation of tissue lipid, staining for which (oil-red O stain) plays a role in diagnosing sebaceous cell carcinoma.

225. b.   This is a feature of basal cell, not sebaceous cell, carcinomas.

226. a.   These are all locations of sebaceous-type glands; Moll's glands are apocrine sweat glands.

227. a.   The syringoma is derived from sweat gland tissue.

228. d.   An alternate name for pilomatrixoma is the "calcifying epithelioma of Malherbe."

229. True.   The hyperpigmentation of ephelis is due to increased melanin content of normal (or decreased!) numbers of melanocytes.

230. True.   Melanocytes in nevi are referred to as nevus cells to reflect this difference. Nevus cells are rounder, with distinct margins and more abundant, eosinophilic cytoplasm.

231. b.   The opposite is true. They tend to move deeper into the subepithelial space, migrating into the dermis (or conjunctival substantia propria).

232. a. 5.
    b. 1.
    c. 3.
    d. 2.
    e. 4.

233. c.

234. d.   (This would have to be considered grossly descriptive.)

235. d.   Radiation therapy is a very important and effective modality for treating these lesions.

236. a.   Blockage and inflammation of a meibomian gland produces an "internal hordeolum."

237. False.   Blocked glands of Zeis, in particular, can produce an external hordeolum that is purely inflammatory in nature. (Sebum is very irritating to tissues.)   *Zeal granuloma.*

238. c.   These lesions are sometimes acutely inflamed and markedly tender.

239. c.   Xanthelasma tend to be flat, plaque-like lesions, as opposed to nodules.

240. False.   Epibulbar demands are solid choristomas. Adnexal dermoids are generally cystic.

241. d.   Oral mucosal leukoplakic lesions are the other common finding in benign hereditary intraepithelial dyskeratosis--an obscure, dominantly inherited condition found in a paucity of North Carolinians.

242. c.   The grading of epithelial dysplasia is identical, as is the acronym (CIN: conjunctival, corneal, or cervical intraepithelial neoplasia).

243. a. 3.
    b. 1.
    c. 5.
    d. 5.
    e. 2.
    f. 4.

244. c.   The same is true for conjunctival neoplasms.

245. b.   By definition, the neoplasia of the corneal epithelium is not invasive until it has begun to penetrate Bowman's layer.

246. a.   Although the conjunctiva does not have a dermal layer, subepithelial conjunctival nevi occur and are equivalent to dermal nevi of the skin. The nevus cells, with time, migrate down into the substantia propria.

247. d.   Ocular melanocytosis is a congenital blue nevus of the episclera and is most common in whites. When ocular melanocytosis occurs in combination with periocular cutaneous melanosis (nevus of Ota), it is termed oculodermal melanocytosis. This is more common in blacks and Orientals and is nearly always unilateral. Malignant transformation is rare, but it seems to occur almost exclusively in whites.

248. a. Primary acquired melanosis is most frequently found on the bulbar conjunctiva or in the fornices. Nodular thickening is an indication for excisional biopsy.

249. False. Biopsies of conjunctival melanomas are not thought to increase the risk of metastases. Therefore, suspicious melanotic epibulbar lesions should be representatively biopsied, followed by complete excision if found to be malignant.

250. False. Cryotherapy is the most important adjunctive therapy. Occasionally, enucleation or evisceration is required.

251. a. It is difficult to distinguish conjunctival lymphomas from benign reactive lymphoid hyperplasia, but a prominent vascular stroma, numerous follicles, and cellular heterogeneity are all indicative of reactive (non-neoplastic) lesions!

252. False. Over 90% of periocular lymphoid proliferations are B-cell dominated (all have a small subpopulation of polyclonal T-cells).

253. False. Microscopically, lymphomas are characterized by sheets of relatively monotonous cells. Unlike most other malignancies, atypia is not a feature of lymphoma. In fact, mitotic figures are rare in lymphoma and common in reactive lesions.

254. e. In isolated microcornea, the cornea is flatter than normal, resulting in hyperopia.

255. c. Although the anterior segment dysgenesis anomalies were once felt to be a result of mesodermal dysgenesis, it is now believed that the affected tissues are of neural crest origin.

256. b. Schwalbe's line is the termination of the corneal endothelium.

257. a. Posterior embryotoxon is a centrally displaced Schwalbe's line that is visible without gonioscopy.

258. d. Axenfeld's anomaly is the combination of prominent iris processes and posterior embryotoxon. Glaucoma occurs in approximately 50% of cases and the condition is then referred to as Axenfeld's syndrome. *DONT FORGET HYPERTELORISM FACIAL ASSYMETRY HYPOPLASTIC SHOULDERS.*

259. c. Rieger's anomaly includes the components of Axenfeld's anomaly plus atrophy of the iris stroma. Again, glaucoma is present in 50% of cases. The coincidence of glaucoma, however, does not qualify as Rieger's syndrome. This designation is reserved for the additional findings of skeletal, dental, or craniofacial abnormalities. *! Go Figure!*

260. c. An anterior cataract or dislocated lens may be present but is not necessary for the diagnosis.

261. True.

262. c. Congenital glaucoma can be distinguished from birth trauma by the presence of increased intraocular pressure and horizontal (as opposed to vertical) breaks in Descemet's membrane. In corneal birth trauma, residual hypertrophic ridges in Descemet's membrane are often visible even after the corneal edema clears.

263. b. The actinic damage seen in pingueculae results in changes in the subepithelial collagen. Although these fibers stain with some elastin stains, the fibers are not true elastin and will not be degraded by elastase. This finding is known as "elastosis."

264. b. Pterygia invade the cornea down to Bowman's layer, producing fibrovascular ingrowth at this layer. Because excised pterygia can recur with vigor, surgery is indicated only when the visual axis has been obscured or if there is extreme irritation.

265. a. Mitomycin C, beta-irradiation with strontium-90, and conjunctival autotransplantation have all been shown to reduce the recurrence rate of pterygia.

266. b. Amyloid exhibits dichroisim and birefringence when stained with Congo red.

Crystal violet
Thioflavin T
Congo red

267. e. Note that only one polarizing filter is required to elicit dichroism.

268. a. Primary localized amyloidosis consists of conjunctival amyloid plaques, which occur without systemic involvement and without a local cause.

269. b. Primary systemic amyloidosis produces ecchymotic, waxy eyelid papules. Other ocular structures may also be infiltrated, including vitreous and uveal tract.

270. a. The white limbal girdle of Vogt consists of white fleck-like deposits at the nasal and temporal limbus. It consists of subepithelial elastotic degeneration and is sometimes accompanied by calcium deposition.

271. a. The lipid deposition in arcus senilis tends to occur at the superior and inferior poles (where the local temperature is highest) and then spreads into the palpebral fissure. In the setting of high-grade carotid stenosis, the ipsilateral eye is protected from lipid deposition.

272. True. The guttae in Fuchs' dystrophy as well as Hassall-Henle bodies result from dysfunctional production of basement membrane by endothelial cells.

273. False. Hassall-Henle warts are normal aging changes found in the peripheral cornea. Similar changes in the central cornea are known as corneal guttae, and these may be forerunners of corneal edema.

274. c. Cornea farinata is a condition that is characterized by asymptomatic tiny deep stromal opacities that are best viewed by retroillumination. Corneal guttae are at the level of the corneal endothelium.

275. a. Although any of the causes listed may produce calcific band keratopathy, chronic ocular inflammation is the most common. Juvenile rheumatoid arthritis is the certainly the most common (sarcoidosis is probably the second most common).

276. d. Band keratopathy starts at the horizontal periphery. It may spread centrally to form a horizontal band. Occasionally, it starts paracentrally. It is always in Bowman's zone.

277. d. The urate form is much less common and may be associated with gout or hyperuricemia.

278. True. Actinic damage, age, genetic predisposition, and other environmental factors are thought to contribute to spheroidal degeneration, pterygia, and pingueculae.

279. d. Salzmann's nodular degeneration, spheroidal degeneration, and Coats' white ring are corneal degenerations that typically do not involve neovascularization. (However, if located peripherally, each of the three may have surface neovascularization.)

280. b.   The variety of Mooren's ulcer that occurs in young black men is usually more aggressive and responds poorly to medical or surgical management. Perforation is more common in this group. It is felt that some patients in this group may have developed the corneal ulceration as a result of antigen-antibody reactions to helminthic toxins. The toxins may get deposited during the blood-borne phase of certain parasitic infections.

281. a. 1.
     b. 2.
     c. 3.
     d. 1.
     e. 2.
     f. 1.
     g. 1.
     h. 2.
     i. 4.
     j. 2.
     k. 1.

In general, lipid is more prominent in Terrien's degeneration. Terrien's is more commonly bilateral than Mooren's. However, the aggressive form of Mooren's ulcer seen in young black men is usually bilateral. The eponym Mooren's ulcer is applied only to typical <u>isolated</u> peripheral ulcerative keratitis--that is, no associated autoimmune disorder.

282. e.   A wide variety of systemic inflammatory diseases may be associated with peripheral ulcerative keratitis. Most have a prominent vasculitic component.

283. False.   Senile furrow degeneration is not associated with scleral weakness or melting. The thinning is generally mild with intact epithelium.

284. a. 2.
     b. 1.
     c. 1.
     d. 2.
     e. 1.
     f. 2.
     g. 3.
     h. 1.
     i. 3.
     j. 3.

Degenerations nearly always progress, while dystrophies are generally non-progressive or very slowly progressive. Lipid, amyloid, mucopolysaccharide, hyaline, and cholesterol deposition may be seen in both dystrophic and and degenerative processes.

285. False.   The widely accepted classification scheme for corneal dystrophies is based on the layer of cornea involved (i.e., epithelium, Bowman's zone, stroma, Descemet's membrane, endothelium).

286. b.   Both congenital and acquired (degenerative) forms of map-dot-fingerprint dystrophy may be seen. The latter may develop in the setting of recurrent erosions associated with trauma, contact lens use, or chronic blepharoconjunctivitis. Reis-Bückler's dystrophy involves Bowman's zone, while lattice and central cloudy dystrophies are stromal dystrophies.

287. d.   Dots seen in anterior membrane dystrophy are clumps of degenerated epithelial cells and basement membrane material within the epithelium. They are also known as microcysts. Cogan's microcystic edema is the eponym for the pure "dot" form of this disorder.

288. e.   Successful treatment is generally targeted toward stimulating production of new, healthier basement membrane material via epithelial removal or stimulation (debridement or puncture), occlusion therapy (patching, contact lenses, lubrication), and/or epithelial dehydration (for recurrent erosions).

289. b.   Epithelial cysts are seen in both map-dot-fingerprint and Meesman's dystrophies. The cysts in the former are translucent or opaque and represent degenerated epithelial cells and basement membrane. Those of Meesman's dystrophy are transparent and are filled with PAS-positive material known as "peculiar substance." Fibrocellular invasion of Bowman's zone (pannus) is typical of Reis-Bückler's; hyaline stromal deposits are seen in granular dystrophy. Congophilic stromal deposits are the hallmark of lattice dystrophies.

290. b.   Symptoms in Meesman's dystrophy are usually mild and relate to blurry vision and irritation. Central cloudy dystrophy is usually silent.

291. b.   Recurrent erosions and anterior corneal scarring lead to visual loss in Reis-Bückler's dystrophy sooner and to a greater degree than in the others. Pre-Descemet's dystrophy is usually clinically silent, like central cloudy dystrophy.

292. c.   In granular dystrophy, recurrent erosions are seen, but much less commonly than for the anterior dystrophies or lattice dystrophy. Transmission is autosomal dominant. Visual acuity is generally affected, but not until later in life (fifth decade or later). Stromal deposits of hyaline are diagnostic and may be associated with amyloid deposits in certain subtypes (Avellino variant).

293. b.   Macular dystrophy may have focal granular-like deposits but differs from granular dystrophy in several ways. First, the intervening stroma is cloudy. Second, the peripheral cornea is involved much earlier in macular dystrophy. Third, macular dystrophy is inherited recessively, so that parents or offspring are unlikely to be involved, while siblings are likely to be involved. Patients with macular dystrophy have a deficiency in enzymatic synthesis of keratan sulfate, and serum levels are typically depressed. The mnemonic for stromal dystrophies (Dystrophy, Deposit, Stain) is:

Erosions Rare in Macular and Granular. Than Lattice. Macular Erosions Are less Frequent than granular erosions. Similar pattern exists for Recurrence, lattice > Granular? Reis buck > lattice, > Macular

Marilyn Monroe Always Gets Her Man in Los Angeles County.

Marilyn (Macular) Monroe (Mucopolysaccharide) Always (Alcian blue)

Gets (Granular) Her (Hyaline) Man (Masson trichrome) in

Los (Lattice) Angeles (Amyloid) County (Congo red).

294. d.   Lattice dystrophy may also have granular deposits but also features linear, branching (lattice) deposits. Both types of deposits are amyloid and will demonstrate birefringence and dichroism when stained with Congo red. In type I, as in this patient, the deposits are randomly distributed, greater centrally. This form is localized. In type II, the deposits are along the course of the corneal nerves, so are denser peripherally. Type II is seen only in familial amyloidotic polyneuropathy type IV (Meretoja's syndrome) and is associated with cranial nerve palsies and dry, redundant skin. Like granular dystrophy, lattice dystrophies are inherited dominantly. This is the stromal dystrophy most likely to be associated with recurrent erosions.

295. b.   Central crystalline dystrophy of Schnyder represents intrastromal accumulation of cholesterol crystals. Like xanthelasma, a minority of patients have systemic hyperlipidemia.

296. c.   This disorder may be highly asymmetric or unilateral and associated with a wide range of ocular or systemic disorders. Tiny flecks are visible in corneal stroma. Vision is not affected.

297. d.   Central cloudy dystrophy is nearly always clinically silent.

298. True. Both corneal guttae and macular drusen represent focal accumulations of basement membrane produced by a cellular monolayer undergoing senescence, at a normal or accelerated rate.

299. b.   Symptoms of Fuchs' dystrophy are typically worse in the morning, when the corneal epithelium is more hydrated. Mild corneal stromal edema may be silent in the setting of visually significant cataract, so that triple procedures, (penetrating keratoplasty, cataract extraction, intraocular lens placement) may be indicated despite asymptomatic corneal changes (with preexistent corneal edema, further decompensation is almost certain). If there are no signs (as opposed to symptoms) of corneal decompensation (stromal or epithelial edema), then cataract extraction and intraocular lens implantation may be undertaken alone.

300. a.   In the setting of normal corneal diameters, glaucoma is less likely. Congenital hereditary endothelial dystrophy presents like congenital glaucoma, except the corneal diameters and IOP are normal. In congenital hereditary stromal dystrophy, the clinical appearance is similar, except the stroma is normal thickness (but diffusely hazy), and the epithelium is spared.

301. e.   This bilateral disorder presenting in a young man is less likely to be ICE than posterior polymorphous dystrophy (PPMD). Transmission is autosomal dominant, but expression is highly variable and asymmetric. Clinical findings may be similar to ICE. Histopathologically, the disorder may simulate epithelial downgrowth, but the cell of origin is the corneal endothelial cell.

302. b.   See answer 301.

303. d.   The earliest stage of keratoconus is progressive myopia with high astigmatism. Exactly when an eye may be declared to have keratoconus is a matter of opinion.

304. b.   Corneal thinning, myopia, and astigmatism are most likely to progress significantly during adolescence, although progression can occur at any time.

305. a. 3.
     b. 1.
     c. 4.
     d. 2.

306. a.   Acute hydrops reflects sudden stromal edema associated with an acute break in Descemet's membrane. Pain may be severe, but frequently the only symptom is blurry vision. Once the break in Descemet's membrane spontaneously seals (in 6-10 weeks), the stromal edema clears. Residual scarring may or may not require penetrating keratoplasty.

307. c.   Rigid gas-permeable contact lenses are the optical correction of choice in keratoconus, since these are the most successful at eradicating irregular astigmatism.

308. False. A satisfactory optical outcome in surgery for keratoglobus is more difficult to obtain than for keratoconus.

309. c.   Higher corneal protrusion above the area of corneal thinning makes fitting very difficult in pellucid degeneration. Scleral contact lenses have been tried with some success.

310. a. 3.
     b. 1.
     c. 2.
     d. 1.
     e. 2.
     f. 3.
     g. 1.
     h. 1.
     i. 3.
     j. 2.

311. c.   Typically, tear volume is deficient in dry eye syndrome (inadequate aqueous phase), but an important subset of patients have problems with surface wetting due to deficiencies of the other phases (mucus problems in keratinizing disorders, lipid problems in blepharitis). Schirmer's testing in these cases may be normal or supranormal despite a history and examination suggestive of dry eye. Tear breakup time is frequently the important clue.

312. False. Topical anesthesia eliminates reflex tearing so that a reliable estimate of basal tear secretion may be made.

313. True.   Without anesthesia, at least 15 mm of the paper strip should be moistened after 5 minutes.

314. a. 1.   f. 1.   Herpes - pap
     b. 2.   g. 1.
     c. 2.   h. 2.
     d. 1.   i. 3.
     e. 2.   j. 2.

315. b.   See answer 311.

316. c.   Blepharoconjunctivitis may produce a syndrome similar to dry eye syndrome, except symptoms are typically worse in the morning. In dry eye syndrome, symptoms are worse in the evening. Chalazia are associated with chronic blepharoconjunctivitis, not dry eye syndrome.

317. b.   The most frequent association is classic rheumatoid arthritis.

318. e.   The definition of secondary Sjögren's syndrome is sicca complex plus coexistent autoimmune disease. Autoantibodies may be more prevalent and at higher concentrations in primary disease (no systemic disorder), but this is not a reliable differentiating feature. Dry mouth is a feature of both types. While HLA-Dw3 may be seen more commonly in primary disease, this is also not foolproof.

319. a.   A variety of autoimmune diseases have been reported to develop following chronic primary Sjögren's syndrome. There is no known association with epithelial lacrimal gland neoplasms.

320. d.   Punctal occlusion is safe and effective therapy for severe dry eye syndrome. Epiphora is the most likely adverse effect, so a graded, stepwise approach is generally taken. Temporary occlusion of inferior puncta allows assessment of response prior to permanent occlusion.

321. a.   In OCP, a deficient mucus phase leads to tear dysfunction. In Bell's palsy, there is exaggerated drying due to exposure and lagophthalmos. Oral contraceptives have been associated with decreased aqueous tear production. Herpes zoster renders a cornea hypesthetic with impaired reflex tearing and drying.

322. True.   In both disorders, the interpalpebral cornea is the area affected earliest and most severely.

323. True.   Like exposure keratopathy, neurotrophic keratopathy affects the interpalpebral zone preferentially, since this is the area of greatest exposure and drying.

324. c.   The combination of corneal hypesthesia and exposure/lagophthalmos is nearly always disastrous for the corneal surface. Lateral tarsorrhaphy is probably advisable before irreversible, destructive changes can commence. Remember:

Five (V) + Seven (VII) = T

That is,

Vth nerve (hypesthesia) plus VIIth (exposure) dysfunction equals Tarsorrhaphy.

325. b.   Comedones are not a feature of rosacea dermatitis. This differentiates acne rosacea from acne vulgaris.

326. a.   Anterior uveitis is uncommon. The other external manifestations are common, but the most common, by far, is meibomitis.

327. True.   This reflects deficient tear function secondary to decreased lipid secretion by damaged meibomian glands.

328. e.   *Demodex folliculorum* may play an adjuvant role in what is primarily a type IV hypersensitivity reaction to unknown stimuli.

329. c.   Potent steroids may precipitate melting in eyes with rosacea keratitis. Any steroid preparation should probably be avoided in the setting of frank corneal ulceration. Once epithelial continuity has been restored and secondary infection adequately treated (hygeine, antibiotic ointments, oral teracycline), mild steroid preparations are probably safe but must be used with adequate surveillance.

330. d.   Erythema multiforme minor is strictly a skin disease. The systemic variety (erythema multiforme major) has mucous membrane ulceration, as well as dermatitis, and is life-threatening (20% systemic mortality from secondary infection).

331. d.   Recent sulfonamide use is the clearest association. Postinfectious etiologies have also been recognized (HSV, adenovirus, mycoplasma).

332. False. Mucuos membrane lesions are bullous. Skin lesions are macular and consist of a "target" lesion--red center, inner pale annulus, outer red annulus.

333. d. Some experts feel that lysis of symblepharons may lead to secondary infection and/or worsened scarring. In addition, despite vigorous attempts, subconjunctival scarring may still occur.

334. b. Oral and conjunctival epithelia are the most frequently involved, with a slight preponderance of the latter.

335. False. Erythema multiforme is a vasculitic process. OCP features deposition of immunoglobulin and complement in the basement membranes of skin and mucous membranes, with subsequent bulla formation.

336. e. The inferior fornix is generally the most rewarding area of the eye to examine in OCP. Here, subepithelial fibrosis and fornix foreshortening may be seen to precede symblepharon formation. The superior tarsus may show subconjunctival scarring.

337. d. This is in distinction to pemphigus, in which epithelial acantholysis and intraepithelial bullae are characteristic features.

338. False. Dapsone is an acceptable first choice in mild to moderate cases in patients with no evidence of glucose-6-phosphate dehydrogenase deficiency (in whom dapsone can cause a fatal hemolytic anemia). The most reliable prognostic indicator for long-term outcome in OCP is the severity and rapidity of active inflammation. Thus, severe cases should be treated with more potent immunosuppressive agents from the outset, such as cyclophosphamide (Cytoxan).

339. e. Areas of metaplastic keratinization of the conjunctiva within the exposure zone are known as Bitot's spots. Secondary infection by xerosis bacilli (*Corynebacterium xerosis*) is common. A peripheral retinopathy of minimal functional significance has also been described. Keratomalacia, diffuse corneal necrosis and melting, is the most disastrous of manifestations.

340. a. Any deficiency of fat absorption may lead to hypovitaminosis A. Chronic alcoholics with very poor nutrition should be suspected of relative hypovitaminosis A and undergo serum vitamin A level testing in the setting of bilateral dry eye or corneal ulceration.

341. e. The history is most compatible with recurrent erosion syndrome. Predisposing factors are numerous and include previous corneal abrasion, particularly recalcitrant ones; contact lens use; anterior corneal dystrophies (map-dot-fingerprint, Reis-Bückler); and diabetes mellitus (defective basal epithelial adherence).

342. c. Hypertonic saline may be useful in maintaining epithelial deturgescence and enhancing adherence but must be used for several (4-6) months if it is to have long-term effect.

343. e. Ligneous deposits nearly always recur after excision if the disease process remains active.

344. a. Type III (Sanfilippo's syndrome) is virtually never associated with corneal clouding. Type II (Hunter's syndrome) is rarely associated with corneal clouding (only adults with the milder variety). Type II is inherited on an X-linked recessive basis.

Cornea and External Disease

345. c. The findings are indistinguishable from medication-induced vortex keratopathy.

346. b. Fabry's disease is an X-linked recessive disorder featuring accumulation of cerebrosides in the cardiovascular system and kidneys. Affected male patients develop renal failure, but female carriers do not.

347. c. Three forms of cystinosis are recognized. The infantile form is the most severe, followed by the juvenile or adolescent form. Renal failure is expected in both. The adult form is mild (renal failure is unusual). Monoclonal gammopathies may be associated with corneal crystals, with immunoglobulin deposits in the peripheral cornea. PUD is not associated with cystinosis or myeloma. Bietti's crystalline dystrophy features crystalline keratopathy and a pigmentary retinopathy.

348. b. In tyrosinemia, elevated serum tyrosine levels lead to lysosomal instability with dermal and ocular inflammation, as well as mental retardation. Nonstaining pseudodendrites may recur and be misdiagnosed as HSV.

349. d. Of the agents known to cause vortex keratopathy, only chlorpromazine is associated with pigmentary retinopathy. The two are generally independent. (Chloroquine can cause a bull's-eye maculopathy, as well.)

350. d. The earliest sign of copper deposition in Descemet's membrane (Kayser-Fleischer ring) is detectable only at the far periphery with gonioscopy. Slit-lamp examination alone is insufficient.

351. e. Like the sunflower cataract of Wilson's disease, copper accumulation in Descemet's membrane may be seen in chalcosis and other specific cholestatic disorders.

352. a. 7.
b. 2.
c. 6.
d. 3.
e. 8.
f. 4.
g. 5.
h. 1.

353. d.

354. b.

355. d. Other favorable factors include lack of neovascularization, lack of inflammation, and no history of previous graft failure.

356. e. Other unfavorable factors include youth, larger grafts, and glaucoma.

357. c. Most IOLs capable of causing corneal decompensation can also cause chronic intraocular inflammation and secondary cystoid macular edema.

358. a. Indirect miotics like phospholine are generally stopped several weeks before surgery, to stabilize the blood-aqueous barrier and allow repletion of serum cholinesterase. Hypotensive maneuvers like the Honan balloon and mannitol lower the incidence of vitreous loss. Pilocarpine preoperatively protects the lens from incidental damage.

359. True.　Aphakic globes have lower rigidity and structural integrity, leading to collapse and vitreous presentation. A support ring helps avoid this.

360. False.　The main advantage of smaller donor size is decreased risk of rejection, while the main disadvantage is increased central astigmatism. For larger grafts, the opposite is true.

361. True.　Donor buttons that are larger than the host bed are believed to generate centrifugal radial forces that tend to keep the anterior chamber angle open. Smaller buttons are more likely to lead to collapse and peripheral anterior synechiae.

362. a.　Smaller-than-host donor buttons tend to be flatter and thus more hyperopic than the larger-than-host buttons. This effect helps to neutralize part of the high myopia seen in eyes with keratoconus.

363. a.

364. c.　Keratoscopy gives qualitative information regarding corneal topography when the surface is too irregular to permit quantification with keratometry.

365. False.　If the ACIOL is of a style known to be associated with corneal decompensation or cystoid macular edema, it should be replaced at the time of PK. If the keratopathy is primarily due to corneal failure rather than the IOL, it need not be replaced.

366. False.　Cataract extraction after PK increases the risk of graft rejection or failure. If possible, these procedures are generally performed simultaneously (when indicated).

367. e.　In the setting of corneal edema and cataract, the triple procedure is probably advisable. Guttae alone are not a sufficient indication for this procedure. There should be stromal or epithelial edema before it is undertaken.

368. b.　See answer 367.

369. b.　Ocular surgery may precipitate increased disease activity in OCP. Once the other disorders have become quiescent, they typically remain so.

370. c.　Preexistent epithelial and/or surface disorders predispose the graft to chronic epithelial defects. Keratoconus has an excellent prognosis after PK.

371. d.　Unless the donor endothelium is unhealthy or damaged at the time of transplantation (primary graft failure), the findings of Fuchs' dystrophy do not recur. Primary is different than true recurrence, which has been reported several times for each of the other disorders.

372. d.　This complication can frequently be controlled with selective suture removal, but in some cases, refractive surgery is necessary.

373. c.　Frequently, prolonged topical and systemic antibiotic therapy is necessary, with or without surgical therapy (lamellar or penetrating excision). This infectious crystalline keratopathy (IKC) is closely associated with keratoplasty and topical steroid use.

374. a.　Immunologic graft failure never presents within 24 hours of transplantation.

375. d.　Type II mechanisms are also important.

376. a. In first-time grafts, rejection rarely, if ever, presents within the first 10 days postoperatively. It is possible, however, with subsequent grafts in sensitized patients. Graft rejection should spare the host bed, unlike glaucoma. A linear array of KPs, the Khoudadoust line, may be seen in the earlier phases of immunologic rejection but is not universal.

377. e. Epithelial rejection is typically mild and of no long-term significance, as host epithelium quickly populates the donor surface. Endothelial rejection is of far greater visual significance and may be precipitated by seemingly innocuous events, all of which stimulate ocular inflammation.

378. b. Actually, lamellar keratoplasty is technically more difficult! The interface frequently becomes cloudy, but rejection is less common than with penetrating surgery.

379. d. Lattice dystrophy typically involves the deeper stroma, so lamellar surgery is not definitive.

380. d. The absence of significant heat release makes adhesives safer and more reliable.

381. d. A conjunctival flap will not provide an adequate seal over an underlying fistula or perforation. The "hole" must be closed with a tectonic graft (full-thickness or lamellar, with sclera or cornea) before a flap may be advanced.

382. b. The multiple subepithelial infiltrates seen in color plate 13 are most typical of the postinfectious stage of epidemic keratoconjunctivitis (EKC). The history and findings are most consistent with this as well. EKC can be membranous in severe cases. The infiltrates themselves are felt to represent hypersensitivity reactions to viral antigens, without active microbial replication. Topical corticosteroids are quite helpful in controlling potentially disabling photophobia and pain but can lead to a medication-dependent state requiring months or years to reverse. Subepithelial infiltrates hat may be indistiguishable from those of EKC may be seen in Thygeson's disease. In the latter, there is no conjunctivitis prior to the corneal manifestations.

383. a. This patient has band keratopathy. The most frequent etiology of findings as severe as this is chronic intraocular inflammation, particularly juvenile rheumatoid arthritis (JRA). Other uveitides implicated in band keratopathy include sarcoidosis and syphilis. Systemic metabolic disorders including hypercalcemia of any etiology and hyperuricemia, with or without gouty arthritis, are also clearly associated with band keratopathy. Uveitides related to HLA type (HLA-B27 uveitis, Reiter's syndrome, Behçet's disease, birdshot chorioretinopathy) are less commonly associated with band keratopathy.

384. c. The time of onset (only a few weeks after excision) and appearance of the lesion are most suggestive of a pyogenic granuloma--essentially hypertrophic granulation tissue. The lesions are neither pyogenic (copious neutrophils) nor granulomatous; instead, they feature abundant immature vascular channels in a matrix of ground substance secreted by active fibroblasts. Intensive topical steroids are typically curative.

References

1. Belin, Michael. "Section 8: External Disease and Cornea." in F.M. Wilson (ed.). <u>Basic and Clinical Science Course</u>. San Francisco: American Academy of Ophthalmology, 1991-1992.

2. Smolin, Gilbert, and Thoft, Richard (eds.). <u>The Cornea</u>. Boston: Little, Brown and Company, 1983.

8: Intraocular Inflammation and Uveitis

1. T or F -- Passive immunization confers immunity that is longer lasting than that offered by active immunization.

2. Which cellular member of the lymphoreticular system has cytotoxic activity without any previous exposure to antigen, even across organ strains and species barriers?

   a. T-lymphocytes.
   b. B-lymphocytes.
   c. plasma cells.
   d. killer cells.
   e. natural killer (NK) cells.

3. Which cellular component of the lymphoreticular system has cytotoxic activity that is antibody-dependent?

   a. T-lymphocytes.
   b. B-lymphocytes.
   c. plasma cells.
   d. killer cells.
   e. natural killer cells.

4. The most likely human fetal analog of the bursa of Fabricius in birds is thought to be the:

   a. thymus.
   b. spleen.
   c. liver.
   d. lymph nodes.
   e. colon.

5. The class of antigen most typically responsible in immune responses is/are:

   1. protein.
   2. lipid.
   3. polysaccharide.
   4. nucleic acid.

   a. 1, 2, and 3.
   b. 1 and 3.
   c. 2 and 4.
   d. 4 only.
   e. 1, 2, 3, and 4.

6. The first cell that an antigen typically contacts in the cascade of immune response is the:

    a. NK cell.
    b. T-lymphocyte.
    c. B-lymphocyte.
    d. plasma cell.
    e. macrophage.

7. Typically, the first class of antibody produced against a newly encountered antigen is:

    a. IgA.
    b. IgD.
    c. IgE.
    d. IgG.
    e. IgM.

8. Typically, the antibody class produced to an antigen previously exposed to the immune system is:

    a. IgA.
    b. IgD.
    c. IgE.
    d. IgG.
    e. IgM.

9. T or F -- Class I cell surface antigens are typically expressed on the cell surfaces of all nucleated human cells.

10. T or F -- Class II cell surface antigens are typically expressed on the cell surfaces of all nucleated human cells.

11. The major histocompatibility antigen complex in humans (human leukocyte antigen, or HLA system) is coded for by genes located on chromosome:

    a. 6.
    b. 11.
    c. 13.
    d. 18.
    e. 21.

12. Which of the following is/are examples of homologous antigens?

        1. ABO blood groups.
        2. HLA, class I.
        3. Rh blood group.
        4. cardiolipin.

  a. 1, 2, and 3.
  b. 1 and 3.
  c. 2 and 4.
  d. 4 only.
  e. 1, 2, 3, and 4.

13. T or F -- HLA-B27 is associated with uveitis in whites, while HLA-B8 is associated with uveitis in blacks.

14. Which one of the following HLA markers is associated with the presumed ocular histoplasmosis syndrome (POHS)?

  a. A29.
  b. B5.
  c. B7.
  d. B8.
  e. B27.

15. T or F -- The variable regions of the immunoglobulin molecule are the amino termini of both the light and heavy chains.

16. Arrange the following immunoglobulin classes in order of serum concentration, from most abundant (1) to least abundant (5).

  a. IgA.   1.
  b. IgD.   2.
  c. IgE.   3.
  d. IgG.   4.
  e. IgM.   5.

17. Which immunoglobulin class has the highest individual molecular weight?

  a. IgA.
  b. IgD.
  c. IgE.
  d. IgG.
  e. IgM.

18. Which immunoglobulin molecule has the longest serum half-life?

   a. IgA.
   b. IgD.
   c. IgE.
   d. IgG.
   e. IgM.

19. Which is the only immunoglobulin class to cross the human placenta?

   a. IgA.
   b. IgD.
   c. IgE.
   d. IgG.
   e. IgM.

20. Which immunoglobulin classes may exist in polymer form?

   1. IgA.
   2. IgD.
   3. IgM.
   4. IgG.

   a. 1, 2, and 3.
   b. 1 and 3.
   c. 2 and 4.
   d. 4 only.
   e. 1, 2, 3, and 4.

21. Which antibody classes fix complement?

   1. IgA.
   2. IgM.
   3. IgD.
   4. IgG.

   a. 1, 2, and 3.
   b. 1 and 3.
   c. 2 and 4.
   d. 4 only.
   e. 1, 2, 3, and 4.

22. T or F -- Secretory immunoglobulin contains alpha heavy chain and is secreted by the plasma cell as a dimer.

23. Which immunoglobulin class is probably the oldest phylogenetically?

    a. IgA.
    b. IgD.
    c. IgE.
    d. IgG.
    e. IgM.

24. Which of the following immunoglobulin classes is/are important in antigen reception at the surface of lymphocytes in primary immune responses?

                    1. IgD.
                    2. IgG.
                    3. IgM.
                    4. IgE.

    a. 1, 2, and 3.
    b. 1 and 3.
    c. 2 and 4.
    d. 4 only.
    e. 1, 2, 3, and 4.

25. Which of the following immunoglobulin classes is/are important in antigen reception at the lymphocyte cell surfaces for anamnestic immune responses?

                    1. IgD.
                    2. IgG.
                    3. IgM.
                    4. IgE.

    a. 1, 2, and 3.
    b. 1 and 3.
    c. 2 and 4.
    d. 4 only.
    e. 1, 2, 3, and 4.

26. Which complement component is present in the highest serum concentrations?

    a. C1q.
    b. C3.
    c. C4.
    d. C5.
    e. C9.

27. Which of the following hypersensitivity reaction types involve the participation of antibody?

　　　　　　　　　　　　1. type I.
　　　　　　　　　　　　2. type II.
　　　　　　　　　　　　3. type III.
　　　　　　　　　　　　4. type IV.

　　a. 1, 2, and 3.
　　b. 1 and 3.
　　c. 2 and 4.
　　d. 4 only.
　　e. 1, 2, 3, and 4.

28. T or F -- The cyclo-oxygenase pathway leads to the production of prostaglandins, thromboxane, and prostacyclins, while the lipoxygenase pathway leads to the production of leukotrienes.

29. T or F -- In the classic wheal-and-flare reaction, edema and tissue infiltration with circulating inflammatory cells are prominent findings.

30. T or F -- Cytotoxicity is strictly complement-dependent.

31. T or F -- Neutrophil inhibitors, such as nitrogen mustard, will block the manifestations of an Arthus reaction.

32. T or F -- Interleukins are immune upregulators produced by white blood cells and fibroblasts.

33. Graves' disease is a manifestation of what type of hypersensitivity?

　　a. type I.
　　b. type II.
　　c. type III.
　　d. type IV.
　　e. type V.

34. In the left column are listed various hypersensitivity reactions with ocular manifestations. In the right column are listed the hypersensitivity reaction types. Assign a reaction type to each condition.

a. idiopathic scleritis.
b. Mooren's ulcer.
c. tuberculous leprosy.
d. giant papillary conjunctivitis.
e. interstitial keratitis.
f. atopic keratoconjunctivitis.
g. sarcoidosis.
h. retinal vasculitis.
i. corneal graft rejection.
j. phlyctenulosis.

1. type I.
2. type II.
3. type III.
4. type IV.
5. type V.

35. Which immunoglobulin has not been detected in tear samples?

a. IgA.
b. IgD.
c. IgE.
d. IgG.
e. IgM.

36. Wessely rings are a manifestation of what type hypersensitivity?

a. type I.
b. type II.
c. type III.
d. type IV.
e. type V.

37. What percentage of patients with ankylosing spondylitis possess the HLA-B27 gene?

a. 10%.
b. 25%.
c. 50%.
d. 75%.
e. over 90%.

38. The Dalen-Fuchs nodule may be seen in which of the following conditions?

1. sympathetic ophthalmia.
2. tuberculous choroiditis.
3. Vogt-Koyanagi-Harada (VKH) syndrome.
4. Behçet's disease.

a. 1, 2, and 3.
b. 1 and 3.
c. 2 and 4.
d. 4 only.
e. 1, 2, 3, and 4.

39. The most common cause of anterior uveitis in the adult population is:

   a. herpes simplex keratouveitis.
   b. herpes zoster keratouveitis.
   c. syphilitic uveitis.
   d. HLA-B27 iridocyclitis.
   e. idiopathic iridocyclitis.

40. The most common cause of posterior uveitis in the adult population is:

   a. toxocariasis.
   b. sarcoidosis.
   c. toxoplasmosis.
   d. idiopathic posterior uveitis.
   e. tuberculosis.

41. A low-grade uveitis associated with nongranulomatous keratic precipitates (KP) distributed diffusely on the corneal endothelium (i.e., both upper and lower cornea) should suggest the diagnosis of:

   a. syphilitic uveitis.
   b. HLA-B27 uveitis.
   c. Fuchs' iridocyclitis.
   d. sarcoidosis.
   e. idiopathic iridocyclitis.

42. Match the iris nodule characteristic in the left column with the type of nodule listed in the right column.

   a. occur at the pupillary border.
   b. are gray or white in appearance.
   c. occur within the iris stroma.
   d. may be associated with posterior synechiae.
   e. may be associated with granulomatous or nongranulomatous uveitis.
   f. are associated only with granulomatous uveitis.

   1. Busacca nodule.
   2. Koeppe nodule.
   3. both 1 and 2.
   4. neither 1 nor 2.

43. Which of the following conditions may be associated with iris nodules and skin findings?

   1. sarcoidosis.
   2. juvenile xanthogranuloma.
   3. neurofibromatosis.
   4. pseudoxanthoma elasticum.

   a. 1, 2, and 3.
   b. 1 and 3.
   c. 2 and 4.
   d. 4 only.
   e. 1, 2, 3, and 4.

44. The most common cause of decreased vision in chronic peripheral uveitis is:

    a. occluded pupil.
    b. posterior subcapsular cataract.
    c. vitritis.
    d. cystoid macular edema.
    e. papillitis with optic atrophy.

45. The prevalence of HLA-B27 in the general population is:

    a. less than 5%.
    b. 10%.
    c. 25%.
    d. 50%.
    e. 75%.

46. T or F -- After juvenile rheumatoid arthritis (JRA), the second most frequent "etiology" for nonidiopathic iritis is HLA-B27 associated uveitis.

47. Which of the following conditions are associated with the HLA-B27 genotype?

                    1. inflammatory bowel disease.
                    2. Reiter's syndrome.
                    3. ankylosing spondylitis.
                    4. psoriatic arthritis.

    a. 1, 2, and 3.
    b. 1 and 3.
    c. 2 and 4.
    d. 4 only.
    e. 1, 2, 3, and 4.

48. What is the probability, given HLA-B27 genotype, of sacroiliac disease?

    a. less than 5%.
    b. 10%.
    c. 25%.
    d. 50%.
    e. 75%.

49. The most important component of long-term therapy in a young man who is HLA-B27 positive is:

    a. recurrent annual visual acuity testing.
    b. annual tonometry.
    c. systemic (oral) nonsteroidal anti-inflammatory therapy.
    d. physical therapy.
    e. cardiac ultrasonography.

50. Which one of the following concerning Reiter's syndrome is false?

   a. It affects men more frequently than women.
   b. It may follow a bout of either urethritis or dysentery.
   c. The majority of patients are HLA-B27 positive.
   d. The most common eye finding is an acute nongranulomatous anterior uveitis.
   e. The characteristic skin finding is a rash similar to pustular psoriasis.

51. T or F -- Acute anterior uveitis is more likely to develop in patients with ulcerative colitis than in patients with Crohn's disease.

52. T or F -- Acute anterior uveitis commonly develops in conjunction with both psoriasis and psoriatic arthritis.

53. Which one of the following concerning Behçet's disease is false?

   a. The disease is more common in the Far East than in the Occident.
   b. The classic acute uveitis of Behçet's disease is typically associated with a hypopyon.
   c. Anterior uveitis is more common in Behçet's disease than posterior uveitis.
   d. Characteristic aphthous ulcers develop on mucous membranes, including the mouth and genital tract.
   e. A potentially lethal systemic vasculitis may be successfully treated with colchicine.

54. T or F -- The uveitis that accompanies glaucomatocyclitic crisis is typically very mild, with only a few or no KP.

55. T or F -- The uveitis-glaucoma-hyphema syndrome is generally caused by posterior chamber intraocular lenses that are inappropriately sized or have closed loops.

56. Which one of the following concerning Kawasaki disease is false?

   a. The vast the majority of affected patients are children under the age of 10 years.
   b. The hallmark of the eye findings is a bilateral conjunctival congestion that spares the limbus.
   c. The hallmark of the dermatologic findings is a shedding rash affecting the extremities.
   d. Painful swelling of cervical lymph nodes is commonly present.
   e. A mild bilateral anterior uveitis may accompany the conjunctival injection but is not present in all cases.

57. T or F -- Unlike most other uveitides, herpetic uveitis is frequently accompanied by elevated intraocular pressure.

58. T or F -- The iris atrophy of herpes simplex uveitis tends to be segmental, while that of herpes zoster uveitis tends to be patchy.

59. In order to be appropriately termed "chronic," a uveitis must last at least:

    a. 2 weeks.
    b. 4 weeks.
    c. 6 weeks.
    d. 8 weeks.
    e. 12 weeks.

60. Which one of the following concerning uveitis associated with juvenile rheumatoid arthritis is false?

    a. The majority of affected children are girls.
    b. The majority of affected children have pauciarticular arthritis.
    c. The majority of affected children will be antinuclear antibody (ANA) positive.
    d. The majority of affected children will be rheumatoid factor (RF) positive.
    e. The onset of anterior uveitis in the third decade of life of a patient with a remote history of pediatric arthritis does not preclude the diagnosis of JRA.

61. T or F -- The diagnosis of JRA is often made incidentally because of its insidious progress.

62. T or F -- An ocular condition identical to the uveitis associated with JRA may be seen in children who never develop arthritis.

63. All of the following are considered clinical hallmarks of Fuchs' heterochromic iridocyclitis except:

    a. diffuse atrophy of the iris stroma.
    b. gelatinous KP with filamentous interconnections.
    c. mild or minimal anterior chamber reaction.
    d. anterior and posterior synechialization.
    e. cataract rapidly progressing from posterior subcapsular to complete "white-out."

64. T or F -- In Fuchs' heterochromic iridocyclitis, the cataractous eye typically has the lighter colored iris.

65. T or F -- In Fuchs' heterochromia, the long-term vision-limiting complication is generally band keratopathy.

66. Which one of the following concerning the manifestations of sarcoidosis is false?

    a. The uveitis may be granulomatous or nongranulomatous.
    b. A classic orbit/adnexal finding is bilateral painless enlargement of the lacrimal gland.
    c. The most commonly involved organ system is pulmonary.
    d. "Candle-wax" drippings are actually irregular granulomas along retinal venules.
    e. The anterior uveitis of sarcoidosis is non-scarring (i.e., few or no synechiae).

67. Laboratory tests that are helpful in the evaluation of the patient with suspected sarcoidosis include:

1. angiotensin converting enzyme (ACE).
2. serum lysozyme (muramidase).
3. chest x-ray.
4. antineutrophil cytoplasmic antibody assay (ANCA).

a. 1, 2, and 3.
b. 1 and 3.
c. 2 and 4.
d. 4 only.
e. 1, 2, 3, and 4.

68. T or F -- The key histopathologic feature separating the tubercles of sarcoidosis from those of tuberculosis is the presence of caseation in the former.

69. T or F -- Seventh nerve palsy in neurosarcoidosis is secondary to primary, granulomatous neuritis.

70. Which one of the following concerning congenital syphilis is true?

a. The interstitial keratitis of congenital syphilis is generally bilateral and asymptomatic.
b. Syphilitic interstitial keratitis is a direct manifestation of active corneal infection.
c. The chorioretinitis of congenital syphilis is generally bilateral and nonprogressive.
d. The findings of syphilitic interstitial keratitis mandate a full course of treatment for neurosyphilis.
e. Serologic testing of congenital syphilis is generally not rewarding.

71. Which one of the following concerning acquired ocular syphilis is false?

a. The eye may be involved in either secondary or tertiary syphilis.
b. Ocular findings may include iris nodules or vascularized papules.
c. The end stage of retinal vasculitis and inflammation may resemble retinitis pigmentosa.
d. Treatment of syphilitic uveitis is identical to that of neurosyphilis.
e. The FTA-ABS is a useful measure of disease response to therapy.

72. Which one of the following concerning Lyme disease is false?

a. The earliest eye finding is typically a follicular conjunctivitis.
b. The most common eye finding is a chronic iridocyclitis with vitreous cells.
c. Current serologic tests for Lyme disease are approaching greater than 90% sensitivity.
d. The other organ systems commonly affected by Lyme disease include skin, central nervous system, cardiovascular, and musculoskeletal systems.
e. Recommended therapy includes either oral tetracycline or oral penicillin, with intravenous antibiotics reserved for neurologic involvement or multiple recurrences.

73. Which one of the following concerning ocular tuberculosis (TB) is true?

   a. TB is the second most common cause of uveitis in the United States.
   b. The ocular inflammation associated with TB reflects a hypersensitivity reaction without active infection.
   c. Skin testing is valuable in the diagnosis of tuberculous uveitis but may need to be repeated with higher concentrations of PPD.
   d. Eye disease is never seen in the setting of a normal chest x-ray.
   e. Treatment of choice for tuberculous uveitis is topical and/or systemic corticosteroid.

74. Which one of the following concerning pars planitis is false?

   a. The majority of patients have unilateral involvement.
   b. The majority of patients are under the age of 30 years.
   c. The most common cause of visual reduction is cystoid macular edema.
   d. It may be associated with systemic condition such as Lyme disease, sarcoidosis, and multiple sclerosis.
   e. Systemic immunosuppressives and pars plana vitrectomy may play a role in disease control.

75. Arrange the three etiologies of exogenous endophthalmitis in order of decreasing frequency (1 being the most frequent and 3 being the least frequent):

   a. postoperative (cataract) endophthalmitis.   1.
   b. bleb-associated endophthalmitis.   2.
   c. post-traumatic endophthalmitis.   3.

76. T or F -- The most frequent source of contaminating organisms in postoperative endophthalmitis is incompletely sterilized surgical instrumentation.

77. T or F -- Pain is a sine qua non of endophthalmitis.

78. The organism most commonly isolated in bleb-associated endophthalmitis is:

   a. *Staphylococcus aureus.*
   b. *Staphylococcus epidermidis.*
   c. *Propionibacterium acnes.*
   d. *Streptococcus* species.
   e. *Hemophilus influenzae.*

79. T or F -- Postoperative endophthalmitis develops only after penetrating ocular surgery.

80. The organism(s) implicated in the pathogenesis of chronic postoperative endophthalmitis include:

> 1. *S. epidermidis.*
> 2. *Candida* species.
> 3. *P. acnes.*
> 4. *Serratia* species.

   a. 1, 2, and 3.
   b. 1 and 3.
   c. 2 and 4.
   d. 4 only.
   e. 1, 2, 3, and 4.

81. Which endophthalmitis has the worst prognosis?

   a. acute postoperative endophthalmitis.
   b. chronic postoperative endophthalmitis.
   c. post-traumatic endophthalmitis.
   d. bleb-associated endophthalmitis.
   e. endogenous *Candida* endophthalmitis.

82. The organism responsible for approximately 25% of post-traumatic endophthalmitis is:

   a. *S. aureus.*
   b. *S. pneumoniae.*
   c. *Aspergillus.*
   d. *Acanthamoeba.*
   e. *Bacillus cereus.*

83. The organism with the poorest prognosis in post-traumatic endophthalmitis is:

   a. *S. aureus.*
   b. *S. pneumoniae.*
   c. *Aspergillus.*
   d. *Acanthamoeba.*
   e. *B. cereus.*

84. The organism(s) most commonly implicated in post-traumatic endophthalmitis is/are:

> 1. *Bacillus* species.
> 2. *H. influenzae.*
> 3. *S. epidermidis.*
> 4. *S. pneumoniae.*

   a. 1, 2, and 3.
   b. 1 and 3.
   c. 2 and 4.
   d. 4 only.
   e. 1, 2, 3, and 4.

85. A patient with known colon cancer presents with a painful, red, chemotic eye with hypopyon and vitritis. The diagnosis of endogenous endophthalmitis is made. What agent(s) is/are most likely to be implicated?

    1. *Clostridium* species.
    2. *Pseudomonas* species.
    3. *Streptococcus bovis.*
    4. *B. cereus.*

a. 1, 2, and 3.
b. 1 and 3.
c. 2 and 4.
d. 4 only.
e. 1, 2, 3, and 4.

86. Which one of the following concerning fungal endophthalmitis is false?

a. *Candida* is the most common etiology.
b. The classic vitritis follows an earlier retinochoroiditis.
c. The majority of patients with endogenous *Candida* endophthalmitis will have positive blood cultures.
d. Approximately 10% of patients with candidemia will eventually develop endophthalmitis.
e. *Candida* endophthalmitis is an uncommon manifestation of AIDS.

87. T or F -- The most helpful finding distinguishing true infectious endophthalmitis from exaggerated inflammation following trauma or intraocular surgery is vitritis out of proportion to anterior chamber reaction in the former.

88. Signs and/or symptoms typical of the onset of posterior uveitis include:

    1. floaters.
    2. cilary flush.
    3. scotomata.
    4. brow pain.

a. 1, 2, and 3.
b. 1 and 3.
c. 2 and 4.
d. 4 only.
e. 1, 2, 3, and 4.

89. Which one of the following concerning toxoplasmosis is true?

a. The manifestations are always strictly posterior.
b. The retinal vessels are always spared in ocular toxoplasmosis.
c. ELISA testing for antitoxoplasma antibodies is important in the diagnosis of atypical lesions.
d. Vitritis is a sine qua non of ocular toxoplasmosis.
e. The definitive hosts of *Toxoplasma gondii* are mainly small rodents.

90. Potential adverse affects of the pharmacologic management of toxoplasmosis include all of the following except:

   a. pseudomembranous colitis.
   b. Stevens-Johnson syndrome.
   c. aggravation of diabetes mellitus.
   d. microcytic anemia.
   e. aplastic anemia.

91. Which one of the following regarding onchocerciasis is false?

   a. Humans are the only definitive host for the causative organism, *Onchocerca volvulus*.
   b. Skin findings are rare in this condition.
   c. Microfilariae, released by adult worms, penetrate the eye by both direct invasion and hematogenous spread.
   d. Microfilariae may be seen swimming in the anterior chamber and may induce a severe anterior uveitis with glaucoma and cataract.
   e. Chorioretinal and optic atrophy are common in advanced disease.

92. T or F -- Like onchocerciasis, the pathology of cysticercosis is often dramatically worsened by death of the organism.

93. Which of the following constitute risk factors for *Candida* endophthalmitis?

   1. recent total parenteral nutrition.
   2. intravenous drug abuse.
   3. recent chemotherapy.
   4. AIDS.

   a. 1, 2, and 3.
   b. 1 and 3.
   c. 2 and 4.
   d. 4 only.
   e. 1, 2, 3, and 4.

94. Which one of the following concerning cytomegalovirus (CMV) infection is false?

   a. The congenital form may be heralded by fever, pneumonia, or hepatosplenomegaly.
   b. The eye findings in congenital disease include cataract and peripheral retinal lesions, both atrophic and hyperpigmented.
   c. Retinal detachment is uncommon in CMV retinitis.
   d. Posterior segment involvement generally starts as a retinitis and secondarily involves the choroid.
   e. Viral inclusions may be seen both within the nucleus and cytoplasm of affected retinal cells.

95. T or F -- The retinitis of the maternal rubella syndrome is generally benign.

96. T or F -- Like congenital syphilitic retinopathy, congenital measles (rubeola) retinopathy is generally benign but may progress to a secondary pigmentary degeneration with a poor prognosis.

97. Which one of the following concerning acute multifocal posterior placoid pigment epitheliopathy (AMPPPE) is false?

    a. The condition has only ocular manifestations.
    b. It typically affects patients under the age of 30.
    c. There may be a mild or moderate anterior nongranulomatous uveitis.
    d. The fundus lesions generally have indistinct borders with minimal elevation.
    e. Angiographic findings include early hypofluorescence and late hyperfluorescence.

98. Which one of the following concerning acute retinal necrosis is false?

    a. Anterior segment inflammation is variable.
    b. Posterior segment inflammation is generally heavy.
    c. The periphery of the retina is affected earlier and more severely than the posterior pole.
    d. Retinal detachment occurs in up to three-quarters of cases.
    e. Like other viral retinitides, affected patients are usually immunosuppressed.

99. T or F -- The fungus *Nocardia asteroides* may cause uveal inflammation as part of a systemic hematogenously spread infection dominated by the presence of multiple abscesses.

100. Which of the following concerning ocular toxocariasis is/are true?

    1. The definitive host for the parasite is the dog or cat.
    2. Ingested ova initially take up residence in the liver and lung.
    3. Manifestations may include chronic endophthalmitis, localized macular granuloma, or localized peripheral granuloma.
    4. Inflammation is almost always unilateral.

    a. 1, 2, and 3.
    b. 1 and 3.
    c. 2 and 4.
    d. 4 only.
    e. 1, 2, 3, and 4.

101. Which of the following concerning the presumed ocular histoplasmosis syndrome is/are true?

1. The maculopathy generally precedes the formation of peripheral "histo spots."
2. The vitritis associated with the condition may decrease vision.
3. Fundus lesions in their acute phase represent a retinitis with a secondary choroidal reaction.
4. A patient with a macular histo spot has about a 1 in 4 chance of active maculopathy over the next 3 years.

a. 1, 2, and 3.
b. 1 and 3.
c. 2 and 4.
d. 4 only.
e. 1, 2, 3, and 4.

102. Which of the following concerning sympathetic ophthalmia is/are true?

1. The anterior uveitis associated with sympathetic ophthalmia is nearly always non-granulomatous.
2. The shortest reported interval between injury or surgery and the onset of sympathetic ophthalmia is between 1 and 2 weeks.
3. The histopathologic features of the uveitis are consistent with discrete granulomatous inflammation.
4. Granulomatous optic neuritis is commonly seen.

a. 1, 2, and 3.
b. 1 and 3.
c. 2 and 4.
d. 4 only.
e. 1, 2, 3, and 4.

103. Which of the following findings in a patient with bilateral granulomatous uveitis establish(es) the diagnosis of Vogt-Koyanagi-Harada (VKH) syndrome, rather than sympathetic ophthalmia (SO)?

1. vitiligo.
2. cerebrospinal fluid (CSF) pleocytosis.
3. poliosis.
4. histopathology revealing involvement of the choriocapillaris by the inflammatory process.

a. 1, 2, and 3.
b. 1 and 3.
c. 2 and 4.
d. 4 only.
e. 1, 2, 3, and 4.

104. Select the retinochoroidopathy with each of the following characteristics.

1. Presents with blurry central vision.
2. Presents with nyctalopia and/or decreased colored vision.
3. Extends contiguously from the disc.
4. Retinal vessels may be sheathed.
5. Angiography reveals pronounced perifoveal capillary leakage with cystoid macular edema (CME).
6. Epiretinal membrane is common.
7. Electroretinogram (ERG) is abnormal.
8. No clear HLA association.
9. Associated strongly with HLA-A29.
10. Associated with choroidal neovascularization.

a. serpiginous choroidopathy.
b. birdshot chorioretinitis.
c. both.
d. neither.

105. Periocular steroid injection should be avoided in which of the following conditions?

1. Pars planitis associated with sarcoidosis and cystoid macular edema.
2. Necrotizing scleritis associated with rheumatoid arthritis.
3. CME following cataract surgery
4. Ocular toxoplasmosis.

a. 1, 2, and 3.
b. 1 and 3.
c. 2 and 4.
d. 4 only.
e. 1, 2, 3, and 4.

106. In the left column are listed characteristics associated with the cytotoxic agents listed in the right column. Match the correct agent with its characteristics. (Note that the agents may be assigned to more than one characteristic and that each characteristic may be associated with more than one agent.)

1. DNA cross-linking agent.
2. purine analog.
3. folate analog.
4. associated with hepatotoxicity.
5. associated with azoospermia.
6. associated with hemorrhagic cystitis.
7. associated with hemolytic anemia.
8. associated with renal failure.
9. useful in the treatment of sympathetic ophthalmia, VKH syndrome, and ocular cicatricial pemphigoid (OCP).
10. potent suppressor of interleukin-2 production.
11. useful in the treatment of mild to moderate OCP.
12. useful in the treatment of sympathetic ophthalmia, VKH, Behçet's disease, and corneal graft rejection.

a. chlorambucil (Leukeran).
b. azathioprine (Imuran).
c. methotrexate.
d. cyclophosphamide (Cytoxan).
e. cyclosporine.
f. dapsone.

107. Assuming all inflammation has been quiescent for several months, visually significant cataract associated with chronic/recurrent uveitis may be successfully managed with extracapsular cataract extraction and posterior chamber intraocular lens (IOL) implantation in which of the following disorders?

1. idiopathic iritis.
2. sarcoidosis.
3. HLA-B27 associated uveitis.
4. juvenile rheumatoid arthritis (JRA).

a. 1, 2, and 3.
b. 1 and 3.
c. 2 and 4.
d. 4 only.
e. 1, 2, 3, and 4.

108. Which of the following are common hematologic findings in patients with AIDS?

> 1. lymphocytopenia.
> 2. hypergammaglobulinemia.
> 3. increased suppressor T-cells, relative to helper T-cells.
> 4. granulocytopenia.

a. 1, 2, and 3.
b. 1 and 3.
c. 2 and 4.
d. 4 only.
e. 1, 2, 3, and 4.

109. What percentage of patients with full-blown AIDS will develop some ocular abnormality?

a. 5%.
b. 10%.
c. 25%.
d. 50%.
e. at least 65%.

110. T or F -- Cotton-wool spots, the most common ocular manifestation of HIV infection, are probably due to immune complex pathophysiology.

111. The most common intraocular infection associated with HIV infection is:

a. toxoplasmosis.
b. acute retinal necrosis secondary to herpes simplex virus.
c. pneumocystis choroiditis.
d. CMV retinitis.
e. syphilitic uveitis.

112. T or F -- CMV retinitis is typically seen in the later stages of AIDS.

113. T or F -- Ocular toxoplasmosis in AIDS is similar in every way to other forms of acquired ocular toxoplasmosis, except for being slightly more severe.

114. Which of the following is believed to be a significant risk factor for the development of *Pneumocystis* choroiditis?

a. active *Pneumocystis carinii* pneumonia (PCP).
b. concurrent treatment with aerosolized pentamidine.
c. severe cachexia.
d. absolute lymphocyte count below 500 cells/mm^3.
e. concurrent syphilitic uveitis.

115. Which of the following conditions developing in a healthy man in his 20s or 30s should raise suspicion of coincident HIV infection?

       1. acute retinal necrosis.
       2. syphilitic uveitis.
       3. herpes simplex keratitis.
       4. herpes zoster ophthalmicus.

a. 1, 2, and 3.
b. 1 and 3.
c. 2 and 4.
d. 4 only.
e. 1, 2, 3, and 4.

116. Which of the following foci may harbor the development of ocular Kaposi's sarcoma?

       1. eyelid skin.
       2. choroid.
       3. conjunctiva.
       4. orbit.

a. 1, 2, and 3.
b. 1 and 3.
c. 2 and 4.
d. 4 only.
e. 1, 2, 3, and 4.

Answers

1. False.   Passive immunization (parenteral administration of antibody) confers immediate but short-lived protection, while active immunization (vaccination with active or inactivated immunogens) confers protection that lasts months to years.

2. e.   These cells are a distinct class of T-cells that have the ability to lyse a wide variety of cell types. It is felt that they represent the front-line defense against infections and neoplasia.

3. d.   Killer, or K, cells require antibody to effect cell death through so-called antibody-dependent cellular cytotoxicity (ADCC).

4. c.   The exact location of B-lymphocyte maturation in utero is not firmly established. The most likely analog (human) of the avian bursa of Fabricius is thought to be the fetal liver, where lymphoid stem cells give rise to B-cell progenitors.

5. b.   Typically, lipids and nucleate acids are not antigenic but may become so if coupled with proteins or polysaccharides.

6. e.   Macrophages initiate the immune cascade by "phagocytosing" antigen and presenting it to T-cells.

7. e.   IgM peaks earlier and disappears earlier than IgG during the primary immune response.

8. d.   IgG is the major antibody formed following exposure to an antigen that has previously been encountered.

9. True.   Class I molecules are found on all nucleated human cells. The subregions A, B, and C within the HLA system are responsible for their genetic coding.

10. False.   Class II molecules are found only on monocytes, B-cells, and some activated T-cells. The Dr, Dp, and Dq regions code for these antigens.

11. a.   The HLA complex governs immune response and surveillance.

12. a.   Cardiolipin represents a <u>heterologous</u> antigen, or an antigen that is found in phylogenetically unrelated species. Cardiolipin is found in beef heart, plants, and spirochetes. ABO, Rh, and HLA antigens are found only in humans.

13. True.

14. c.   Other HLA associations include:
    A29   Birdshot chorioretinitis.
    B5   Behçet's disease (in Orientals only).
    B7   POHS.
    B8   Uveitis in blacks.
    B27   Idiopathic iritis, psoriatic arthritis, inflammatory bowel disease, ankylosing spondylitis, Reiter's syndrome, and juvenile rheumatoid arthritis, subtype V.

Bil — sympathetic ophthalmia

DRW54 — VKH

15. True.   The carboxy termini form the constant portion of the antibody molecule.

16. 1. IgG (1.0-1.4 gm/100 ml).
    2. IgA (0.2-0.3 gm/100 ml).
    3. IgM (0.04-0.15 gm/100 ml).
    4. IgD (about 0.003 gm/100 ml).
    5. IgE (about 0.00007 gm/100 ml).

17. e.   IgM is made of five units of the size of one IgG.

18. d.   IgG has the longest half-life, 21 to 23 days. IgA is second at about 6 days, followed by IgM (5 days), IgD (3 days), and IgE (2 days).

19. d.   IgG transfer occurs both passively and by active transport. (Minimal amounts of IgA may also cross by passive diffusion.)

20. b.   IgA may exist in a dimeric form (2 subunits), especially when secreted. IgM is produced as a pentamer (5 subunits).

21. c.   IgA and IgE may play a role in activating the "alternative" pathway, but neither directly binds complement components nor initiates the complement cascade like IgG and IgM.

22. True.   Two IgA molecules require two extra, nonimmunoglobulin proteins to form true secretory immunoglobulin. The first is the "J-chain" provided by the plasma cell. The dimer is secreted, and as it passes through the epithelium, "secretory piece" is added to form definitive secretory immunoglobulin.

23. e.   IgM or IgM-like immunoglobulins tend to be the only type present in organisms with the most "rudimentary" immune systems (relative to mammals).

24. a.   IgM, IgG, and IgD can be demonstrated on the surface of "virgin" B lymphocytes and are involved with binding antigen, leading to the activation of the cells, and confer the capability for anamnestic responses.

25. c.   Following initial exposure to an antigen, IgG will be produced in great abundance and may thereafter participate in the re-identification of the antigen, as well as response to it. IgE, after initial sensitization, binds to mast cell surfaces. Cross-linking by antigen of bound IgE molecules leads to histamine release (type I hypersensitivity).

26. b.   C3 is present at close to 1 mg/ml.

27. a.   Type I reactions involve cross-linking of IgE bound to mast cells and basophils. Type II reactions frequently feature IgG or IgM interaction with either cytotoxic cells or circulating immunoglobulins and antigens and the subsequent deposition of those complexes. (Note that some type II processes are not strictly antibody dependent.) Type III reactions result from antigen-antibody complex formation.

28. True.   Cyclo-oxygenase inhibitors (nonsteroidal agents) block production of all three endproducts. The search for a clinically useful selective lipoxygenase inhibitor continues.

29. False.   While edema occurs as a result of the effects of vasoactive substances released during mast cell and basophil activation, inflammatory cell infiltration of the affected area does not occur in the acute phase of type I reactions.

30. False.   Cytotoxic T-cells and killer cells may be involved without complement playing a role; also, macrophages may ingest target cells marked with antibody--again without complement involvement.

31. True.   The Arthus reaction (type III) results from formation of antigen-antibody complexes in tissue. Neutrophils are the key players in effecting subsequent tissue damage.

32. True.   Interleukins are products of activated monocytes, lymphocytes, and activated fibroblasts, which in general seem to upregulate cellular immunity. Fibroblasts also produce interferons, as do lymphocytes, which may augment or suppress cellular immune response.

33. e.   Graves' disease and myasthenia gravis are excellent examples of type V hypersensitivity. In these conditions, antibodies react with cell surface receptors and either stimulate or depress cellular function.

34. a. 3.   Note that corneal graft rejection may involve type II mechanisms as well.
    b. 2.
    c   4.
    d. 1.
    e. 4.
    f. 1.
    g. 4.
    h. 3.
    i. 4.
    j. 4.

35. b.   All major immunoglobulins classes except IgD have been detected in human tears. IgA (secretory immunoglobulin) is the primary immunoglobulin in tears.

36. c.   Wessely rings, also known as immune rings, are ring infiltrates of the corneal stroma, parallel to the limbus. Some corneal rings are probably formed as antigen from a corneal infiltrate encounters antibody from peripheral corneal blood vessels.

37. e.   In one study, 50% of iritis patients from a uveitis clinic were HLA-B27 positive.

38. a.   Dalen-Fuchs nodules are focal accumulations of epithelioid-like cells between Bruch's membrane and the retinal pigment epithelium (RPE). They may include depigmented RPE cells. They are classically associated with sympathetic ophthalmia and VKH syndrome. They may also be found in tuberculous choroiditis and sarcoidosis.

39. e.   According to Henderley et al. (1987), idiopathic iridiocyclitis was the most common cause of anterior uveitis, making up 12.1% of all uveitis cases. HLA-B27 iridocyclitis (3.0%) and juvenile rheumatoid arthritis (2.8%) were second and third, respectively.

40. c.   Toxoplasmosis is the most common cause of posterior uveitis. Henderley et al. (1987) showed it represented 7.0% of total uveitis cases, followed by retinal vasculitis (6.8%).

41. c. The differential diagnosis of diffusely distributed keratic precipitates includes Fuchs' heterochromic iridocyclitis, and rarely sarcoidosis, syphilis, and toxoplasmosis. The diffuse distribution, along with a gelatinous, stellate appearance, makes the KP of Fuchs' iridocyclitis distinctive.

42. a. 2. One suggested mnemonic is **P** for **P**upil margin and for Koe**PP**e.
    b. 3.
    c. 1.
    d. 2.
    e. 2.
    f. 1.

43. a. Iris granulomas and Koeppe and Busacca nodules may appear as iris nodules in ocular sarcoidosis. Juvenile xanthogranuloma features yellow iris nodules, appearing during childhood and associated with spontaneous hyphema. Juvenile xanthogranuloma most frequently involves the skin. Raised orange lesions are typical. In neurofibromatosis, Lisch nodules, actually clusters of nevus cells, are definitive. Cutaneous neurofibromatous, café au lait spots, and Lisch nodules are all important diagnostic criteria. Pseudoxanthoma elasticum is associated with "chicken skin" of the head and neck, but no iris nodules.

44. d. Macular edema, followed by cataract, is the most consistent cause of decreased vision in pars planitis. Cystoid macular edema is a problem in anterior or posterior uveitis much less frequently.

45. a. The HLA antigens are determined by a series of four gene loci located on chromosome 6. HLA-B27 is present in 1.4 to 6.0% of the general population.

46. False. HLA-B27 disease is more common than JRA (the most common cause of nonidiopathic disease).

47. e. One subtype of JRA is also associated with HLA-B27 and is probably a pediatric variant of ankylosing spondylitis.

48. c. Up to 25% of individuals with HLA-B27 develop sacroiliac disease. Symptoms of sacroiliac disease may subtle. Personal or family history of back problems in patents with iritis should prompt the physician to obtain sacroiliac radiographs.

49. d. Asymptomatic sacroiliac disease can be seen in patients with HLA-B27 spondylitis, particularly in young men. Since irreversible damage may occur before the onset of significant symptoms and simple physical therapy is effective in limiting disability, physical therapy, consisting of back flexibility and stretching exercises, is recommended in young men who are found to be HLA-B27 positive.

50. d. The most common eye finding in Reiter's syndrome is a nonspecific conjunctivitis. Nongranulomatous iritis, which can be bilateral and chronic, is less common.

51. True. Although it is associated with both forms of inflammatory bowel disease, iritis occurs in over 10% of patents with ulcerative colitis, but in less than 3% of patients with Crohn's disease.

52. False. Acute anterior uveitis is associated with psoriatic arthritis, but usually not with psoriasis without arthritis.

53. c. Posterior uveitis, which can include retinal vasculitis, retinal hemorrhages, and retinal necrosis, is more common than anterior uveitis in Behçet's disease.

54. True. Mild anterior uveitis with nonspecific symptoms is common in glaucomatocyclitic crisis (Posner-Schlossman syndrome). Although the symptoms may be mild, intraocular pressure may be markedly elevated during the recurrent episodes, which may last several days.

55. False. Older anterior chamber intraocular lenses, some of which were poorly sized or manufactured, have been found to cause the uveitis-glaucoma-hyphema syndrome due to chronic irritation of the iris root. The condition has also been rarely described with more modern posterior chamber lens styles, as well.

56. d. The lymphadenopathy of Kawasaki disease is typically painless. Although the vast majority of patients recover without complication, approximately 3% of children with Kawaski disease develop acute coronary arteritis, which may lead to myocardial infarction and death.

57. True. Herpetic uveitis is more commonly associated with elevation of intraocular pressure than other types of uveitis. The differential diagnosis of uveitic glaucoma also includes sarcoidosis, zoster, Fuchs' iridocyclitis, and rarely toxoplasma, syphilis, and sympathetic ophthalmia.

58. False. Segmental iris atrophy is more characterisitic of herpes zoster (due to a segmental iris vasculitis). With herpes simplex, patchy iris atrophy near the pupillary margin is more common.

59. c. Inflammation of the uveal tract lasting longer than 6 weeks is defined as chronic uveitis.

60. d. Rheumatoid factor is typically absent in patients with uveitis secondary to juvenile rheumatoid arthritis. Also, patients with polyarticular JRA are less likely to develop uveitis than those with pauciarthicular (fewer than five joints) or monoarticular disease.

61. True. The iritis in juvenile rheumatoid arthritis has been discovered on routine school eye examinations. The eye can be white and quiet, and the symptoms are often mild.

62. True. A chronic iridocyclitis indistinguishable from JRA, but without arthritis, occurs primarily in young girls.

63. d. For unknown reasons, synechiae are unusual in Fuchs' heterochromic iridocyclitis. Some experts question the "inflammatory" nature of this fascinating disorder.

64. True. The lighter colored eye is usually (but not always) the eye affected with Fuchs' heterochromic iridocyclitis. (Chronic inflammation causes stromal atrophy and melanocyte loss leading to the lighter color.) In some brown eyes, however, iris stromal atrophy causes the involved eye to appear more brown, or darker.

65. False. Cataracts and glaucoma are more common long-term complications in Fuchs' heterochromia.

66. e. Posterior and anterior synechiae can be extensive in sarcoidosis. Although the iridocyclitis in sarcoidosis is classically granulomatous, it can also be non-granulomatous.

67. a. An elevated angiotension converting enzyme level (ACE) and abnormal chest x-ray (hilar and/or mediastinal adenopathy) are likely to be found in sarcoidosis. Elevated serum lysozyme is more sensitive but less specific. Gallium scan may also be helpful in the diagnosis. The antineutrophil cytoplasmic antibody assay (ANCA) is useful in diagnosing Wegener's granulomatosis, not sarcoidosis.

68. False. Caseation is the hallmark of tuberculosis. Sarcoidosis features noncaseating granulomas.

69. False. Parotid gland infiltration compresses the facial nerve as an innocent bystander (remember that the terminal branches of the facial nerve arborize within the substance of the parotid gland).

70. c. Interstitial keratitis (IK) usually produces intense pain and photophobia. The immune response in interstitial keratitis is felt to be an immune response to treponemal antigens (and not live organisms). Standard regimens for neurosyphilis are sufficient for luetic IK. Although the RPR and VDRL may be negative in congenital syphilis, the FTA-ABS is usually positive.

71. e. While nontreponemal tests such as the VDRL and RPR titers decrease with successful syphilis treatment, the FTA-ABS titer usually does not decrease after treatment.

72. c. Lyme immunofluorescent antibody titers and ELISA for IgM and IgG are positive in only 40 to 60% of cases.

73. c. Tuberculosis is an uncommon, but increasingly frequent, cause of uveitis in the United States. Tuberculous bacilli may be found histopathologically in eyes with tuberculous uveitis. Tuberculous uveitis may be present even with a normal PPD and normal chest x-ray. For these cases, a second strength (250 tuberculin units) skin test may be positive. Systemic corticosteroids may cause a dangerous flare-up in otherwise quiescent tuberculosis.

74. a. Eighty percent of cases of "peripheral" or intermediate uveitis are bilateral. Vitrectomy may be helpful in clearing media opacities and alleviating vitreous traction, but chronic cystoid macular edema is often vision limiting. Hypotony due to chronic ciliary body inflammation aggravates this.

75. 1. c.
    2. b.
    3. a.

76. False. Postoperative endophthalmitis usually results from wound contamination by the patient's lids and conjunctiva, generally with endogenous flora.

77. False. Three common signs of endophthalmitis are decreased vision, hypopyon, and vitritis. Pain is variable; if endophthalmitis is painful, the resolution of pain may indicate improvement of the endophthalmitis.

78. b. Acute bleb-associated endophthalmitis can occur at any time following successful filtration surgery. Pneumococcus and other strep species are the most frequent pathogens, followed by *H. influenzae*.

79. False. Although prolonged, complicated, invasive surgeries have higher incidence of postoperative endophthalmitis, even surgeries that do not include ocular penetration, such as pterygium excision and strabismus surgeries, may be associated with endophthalmitis.

80. a. *Serratia* species produce severe acute postoperative endophthalmitis. Certain organisms are clearly implicated in chronic postoperative endophthalmitis and are associated with typical time courses:

    S. epidermidis - within 6 weeks
    Candida species - 1 to 3 months
    P. acnes - 3 months to 2 years

81. c. Post-traumatic endophthalmitis incurs a poor prognosis, with less than 10% retaining vision better than 20/400.

82. e. Post-traumatic endophthalmitis has a uniquely high percentage of *Bacillus* species, especially *B. cereus*, represented etiologically. Estimates have ranged from 20 to 25%, and the organisms seem to be particularly associated with retained metallic foreign bodies, as well as farm or soil-related injuries. Of slightly greater incidence is *S. epidermidis* (about 30% of post-traumatic endophthalmitis).

83. e. *B. cereus* may be the single most destructive organism encountered in ocular infections. The organism's enzymes and exotoxins can produce unsalvageable destruction within 24 hours. Of interest, *B. cereus* and *Clostridium* are two organisms capable of producing systemic, constitutional symptoms from endophthalmitis.

84. b. Two to 7% of ocular penetrating injuries are complicated by post traumatic endophthalmitis. *S. epidermidis* is the most common pathogen, followed by *Bacillus* species (see answer 83).

85. b. Curiously, intestinal malignancies have been associated with endogenous endophthalmitis from *Clostridium* and *S. bovis*.

86. c. The majority of fungal endogenous endophthalmitis occurs without evidence of fungemia.

87. True. Considerable inflammation can occur postoperatively, but vitritis out of proportion to anterior chamber reaction should provoke suspicion of infectious endophthalmitis.

88. b. Gradually decreased vision, floaters, and scotomata are common symptoms of posterior uveitis. Ciliary flush and spasm with browache are more typical of anterior uveitis.

89. c. Granulomatous inflammation of the anterior segment can occur in toxoplasmosis. Perivasculitis near active retinal lesions is common (Kyreleis arteriolitis). The classic lesion of toxoplasmosis is exudative focal retinitis. The definitive host for *T. gondii* is the cat, where it is found as an intestinal parasite. (The gondi is a small South American rodent, which is an important intermediate host in that region of the world.)

90. d.   Clindamycin is clearly associated with pseudomembranous colitis. Sulfa drugs can cause Stevens-Johnsons syndrome, as well as either hemolytic or aplastic anemia. Pyrimethamine can cause aplastic anemia. Steroid therapy can aggravate diabetes.

91. b.   The larvae of *O. volvulus* form subcutaneous nodules when they develop into mature worms.

92. True.   Death of the larvae produces a severe inflammatory reaction, with granulomatous inflammation seen around the necrotic organism.

93. a.   Iatrogenic immunosuppression, intravenous drug abuse, and indwelling intravenous catheters for hyperalimenation are risk factors for candidal infections. *Candida* endophthalmitis is uncommon in AIDS (mucocutaneous candidiasis is common).

94. c.   Ocular infection by CMV may cause exudative or rhegmatogenous retinal detachments, with holes in the area of retinal necrosis.

95. True.   Vision and electrophysiologic testing are usually normal after rubella retinitis.

96. True.   Congenital measles can cause a retinitis with blindness 6 to 12 days after the measles rash appears. Infants usually recover fully, but some progress to secondary pigmentary degeneration with poor prognosis.

97. a.   AMPPPE is believed to follow a prodromal influenza-like illness and has been associated with a cerebral vasculitis.

98. e.   Patients with acute retinal necrosis (ARN) are usually otherwise healthy and not debilitated, as opposed to the typical patient with viral (CMV) retinitis. (Severe, bilateral ARN has been described in patients with AIDS.)

99. False.   Systemic infection with *Nocardia* is characterized by pneumonia and disseminated abscesses. *Nocardia* is a filamentary bacterium.

100. e.   *Toxocara canis* is an intestinal parasite of dogs and cats. Dogs are more commonly implicated in human infections. After ingestion of ova, larvae are spawned which will penetrate the intestinal wall and take up residence in the liver and lungs. From there, larvae can disseminate to any organ, including the eye. Eye involvement is usually unilateral.

101. d.   Peripheral histo spots begin to appear around adolescence. The maculopathy usually does not appear until the 20s. The early stage of the disease is thought to be a choroiditis. Vitreous cells are not seen in POHS. Visual complaints are caused by the maculopathy.

102. c.   Sympathetic ophthalmia is a granulomatous panuveitis. Histologically, the granulomatous inflammation of the uvea is diffuse. The granulomatous process can extend into scleral canals and the optic nerve.

103. c.   While vitiligo and poliosis are classic for VKH, they have also been reported in SO. The same is true of sensorineural hearing loss and CSF pleocytosis. VKH syndrome may also feature other central nervous system signs such as nuchal rigidity, fever, , coma, and seizures. In the VKH syndrome, the chronic diffuse granulomatous uveitis involves the choriocapillaris, whereas in SO, this layer is spared. Obviously, the two diseases overlap considerably.

104. 1. c.   Blurry vision is more likely to be the presenting symptom in serpiginous
     2. b.   but may also be seen in birdshot, due to CME. Serpiginous lesions may spread
     3. a.   contiguously, but birdshot lesions are usually scattered. Retinal vessels may be
     4. c.   sheathed in both conditions. In birdshot, angiography reveals pronounced
     5. b.   perifoveal capillary leakage and CME. Epiretinal membranes are common
     6. b.   in birdshot, and the ERG is reduced or extinguished late in its course.
     7. b.   HLA-A29 has been detected in over 80% of patients with birdshot,
     8. a.   whereas there is no clear HLA association with serpiginous (one report showed
     9. b.   an association with HLA-B7) Both serpiginous and birdshot may be associated
    10. c.   with choroidal neovascularization.

105. c.   Periocular steroid injection may exacerbate *Toxoplasma* retinitis and lead to further
          melting in necrotizing scleritis.

106. 1. d, a.   Alkylating agents function by cross-linking DNA. Alkylating agents
     2. b.   in this list are cyclophosphamide and chlorambucil. Methotrexate (and rarely
     3. c, a,   cyclosporine and chlorambucil) are associated with hepatotoxicity. Sperm
        e.   banking is recommended before chlorambucil therapy. Dapsone is associated
     4. e.   with hemolytic anemia in patients with glucose-6-phosphate dehydrogenase
     5. a.   (G6PD) deficiency. Cyclosporine is strongly associated with renal failure.
     6. d.   Cyclophosphamide is useful in the treatment of VKH syndrome, OCP,
     7. f.   and sympathetic ophthalmia. Cyclosporine is a potent suppressor of interleukin-2
     8. e.   production and is useful in the treatment of SO, VKH, Behçet's disease, and
     9. d.   corneal graft rejection. Through an unknown mechanism, dapsone is useful
    10. e.   in the treatment of mild to moderate OCP.
    11. f.
    12. e.

107. a.   If inflammation has been well-controlled for at least 3 months prior to surgery,
          extracapsular cataract extraction with posterior chamber intraocular lens implantation
          may be successful in many types of uveitic cataract. Patients with cataract secondary
          to chronic uveitis associated with JRA should not undergo IOL implantation after
          extracapsular cataract extraction. Persistent postoperative uveitis aggravated by an
          IOL can be devastating.

108. a.   AIDS patients exhibit absolute lymphocytopenia, <u>elevated</u> immunoglobulin
          (especially IgA and IgG), and increased suppressor T-cell counts, particularly relative
          to helper T-cells. Although there is an absolute lymphocytopenia, there may be no
          leukocytopenia or granulocytopenia.

109. e.   Over 65% of patients with AIDS develop some ocular abnormality. One series
          reported up to 92% of patients with AIDS will develop cotton-wool spots.

110. True.   Cotton-wool spots in AIDS are similar to those seen in diseases associated with
             microvascular occlusive disease or circulating immune complexes. Fluorescein
             angiography shows foci of retinal capillary nonperfusion, and histopathologic studies
             show cytoid bodies in the nerve fiber layer.

111. d.   CMV retinitis, along with *Pneumocystis carinii* pneumonia and Kaposi's sarcoma,
          was one of recognized early in the course of the epidemic as a defining feature of the
          disease.

112. True. The occurrence of CMV retinitis is an AIDS patient is thought to be confer a poor prognosis since many patients die within months after onset of retinitis. Yet, the mean survival of patients with AIDS and newly diagnosed CMV retinitis is gradually increasing (9 to 12 months).

113. False. Usually, cases of ocular toxoplasmosis in AIDS patients do not show the typical fundus scar of a previous infection. Primary ocular toxoplasmosis, associated with CNS toxo, is more common in patients with AIDS.

114. b. *Pneumocystis* choroiditis is seen particularly in patients receiving aerosolized pentamidine. Histopathologically, the lesions in the choroid contain cysts or trophozoites of *Pneumocystis carinii*.

115. c. The development of herpes zoster ophthalmicus in a young and otherwise healthy patient should raise the suspicion of immunocompromise (leukemia, chemotherapy, AIDS). Sexually transmitted diseases tend to occur together. This is particularly true of syphilis and HIV. If a clinician obtains serologic studies for one disorder (lues or AIDS), he or she should strongly consider testing for the other, as well (joint FTA-ABS and anti-HIV titers).

116. b. Kaposi's sarcoma may be noted on the eyelid skin or conjunctiva. Skin lesions usually appear as nontender, elevated, purple nodules. Conjunctival involvement is manifested by red subconjunctival masses. The orbit and choroid lack lymphatics, the probable origin of Kaposi's. Thus, they are spared.

References

1. Weinberg, Robert. "Section 9: Intraocular Inflammation and Uveitis." in F.M. Wilson (ed.). Basic and Clinical Science Course. San Francisco: American Academy of Ophthalmology, 1991-1992.

2. Nussenblatt, Robert, and Palestine, Alan. Uveitis: Fundamentals and Clinical Practice. Chicago: Year Book Medical Publishers, Inc., 1989.

9: Glaucoma, Lens, and Anterior Segment Trauma

1. Which of the following are primary determinants of intraocular pressure?

> 1. episcleral venous pressure.
> 2. rate of aqueous humor secretion.
> 3. aqueous humor outflow facility.
> 4. relative pupillary block.

   a. 1, 2, and 3.
   b. 1 and 3.
   c. 2 and 4.
   d. 4 only.
   e. 1, 2, 3, and 4.

2. Which of the following concerning the production of aqueous humor is/are true?

> 1. The active transport component is independent of intraocular pressure, while the ultrafiltration component decreases as intraocular pressure decreases.
> 2. Aqueous humor formation is probably based on active ionic secretion with secondary passive fluid movement.
> 3. Aqueous humor formation is entirely dependent upon adenosine triphosphatase (ATPase) activity.
> 4. Aqueous humor formation diminishes considerably during night-time.

   a. 1, 2, and 3.
   b. 2 and 3.
   c. 2 and 4.
   d. 4 only.
   e. 1, 2, 3, and 4.

3. T or F -- Approximately 1% of the anterior chamber volume turns over every minute.

4. Which of the following factors are associated with a decrease in aqueous humor formation?

        1. inflammation.
        2. surgery.
        3. trauma.
        4. age.

    a. 1, 2, and 3.
    b. 1 and 3.
    c. 2 and 4.
    d. 4 only.
    e. 1, 2, 3, and 4.

5. T or F -- The trabecular meshwork functions like a one-way valve.

6. Uveoscleral outflow accounts for what percentage of total aqueous outflow facility?

    a. less than 5%.
    b. 5 to 10%.
    c. 10 to 20%.
    d. 25 to 50%.
    e. 50 to 75%.

7. T or F -- Miotics decrease uveoscleral outflow facility.

8. The mean value for outflow facility in normal eyes is:

    a. 0.05 µl/min/mm Hg.
    b. 0.15 µl/min/mm Hg.
    c. 0.28 µl/min/mm Hg.
    d. 0.48 µl/min/mm Hg.
    e. 1.00 µl/min/mm Hg.

9. T or F -- The normal range for episcleral venous pressure is 4 to 8 mm Hg.

10. T or F -- In chronic elevation of episcleral venous pressure, each 1 mm Hg alteration in episcleral venous pressure will lead to a 1 mm Hg alteration in intraocular pressure (IOP).

11. T or F -- Intraocular pressure (IOP) is distributed along a gaussian curve.

12. T or F -- The typical range of diurnal fluctuation in IOP ranges from 2 to 6 mm Hg.

13. T or F -- The timing of diurnal IOP fluctuations varies from person to person.

14. T or F -- The general pattern of diurnal fluctuation in IOP in a patient with open-angle glaucoma shows a consistently elevated IOP with less variability.

15. Which one of the following concerning Goldmann applanation tonometry is false?

    a. It is based on the Fick principle, which holds that the pressure inside an ideal sphere is equal to the force required to flatten the sphere divided by the area of flattening.
    b. The diameter of flattening, 3.06 mm, is based on counterbalancing the corneal resistance and the capillary attraction of tears for the tonometer head.
    c. The intraocular pressure on the Goldmann scale is equal to the force required to flatten the cornea multiplied by 10.
    d. Like Schiotz tonometry, applanation tonometry reflects ocular rigidity.
    e. Goldmann tonometer tip alignment is important in accurately determining intraocular pressure in eyes with high degrees of corneal astigmatism.

16. T or F -- The Perkins tonometer may only be used on supine patients.

17. Which of the following tonometers is/are particularly useful with dense central corneal scarring or edema?

                1. Mackay-Marg.
                2. Goldmann.
                3. Pneumotonometry.
                4. Perkins.

    a. 1, 2, and 3.
    b. 1 and 3.
    c. 2 and 4.
    d. 4 only.
    e. 1, 2, 3, and 4.

18. Which of the following may be accompanied by a falsely low Schiotz IOP measurement?

                1. myopia.
                2. proptosis.
                3. a history of eye surgery.
                4. inadvertent digital pressure on the eyelids while applanating.

    a. 1, 2, and 3.
    b. 1 and 3.
    c. 2 and 4.
    d. 4 only.
    e. 1, 2, 3, and 4.

19. Which of the following are important historical factors in evaluating a patient who may have early glaucoma?

        1. history of eye surgery.
        2. history of eye trauma.
        3. family history of eye diseases.
        4. history of difficulty with near vision.

a. 1, 2, and 3.
b. 1 and 3.
c. 2 and 4.
d. 4 only.
e. 1, 2, 3, and 4.

20. The anterior chamber angle structures may not be directly visualized because:

a. there is total internal reflection at the aqueous-corneal endothelial interface.
b. there is excessive scattering of light reflected from the angle off of the iris.
c. opaque sclera overhangs the anterior chamber angle sufficiently to preclude direct visualization.
d. there is total internal reflection at the cornea-air interface.
e. the anterior chamber angle can be directly visualized, with a sufficiently oblique angle of view.

21. Which of the following gonioscopic methods is direct?

        1. Sussman.
        2. Goldmann.
        3. Zeiss.
        4. Koeppe.

a. 1, 2, and 3.
b. 1 and 3.
c. 2 and 4.
d. 4 only.
e. 1, 2, 3, and 4.

22. Which method of gonioscopy is considered best for evaluating a patient with potential traumatic (angle-recession) glaucoma?

a. Goldmann.
b. Koeppe.
c. Zeiss.
d. Sussman.
e. any of the above.

23. Which gonioscopic method is least likely to distort the anterior chamber anatomy and lead to an incorrect diagnosis?

   a. Goldmann.
   b. Koeppe.
   c. Zeiss.
   d. Sussman.
   e. any of the above.

24. T or F -- Posterior digital pressure on a Goldmann lens will tend to narrow the angle.

25. T or F -- Compression gonioscopy with the Goldmann contact lens is useful in distinguishing appositional angle closure from synechial angle closure.

26. T or F -- The superior portion of the angle is generally the easiest for distinguishing landmarks.

27. T or F -- A grade IV angle is less likely to undergo spontaneous closure than a grade I angle.

28. Which of the following conditions may be associated with blood in Schlemm's canal?

   1. carotid-cavernous fistula.
   2. severe thyroid eye disease.
   3. excessive digital pressure on a Goldmann gonioscopic lens.
   4. ocular hypotony.

   a. 1, 2, and 3.
   b. 1 and 3.
   c. 2 and 4.
   d. 4 only.
   e. 1, 2, 3, and 4.

29. Abnormally heavy trabecular meshwork pigmentation is associated with:

   1. pseudoexfoliation.
   2. pigment dispersion.
   3. previous trauma or surgery.
   4. anterior segment dysgenesis.

   a. 1, 2, and 3.
   b. 1 and 3.
   c. 2 and 4.
   d. 4 only.
   e. 1, 2, 3, and 4.

30. Which one of the following concerning glaucoma and the optic nerve head is true?

    a. The nerve fibers in the papillomacular bundle are more susceptible to the early effects of elevated intraocular pressure (IOP).
    b. All four layers of the optic nerve head are supplied by the short posterior ciliary arteries.
    c. The earliest histologic changes in glaucoma occur at the level of the lamina cribrosa.
    d. It is rare to have significant axonal drop out from glaucoma without an accompanying visual field defect.
    e. Reversal of cupping may be seen in both pediatric and adult glaucomas but is more common in the latter.

31. T or F -- The mechanical theory of glaucomatous damage of the optic nerve states that pressure-induced distortion of optic nerve head blood vessels leads to hypoperfusion and axonal loss.

32. Which of the following signs is accompanied by the worst prognosis for the development or progression of glaucomatous visual field loss?

    a. generalized enlargement of both optic cups.
    b. exposure of the lamina cribrosa.
    c. baring of circumlinear vessels.
    d. focal loss neural rim tissue.
    e. splinter hemorrhage at the disc margin.

33. Which one of the following statements concerning perimetry is true?

    a. In static perimetry, the stimulus intensity is held constant (static) and moved centrally until it is detected.
    b. Kinetic perimetry is most useful for quantifying and tracking visual field changes in a patient with established glaucoma.
    c. Early, specific signs of glaucoma include generalized constriction of isopters and baring of the blind spot.
    d. For a visual field defect to be classified as glaucomatous, it should have corresponding optic nerve head abnormalities.
    e. Vertical steps, i.e., sensitivity discrepancy across the vertical meridian, are sensitive early signs of glaucomatous visual field loss.

34. A 64-year-old black man with a history of open-angle glaucoma presents with a Goldmann visual field documenting a superior nasal step to the I4e isopter OD. When he returns with a deteriorated visual field 1 year later, the most likely form of deterioration is:

    a. an inferior Bjerrum scotoma.
    b. a superior paracentral scotoma.
    c. an inferior nasal step.
    d. encroachment of his superior nasal step toward fixation.
    e. a superotemporal wedge defect.

35. Which one of the following visual field patterns will most quickly progress to loss of fixation?

   a. central 5-degree island.
   b. a large superior nasal step encroaching on fixation (less than 10 degrees).
   c. superior and inferior nasal steps encroaching to 20 degrees.
   d. superior and inferior paracentral scotomas with no other defects.
   e. split fixation to the I4e isopter.

36. T or F -- Static perimetry may be considered abnormal if a single testing point is depressed 10 dB or a cluster of three adjacent points is depressed 5 dB from a population of age-matched normal patients.

37. Which of the following features would raise doubt about the diagnosis of glaucomatous optic nerve damage?

   1. pallor out of proportion to cupping.
   2. markedly asymmetric color visual loss.
   3. field defects obeying the vertical meridian.
   4. presence of afferent pupillary defect.

   a. 1, 2, and 3.
   b. 1 and 3.
   c. 2 and 4.
   d. 4 only.
   e. 1, 2, 3, and 4.

38. Which of the following concerning open-angle glaucoma is/are true?

   1. The particulate glaucomas constitute the majority of open-angle glaucomas.
   2. Glaucoma is the leading cause of blindness in black patients.
   3. There is an association of glaucoma with hyperopia.
   4. There is a bidirectional association of diabetes and glaucoma.

   a. 1, 2, and 3.
   b. 1 and 3.
   c. 2 and 4.
   d. 4 only.
   e. 1, 2, 3, and 4.

39. A 54-year-old man presents with intraocular pressures (IOP) of 24 mm Hg OD and 26 mm Hg OS. His visual fields and optic nerve heads appear normal. Which of the following clinical features might prompt prophylactic topical treatment?

      1. family history of diabetes.
      2. family history of glaucoma.
      3. hyperopia.
      4. black race.

    a. 1, 2, and 3.
    b. 1 and 3.
    c. 2 and 4.
    d. 4 only.
    e. 1, 2, 3, and 4.

40. Which of the following conditions might be misdiagnosed as normal tension glaucoma on initial evaluation?

      1. parasellar tumors.
      2. methanol toxicity.
      3. arteritic ischemic optic neuropathy.
      4. primary open-angle glaucoma.

    a. 1, 2, and 3.
    b. 1 and 3.
    c. 2 and 4.
    d. 4 only.
    e. 1, 2, 3, and 4.

41. T or F -- Therapy for normal tension glaucoma generally is more aggressive, with a lower target intraocular pressure (IOP) than therapy for POAG.

42. Features that distinguish pseudoexfoliation glaucoma from primary open-angle glaucoma include:

      1. greater sensitivity to laser therapy.
      2. greater degree of interocular asymmetry.
      3. degree of TM pigmentation.
      4. the age of affected patients.

    a. 1, 2, and 3.
    b. 1 and 3.
    c. 2 and 4.
    d. 4 only.
    e. 1, 2, 3, and 4.

43. Which of the following concerning pigmentary glaucoma is/are true?

　　　　　　　　　　1. The sine qua non is the Krukenberg's spindle.
　　　　　　　　　　2. There is an association with myopia.
　　　　　　　　　　3. Women with the disease are younger than men with the disease.
　　　　　　　　　　4. IOP may fluctuate widely in this disorder.

　　　a. 1, 2, and 3.
　　　b. 1 and 3.
　　　c. 2 and 4.
　　　d. 4 only.
　　　e. 1, 2, 3, and 4.

44. Which of the following glaucomas is least likely to respond to medical therapy alone?

　　　a. pseudoexfoliation.
　　　b. pigmentary glaucoma.
　　　c. phacolytic glaucoma.
　　　d. lens particle glaucoma.
　　　e. phacoantigenic glaucoma.

45. T or F -- Fuchs' heterochromic iridocyclitis is a typical rubeotic glaucoma culminating in secondary angle closure.

46. T or F -- Acid burns of the ocular adnexa are more likely to be associated with glaucoma than alkali burns.

47. T or F -- Hemolytic and ghost cell glaucomas both feature acute pressure rises following intraocular hemorrhage.

48. Topical corticosteroids should be used with great caution in patients with:

　　　　　　　　　　1. open-angle glaucoma.
　　　　　　　　　　2. a family history of open-angle glaucoma.
　　　　　　　　　　3. diabetes.
　　　　　　　　　　4. high myopia.

　　　a. 1, 2, and 3.
　　　b. 1 and 3.
　　　c. 2 and 4.
　　　d. 4 only.
　　　e. 1, 2, 3, and 4.

49. T or F -- The most common cause of angle closure is pupillary block.

50. T or F -- In whites, angle closure is more common among women than men.

51. T or F -- Most primary angle-closure glaucoma develops as the pupil dilates to mid-position.

52. Specific signs of previous angle-closure glaucoma include:

    1. small white opacities immediately beneath the anterior capsule of the lens.
    2. optic disc cupping.
    3. patchy iris stromal atrophy.
    4. patchy iris pigment epithelial loss.

a. 1, 2, and 3.
b. 1 and 3.
c. 2 and 4.
d. 4 only.
e. 1, 2, 3, and 4.

53. Which of the following modalities may be successful in breaking an attack of angle-closure glaucoma with pupillary block?

    1. compression gonioscopy.
    2. laser iridotomy.
    3. topical miotic treatment.
    4. oral osmotic agents.

a. 1, 2, and 3.
b. 1 and 3.
c. 2 and 4.
d. 4 only.
e. 1, 2, 3, and 4.

54. T or F -- In primary angle-closure glaucoma, once the attack is broken with laser iridotomy, in the absence of peripheral synechialization, no further intervention is required. (That is, this is a "cure.")

55. Which of the following medications may be associated with the induction or aggravation of angle-closure glaucoma?

    1. pilocarpine.
    2. oral antihistamines.
    3. cyclogyl.
    4. aspirin.

a. 1, 2, and 3.
b. 1 and 3.
c. 2 and 4.
d. 4 only.
e. 1, 2, 3, and 4.

                         Glaucoma, Lens, and Trauma

56. The patient with bilaterally narrow anterior chamber angles and normal IOP should probably undergo which of the following tests?

    a. thymoxamine test.
    b. topical steroid challenge.
    c. oral water challenge.
    d. the prone-dark room test.
    e. careful, depressed dilated examination.

57. A patient with bilaterally narrow anterior chamber angles and elevated IOP should probably undergo which of the following tests?

    a. thymoxamine test.
    b. topical steroid challenge.
    c. oral water challenge.
    d. the prone-dark room test.
    e. careful, depressed dilated examination.

58. Which of the following clinical features might lead to a suspicion of plateau iris in a patient with angle closure?

    1. deep anterior chamber centrally.
    2. young age.
    3. a flat iris plane.
    4. a small anterior segment.

    a. 1, 2, and 3.
    b. 1 and 3.
    c. 2 and 4.
    d. 4 only.
    e. 1, 2, 3, and 4.

59. Which of the following conditions may be associated with pupillary block and secondary angle closure?

    1. previous episodes of a flat anterior chamber.
    2. Marfan's syndrome.
    3. neovascular glaucoma.
    4. pseudophakia.

    a. 1, 2, and 3.
    b. 1 and 3.
    c. 2 and 4.
    d. 4 only.
    e. 1, 2, 3, and 4.

60. Which of the following concerning the iridocorneoendothelial (ICE) syndromes is/are true?

> 1. They are almost always unilateral and affect women more frequently than men.
> 2. In Chandler's syndrome, there may be corneal edema with only modestly elevated or normal IOP.
> 3. Essential iris atrophy features stretch and atrophic iris holes with corectopia.
> 4. The degree of intraocular pressure elevation directly reflects the amount of angle synechialization.

a. 1, 2, and 3.
b. 1 and 3.
c. 2 and 4.
d. 4 only.
e. 1, 2, 3, and 4.

61. T or F -- The pigmented lesions in the Cogan-Reese syndrome represent iris nevi.

62. Which of the following concerning malignant glaucoma (aqueous misdirection syndrome) is/are true?

> 1. It most commonly arises following glaucoma surgery.
> 2. A feature differentiating malignant glaucoma from primary angle closure is the depth of the central portion of the anterior chamber.
> 3. Definitive treatment usually alters the nature of the anterior hyaloid face.
> 4. The initial medical agent of choice is pilocarpine.

a. 1, 2, and 3.
b. 1 and 3.
c. 2 and 4.
d. 4 only.
e. 1, 2, 3, and 4.

63. T or F -- Fibrous downgrowth is generally more aggressive than epithelial downgrowth.

64. T or F -- In angle-closure glaucoma following scleral buckling procedures, a peripheral iridotomy is curative.

65. T or F -- The mechanism of secondary angle closure following panretinal photocoagulation and that seen following central retinal vein occlusion (CRVO) are similar in pathophysiology.

66. Which of the following concerning infantile glaucoma is/are true?

    1. Approximately 50% of cases are primary (i.e., no associated ocular or systemic conditions).
    2. Sixty percent are diagnosed within the first 6 months, and 80% within the first year.
    3. Two-thirds of cases are bilateral and two-thirds of cases affect boys.
    4. In many cases, gonioscopy reveals an immature or dysgenic anterior chamber angle.

a. 1, 2, and 3.
b. 1 and 3.
c. 2 and 4.
d. 4 only.
e. 1, 2, 3, and 4.

67. Findings in an eye with infantile glaucoma that are not seen in eyes with adult forms of glaucoma include:

    1. Haab's striae.
    2. corneal edema.
    3. enlarged corneal diameter.
    4. optic nerve cupping.

a. 1, 2, and 3.
b. 1 and 3.
c. 2 and 4.
d. 4 only.
e. 1, 2, 3, and 4.

68. Which of the following agents diminish intraocular pressure during general anesthesia?

    1. halothane.
    2. enflurane.
    3. isoflurane.
    4. ketamine.

a. 1, 2, and 3.
b. 1 and 3.
c. 2 and 4.
d. 4 only.
e. 1, 2, 3, and 4.

69. T or F -- Like adult forms of glaucoma, infantile glaucoma is often successfully controlled with medical therapy.

70. The proper pediatric dose of acetazolamide (Diamox) is:

   a. 15 mg/kg/day in one dose.
   b. 15 mg/kg/day in three or four divided doses.
   c. 5 mg/kg/day in one dose.
   d. 5 mg/kg/day in three or four divided doses.
   e. 250 mg/day in three or four divided doses.

71. For each of the glaucoma medications that follows, indicate whether it acts to lower IOP by diminishing aqueous humor production, by increasing aqueous humor outflow, or via another mechanism.

   a. timolol.
   b. epinephrine.
   c. acetazolamide.
   d. levobunolol.
   e. apraclonidine.
   f. pilocarpine.
   g. betaxolol.
   h. phospholine.
   i. propine.
   j. mannitol.

   1. decreases aqueous production.
   2. increases outflow facility.
   3. another mechanism.

72. Which of the following medications would be contraindicated in a patient with a history of paroxysmal tachycardia?

   1. propine.
   2. timolol.
   3. epinephrine.
   4. pilocarpine.

   a. 1, 2, and 3.
   b. 1 and 3.
   c. 2 and 4.
   d. 4 only.
   e. 1, 2, 3, and 4.

73. Which agents are relatively contraindicated in patients with a history of depression or other psychiatric illness?

   1. pilocarpine.
   2. timolol.
   3. propine.
   4. acetazolamide.

   a. 1, 2, and 3.
   b. 1 and 3.
   c. 2 and 4.
   d. 4 only.
   e. 1, 2, 3, and 4.

74. Which of the following agents should be used with caution in the patient with narrow angles?

        1. timolol.
        2. epinephrine.
        3. acetazolamide.
        4. apraclonidine.

  a. 1, 2, and 3.
  b. 1 and 3.
  c. 2 and 4.
  d. 4 only.
  e. 1, 2, 3, and 4.

75. The agent most likely to cause topical sensitization and medicamentosa is:

  a. timolol.
  b. betaxolol.
  c. epinephrine.
  d. pilocarpine.
  e. apraclonidine.

76. Which of the following miotics are direct-acting agents?

        1. echothiophate.
        2. carbachol.
        3. demecarium.
        4. pilocarpine.

  a. 1, 2, and 3.
  b. 1 and 3.
  c. 2 and 4.
  d. 4 only.
  e. 1, 2, 3, and 4.

77. Which of the following miotics are indirect-acting agents?

        1. echothiophate.
        2. carbachol.
        3. demecarium.
        4. pilocarpine.

  a. 1, 2, and 3.
  b. 1 and 3.
  c. 2 and 4.
  d. 4 only.
  e. 1, 2, 3, and 4.

78. T or F -- In general, miotics act to lower IOP by moving peripheral iris out of the anterior chamber angle, thus enchancing outflow facility.

79. Which of the following complications of miotic administration are more likely with the indirect agents?

    1. cataractogenesis.
    2. punctal stenosis.
    3. retinal tears and detachment.
    4. bradycardia.

    a. 1, 2, and 3.
    b. 1 and 3.
    c. 2 and 4.
    d. 4 only.
    e. 1, 2, 3, and 4.

80. The side effect of carbonic anhydrase inhibitors that is most commonly encountered is:

    a. gastrointestinal distress.
    b. kidney stones.
    c. anemia.
    d. hypocalcemia.
    e. paresthesias.

81. T or F -- Intravenous mannitol is more effective than intravenous urea in lowering intraocular pressure.

82. T or F -- Osmotic agents are more effective in inflamed eyes, since the blood ocular barrier has been disrupted.

83. Which one of the following concerning YAG laser iridotomy is true?

    a. The incidence of closure of a previously patent iridotomy is higher with YAG iridotomy than with argon iridotomy.
    b. The YAG laser is generally more effective for heavily pigmented irides.
    c. The most frequent significant complication of YAG peripheral iridotomy is cystoid macular edema (CME).
    d. Malignant glaucoma has been reported as a sequela of YAG laser iridotomy.
    e. Unlike argon iridotomies, YAG laser iridotomy rarely induces elevation in intraocular pressure which might threaten vision.

84. T or F -- In infantile glaucoma, the treatment of choice in the setting of a cloudy cornea is goniotomy.

85. The correct spot size for argon laser trabeculoplasty (LTP, ALT) is:

    a. 50 microns.
    b. 100 microns.
    c. 200 microns.
    d. 250 microns.
    e. 500 microns.

86. What proportion of patients with open-angle glaucoma enjoy a substantial drop in intraocular pressure during the first year following argon laser trabeculoplasty?

    a. 20%.
    b. 40%.
    c. 50%.
    d. 80%.
    e. 90%.

87. Relative to patients with primary open-angle glaucoma, which of the following conditions is associated with an equal or better response to argon laser trabeculoplasty?

    1. aphakic glaucoma.
    2. pigmentary glaucoma.
    3. uveitic glaucoma.
    4. pseudoexfoliative glaucoma.

    a. 1, 2, and 3.
    b. 1 and 3.
    c. 2 and 4.
    d. 4 only.
    e. 1, 2, 3, and 4.

88. A 54-year-old white woman presents with glaucomatous optic nerve head changes in each eye and split fixation in her right eye, consistent with her disc findings. Review of her record documents that she has progressively lost visual field and neural rim tissue while running intraocular pressures in the low teens. Gonioscopy has been documented as normal repeatedly. She is currently on maximal tolerated medical therapy and reports subjective decrease in vision in her right eye. A surgical intervention is felt to be the next indicated maneuver. Which procedure might be the one of choice?

    a. combined cataract extraction and trabeculectomy OD.
    b. surgical peripheral iridectomy OD.
    c. posterior lip sclerectomy OD.
    d. trabeculectomy with a seton.
    e. cyclocryotherapy or cyclophotocoagulation.

89. A 63-year-old patient presents 4 days following trabeculectomy for early suture lysis. She complains of severe pain and decreased vision in her operated eye. Examination discloses visual acuity that is slightly lower than her last postoperative checkup, a diffusely shallow anterior chamber, and no view of the posterior segment. There is no excessive anterior chamber inflammation. The most important conditions to be considered in this clinical circumstance include:

> 1. endophthalmitis.
> 2. malignant glaucoma.
> 3. corneal ulcer.
> 4. suprachoroidal hemorrhage.

  a. 1, 2, and 3.
  b. 1 and 3.
  c. 2 and 4.
  d. 4 only.
  e. 1, 2, 3, and 4.

90. The most helpful diagnostic interventions at this point would include:

> 1. anterior chamber paracentesis.
> 2. tonometry.
> 3. corneal scraping and culture.
> 4. B-mode ultrasonography.

  a. 1, 2, and 3.
  b. 1 and 3.
  c. 2 and 4.
  d. 4 only.
  e. 1, 2, 3, and 4.

91. T or F -- The lens arises embryologically from surface ectoderm.

92. Microspherophakia is most often one component of:

  a. Peters' anomaly.
  b. Marfan's syndrome.
  c. Lowe's syndrome.
  d. Alport's syndrome.
  e. Weill-Marchesani syndrome.

93. T or F -- Since microspherophakia may lead to an angle-closure glaucoma with pupillary block, treatment with miotics is helpful until iridotomy can be performed.

94. T or F -- Congenital lens dislocations are commonly inherited on an autosomal dominant basis.

95. T or F -- Dilated examination of a patient with Marfan's syndrome frequently reveals a subluxated lens, upward and outward.

96. All of the following findings might be indicative of an underlying systemic disorder except:

   a. horizontal breaks in Descemet's membrane.
   b. joint laxity and hypermobility.
   c. iris sphincter tears.
   d. localized cortical cataract.
   e. extremely tall habitus and fundus findings consistent with high myopia.

97. Dilated examination reveals a dense white dot on the vitreal surface of the posterior capsule just inferonasal to the center of the posterior capsule. The patient should be advised that:

   a. cataract formation with visual loss is imminent.
   b. she should have a glucose tolerance test immediately.
   c. she should have urinalysis done to detect hematuria and proteinuria.
   d. she has a benign remnant with no significant implications.
   e. she should undergo cataract extraction as soon as possible.

98. T or F -- In young children, polar cataracts are typically unilateral, while nuclear cataracts are typically bilateral.

99. Which of the following forms of infantile/congenital cataract is least likely to affect vision seriously?

   a. complete.
   b. nuclear.
   c. lamellar.
   d. capsular.
   e. polar.

100. The condition seen most commonly in association with congenital/infantile cataracts is:

   a. maternal drug ingestion.
   b. aniridia.
   c. Lowe's syndrome.
   d. persistent hyperplastic primary vitreous (PHPV).
   e. maternal rubella infection.

101. T or F -- The key feature differentiating true galactosemia and galactokinase deficiency is the presence of cataract in the former.

102. Indicate the proper association for each of the following symptoms or signs:

   a. glaucoma.
   b. polar cataracts and lenticonus.
   c. hematuria.
   d. X-linked inheritance pattern.
   e. progressive sensorineural hearing loss.
   f. vestibular dysfunction.
   g. areflexia.
   h. renal tubular acidosis with rickets.
   i. pigmentary retinopathy.

   1. Lowe's syndrome.
   2. Alport's syndrome.
   3. both.
   4. neither.

103. Which of the following syndromes featuring congenital/infantile cataract may be associated with facial abnormalities?

   1. Craniosynostosis.
   2. Hallermann-Streiff syndrome.
   3. Stickler's syndrome.
   4. Alport's syndrome.

   a. 1, 2, and 3.
   b. 1 and 3.
   c. 2 and 4.
   d. 4 only.
   e. 1, 2, 3, and 4.

104. Which of the following conditions are associated with cataracts in juveniles and young adults (with no history of ocular trauma)?

   1. myotonic dystrophy.
   2. neurofibromatosis type 1.
   3. atopic dermatitis.
   4. galactosemia.

   a. 1, 2, and 3.
   b. 1 and 3.
   c. 2 and 4.
   d. 4 only.
   e. 1, 2, 3, and 4.

105. T or F -- Surgical removal of the cataract associated with pseudoexfoliation glaucoma will generally result in resolution of the glaucoma and pseudoexfoliative material.

106. T or F -- The lens of an older patient is more susceptible to the cataractogenic affects of ionizing radiation than the lens of a younger patient.

107. Match the cataract morphologies listed in the left column with the systemic association in the right column.

a. sunflower cataract.
b. oil droplet cataract.
c. snowflake cataract.
d. Christmas tree cataract.

1. diabetes mellitus type 1.
2. myotonic dystrophy.
3. Wilson's disease.
4. galactosemia.

108. A 74-year-old man comes in complaining of difficulty driving due to decreased distance vision. Upon questioning, he has no complaints regarding his near vision. This is most consistent with:

a. nuclear sclerotic cataract.
b. posterior subcapsular cataract.
c. cortical cataract.
d. anterior polar cataract.
e. subluxated lens.

109. T or F -- With many cataract patients, standard acuity testing in a darkened room may considerably overestimate functional acuity.

110. Cataract extraction in patients with pseudoexfoliation syndrome may be more hazardous than in other patients due to:

1. incomplete pupillary dilation.
2. abnormally weak lens zonules.
3. a thickened or "tough" anterior capsule.
4. abnormally thin sclera.

a. 1, 2, and 3.
b. 1 and 3.
c. 2 and 4.
d. 4 only.
e. 1, 2, 3, and 4.

111. Clinical features of particular importance in determining the strategy of cataract extraction include:

1. presence of pseudoexfoliation syndrome.
2. a history of topical steroid use for a previous episode of uveitis.
3. presence of corneal guttae.
4. presence of lattice retinal degeneration.

a. 1, 2, and 3.
b. 1 and 3.
c. 2 and 4.
d. 4 only.
e. 1, 2, 3, and 4.

112. A 73-year-old man reports to the office on his first day following a cataract extraction complaining of severe eye pain. Visual acuity is counting fingers at 3 feet in the involved eye. Slit-lamp examination reveals a diffusely shallow anterior chamber and corneal edema without hypopyon. The next step should be:

a. dilated fundus examination.
b. tonometry.
c. gonioscopy.
d. pachymetry.
e. B-mode ultrasonography.

113. After obtaining an applanation intraocular pressure (IOP) of 42 mm Hg and attempting to examine the fundus unsuccessfully, an ultrasound is obtained that reveals a normal posterior segment. Gonioscopy reveals a completely closed angle. The next intervention should be:

a. surgical revision of the wound.
b. posterior sclerotomy.
c. peripheral iridotomy.
d. dilation with potent cycloplegics.
e. medical treatment with potent miotics.

114. The intervention in question 113 fails. What is the next step?

a. surgical revision of the wound.
b. posterior sclerotomy.
c. peripheral iridotomy.
d. dilation with potent cycloplegics.
e. medical treatment with potent miotics.

115. Vitreous prolapse into the anterior chamber following extracapsular cataract extraction with posterior chamber intraocular lens implantation (ECCE/PCIOL) may lead to which of the following complications?

1. localized or diffused corneal edema.
2. open-angle glaucoma.
3. cystoid macular edema.
4. retinal detachment.

a. 1, 2, and 3.
b. 1 and 3.
c. 2 and 4.
d. 4 only.
e. 1, 2, 3, and 4.

116. Recurrent hyphema weeks to months following uneventful extracapsular cataract extraction with posterior chamber intraocular lens implantation (ECCE/PCIOL) is a rare syndrome whose etiology may be discerned by:

a. tonometry.
b. gonioscopy.
c. dilated fundus examination.
d. wound exploration.
e. ultrasonography.

117. The incidence of visually significant cystoid macular edema (CME) following uncomplicated extracapsular cataract surgery is approximately:

a. less than 1%.
b. 1 to 2%.
c. 3 to 5%.
d. 5 to 10%.
e. 15 to 20%.

118. T or F -- The incidence of angiographic CME is considerably higher than that of visually significant CME.

119. Potential risk factors for CME following cataract surgery include:

1. vitreous proplase into the anterior chamber or wound.
2. malpositioned posterior chamber implants.
3. chronic inflammation or endophthalmitis.
4. corneal decompensation.

a. 1, 2, and 3.
b. 1 and 3.
c. 2 and 4.
d. 4 only.
e. 1, 2, 3, and 4.

120. Risk factors for retinal detachment following cataract extraction include:

1. retinal detachment in the contralateral eye.
2. myopia.
3. lattice retinal degeneration.
4. family history of retinal detachment.

a. 1, 2, and 3.
b. 1 and 3.
c. 2 and 4.
d. 4 only.
e. 1, 2, 3, and 4.

121. Which one of the following is true concerning postoperative endophthalmitis?

   a. It most commonly presents 7 to 10 days postoperatively, and the most common etiologic agent is *Streptococcus*.
   b. It most commonly presents 2 to 5 days postoperatively, and the most common etiologic agent is *Streptococcus*.
   c. It most commonly presents 2 to 5 days postoperatively, and the most common etiologic agent is *Staphylococcus*.
   d. It most commonly presents 7 to 10 days postoperatively, and the most common etiologic agent is *Staphylococcus*.
   e. Agents responsible for these infections are generally part of the surgeon's normal flora.

122. T or F -- The style of anterior chamber intraocular lens implant (ACIOL) currently preferred to minimize complications features closed loops with three or four footplates.

123. Which of the following complications are more frequently seen following cataract surgery in children than in adults?

   1. opacification of posterior capsule.
   2. glaucoma.
   3. retinal detachment.
   4. cystoid macular edema (CME).

   a. 1, 2, and 3.
   b. 1 and 3.
   c. 2 and 4.
   d. 4 only.
   e. 1, 2, 3, and 4.

124. T or F -- Correction of aphakia with spectacles is less successful in children than in adults.

125. The male to female patient ratio in ocular trauma is approximately:

   a. 1:1.
   b. 2:1.
   c. 4:1.
   d. 10:1.
   e. 20:1.

126. The primary ocular manifestation of electrocution injury is:

   a. madarosis.
   b. superficial punctate keratitis.
   c. iritis.
   d. cataract.
   e. pigmentary retinopathy.

127. The initial step in management of chemical burns must be:

a. debridement of foreign particles.
b. copious irrigation.
c. measurement of intraocular pressure.
d. slit-lamp examination.
e. fundus examination.

128. Clinical features used to grade the severity of ocular chemical injuries include:

1. limbal whitening.
2. corneal clarity.
3. extent of epithelial defect.
4. intraocular pressure.

a. 1, 2, and 3.
b. 1 and 3.
c. 2 and 4.
d. 4 only.
e. 1, 2, 3, and 4.

129. Which one of the following concerning hyphema is false?

a. The source of the hemorrhage is typically the major arterial circle of the iris.
b. The incidence of complications from hyphema increases with rebleeding.
c. The most frequent time for rebleeding is between 2 and 5 days after the original injury.
d. Optic nerve atrophy may develop more quickly and at lower intraocular pressure (IOP) in patients with sickle cell disease or trait.
e. Corneal blood staining generally clears rapidly once IOP is normalized.

130. Which of the following constitute(s) indication(s) for intervention (medical or surgical) in lens subluxation or dislocation?

1. polyopia.
2. pupillary block.
3. corneal-lenticular touch.
4. decreased vision.

a. 1, 2, and 3.
b. 1 and 3.
c. 2 and 4.
d. 4 only.
e. 1, 2, 3, and 4.

131. T or F -- Intraocular copper of greater than 85 to 90% purity generally causes an acute inflammatory response, while concentrations less than this are generally inert.

132. T or F -- Iron has an affinity for epithelial cells, while copper tends to deposit in basement membranes.

133. Features of ocular siderosis include all of the following except:

   a. deposits in Descemet's membrane identical to the Kayser-Fleischer ring in Wilson's disease.
   b. iris heterochromia.
   c. brunescent cataract.
   d. miosis.
   e. loss of the B-wave on electroretinography.

134. A 37-year-old man presents with gradual loss of vision affecting his right eye. His past medical and ocular histories are unremarkable. Visual acuity is 20/400 OD and 20/15 OS. The neuromuscular examination is normal. Slit-lamp examination reveals stellate keratic precipitates on the right corneal endothelium, along with a "washed-out" appearing iris stroma, and dense white cataract, as shown in color plate 16. There are trace cells in the aqueous. The left eye is normal (color plate 17). Intraocular pressures are 32 OD and 12 OS. Gonioscopy of the right eye reveals prominent, engorged vessels that bridge the angle without synechiae. Gonioscopy of the left eye is normal. The right fundus cannot be clearly seen due to the cataract. Which one of the following is true regarding this patient?

   a. There was probably an episode of intense intraocular inflammation affecting the right eye in the past.
   b. Antibody titers to herpes zoster virus are likely to be elevated in serum and aqueous humor.
   c. A classic sign of this disorder is hyphema occurring at the beginning of filtration surgery.
   d. The glaucoma is due to typical rubeosis and secondary angle closure.
   e. Cataract surgery will cure the glaucoma.

135. A 48-year-old man presents complaining of difficulty reading. Subjective refraction reveals +0.25 OU, giving 20/15 OU. During the completion of the routine examination, intraocular pressure is measured as 34 OD and 16 OS. Gonioscopy of the right eye is shown in color plate 18, and the left eye is shown in color plate 19. The right optic nerve shows evidence of inferior rim excavation. Which one of the following regarding these findings is false?

   a. This entity is more common in men.
   b. The incidence and severity of the glaucoma in this condition are correlated with the extent of angle abnormalities.
   c. Careful slit-lamp examination may reveal iris abnormalities in the right eye.
   d. The same process will affect the left eye within the next 3 to 5 years.
   e. The patient should undergo careful, dilated, depressed retinal examination.

Answers

1. a.   As with any system of fluid dynamics, the equation

    pressure = flow x resistance

    defines the relationship between these variables. In the eye, the driving pressure for aqueous outflow equals the difference between intraocular pressure (IOP) and episcleral venous pressure (Ve). The outflow facility is the reciprocal of resistance. Therefore,

    IOP - Ve = (aqueous flow/outflow facility), so
    IOP = (aqueous flow/outflow facility) + Ve.

    Aqueous flow, outflow facility, and episcleral venous pressure are thus the primary determinants of intraocular pressure. Relative pupillary block can affect IOP by decreasing outflow facility but is not a primary determinant of IOP.

2. c.   A pressure-independent active transport mechanism and a pressure-dependent ultrafiltration component both contribute to aqueous formation. The active transport component is felt to be the primary mechanism of aqueous production. This requires ATP-ase activity and creates a concentration gradient of certain ions such as sodium chloride or bicarbonate, followed by a passive fluid movement. Ultrafiltration, which is independent of ATP, generally decreases as IOP increases. A diurnal rhythm of aqueous flow has been found to exist, with flow being lower at night.

3. True. The anterior chamber volume is approximately 200 to 250 µl, and the rate of aqueous formation is approximately 2 to 3 µl/minute.

4. e.

5. True. The trabecular meshwork (TM) collapses when intraocular pressure is low, thereby reducing backflow and functioning to an extent as a one-way valve. Also, even at normal IOP, blood cells cannot reflux out of the TM into the anterior chamber.

6. c.   Estimates of this value actually vary, with some being as low as 10%. Twenty percent is probably the upper end of uveoscleral contribution.

7. True. Miotics lower IOP by increasing trabecular outflow facility. Cycloplegic agents and epinephrine have been shown to increase uveoscleral flow, while miotics decrease uveoscleral flow.

8. c.   Outflow facility in normal eyes is approximately 0.28 ± 0.05 µl/min/mm Hg.

9. False. The normal range of episcleral venous pressure is approximately 8 to 12 mm Hg.

10. False. Acute elevation in episcleral venous pressure will generally lead to an abrupt rise in IOP of roughly equal magnitude. Chronic elevation of episcleral venous pressure has a more complex effect on IOP and may result in elevations that are greater, lesser, or equal in magnitude to the rise in episcleral venous pressure.

11. False. The distribution of IOP cannot be predicted by the normal (gaussian) distribution. The use of the mean ± 2 standard deviations as the range of "normal IOP" in the general population is not valid, since the actual distribution is skewed toward higher IOP.

12. True.

13. True.

14. False. Diurnal IOP fluctuation in normal eyes ranges from 2 to 6 mm Hg. Glaucomatous eyes often show a wider range of diurnal variation, sometimes exceeding 20 mm Hg (of fluctuation!). The peak IOP in most individuals occurs during the day, although morning, afternoon, and evening peaks have been demonstrated. Measurement of IOP at different times during the day is useful in evaluating patients with apparent glaucomatous optic nerve damage but with no documented elevation of IOP.

15. d. Unlike Schiotz tonometry, applanation tonometry displaces a very small volume of aqueous humor from the eye and does not significantly increase IOP. For this reason, applanation measurements are essentially independent of ocular rigidity.

16. False. The Perkins tonometer is counterbalanced so that it can be used in the erect or supine position.

17. b. The Mackay-Marg tonometer applanates a very small area of the cornea and is useful in the presence of corneal scars or edema. The pneumatic tonometer is useful for the same reason.

18. a. Schiotz indentation tonometry may give falsely low readings in cases where scleral rigidity is reduced (thyroid disease or any other cause of proptosis, high myopia, previous ocular surgery). *Ar Gas Bubble in eye. Why does Hyperthyroidism ↓ ocular rigidity?*

19. a. A previous history of eye surgery, eye trauma, and a family history of eye diseases are all important factors in evaluating a patient who may have glaucoma. A history of difficulty with near vision suggests presbyopia and is not pertinent in this case.

20. d. The anterior chamber angle cannot be viewed directly through the cornea because there is total internal reflection of light at the cornea-air interface. Gonioscopy replaces this interface with a new cornea-lens interface. The difference in refractive indices is reduced, so total internal reflection does not occur.

21. d. A Koeppe lens is used in direct gonioscopy, while the Sussman, Goldmann, and Zeiss lenses are used in indirect gonioscopy.

22. b. Koeppe gonioscopy is considered best for evaluating a patient with potential angle recession because this system allows easier comparison of one eye to the fellow eye, or one portion of the angle to another.

23. b. The Koeppe lens is least likely to distort the anterior chamber anatomy. Posterior pressure on the Goldmann lens may falsely narrow the angle by indenting the sclera.

24. True. See answer 23.

25. False. Because of their smaller diameters, Zeiss and Sussman lenses may be used in indentation gonioscopy. This maneuver distinguishes appositional angle closure from synechial angle closure by artificially deepening the anterior chamber with digital pressure on the lens. Goldmann lenses are too large for this.

26. False. The inferior angle is wider and is thought to be the easiest portion for distinguishing landmarks.

27. True. Grade IV describes a 45 degree angle between the surface of the trabecular meshwork and the iris while grade I describes a 10 degree angle. Thus, a grade IV angle is less likely to undergo spontaneous closure.

28. e. Blood may enter Schlemm's canal when episcleral venous pressure exceeds intraocular pressure. This may be seen in all of the mentioned conditions.

29. a. Heavy trabecular meshwork pigmentation is not a feature of anterior segment dysgenesis. It should suggest the differential diagnosis of pseudoexfoliation, pigment dispersion, previous inflammation or surgery, or uveal melanoma.

30. c. The earliest detected histologic changes in glaucoma may occur at the level of the lamina cribrosa (compression of laminar collagen). Prelaminar optic nerve is supplied by the choroid and, possibly, central retinal anteriole branches. Up to 50% of the optic nerve axons may be lost without clinically detectable changes on kinetic perimetry. Although reversal of cupping may be seen in both pediatric and adult populations, it is far more likely in the pediatric population.

31. False. This is actually the vascular or ischemic theory of glaucomatous damage. The mechanical theory states that elevated intraocular pressure causes pressure-induced damage of optic nerve axons by compression at the lamina cribrosa.

32. e. Although all the stated answers may be seen with the progression of glaucomatous visual field loss, the appearance of a splinter hemorrhage may be the most specific and worrisome for progressive glaucoma.

33. d. If a patient has glaucomatous visual field-type defects, corresponding optic nerve head abnormalities should exist. Otherwise, alternative etiologies should be considered. In static perimetry, the stimulus is of variable intensity and is kept stationary (static) until it is noticed by the patient. Baring of the blind spot and generalized constriction are not very specific and can be produced by miosis, uncorrected refractive error, aging, and cataract.

34. d. Areas of retina and/or optic nerve damaged by glaucoma are believed to be more vulnerable to ongoing damage at lower IOP. Thus, field defects tend to become more severe with time. New defects may also appear, of course, but generally accompany progression of previous defects.

35. e. A typical pattern of progression is (1) loss near fixation (paracentral scotoma) to (2) split fixation to (3) loss of fixation. Thus, the eye at greatest risk is not one with a 5-degree central field but one with split-fixation in the horizontal meridian.

36. True. Points on the periphery of the visual field are often depressed because of malpositioning of the near add and should be interpreted cautiously.

37. a. It is important to correlate changes in visual field with changes in the optic disc. The following should raise suspicion about the diagnosis of glaucoma: (1) an optic disc that is less cupped than would be expected for observed field loss, (2) pallor of the disc that is more impressive than the cupping, (3) markedly asymmetric dyschromatopsia, or (4) visual field defects uncharacteristic for glaucoma (e.g., respecting the vertical meridian).

38. c. Primary open-angle glaucoma (POAG) is the most common of all glaucomas in the United States (60-70%), affecting 0.5 to 1.0% of people over age 40. POAG occurs more frequently in blacks than in whites and is the leading cause of blindness in blacks. Patients with glaucoma are more likely to have diabetes, and patients with diabetes are more likely to have glaucoma.

39. c. Most authorities agree that treatment of the glaucoma suspect should be limited to patients with a high risk of ultimate damage to the optic nerve due to elevated intraocular pressure. These risk factors include elevated intraocular pressure, positive family history of glaucoma, myopia, diabetes mellitus, cardiovascular disease, race (i.e., blacks), asymmetric cupping, large cups, and early nonspecific visual field changes.

40. e. A diagnosis of normal tension can be made only after other causes of optic neuropathy are eliminated. Although difficult to prove, the situation that may be the one most frequently misdiagnosed an "normal-tension" glaucoma is primary open-angle glaucoma in which IOP fluctuations have obscured the actual nature of the disease. In addition, there are four disorders that feature pseudoglaucomatous optic nerve cupping: (1) chiasmal compression, (2) arteritic anterior ischemic optic neuropathy, (3) methanol toxicity, and (4) hypotension ("shock" optic neuropathy).

41. True. Some experts feel that therapy should be instituted only when progression has been documented. The goal of therapy should be an IOP as low as practical.

42. a. In pseudoexfoliation, fibrillar material similar to elastin is deposited in the anterior segment of the eye. Patients with this glaucoma are often resistant to medical therapy, but laser trabeculoplasty is often very effective. Pseudoexfoliation with glaucoma also differs from POAG in that it is often monocular or asymmetric and has greater pigmentation of the trabecular meshwork, as well as pigment deposited anterior to Schwalbe's line (Sampaolesi's line). There is considerable overlap in the age range of patients affected by each disorder.

43. c. The sine qua non of this condition are radial defects in the iris pigment epithelium. Krukenberg spindles are less specific. Pigmentary glaucoma usually occurs in young myopic males, typically in their third or fourth decades. For obscure reasons, women with the disease tend to be older then men. Exercise or pupillary movements may induce a shower of iris pigment release, with resultant increased IOP.

44. c. Phacolytic glaucoma results when mature or hypermature cataracts leak high-molecular weight proteins through microscopic defects in the capsule. A resultant macrophage response clogs the trabecular meshwork. While medication is used for short-term intraocular pressure control, definitive therapy requires cataract extraction. Other lens-induced conditions may respond to topical steroid.

45. False.   Fuchs' heterochromatic iridocyclitis is considered a secondary open-angle glaucoma. The glaucoma can be difficult to control and does not parallel the degree of inflammation. The rubeosis in this condition is odd--the vessels are particularly prone to bleed but do not induce synechialization.

46. False.   Alkali penetrates ocular tissues rapidly, unlike acid. The glaucoma that results is probably multifactorial, with primary structural damage to the trabecular meshwork, with sclerosis and shrinking accounting for chronic hypertension.

47. False.   In hemolytic glaucoma, hemoglobin-laden macrophages block the trabecular meshwork (TM), while in ghost cell glaucoma, rigid, degenerated khaki-colored red blood cells from the vitreous enter the anterior chamber and obstruct the TM. Hemolytic glaucoma may occur within days of hemorrhage, whereas ghost cell glaucoma is seen weeks to months later.

48. e.   These four groups are at greatest risk of developing a steroid response. The magnitude of the rise in pressure depends on corticosteroid strength and duration of administration.

49. True.   Pupillary block is obstruction of flow of aqueous from posterior to anterior due to a functional block between the lens and iris. It is the most frequent cause of angle-closure glaucoma.

50. True.   Pupillary block is more common in women than in men, but only among whites; in blacks, the occurrence of pupillary block is roughly equal in men and women.

51. False.   Generally, it occurs after full dilation, as the pupil shrinks to mid-position. This is the region of maximal iris-lens contact.

52. b.   The increased intraocular pressure that occurs during an attack of angle closure can cause ischemia of the iris and may produce stromal atrophy. Small anterior subcapsular lens opacites, or glaukomflecken, may also develop as a direct result of pressure-induced lens epithelial death. Optic disc cupping may be seen if the attack is prolonged or severe, but this is not specific.

53. a.   The major goal of treatment of pupillary block is to relieve the block. Compression gonioscopy may "burp" aqueous through the block and open the angle. In some cases, pilocarpine will accomplish this by moving the iris away from the lens. When the intraocular pressure is elevated, however, the iris may not respond to miotics. In such cases, IOP should first be lowered by other medications, such as beta blockers, carbonic anhydrase inhibitors, and/or hyperosmotic agents. Once the IOP is controlled, iridotomy is indicated. Laser iridotomy is the treatment of choice; if this cannot be accomplished, surgical iridectomy should be considered.

54. False.   Angle-closure glaucoma is a <u>bilateral</u> disease, and treatment of the fellow eye with iridotomy must be considered.

55. a.   Both mydriatics and miotics can precipitate angle-closure in eyes with shallow anterior chambers. This is true for both topical medications and systemic drugs that affect the pupil. Examples include <u>antihistamines, which can have anticholinergic</u> activity

ASA has ANTI. PROSTAGLANDIN AFFECTS

56. d.　Angle-closure develops in only a small number of patients with narrow anterior chambers. A number of provocative tests exist to attempt to cause angle-closure in susceptible patients. Perhaps the most predictive is the prone-dark room test. Intraocular pressure is measured before and after 30 to 60 minutes of total dark adaptation attained with the patient prone. Dark will induce pupillary dilation, and prone positioning will move the lens forward. Both tend to increase pupillary block. None of these tests, however, has been evaluated in a prospective study.

57. a.　The patient with very narrow angles and elevated pressure may have "mixed mechanism" glaucoma with partial angle closure due to pupillary block superimposed on open-angle glaucoma. To determine if an angle-closure component is present, the effect of minimizing pupillary block on IOP must be determined. Cholinergic miotics (pilocarpine) will cause miosis and lessen pupillary block but will also exert traction on the trabecular meshwork and lower IOP by this unrelated mechanism. Thymoxamine, a selective alpha-adrenergic antagonist, causes miosis and lessens pupillary block, without affecting outflow facility. A fall in pressure after thymoxamine (lessened pupillary block) implies partial angle closure, and iridotomy is indicated. No change in IOP after thymoxamine-induced miosis implies that an iridotomy may not be helpful.

58. a.　A small anterior segment is not associated with plateau iris.

59. c.　Microspherophakia increases pupillary block. Microspherophakia may occur in association with Marfan's syndrome or as an isolated condition. Neovascular glaucoma typically starts as an open-angle glaucoma with progressive anterior synechialization leading to closure without any obstruction to flow of aqueous through the pupil. The same is true of synechialization following a flat chamber.

60. a.　The glaucoma associated with ICE syndrome is often worse than predicted by the extent of synechiae, likely due to nondetectable endothelialization of the angle.

61. False.　The "nevi" are actually nodular collections of stromal melanocytes, not nevus cells.

62. a.　Initial treatment of ciliary block or malignant glaucoma includes cycloplegia. Definitive therapy in phakic eyes is vitrectomy to alter the anterior vitreous zone. In aphakic or pseudophakic eyes, the anterior vitreous can be disrupted by laser treatment. In primary angle closure, the central chamber is deeper than the peripheral angle due to pupillary block. In malignant glaucoma, vitreous enlargement by aqueous causes the entire chamber to shallow.

63. False.　Epithelial downgrowth is usually more aggressive than fibrous downgrowth.

64. False.　Peripheral iridotomy does not help relieve the glaucoma associated with scleral buckling because the mechanism of angle closure is not pupillary block. Obstruction of venous outflow produces choroidal effusions that cause anterior rotation of the ciliary body and secondary angle closure. If medical management is not effective during the acute period, the buckle may need to be repositioned.

65. False.　Following heavy panretinal photocoagulation, choroidal effusion may cause anterior rotation of the ciliary body resulting in closure of the angle. In CRVO, there may be transudation of serum into the vitreous, driven by the elevated intravascular pressure. This hydration causes vitreous swelling with subsequent secondary angle closure.

66. e. The pathophysiology of this disorder has not been elucidated, but gonioscopy suggests maldevelopment of the anterior chamber angle. In some cases, an imperforate membrane ("Barkan's membrane") occludes the angle.

67. b. Haab's striae are tears in Descemet's membrane resulting from corneal stretching induced by high intraocular pressure. The same phenomenon leads to enlarged corneal diameter. Corneal edema and optic nerve cupping can be seen in adult glaucoma.

68. a. Among these general anesthetic agents, ketamine alone is associated with rises in intraocular pressure (primarily at high doses). Succinylcholine can also elevate IOP. The other agents usually result in a decrease.

69. False. Infantile glaucoma represents a developmental anomaly of the angle structures, with either an intrinsic defect of the trabecular meshwork (TM) or mechanical obstruction of the TM by a membrane. It is not amenable to long-term medical management, although aqueous supressants are useful as a temporizing measure before surgery.

70. b. Caution must be exercised in the use of carbonic anhydrase inhibitors for small children because of their susceptibility to rapid changes in serum pH.

71. a. 1. Mannitol is an osmotic diuretic that decreases vitreous volume by creating
    b. 2. an osmotic gradient between the gel and plasma.
    c. 1.
    d. 1.
    e. 1.
    f. 2.
    g. 1.
    h. 2.
    i. 2.
    j. 3.

    Phospholine iodine works as an inhibitor of cholinesterase.

    Carbachol has a Dual action of both cholinergic and anticholinesterase

72. b. Propine is a pro-drug that is converted to epinephrine by corneal enzymes. Systemic absorption of epinephrine is dramatically reduced, but the drug is still relatively contraindicated in this circumstance, as is epinephrine itself. Timolol, as a beta antagonist, is not a cardio-stimulant (quite the opposite). The same is true of pilocarpine.

73. c. Beta antagonists, in general, can cause fatigue, dizziness, and depression at therapeutic doses. Carbonic anhydrase inhibitors share an ability to cause lethargy, malaise, and depression. Either of these groups should be used with caution in patients with a history of significant depression.

74. c. There is a danger of precipitating angle closure in individuals with very narrow angles through the use of any medication with mydriatic action. In the case of plateau iris with narrow angles, dilation causes the peripheral roll of iris to "bunch up" and obstruct the trabecular meshwork. With narrow angles, mydriasis may increase pupillary block, most commonly as the agent is wearing off.

75. c. Epinephrine has a well-established tendency to provoke irritation and allergic responses. More than one-fifth of patients will eventually experience an adverses local reaction with prolonged use.

    Apraclonidine has allergic side effects

76. c. Direct-acting miotics interact directly with the acetylcholine receptor, while indirect-acting agents increase the activity of native acetylcholine at the synaptic junction (by blocking its enzymatic degradation). Pilocarpine is a purely direct agent, while carbachol is felt to exhibit some of both effects, possibly by being both an acetylcholine analog and a competitive inhibitor for acetylcholinesterase.

77. a. See answer 76.

78. False. This statement is true only for the unusual patient with plateau iris. The primary mode of action is through ciliary muscle contraction. By way of its insertion on the scleral spur, ciliary muscle tightening puts traction on the trabeculum. This apparently increases outflow, possibly by "opening" the intermeshwork spaces or by increasing the size of the surface over which drainage takes place.

79. a. Indirect agents, along with the strongest direct agents, tend to have the most pronounced systemic and ocular side effects. Bradycardia is never seen with any of the miotics.

80. e. Changes in urine pH secondary to carbonic anhydrase inhibitors can predispose a patient to calcium oxalate and calcium phosphate nephrolithiasis. Aplastic anemia is a rare, but potentially lethal side effect related to the sulfa derivation of the drugs. Gastrointestinal distress occurs, but not most commonly. Hypokalemia may occur as a result of the effects on renal ion transport, but hypocalcemia is not seen. Paresthesias are reported by virtually every patient taking these potent agents.

81. True. Mannitol is distributed only in the blood compartment, while urea moves freely in total body water. As a result, mannitol can generate a greater osmotic gradient than urea, since its intravascular concentration remains greater.

82. False. The blood-aqueous barrier allows formation of the gradient necessary to draw fluid from the vitreous. Interruption of this gradient decreases the effectiveness and duration of osmotic effects.

83. d. Argon iridotomies are less likely to close spontaneously than YAG iridotomies Argon laser is often useful for pretreating dark irides before YAG iridotomy, since YAG iridotomy on heavily pigmented irides is difficult. The most common complication of both YAG and argon laser iridotomies is acute glaucoma. Malignant glaucoma has been reported after a variety of seemingly benign ocular laser procedures.

84. False. Goniotomy requires a clear cornea for viewing of the needle knife. Trabeculotomy is the treatment of choice, since an external incision is used and the trabeculotome is rotated into the anterior chamber.

85. a. Argon LTP uses a 50-micron beam with variable power to produce blanching or a tiny bubble at the anterior pigmented edge of TM. This requires 180 degrees of treatment, rather than 360. The mechanism of action is unclear, but outflow facility improves following successful LTP.

86. d. Studies suggest that approximately 80% experience a significant decrease in IOP 1 year after argon LTP.

87. c. LTP response appears to be better for pigmentary glaucoma and pseudoexfoliation and poorer for inflammatory diseases, recessed angles, membranes in angles, young patients with developmental defects, and aphakic eyes.

88. c.   Given the extent of the glaucomatous damage as indicated by split fixation and progression of both fields and disc at low-normal pressures, the maximal decrease in IOP is necessary. Sclerectomy presents the best choice. Peripheral iridectomy would not be appropriate since the angles appear normal, and the likelihood of excellent pressure control after combined procedure is not high enough. Cyclocryotherapy and cyclophotocoagulation are reserved for end-stage disease. Setons (Molteno, Baerveldt, Denver-Krupin) are reserved for special cases because of a higher rate of complication.

89. c.   Post-trabeculectomy pain and decreased vision require evaluation for endophthalmitis, malignant glaucoma, and suprachoroidal hemorrhage. However, a clear anterior chamber makes endophthalmitis less likely.

90. c.   To distinguish malignant glaucoma from suprachoroidal hemorrhage, which usually occurs in a setting of hypotony, tonometry and ultrasonography would be most helpful.

91. True. Optic vesicle formation influences surface ectoderm to form the lens plate, which then forms the lens.

92. e.   Microspherophakia, as its name implies, is characterized by a lens with small diameter, a spherical shape. High ametropia is often found as well. It may occur as an isolated hereditary disorder but most commonly accompanies Weill-Marchesani syndrome, with short stubby fingers, broad hands, and decreased joint mobility.

93. False. Spherical shape increases relative pupillary block by increasing the degree of iris-lens conact. Miotics further exacerbate this by shifting the iris-lens diaphragm forward and further increasing iris-lens contact (as the lens becomes even more spherical). Cycloplegia moves the diaphragm backward and flattens the lens. It is the medical treatment of choice.

94. True. Simple ectopia lentis is usually transmitted in autosomal dominant fashion.

95. True. Superotemporal lens subluxation is typical of Marfan's syndrome. In homocystinuria, the subluxation is typically inferonasal.

96. c.   Iris sphincter tears occur with birth trauma. No systemic disorder would be expected. Horizontal breaks in Descemet's membrane, or Haab's striae, can occur with congenital glaucoma, which has numerous potential systemic associations. Joint laxity suggests Ehlers-Danlos or Marfan's syndromes. Tall habitus suggests Marfan's. Localized cortical cataract can occur with hypocalcemia from parathyroid disorders.

97. d.   Mittendorf's dot is a remnant of the posterior tunica vasculosa lentis and results in a white dot inferonasally on the posterior capsule of the lens.

98. True. Polar cataracts are usually unilateral and cause variable visual impairment. Nuclear cataracts are usually bilateral and often cause severe visual impairment.

99. d.   Capsular cataracts are opacities of the anterior lens capsule and epithelium that do not usually affect vision.

100. e.   Rubella infection is the most common cause of congenital cataracts.

101. False.   Cataracts may occur both in galactosemia (galactose-1-phosphate uridyltransferase deficiency) and galactokinase deficiency. In the latter, however, hepatosplenomegaly, mental retardation, and the other systemic manifestations are not seen.

102. a. 1.   The retinopathy of Alport's syndrome is generally mild and nonprogressive
 b. 2.   and resembles fundus albipunctatus clinically.
 c. 2.
 d. 1.
 e. 2.
 f. 4.
 g. 1.
 h. 1.
 i. 2.

103. a.   In the craniosynostoses, small orbits, proptosis, and cranial changes affect facial structure. Hallermann-Streiff patients typically have mandibular hypoplasia with "bird face." Stickler's syndrome may be associated with many facial abnormalities, including maxillary and mandibular hypoplasia, epicanthus, a long philtrum, and the Pierre-Robin anomaly. Alport's syndrome features hereditary nephritis and cataract with normal facies.

104. b.   Neurofibromatosis type 2, not type 1, may be associated with posterior subcapsular cataracts. Galactosemia usually results in early death unless galactose is removed from the diet.

105. False.   Surgical removal of the lens does not seem to change the course of pseudoexfoliation glaucoma.

106. False.   A younger patient's lens epithelial cells are more actively growing than an older patient's and are thus more susceptible to radiation damage.

107. a. 3.
 b. 4.
 c. 1.
 d. 2.

108. a.   This history is most consistent with nuclear sclerosis. In contrast, patients with posterior subcapsular cataract (PSC) will notice difficulty primarily with reading vision, particularly in bright ambient lighting.

109. True.   Glare can be disabling to patients with PSC. Thus, standard dark room visual acuity may overestimate their functional acuity.

110. a.   Abnormally thin sclera is not a feature of pseudoexfoliation syndrome. The other three options are recognized hazards of cataract surgery in patients with pseudoexfoliation.

111. b.   Careful surgical technique (copious viscoelastic, low ultrasound energies, minimal corneal manipulation) is essential during cataract extraction on eyes with corneal guttae to avoid damage to an already compromised endothelium. While lattice degeneration increases the risk of retinal detachment after cataract extraction, it does not affect surgical strategy.

112. b.   High intraocular pressure secondary to angle closure may be causing severe eye pain and decreased visual acuity.

113. c.   Since pupillary block is probably present, an iridotomy should be performed. Miotics tend to increase postoperative inflammation and should be avoided here.

114. d.   Failure to relieve postoperative angle closure with iridotomy suggests malignant glaucoma, which often responds to potent cycloplegics. If medical management fails, laser treatment to open the anterior hyaloid face, or even pars plana vitrectomy, is necessary.

115. e.

116. b.   A recurrent or delayed hyphema after uncomplicated cataract surgery is usually due to vascularization of the wound or an implant that is rubbing against the iris. Gonioscopy is useful in identifying these vessels. Laser photocoagulation can then be used to ablate the offending vessels.

117. b.   Although angiographically detectable CME is present in 10 to 20% of patients following extracapsular surgery, visual loss only occurs in 1 to 2%. For intracapsular surgery, the percentages are 40 to 60% and 2 to 10%, respectively.

118. True.

119. a.   Vitreomacular traction is felt to be one of the mechanisms of postoperative CME. CME is also felt to be more common with chronic inflammation or malposition of the intraocular lens implant. Corneal decompensation is not thought to be a separate risk factor for CME.

120. a.   Retinal detachment as a complication of cataract surgery usually occurs within 6 months of the surgery or following YAG capsulotomy. It is more common after intracapsular extraction and in cases with vitreous loss. Contralateral retinal detachment, myopia, and peripheral lattice degeneration are risk factors for retinal detachment. A family history of retinal detachment is not felt to be an independent risk factor for aphakic retinal detachment.

121. c.   Postoperative endophthalmitis is usually caused by contamination with bacteria from the patient's normal lid flora. *Staphylococcus epidermidis* is the most common agent.

122. False.   Anterior chamber intraocular lenses with closed support loops are associated with a higher incidence of complications. They are no longer used for this reason.

123. a.   Posterior capsule opacification, glaucoma (angle closure due to excessive inflammation), and retinal detachment (due to vitreous loss) are more common postoperative complications in children undergoing cataract extraction. The incidence of CME is lower in children than in adults.

124. False.   The plasticity of the visual system in children allows them to adapt to the various distortions inherent in aphakic spectacles more readily than adults.

125. c.   Eighty percent of eye injuries occur in males, perhaps in part because half of all eye injuries occur in industrial and construction environments.

126. d.   Electrical injuries to the eye most often involve the cortex of the lens, producing a cataract.

127. b.   The initial treatment of chemical burns is copious irrigation of the affected eye. This should take place at the site of injury if possible; tap water or any nontoxic liquid may be used.

128. a.   A modern grading system has been derived that employs three findings at presentation in order to prognosticate regarding long-term outcome: (1) extent of epithelial defect, (2) corneal stromal haze, and (3) limbal ischemia. The last of the three is probably the most important, since healing following chemical injury is dependent on limbal blood flow. Elevated intraocular pressure is a poor prognostic factor but not part of the grading system.

129. e.   Corneal blood staining is a complication of hyphema that may take years to clear. The blood staining clears in a centripetal pattern (starting at the periphery). Blacks with hyphema should be checked for sickle cell disease or trait, as the sickled cells may become trapped in the trabecular meshwork, raising the intraocular pressure. Furthermore, the optic nerve is more susceptible to atrophy in sickle cell patients, even at relatively mild elevations of intraocular pressure. This probably reflects poor optic disc perfusion (due to higher blood viscosity).

130. a.   Polyopia, pupillary block, and corneal-lenticular touch are indications for medical or surgical intervention in lens subluxation. Decreased vision can often be corrected solely with an aphakic refraction.

131. False.   While intraocular foreign bodies containing greater than 90% copper generally cause an acute inflammatory response, concentrations of 70% to 90% cause chalcosis. Manifestations include a copper ring (identical to the Kayser-Fleischer ring in Wilson's disease) and anterior subcapsular cataract. Concentrations less than 70% are generally well tolerated; however, other factors such as location and fibrous encapsulation modulate the tissue reaction.

132. True.   Copper accumulates in Descemet's membrane, the lens capsule, and other basement membranes, while iron accumulates in basal epithelial cells.

133. a.   The deposit of metal in Descemet's membrane occurs with <u>copper</u> foreign bodies, not siderosis bulbi.

134. c. The constellation of heterochromia iridis (compare color plates 16 and 17 carefully), gelatinous-stellate keratic precipitates, mild anterior chamber reaction, distinctive rubeosis, and ipsilateral cataract and glaucoma is nearly pathognomonic for Fuchs' heterochromatic iridocyclitis. If inflammation is severe, another diagnosis should be sought. The iris atrophy in Fuchs' is generally diffuse and stromal, while that of herpes zoster iritis is typically sectoral with pigment epithelial involvement. The rubeosis is distinctive because the vessels are typically quite fine and rarely induce synechiae or angle closure. The vessels are also quite fragile, and spontaneous or iatrogenic hyphema (as the paracentesis is performed at filtration surgery) is a classic sign. The mechanism for the glaucoma is poorly understood. Cataract surgery is usually indicated for visual rehabilitation; it has little or no effect on the glaucoma. In fact, in many patients, intraocular pressure does not go up for many months or years after cataract extraction.

135. d. Assuming the left angle is normal, this patient can be diagnosed with angle recession (post-traumatic) glaucoma affecting the right eye. Since men are involved with ocular trauma as much as nine times as frequently as women, this glaucoma is far more common in men. The lifetime risk for developing glaucoma seems to be correlated with the amount of angle recession and is estimated to be approximately 10% in patients with 180 degrees of involved angle. Iris sphincter tears, Vossius' ring, and posterior subcapsular cataract may all be seen in conjunction with the disorder. Retinal dialysis must be ruled out in the post-traumatic period by careful, dilated and depressed retinal examination. While the disorder may be bilateral if the contralateral eye is traumatized, it is much more commonly unilateral.

References

1. Kass, Michael. "Section 10: Glaucoma, Lens, and Anterior Segment Trauma." in F.M. Wilson (ed.). Basic and Clinical Science Course. San Francisco: American Academy of Ophthalmology, 1991-1992.

2. Epstein, David (ed.). Chandler and Grant's Glaucoma. Philadelphia: Lea and Febiger, 1986.

3. Ritch, Robert; Shields, M. Bruce; and Krupin, Theodore (eds.). The Glaucomas. St. Louis: C.V. Mosby Company, 1989.

10: Retina and Vitreous

1. Effects of acute or chronic systemic hypertension on the retinal vascular system include all of the following except:

   a. focal or generalized vasoconstriction.
   b. breakdown of the blood-retinal barrier with subsequent hemorrhage and exudate.
   c. thickening of venous walls with secondary nicking of arterioles.
   d. histopathologic evidence of endothelial hyperplasia.
   e. development of micro- and macroaneurysms.

2. Which of the following concerning blood pressure-induced choroidal disease is false?

   a. The important pathophysiology leads to occlusion of the the choriocapillaris.
   b. Elschnig spots are characteristic.
   c. Exudative retinal detachment may develop as a secondary manifestation.
   d. Hypertensive choroidopathy is associated with chronic elevation in systemic blood pressure.
   e. Hypertensive choroidopathy may be associated with acute elevations in intraocular pressure.

3. Which of the following concerning the incidence and prevalence of diabetic retinopathy is/are true?

   1. Approximately 25% of the diabetic population has some degree of retinopathy.
   2. The incidence of any degree of retinopathy after 7 to 10 years of diabetes is approximately 50%.
   3. Approximately 5% of all diabetic patients have proliferative retinopathy.
   4. The incidence of proliferative retinopathy after 25 years of diabetes is approximately 25%.

   a. 1, 2, and 3.
   b. 1 and 3.
   c. 2 and 4.
   d. 4 only.
   e. 1, 2, 3, and 4.

4. Abnormalities in retinal physiology felt to be important in the early stages of diabetic retinopathy include:

      1. impaired photopigment recycling and metabolism.
      2. impaired autoregulation of retinal blood flow.
      3. impaired retrograde axoplasmic transport.
      4. breakdown in the blood-retinal barrier.

    a. 1, 2, and 3.
    b. 1 and 3.
    c. 2 and 4.
    d. 4 only.
    e. 1, 2, 3, and 4.

5. T or F -- Evidence of breakdown in the blood-retinal barrier in diabetic patients may be detected prior to the onset of clinical retinopathy.

6. T or F -- The abnormalities in the blood-retinal barrier in diabetics are believed to be due to loss of tight junctions between retinal pigment epithelial cells.

7. Histopathologic features seen in the retinal vasculature of patients with early diabetic retinopathy include:

      1. loss of arteriolar pericytes.
      2. thickening of endothelial basement membranes.
      3. capillary closure and/or nonperfusion.
      4. medial hyperplasia.

    a. 1, 2, and 3.
    b. 1 and 3.
    c. 2 and 4.
    d. 4 only.
    e. 1, 2, 3, and 4.

8. T or F -- In diabetes, the visual prognosis for diffuse macular edema is better than for focal macular edema.

9. According to the Early Treatment for Diabetic Retinopathy Study (ETDRS), which of the following is/are indication(s) for treatment of diabetic macular edema?

1. retinal thickening within the temporal arcades.
2. hard exudate within 500 microns of the center of the fovea with adjacent thickening of the retina.
3. extensive foveal and parafoveal nonperfusion on fluorescein angiography.
4. an area of retinal thickening equal to or greater than 1 disc area any part of which lies within 1 disc diameter of the center of the fovea.

a. 1, 2, and 3.
b. 1 and 3.
c. 2 and 4.
d. 4 only.
e. 1, 2, 3, and 4.

10. Which of the following is a poor prognostic sign in a patient with nonproliferative diabetic retinopathy?

a. extensive blot hemorrhages.
b. extensive microaneurysms.
c. extensive intraretinal microvascular abnormalities (IRMA).
d. extensive exudate.
e. neovascularization of the disc.

11. In untreated eyes with preproliferative disease, the probability of progression to proliferative retinopathy over 2 years is approximately:

a. 5%.
b. 10%.
c. 25%.
d. 50%.
e. 75%.

12. T or F -- Retinal neovascularization must extend internal to the internal limiting membrane.

13. T or F -- Rhegmatogenous retinal detachment is uncommon in proliferative diabetic retinopathy.

14. Which of the following concerning metabolic control of diabetes and its end-organ manifestations is/are true?

1. Rapid normalization and tight control of blood sugar after a period of prolonged hyperglycemia may induce a deterioration in retinopathy.
2. Blood pressure control is probably important in slowing the progression of diabetic retinopathy.
3. The Diabetes Control and Complications Trial (DCCT) may answer the controversial question regarding the effect of blood sugar control on progression of retinopathy.
4. Animal models such as the galactosemic dog are critical in investigating metabolic control on diabetic retinopathy.

a. 1, 2, and 3.
b. 1 and 3.
c. 2 and 4.
d. 4 only.
e. 1, 2, 3, and 4.

15. Which of the following are favorable clinical prognostic features for visual stabilization following laser treatment of diabetic macular edema?

1. macular nonperfusion.
2. cystoid macular edema.
3. extensive hard exudate within the fovea.
4. focal leakage and thickening.

a. 1, 2, and 3.
b. 1 and 3.
c. 2 and 4.
d. 4 only.
e. 1, 2, 3, and 4.

16. T or F -- Laser treatment of diabetic macular edema more frequently leads to resolution of retinal exudate than retinal thickening.

17. T or F -- The Early Treatment of Diabetic Retinopathy Study (ETDRS) showed that laser treatment of clinically significant diabetic macular edema leads to an improvement in vision in twice as many treated patients as untreated patients.

18. T or F -- The Diabetic Retinopathy Study (DRS) showed that panretinal photocoagulation (PRP) could reduce the incidence of severe visual loss in certain patients by over 50%.

19. High-risk characteristics of proliferative retinopathy mandating immediate PRP include:

    1. neovascularization of the disc covering greater than half of its area, only if associated with vitreous hemorrhage.
    2. any neovascularization elsewhere.
    3. severe neovascularization elsewhere.
    4. moderate to severe neovascularization elsewhere, only if associated with vitreous hemorrhage.

a. 1, 2, and 3.
b. 1 and 3.
c. 2 and 4.
d. 4 only.
e. 1, 2, 3, and 4.

20. Adverse effects of PRP may include which of the following?

    1. decreased night vision.
    2. angle-closure glaucoma.
    3. retinal detachment.
    4. central scotoma.

a. 1, 2, and 3.
b. 1 and 3.
c. 2 and 4.
d. 4 only.
e. 1, 2, 3, and 4.

21. Which one of the following concerning hemoglobinopathy and retinopathy is false?

a. The incidence of sickle cell disease in the black population is less than 1%.
b. The incidence of sickle cell trait in the black population is approximately 8%.
c. The incidence of SC disease in the black population is less than 0.5%.
d. Fortunately, retinopathy has never been reported in patients with sickle cell trait.
e. The ocular findings of sickle cell disease are not limited to the retina.

22. T or F -- Like diabetic retinopathy, the earliest pathophysiologic changes in proliferative sickle cell retinopathy include capillary closure and drop out.

23. T or F -- Like diabetic retinopathy, sickle cell retinopathy may have both nonproliferative and proliferative forms.

24. Which of the following is/are common manifestations of nonproliferative sickle cell retinopathy?

        1. salmon patches.
        2. iridescent deposits.
        3. black sunbursts.
        4. preretinal hemorrhage.

  a. 1, 2, and 3.
  b. 1 and 3.
  c. 2 and 4.
  d. 4 only.
  e. 1, 2, 3, and 4.

25. Which of the following may be causes of visual loss in sickle cell disease?

        1. vitreous hemorrhage.
        2. parafoveal capillary nonperfusion.
        3. retinal detachment.
        4. choroidal neovascularization.

  a. 1, 2, and 3.
  b. 1 and 3.
  c. 2 and 4.
  d. 4 only.
  e. 1, 2, 3, and 4.

26. T or F -- Angioid streaks have been associated with both sickle cell disease and sickle cell trait.

27. T or F -- Patients with sickle cell hemoglobinopathy are more prone to develop retinal arterial occlusions, both central and branch.

28. T or F -- The retinopathy of sickle cell disease (SS) is generally worse than that of SC or Sickle-cell thalassemia (SThal) disease.

29. Modalities useful in the treatment of proliferative sickle cell retinopathy include:

        1. pars plana vitrectomy with endolaser.
        2. scatter photocoagulation in the region of a neovascular frond.
        3. feeder-vessel photocoagulation.
        4. macular grid photocoagulation.

  a. 1, 2, and 3.
  b. 1 and 3.
  c. 2 and 4.
  d. 4 only.
  e. 1, 2, 3, and 4.

30. The American Academy of Pediatrics defines an infant at high risk for developing retinopathy of prematurity (ROP) as one who has received any oxygen and is:

> 1. less than 2000 gm (4 lb. 7 oz.) at birth.
> 2. born to a diabetic mother.
> 3. less than 36 weeks' gestation at birth.
> 4. a victim of another perinatal complication, such as necrotizing enterocolitis or intraventricular hemorrhage.

    a. 1, 2, and 3.
    b. 1 and 3.
    c. 2 and 4.
    d. 4 only.
    e. 1, 2, 3, and 4.

31. T or F -- The temporal retina is vascularized at 36 weeks' gestation, approximately 4 weeks before the nasal retina.

32. Spontaneous regression of retinopathy of prematurity occurs in approximately what percentage of infant eyes?

    a. 5%.
    b. 10%.
    c. 25%.
    d. 50%.
    e. greater than 75%.

33. Which of the following descriptions of severity of retinopathy of prematurity (ROP) is correct?

    a. stage 1: presence of a demarcation line having width and height (protruding into the vitreous).
    b. stage 2: an elevated demarcation line with preretinal fibrovascular proliferation.
    c. stage 3: a demarcation line having width and height (protuding into the vitreous cavity).
    d. stage 4: total retinal detachment.
    e. stage 5: total retinal detachment.

34. T or F -- The development of ROP requires the exposure of an immature retinal vascular system to some supplemental oxygen.

35. Which of the following criteria are part of the definition of a "high-risk" eye by the Cryo-ROP Treatment Trial?

    1. at least stage 3 disease.
    2. plus disease.
    3. 5 continuous clock hours or 8 interrupted clock hours of disease retina.
    4. rush disease.

    a. 1, 2, and 3.
    b. 1 and 3.
    c. 2 and 4.
    d. 4 only.
    e. 1, 2, 3, and 4.

36. Which of the following are considered necessary, but not sufficient, for the development of ROP?

    1. prematurity.
    2. supplemental oxygen exposure.
    3. low birth weight.
    4. immature retinal vascular system.

    a. 1, 2, and 3.
    b. 1 and 3.
    c. 2 and 4.
    d. 4 only.
    e. 1, 2, 3, and 4.

37. Which of the following concerning branch retinal vein occlusion (BRVO) is/are true?

    1. The inferotemporal quadrant is the most commonly affected.
    2. The actual site of focal occlusion is an arterial-venous crossing.
    3. BRVO is associated with primary open-angle glaucoma (POAG).
    4. BRVO is associated with systemic hypertension.

    a. 1, 2, and 3.
    b. 1 and 3.
    c. 2 and 4.
    d. 4 only.
    e. 1, 2, 3, and 4.

38. Common complications of BRVO include:

       1. macular edema.
       2. macular nonperfusion.
       3. neovascularization elsewhere.
       4. rubeotic glaucoma.

    a. 1, 2, and 3.
    b. 1 and 3.
    c. 2 and 4.
    d. 4 only.
    e. 1, 2, 3, and 4.

39. T or F -- The Branch Vein Occlusion Study (BVOS) documented recovery of a final visual acuity of 20/40 or better in nearly twice as many patients treated with argon macular grid laser (compared to those who were untreated).

40. Other conclusions of the Branch Vein Occlusion Study (BVOS) include which of the following?

       1. Quadrantic scatter photocoagulation reduces the risk of vitreous hemorrhage in eyes with established neovascularization.
       2. Quadrantic scatter photocoagulation reduces the risk of developing neovascularization if the area of retina affected by the vein occlusion is at least 5 disc diameters in size.
       3. Large areas of nonperfusion were a significant risk factor for the development of neovascularization.
       4. Quadrantic scatter photocoagulation should be used in patients with greater than 5 disc areas of nonperfusion.

    a. 1, 2, and 3.
    b. 1 and 3.
    c. 2 and 4.
    d. 4 only.
    e. 1, 2, 3, and 4.

41. T or F -- Nonischemic and ischemic central retinal vein occlusions should probably be considered as separate pathophysiologic disorders.

42. Which of the following would define a central retinal vein occlusion (CRVO) as nonischemic?

    a. mild vessel dilatation.
    b. mild disc edema.
    c. lack of significant parafoveal leakage on fluorescein angiography.
    d. lack of significant nonperfusion on fluorescein angiography.
    e. visual acuity better than 20/60.

43. T or F -- Nearly one-half of nonischemic CRVO resolve entirely without treatment.

44. Which of the following systemic disorders may be associated with CRVO?

        1. diabetes.
        2. multiple myeloma.
        3. hypertension.
        4. syphilis.

a. 1, 2, and 3.
b. 1 and 3.
c. 2 and 4.
d. 4 only.
e. 1, 2, 3, and 4.

45. T or F -- CRVO may be induced by acute angle-closure glaucoma.

46. T or F -- CRVO may induce acute angle-closure glaucoma.

47. Important markers of ischemic CRVO include all of the following except:

a. numerous cotton-wool spots.
b. extreme venous dilation.
c. retinal hemorrhages in all four quadrants.
d. extensive nonperfusion on fluorescein angiography.
e. b/a wave ratio < 1.0 on dark-adapted electroretinography.

48. Venous stasis retinopathy (carotid occlusive retinopathy) and CRVO share which of the following features?

        1. venous dilation.
        2. cotton-wool spots.
        3. mid-peripheral blot retinal hemorrhages.
        4. diminished central retinal arterial pressure.

a. 1, 2, and 3.
b. 1 and 3.
c. 2 and 4.
d. 4 only.
e. 1, 2, 3, and 4.

49. T or F -- Regardless of etiology, the final clinical manifestation of precapillary arteriolar occlusion is the cherry-red spot.

50. Branch retinal arterial occlusion (BRAO) may be associated with which of the following?

    1. mitral valve prolapse.
    2. cardiac myxoma.
    3. systemic lupus erythematosus.
    4. intravenous drug abuse.

a. 1, 2, and 3.
b. 1 and 3.
c. 2 and 4.
d. 4 only.
e. 1, 2, 3, and 4.

51. T or F -- Compared to ischemic CRVO, central retinal arterial occlusion (CRAO) has a better visual prognosis (i.e., a larger percentage of patients with final visual acuity of 20/400 or better).

52. Irreversible structural damage occurs in the retina after what duration of total ischemia?

a. 15-20 minutes.
b. 30-40 minutes.
c. 45-60 minutes.
d. 90-100 minutes.
e. 120 minutes.

53. Which of the following concerning idiopathic juxtafoveal telangiectasis is/are true?

    1. Of the four subtypes, only one seems to fall within the spectrum of Coats' disease.
    2. The histopathology of the adult forms of the disorder resembles diabetic retinopathy.
    3. Visual loss is generally due to macular edema and/or exudate.
    4. The risk of retinal neovascularization, as with diabetic retinopathy, may be lessened with scatter photocoagulation.

a. 1, 2, and 3.
b. 1 and 3.
c. 2 and 4.
d. 4 only.
e. 1, 2, 3, and 4.

54. Which of the following concerning idiopathic primary retinal vasculitis (Eales' disease) is/are true?

    1. It is primarily a disease of childhood and young adulthood, more commonly affecting girls.
    2. It may be associated with tuberculous infection.
    3. It is generally unilateral.
    4. It may be associated with epistaxis and a cerebral vasculitis.

a. 1, 2, and 3.
b. 1 and 3.
c. 2 and 4.
d. 4 only.
e. 1, 2, 3, and 4.

55. Retinal vasculitis may be associated with which of the following disorders?

    1. systemic lupus erythematosus.
    2. multiple sclerosis.
    3. polyarteritis nodosa.
    4. intravenous drug abuse.

a. 1, 2, and 3.
b. 1 and 3.
c. 2 and 4.
d. 4 only.
e. 1, 2, 3, and 4.

56. Which of the following regarding arterial macroaneurysms of the retina is/are true?

    1. They are generally associated with hypertension and are more frequent in older women.
    2. Visual loss is always due to associated macular edema.
    3. Laser treatment may be applied in the region of the macroaneurysm to reduce macular edema.
    4. Direct treatment of the macroaneurysm is most effective for reducing associated macular edema.

a. 1, 2, and 3.
b. 1 and 3.
c. 2 and 4.
d. 4 only.
e. 1, 2, 3, and 4.

57. Which one of the following concerning aphakic or pseudophakic cystoid macular edema is false?

   a. The incidence is lower with extracapsular surgery compared to intracapsular surgery.
   b. Intraocular lens implantation decreases the incidence of CME following cataract surgery.
   c. The presence of an intact posterior capsule is associated with a lower incidence of CME.
   d. Seventy-five percent of cases spontaneously regress within 6 months.
   e. Topical nonsteroidal anti-inflammatory medications have been shown to reduce the incidence as well as to improve vision in CME following cataract surgery.

58. Which one of the following concerning Coats' disease (retinal telangiectasis) is false?

   a. The male to female ratio is approximately 7:1.
   b. It is primarily a disease of childhood, although adults may be affected.
   c. Inheritance is autosomal dominant with incomplete penetrance.
   d. Patients whose disease has an onset before 4 years of age follow a more fulminant course.
   e. Treatment alternatives include photocoagulation and cryotherapy.

59. T or F -- Pathologically, the vascular lesion of von Hippel's disease is a cavernous hemangioma.

60. T or F -- Rhegmatogenous retinal detachment is uncommon in retinitis pigmentosa.

61. Findings in a patient with angiomatosis retinae (von Hippel's disease) may include all of the following except:

   a. café au lait spots.
   b. pancreatic and renal cysts.
   c. hemangioblastomas of the brainstem.
   d. renal cell carcinoma.
   e. pheochromocytoma.

62. T or F -- An ophthalmologist treating a retinal hemangioma may expect temporary worsening of exudation following successful treatment.

63. T or F -- Both congenital arteriovenous malformations of the retina (racemose angioma) and cavernous hemangiomas of the retina are distinquished from the vascular malformations of von Hippel's disease by the lack of exudation and subretinal fluid.

64. T or F -- The most common complication of retinal cavernous hemangioma is vitreous hemorrhage.

65. Which of the following constitutes the histoanatomic definition of the macula?

   a. the area of the retina with increased xanthophyll pigment concentration.
   b. the area of the retina whose ganglion cell layer is more than one cell thick.
   c. the area of the retina whose innermost layer is the outer plexiform layer.
   d. the area of the retina with the tallest retinal pigment epithelial cells.
   e. the area of the retina within the temporal arcades.

66. Which is the outermost layer supplied by the central retinal circulation?

   a. ganglion cell layer.
   b. inner plexiform layer.
   c. inner nuclear layer.
   d. outer plexiform layer.
   e. outer nuclear layer.

67. Which is the correct order of the five layers of Bruch's membrane (from retina toward sclera)?

   a. retinal pigment epithelium (RPE) basement membrane, inner collagenous zone, elastic layer, outer collagenous zone, and choriocapillaris basement membrane.
   b. RPE basement membrane, elastic layer, inner collagenous zone, outer collagenous zone, and choriocapillaris basement membrane.
   c. elastic layer, RPE basement membrane, inner collagenous zone, outer collagenous zone, and choriocapillaris basement membrane.
   d. inner collagenous zone, elastic layer, outer collagenous zone, RPE basement membrane, and choriocapillaris basement membrane.
   e. RPE basement membrane, inner collagenous zone, elastic layer, choriocapillaris basement membrane, and outer collagenous zone.

68. T or F -- Changes in the RPE and Bruch's membrane seen with aging may be due to an accumulation of metabolic breakdown products from the photoreceptor outer segments.

69. T or F -- The RPE acts as a depot for dietary and excess vitamin A (retinol).

70. T or F -- Hypertrophy of the RPE generally leads to a flat jet-black subretinal lesion, while hyperplasia most frequently leads to intraretinal bone spicule pigment deposition.

71. Which one of the following concerning fluorescein angiography and the blood-ocular barriers is true?

   a. Fluorescein is a large-molecular-weight compound normally confined to the intravascular space.
   b. Fluorescein absorbs light in the yellow-green range, 530 nm.
   c. After stimulation, fluorescein emits light in the blue range, 490 nm.
   d. The "red-free" filter is the initial filter through which white light passes before entering the eye.
   e. The most dreaded complication of fluorescein angiography is anaphylactic shock.

72. Which of the following concerning the characteristics of hyperfluorescence patterns on fluorescein angiography is/are true?

1. Staining generally refers to the uptake of fluorescein by solid collagenous tissue.
2. Transmitted fluorescence, or a window defect, generally implies a focal defect in the retinal pigment epithelium.
3. Pooling implies collections of fluorescein within fluid-filled spaces.
4. True leakage consists of early hyperfluorescence that diminishes in late views.

a. 1, 2, and 3.
b. 1 and 3.
c. 2 and 4.
d. 4 only.
e. 1, 2, 3, and 4.

73. Which of the following features are considered necessary for the development of retinal neovascularization?

1. production of a local angiogenic factor.
2. some source of endothelial cells capable of replication and migration.
3. a structural scaffold for vascular growth, presumably posterior cortical vitreous.
4. a focal defect in the internal limiting membrane.

a. 1, 2, and 3.
b. 1 and 3.
c. 2 and 4.
d. 4 only.
e. 1, 2, 3, and 4.

74. Which of the following may lead to visual loss in choroidal neovascularization?

1. focal subretinal exudate.
2. subretinal hemorrhage.
3. sensory retinal detachment .
4. photoreceptor atrophy.

a. 1, 2, and 3.
b. 1 and 3.
c. 2 and 4.
d. 4 only.
e. 1, 2, 3, and 4.

75. Which of the following concerning central serous retinopathy (CSR) is/are true?

   1. The classic fundus finding is a small serous detachment of the macula, although serous detachment of the pigment epithelium may also be seen.
   2. Fluorescein angiography performed at presentation will show a smokestack pattern of leakage 90% of the time.
   3. Affected patients over 45 years of age may be in a more aggressive subgroup.
   4. Laser photocoagulation of fluorescein leakage sites leads to improved final Snellen visual acuity.

   a. 1, 2, and 3.
   b. 1 and 3.
   c. 2 and 4.
   d. 4 only.
   e. 1, 2, 3, and 4.

76. T or F -- Eighty to 90% of cases of CSR will spontaneously resolve, but 40 to 50% will recur.

77. Patients who should be considered for laser treatment of CSR include:

   1. a patient whose sensory retinal detachment has persisted greater than 6 weeks.
   2. monocular patient with occupational visual needs.
   3. a patient with pigment epithelial detachment and surrounding sensory retinal detachment.
   4. a patient whose prior episodes of CSR have been associated with permanently decreased acuity.

   a. 1, 2, and 3.
   b. 1 and 3.
   c. 2 and 4.
   d. 1 and 3.
   e. 1, 2, 3, and 4.

78. Match the types of drusen listed on the left with the histopathologic findings on the right.

a. hard (nodular) drusen.
b. diffuse (confluent) drusen.
c. soft drusen.
d. calcific drusen.

1. small localized pigment epithelial detachment associated with a thickened inner Bruch's membrane.
2. nodular excrescenses between the inner collagenous layer of Bruch's membrane and the RPE basement membrane associated with dystrophic calcification.
3. broad thickening of the inner collagenous layer of Bruch's membrane.
4. nodular excrescences of membranaceous debris between the RPE basement membrane and inner Bruch's membrane.

79. T or F -- The feature necessary and sufficient for the diagnosis of age-related macular degeneration (AMD) is the presence of at least one type of drusen.

80. Risk factors for progressive visual loss in AMD include all of the following except:

a. hyperopia.
b. smoking.
c. light iris color.
d. hypertension.
e. family history of visual loss due to AMD.

81. Which of the following concerning the classification of AMD is/are true?

1. "Dry" AMD accounts for 90% of all patients affected by this disorder.
2. "Wet" AMD accounts for 90% of all patients with severe visual loss (worse than 20/200) who are affected by this disorder.
3. Patients with either pigment epithelial detachment or choroidal neovascularization should be considered as part of the wet variety.
4. In patients with dry AMD, those with central geographic atrophy generally preserve the best visual acuity.

a. 1, 2, and 3.
b. 1 and 3.
c. 2 and 4.
d. 1 and 3.
e. 1, 2, 3, and 4.

82. T or F -- Pigment epithelial detachment (PED) in a patient under the age of 50 years generally has a better prognosis than in a patient over the age of 50 years.

83. Argon laser photocoagulation for exudative AMD has been shown to be effective in reducing the rate of severe visual loss or preserving visual function among which categories of the disease?

1. extrafoveal (greater than 200 microns from the center of foveal avascular zone) choroidal neovascularization (CNV).
2. juxtafoveal CNV (1 to 199 microns from the center of the foveal avascular zone).
3. subfoveal CNV.
4. juxtafoveal PED.

a. 1, 2, and 3.
b. 1 and 3.
c. 2 and 4.
d. 4 only.
e. 1, 2, 3, and 4.

84. Which of the following factor(s) support an etiologic connection between ocular *Histoplasma* infection and the presumed ocular histoplasmosis syndrome (POHS)?

1. Over 90% of patients with POHS will have a positive histoplasmin skin reaction.
2. The highest prevalence of POHS is among the populations of the southwest states such as New Mexico, Arizona, and California.
3. *Histoplasma* organisms have been recovered from the human choroid.
4. Systemic treatment with antifungal agents leads to resolution of the ocular findings.

a. 1, 2, and 3.
b. 1 and 3.
c. 2 and 4.
d. 4 only.
e. 1, 2, 3, and 4.

85. Accepted methods of treatment of ocular POHS include:

1. systemic antifungal medications.
2. corticosteroids.
3. cryotherapy.
4. argon laser photocoagulation.

a. 1, 2, and 3.
b. 1 and 3.
c. 2 and 4.
d. 4 only.
e. 1, 2, 3, and 4.

86. The best predictor of future contralateral macular disease in a patient with a disciform macular scar from POHS is the presence or absence of:

    a. a focal macular scar in the better eye.
    b. peripapillary scarring in the better eye.
    c. active vitritis in the better eye.
    d. symmetric peripheral punched-out lesions of each eye.
    e. antihistoplasma antibodies.

87. Which of the following concerning angioid streaks is/are true?

    1. They always extend in continuity from the optic nerve head.
    2. They appear as window defects on fluorescein angiography.
    3. The typical pattern forms concentric circles around the optic nerve head.
    4. Histopathologically, they represent discontinuities in a thickened, abnormal Bruch's membrane.

    a. 1, 2, and 3.
    b. 1 and 3.
    c. 2 and 4.
    d. 4 only.
    e. 1, 2, 3, and 4.

88. Systemic disorders associated with angioid streaks include:

    1. Paget's disease of bone.
    2. pseudoxanthoma elasticum.
    3. Ehlers-Danlos syndrome.
    4. high myopia.

    a. 1, 2, and 3.
    b. 1 and 3.
    c. 2 and 4.
    d. 4 only.
    e. 1, 2, 3, and 4.

89. Idiopathic epiretinal membranes are bilateral in what proportion of affected patients?

    a. 5%.
    b. 20%.
    c. 50%.
    d. 75%.
    e. 100%.

90. T or F -- The majority of patients with idiopathic epiretinal membranes maintain vision better than 20/50.

91. T or F -- Pars plana vitrectomy and intraocular gas injection may be helpful in patients with established full-thickness macular holes.

92. Idiopathic macular holes are bilateral in what proportion of affected patients?

   a. 5%.
   b. 25%.
   c. 50%.
   d. 75%.
   e. 100%.

93. The lesion that is felt to be the immediate precursor to a full-thickness macular hole is:

   a. a partial posterior vitreous detachment.
   b. a macular cyst.
   c. a sensory retinal detachment involving the fovea.
   d. a pigment epithelial detachment under the fovea.
   e. Watzke's sign.

94. Which of the following concerning ocular toxicity of chloroquine and hydroxychloroquine is/are true?

   1. Only chloroquine has been clearly associated with retinal toxicity.
   2. Chloroquine may be associated with a vortex keratopathy.
   3. The most sensitive parameter for detecting chloroquine retinopathy is the electro-oculogram (EOG).
   4. Important tests in the evaluation for subclinical chloroquine retinopathy include color vision testing and threshold central visual field testing.

   a. 1, 2, and 3.
   b. 1 and 3.
   c. 2 and 4.
   d. 4 only.
   e. 1, 2, 3, and 4.

95. T or F -- Cessation of chloroquine treatment in a patient with established chloroquine retinopathy should lead to rapid reversal of the retinal findings.

96. T or F -- Both antimalarial agents (e.g., chloroquine) and antipsychotics (e.g., thioridazine) may cause peripheral pigmentary retinopathy with electroretinographic (ERG) abnormalities.

97. T or F -- Both thioridazine (Mellaril) and chlorpromazine (Thorazine) may lead to abnormal pigment deposition in eyelids, cornea, lens, and retina.

98. T or F -- All of the mucopolysaccharidoses (MPS) are autosomal dominant disorders except type II, which is X-linked recessive.

99. Corneal clouding is a common manifestation of which of the following MPS?

> 1. Type I-H (Hurler's syndrome).
> 2. Type II (Hunter's syndrome).
> 3. Type I-S (Scheie's syndrome).
> 4. Type III (Sanfilippo's syndrome).

a. 1, 2, and 3.
b. 1 and 3.
c. 2 and 4.
d. 4 only.
e. 1, 2, 3, and 4.

100. A pigmentary retinopathy indistinguishable from typical retinitis pigmentosa (RP) may be seen in which of the MPS?

> 1. Type I-H (Hurler's syndrome).
> 2. Type II (Hunter's syndrome).
> 3. Type III (Sanfilippo's syndrome).
> 4. Type IV (Morquio's syndrome).

a. 1, 2, and 3.
b. 1 and 3.
c. 2 and 4.
d. 4 only.
e. 1, 2, 3, and 4.

101. Optic atrophy may be seen in which of the following MPS?

> 1. Type II (Hunter's syndrome).
> 2. Type III (Sanfilippo's syndrome).
> 3. Type IV (Morquio's syndrome).
> 4. Type VII (Sly's syndrome).

a. 1, 2, and 3.
b. 1 and 3.
c. 2 and 4.
d. 4 only.
e. 1, 2, 3, and 4.

102. T or F -- Gangliosides are sphingolipids found only in the central nervous system, while cerebrosides are sphingolipids found throughout the body.

103. Which of the following disorders may be associated with a cherry-red spot?

        1. Tay-Sachs disease.
        2. Sandhoff's disease.
        3. Niemann-Pick disease.
        4. Fabry's disease.

a. 1, 2, and 3.
b. 1 and 3.
c. 2 and 4.
d. 4 only.
e. 1, 2, 3, and 4.

104. T or F -- In Fabry's disease, the leading cause of death is myocardial infarction.

105. Manifestations of Fabry's disease include:

        1. cornea verticillata.
        2. spoke-like posterior subcapsular cataract.
        3. conjunctival and retinal telangiectases.
        4. pigmentary retinopathy.

a. 1, 2, and 3.
b. 1 and 3.
c. 2 and 4.
d. 4 only.
e. 1, 2, 3, and 4.

106. Which of the following concerning cystinosis is/are true?

        1. Each of the three classes of cystinosis is associated with corneal crystals and photophobia.
        2. Each of the three classes of cystinosis is associated with a pigmentary retinopathy.
        3. Cysteamine administered topically may reduce the corneal crystal load and associated photophobia.
        4. Pigmentary retinopathy found in cystinosis is slowly progressive.

a. 1, 2, and 3.
b. 1 and 3.
c. 2 and 4.
d. 4 only.
e. 1, 2, 3, and 4.

107. What radiation dosage level may be considered a threshold for the development of radiation retinopathy?

    a. 500 rads.
    b. 1000 rads.
    c. 3000 rads.
    d. 5 gray.
    e. 15 gray.

108. Which one of the following concerning solar retinopathy is false?

    a. It is generally associated with sun gazing and, less commonly, arc welding.
    b. The lesion is a photochemical and photothermal insult to the RPE.
    c. Visual acuity loss is generally severe, in the hand motions to counting fingers range.
    d. Most patients recover near normal acuity over several months.
    e. The lesion appears as a small yellow white spot in the center of the fovea which fades over time.

109. Which of the following concerning the distribution of photoreceptors in the normal human retina is true?

    1. The ratio of rods to cones is approximately 4:1.
    2. The numbers of rods and cones in the macula (central 18 degrees) is equal.
    3. Cone density is maximal in a ring 20 to 40 degrees eccentric to the foveola.
    4. Forty percent of cones lie outside the macula.

    a. 1, 2, and 3.
    b. 1 and 3.
    c. 2 and 4.
    d. 4 only.
    e. 1, 2, 3, and 4.

110. Listed in the left column are photoreceptor types. In the right column are listed the wavelengths of maximum spectral sensitivity for a specific photoreceptor type. Match the appropriate spectral sensitivity peak with photoreceptor type.

    a. rods.   1. 505 nm.
    b. blue cones.   2. 575 nm.
    c. green cones.   3. 545 nm.
    d. red cones.   4. 445 nm.

111. Match the flash electroretinogram (ERG) component in the left column with the cell of origin in the right column.

    a. early receptor potential.
    b. a-wave.
    c. oscillatory potentials.
    d. b-wave.
    e. c-wave.

    1. retinal pigment epithelium (RPE).
    2. photoreceptor outer segments.
    3. Müller cells.
    4. photoreceptor cell bodies.
    5. amacrine cells.

112. T or F -- A blue flash of light in a dark-adapted patient will generate an ERG with rod input only.

113. T or F -- A blue flash of light in a light-adapted patient will generate an ERG with cone input only.

114. In order to truly isolate cone function, it is necessary to present a light stimulus as flicker-flash at what minimum frequency?

    a. 5 Hz.
    b. 10 Hz.
    c. 15 Hz.
    d. 20 Hz.
    e. 40 Hz.

115. The key feature on electroretinography distinguishing focal or nonprogressive retinal disease from a diffuse progressive degeneration is an abnormality in the:

    a. early receptor potential.
    b. a-wave amplitude.
    c. b-wave implicit time.
    d. b-wave amplitude.
    e. c-wave amplitude.

116. T or F -- Increasing the intensity of the stimulus flash in a scotopic ERG will result in a decrease in both implicit time and amplitude of the b-wave.

117. Which of the following disorders may be considered forms of congenital stationary night blindness (congenital stationary night blindness)?

    1. Oguchi's disease.
    2. choroideremia.
    3. fundus albipunctatus.
    4. fundus flavimaculatus.

    a. 1, 2, and 3.
    b. 1 and 3.
    c. 2 and 4.
    d. 4 only.
    e. 1, 2, 3, and 4.

118. Match the appropriate stimulus parameters (1-3) with the waveforms from a healthy eye below.

1. photopic (white flash in a light-adapted state).
2. scotopic (blue flash in a dark-adapted state).
3. dark-adapted bright flash (bright white flash in a dark-adapted state).

a.

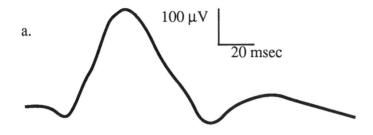

100 μV

20 msec

b.

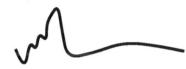

c.

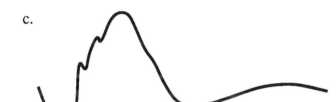

119. Match the waveform sets (a-c) shown below with the appropriate disorder (1 - 3).

1. congenital achromatopsia.
2. progressive rod-cone degeneration.
3. congenital stationary night blindness.

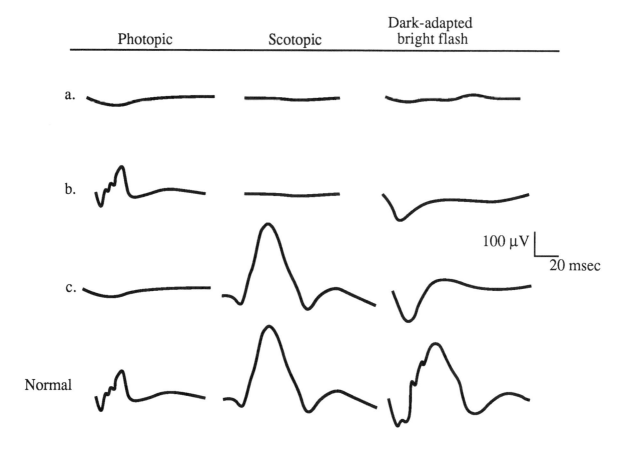

120. Which of the following concerning electro-oculography (EOG) is/are true?

1. The corneal surface or vitreal space is positive relative to sclera.
2. Amplitudes generally diminish with light-adaptation and increase with dark-adaptation.
3. Amplitudes are typically measured by alternating lateral gaze from left to right.
4. An EOG is generally considered abnormal if the dark-peak to light-trough is less than 1.75.

a. 1, 2, and 3.
b. 1 and 3.
c. 2 and 4.
d. 4 only.
e. 1, 2, 3, and 4.

121. Electro-oculography (EOG) and electroretinography (ERG) are similar depressed for all of the following except:

    a. choroideremia.
    b. gyrate atrophy.
    c. Oguchi's disease.
    d. Best's disease.
    e. X-linked recessive retinitis pigmentosa.

122. The electro-oculogram (EOG) may be valuable in evaluating patients with potential retinal toxicity from:

    a. ultraviolet light.
    b. chloroquine.
    c. phenothiazines.
    d. isoniazid.
    e. amiodarone.

123. After dark adaptation, how much more sensitive are rods than cones?

    a. 10 times (1 log unit).
    b. 100 times (2 log units).
    c. 1000 times (3 log units).
    d. 10,000 times (4 log units).
    e. 100,000 times (5 log units).

124. Match the chromosomal location of the genes responsible for the photopigments of each photoreceptor type.

    a. rods (rhodopsin).   1. X chromosome.
    b. s-cones (blue).   2. Y chromosome.
    c. m-cones (green).   3. chromosome 3.
    d. l-cones (red).   4. chromosome 7.

125. T or F -- A ganglion cell whose receptive field consists of an off-center on-surround will increase its firing rate if stimulation to its central photoreceptors is diminished.

126. T or F -- The Purkinje shift refers to the enhancement in light sensitivity during dark adaptation (the shift from cone threshold sensitivity to rod threshold sensitivity).

127. T or F -- A red cone attached directly to a ganglion cell could induce a high rate of ganglion cell firing if appropriately stimulated with monochromatic green light.

128. Match the type of color vision defect in the right-hand column with the most typical characteristics listed in left-hand column.

a. red-green axis.
b. blue-yellow axis.
c. males affected much more frequently than females.
d. males and females affected equally.
e. may be slowly progressive.
f. generally nonprogressive.
g. generally symmetric.
h. generally unilateral or asymmetric.
i. generally associated with some demonstrable pathology on examination.
j. generally an otherwise normal eye examination.
k. generally no genetic pattern.
l. transmitted as an X-linked recessive trait.
m. deep blue is perceived as gray.
n. deep blue is perceived as purple.

1. congenital dyschromatopsia.
2. acquired dyschromatopsia.
3. both.
4. neither.

129. The most common pattern of congenital dyschromatopsia is:

a. deuteranomaly.
b. protanomaly.
c. protanopia.
d. deuteranopia.
e. tritanopia.

130. Which forms of congenital dyschromatopsia are accompanied by abnormally low visual acuity?

1. protanopia.
2. blue cone monochromatism.
3. red cone monochromatism.
4. rod monochromatism.

a. 1, 2, and 3.
b. 1 and 3.
c. 2 and 4.
d. 4 only.
e. 1, 2, 3, and 4.

131. Which of the following help to distinguish between rod monochromats and blue cone monochromats?

        1. specific vision color testing.
        2. the presence or absence of nystagmus.
        3. careful family history.
        4. ERG waveforms.

a. 1, 2, and 3.
b. 1 and 3.
c. 2 and 4.
d. 4 only.
e. 1, 2, 3, and 4.

132. Which of the following color vision tests detect both red-green and blue-yellow defects?

        1. Hardy-Rand-Rittler plates.
        2. Farnsworth-Munsell 100 test.
        3. Farnsworth panel D-15 test.
        4. Ishihara plates.

a. 1, 2, and 3.
b. 1 and 3.
c. 2 and 4.
d. 4 only.
e. 1, 2, 3, and 4.

133. Match the approximate rates of occurrence of retinitis pigmentosa (RP) with each type of RP.

a. 5 to 10% (of all RP patients).   1. simplex type.
b. 15 to 20% (of all RP patients).   2. autosomal recessive.
c. 20 to 25% (of all RP patients).   3. X-linked recessive.
d. 45 to 50% (of all RP patients).   4. autosomal dominant.

134. In the left-hand column are listed systemic disorders associated with pigmentary retinopathies. Match each of these with the appropriate manifestations listed in the right-hand column.

a. myotonic dystrophy.
b. olivopontocerebellar degeneration.
c. Stickler's syndrome.
d. Bassen-Kornzweig syndrome.
e. Bardet-Biedl syndrome.
f. DIDMOAD syndrome.
g. Kearns-Sayre syndrome.
h. Refsum's disease.

1. progressive external ophthalmoplegia associated with heart block.
2. diabetes mellitus diabetes insipidus, optic atrophy, and neurosensory deafness.
3. cerebellar ataxia with or without external ophthalmoplegia.
4. high myopia, vitreoretinal degeneration, facial anomalies, and nonerosive peripheral arthropathy.
5. partial deafness, cerebellar ataxia, and elevations of phytanic acid.
6. frontal bossing, testicular atrophy, muscle wasting, Christmas tree cataract.
7. mild mental retardation, obesity, hypogonadism, polydactyly.
8. abetalipoproteinemia, anemia, celiac sprue.

135. T or F -- The vast majority of severe hearing loss associated with retinitis pigmentosa (RP) is congenital.

136. Which one of the following concerning congenital retinitis pigmentosa (RP) is false?

a. In Leber's congenital amaurosis, the infant is typically blind at birth.
b. In Leber's congenital amaurosis, the electroretinogram is typically nonrecordable at birth.
c. In Leber's congenital amaurosis, the fundus examination is typically normal at birth.
d. A variety of congenital RP is associated with macular coloboma and skeletal abnormalities.
e. The most common pattern of inheritance in congenital RP is autosomal dominant.

137. T or F -- Usher's syndrome describes any combination of pigmentary retinopathy and partial or complete deafness.

138. T or F -- Many patients with Usher's syndrome may have cerebellar and/or vestibular abnormalities.

139. Preservation of central acuity past the age of 45 years in a patient with a retinal degeneration and an X-linked inheritance pattern suggests the diagnosis of:

a. recessive cone-rod degeneration.
b. gyrate atrophy.
c. Refsum's disease.
d. choroideremia.
e. Usher's syndrome type I.

140. T or F -- Bone spicule pigmentation is unusual in choroideremia.

141. Which of the following concerning gyrate atrophy is/are true?

1. It is inherited on a X-linked recessive basis.
2. There is a systemic deficiency in ornithine aminotransferase activity.
3. Serum abnormalities include hyperornithinemia and hyperlysinemia.
4. Life span is normal in this disorder.

a. 1, 2, and 3.
b. 1 and 3.
c. 2 and 4.
d. 4 only.
e. 1, 2, 3, and 4.

142. Which of the following concerning fundus flavimaculatus is/are true?

1. The pisciform lesions seen in the posterior fundus represent lipofuscin deposits within hypertrophied RPE cells.
2. The most common mode of inheritance is autosomal recessive.
3. Visual acuity loss may be mild or severe depending on the extent of macular involvement.
4. The degree of ERG abnormality parallels the amount of fundus involvement.

a. 1, 2, and 3.
b. 1 and 3.
c. 2 and 4.
d. 4 only.
e. 1, 2, 3, and 4.

143. Which of the following regarding familial drusen (Doyne's honeycomb dystrophy) is/are true?

    1. The initial fundus manifestations generally appear in the third decade.
    2. Most cases are diagnosed in the third decade.
    3. There are both atrophic (dry) and exudative (wet) forms of the disease.
    4. The ERG is generally markedly depressed.

a. 1, 2, and 3.
b. 1 and 3.
c. 2 and 4.
d. 4 only.
e. 1, 2, 3, and 4.

144. Which of the following is considered the hallmark of fundus albipunctatus?

a. loss of dark adaptation with relative preservation of color vision and visual field.
b. loss of the scotopic ERG with preservation of cone responses.
c. normalization of scotopic ERG after 4 to 8 hours of dark adaptation.
d. punctate yellow/white deposits scattered throughout the equatorial and peripheral fundus.
e. the Mizuo phenomenon.

145. T or F -- In Best's disease, the macular appearance is considerably worse than the visual acuity.

146. T or F -- In Stargardt's disease, the macular appearance is considerably worse than the visual acuity.

147. The Mizuo phenomenon is a feature of which of the following disorders?

    1. Oguchi's disease.
    2. fundus albipunctatus.
    3. X-linked cone dystrophy.
    4. fundus flavimaculatus.

a. 1, 2, and 3.
b. 1 and 3.
c. 2 and 4.
d. 4 only.
e. 1, 2, 3, and 4.

148. Symptoms of cone degeneration include which of the following?

    1. loss of visual acuity.
    2. photophobia.
    3. progressive dyschromatopsia.
    4. difficulty driving at night.

    a. 1, 2, and 3.
    b. 1 and 3.
    c. 2 and 4.
    d. 4 only.
    e. 1, 2, 3, and 4.

149. Match the characteristics listed in the left-hand column with the type of retinoschisis listed in the right-hand column.

    a. schisis cavity most commonly located inferotemporally.
    b. schisis cavity located in the fovea.
    c. schisis cavity arises within the nerve fiber layer.
    d. schisis cavity arises within the outer plexiform layer.
    e. frequently presents with vitreous hemorrhage.
    f. frequently an incidental finding.
    g. reticular pattern associated with retinal detachment.
    h. may be associated with a panretinal degeneration.
    i. no known inheritance pattern.

    1. juvenile retinoschisis.
    2. degenerative retinoschisis.
    3. both.
    4. neither.

150. The differential diagnosis of peripheral pigmentary retinopathy includes:

    1. syphilitic chorioretinitis.
    2. prior exudative retinal detachment.
    3. phenothiazine toxicity.
    4. ophthalmic artery occlusion.

    a. 1, 2, and 3.
    b. 1 and 3.
    c. 2 and 4.
    d. 4 only.
    e. 1, 2, 3, and 4.

151. Fundus abnormalities associated with congenital stationary night blindness (CSNB) may be seen in:

        1. autosomal dominant CSNB.
        2. fundus albipunctatus.
        3. autosomal recessive CSNB.
        4. Oguchi's disease.

  a. 1, 2, and 3.
  b. 1 and 3.
  c. 2 and 4.
  d. 4 only.
  e. 1, 2, 3, and 4.

152. Foveal hypoplasia may be associated with which of the following disorders?

        1. albinism.
        2. congenital cytomegalovirus disease.
        3. aniridia.
        4. Leber's congenital amaurosis.

  a. 1, 2, and 3.
  b. 1 and 3.
  c. 2 and 4.
  d. 4 only.
  e. 1, 2, 3, and 4.

153. Which one of the following concerning Stargardt's disease is false?

  a. It is generally inherited on an autosomal dominant basis.
  b. It may be associated with peripheral flecks indistinguishable from fundus flavimaculatus.
  c. In its early stages, the maculopathy has a beaten metal appearance, similar to cone-rod dystrophy.
  d. In fundus flavimaculatus, the fluorescein angiogram may reveal a "dark choroid."
  e. The terminal stages of the maculopathy resemble central areolar choroidal dystrophy.

154. T or F -- In typical vitelliform dystrophy, it is unusual for visual acuity to deteriorate beyond 20/200.

155. Which of the following regarding Best's vitelliform dystrophy is/are true?

    1. The general mode of inheritance is autosomal dominant.
    2. Because of its profound effect on visual acuity, the "egg yolk" stage of the disease is frequently found at presentation.
    3. Histopathology reveals abnormal accumulation of lipofuscin within the retinal pigment epithelium and choroid.
    4. The amount of lipofuscin accumulation in an "egg yolk lesion" is proportionally reflected in the EOG.

    a. 1, 2, and 3.
    b. 1 and 3.
    c. 2 and 4.
    d. 4 only.
    e. 1, 2, 3, and 4.

156. T or F -- The adult type of vitelliform macular dystrophy features egg yolk lesions that are smaller than those of classic Best's disease.

157. T or F -- Adult vitelliform macular dystrophy (foveomacular dystrophy) may involve regions other than the fovea, but never simultaneously.

158. Which of the following concerning pattern dystrophies of the retinal pigment epithelium is/are true?

    1. Visual acuity is generally well preserved until late in life.
    2. Clinical examination generally discloses more abnormalities than can be documented with fluorescein angiography.
    3. The ERG is generally normal.
    4. The EOG is generally normal.

    a. 1, 2, and 3.
    b. 1 and 3.
    c. 2 and 4.
    d. 4 only.
    e. 1, 2, 3, and 4.

159. Albinism and albinoidism share which of the following features?

    1. iris transillumination.
    2. markedly decreased vision.
    3. blond fundi.
    4. nystagmus.

    a. 1, 2, and 3.
    b. 1 and 3.
    c. 2 and 4.
    d. 4 only.
    e. 1, 2, 3, and 4.

160. Abnormalties in the visual pathways of patients with true albinism include:

    1. reduced number of ganglion cells.
    2. inappropriate decussation of temporal retinal nerve fibers.
    3. grossly hypoplastic lateral geniculate nuclei.
    4. foveal hypoplasia.

    a. 1, 2, and 3.
    b. 1 and 3.
    c. 2 and 4.
    d. 4 only.
    e. 1, 2, 3, and 4.

161. T or F -- Albinism and albinoidism may be distinguished on the basis of inheritance.

162. The only form of true albinism that is not inherited on an autosomal recessive basis is:

    a. Hermansky-Pudlak syndrome.
    b. tyrosinase-positive oculocutaneous albinism.
    c. Nettleship-Falls ocular albinism.
    d. Chédiak-Higashi syndrome.
    e. yellow-mutant variety of oculocutaneous albinism.

163. Which forms of true albinism are potentially lethal?

    1. tyrosinase-positive.
    2. Chédiak-Higashi syndrome.
    3. yellow-mutant variety.
    4. Hermansky-Pudlak syndrome.

    a. 1, 2, and 3.
    b. 1 and 3.
    c. 2 and 4.
    d. 4 only.
    e. 1, 2, 3, and 4.

164. Disadvantages of xenon arc photocoagulation include:

    1. expensive, sophisticated machinery.
    2. unfocused white light emission.
    3. inability to generate large amounts of power.
    4. considerable amount of emitted blue light.

    a. 1, 2, and 3.
    b. 1 and 3.
    c. 2 and 4.
    d. 4 only.
    e. 1, 2, 3, and 4.

165. Which laser is least absorbed by hemoglobin or red blood cells (RBCs)?

    a. xenon arc.
    b. argon blue-green.
    c. argon green.
    d. krypton red.
    e. tunable dye.

166. Which laser is best for retinal photocoagulation in the setting of dense cataract or vitreous hemorrhage?

    a. xenon arc.
    b. argon blue-green.
    c. argon green.
    d. krypton red.
    e. tunable dye.

167. T or F -- Decreasing the spot size of an argon laser burn increases the energy delivered per unit area.

168. To decrease the pain associated with laser photocoagulation, which parameter of treatment should be changed?

    a. duration of treatment.
    b. spot size.
    c. wavelength.
    d. type of laser.
    e. power.

169. Which of the following are potential complications of fundus photocoagulation?

    1. choroidal neovascularization.
    2. traction retinal detachment.
    3. epiretinal membrane.
    4. angle-closure glaucoma.

    a. 1, 2, and 3.
    b. 1 and 3.
    c. 2 and 4.
    d. 4 only.
    e. 1, 2, 3, and 4.

170. Points of firm vitreoretinal attachment include:

> 1. the vitreous base.
> 2. the edge of retinal scars.
> 3. the edge of lattice retinal degeneration.
> 4. over the vortex veins.

a. 1, 2, and 3.
b. 1 and 3.
c. 2 and 4.
d. 4 only.
e. 1, 2, 3, and 4.

171. T or F -- The prevalence of posterior vitreous detachment (PVD) is higher after intracapsular cataract surgery than after extracapsular cataract surgery.

172. What proportion of patients with an acute symptomatic PVD have a retinal tear?

a. 5%.
b. 10%.
c. 25%.
d. 50%.
e. 75%.

173. What proportion of patients with acute symptomatic PVD and associated vitreous hemorrhage have a retinal tear?

a. 5%.
b. 10%.
c. 25%.
d. 50%.
e. 75%.

174. T or F -- The majority of retinal dialyses occur in the inferotemporal quadrant.

175. T or F -- The majority of superonasal retinal dialyses will be associated with a clear history of head or eye trauma.

176. The prevalence of lattice retinal degeneration in the adult population is approximately:

a. 5%.
b. 10%.
c. 25%.
d. 50%.
e. 75%.

177. The prevalence of lattice retinal degeneration in patients with rhegmatogenous retinal detachment is approximately:

 a. 5%.
 b. 10%.
 c. 25%.
 d. 50%.
 e. 75%.

178. T or F -- In lattice retinal degeneration, histopathology reveals abnormally strong vitreoretinal attachments over the affected retina.

179. Which of the following conditions are felt to increase the risk of rhegmatogenous retinal detachment (RRD)?

 1. lattice degeneration.
 2. oral pearls.
 3. meridional complexes.
 4. cobblestone degeneration.

 a. 1, 2, and 3.
 b. 1 and 3.
 c. 2 and 4.
 d. 4 only.
 e. 1, 2, 3, and 4.

180. The incidence of cobblestone degeneration in the adult population is approximately:

 a. 5%.
 b. 10%.
 c. 25%.
 d. 50%.
 e. 75%.

181. In what proportion of RRD can a retinal break not be found?

 a. 1%.
 b. 3%.
 c. 5%.
 d. 10%.
 e. 20%.

182. Findings consistent with RRD rather than exudative or tractional detachment include:

    1. shifting fluid.
    2. "tobacco dust."
    3. smooth, domed appearance of the retina.
    4. undulation of the retina with eye movements.

    a. 1, 2, and 3.
    b. 1 and 3.
    c. 2 and 4.
    d. 4 only.
    e. 1, 2, 3, and 4.

183. The most common cause of redetachment following initially successful surgical repair of rhegmatogenous retinal detachment is:

    a. occult retinal breaks.
    b. new retinal breaks.
    c. inadequate retinopexy.
    d. proliferative vitreoretinopathy.
    e. failure to relieve vitreoretinal traction adequately.

184. Prognostic factors favoring an excellent outcome after surgery for RRD include:

    1. aphakic detachment.
    2. retinal detachment associated with choroidal detachment.
    3. retinal detachments with breaks larger than 180 degrees.
    4. retinal dialyses.

    a. 1, 2, and 3.
    b. 1 and 3.
    c. 2 and 4.
    d. 4 only.
    e. 1, 2, 3, and 4.

185. The key prognostic factor in predicting postoperative visual acuity following surgical repair of RRD is:

    a. the size of the largest retinal break.
    b. the number of retinal breaks.
    c. the presence and duration of macular detachment.
    d. the presence or absence of lattice degeneration.
    e. the presence or absence of myopia.

186. The finding most frequently associated with degenerative retinoschisis is:

    a. degenerative cystoid degeneration.
    b. bullous retinoschisis.
    c. reticular retinoschisis.
    d. rhegmatogenous retinal detachment.
    e. retinal dialysis.

187. Which of the following concerning retinoschisis is/are true?

    1. Typical degenerative retinoschisis is associated with an increased risk of retinal detachment.
    2. The majority of patients with retinoschisis are hyperopic.
    3. The scotoma associated with retinoschisis is identical to that associated with RRD.
    4. Retinoschisis is bilateral in the majority of patients.

    a. 1, 2, and 3.
    b. 1 and 3.
    c. 2 and 4.
    d. 4 only.
    e. 1, 2, 3, and 4.

188. T or F -- Simple retinoschisis (no retinal detachment) may be associated with a demarcation line.

189. T or F -- Retinal detachment associated with retinoschisis requires holes in both the inner and outer walls of the schisis cavity.

190. Match the funduscopic findings of retinal detachment in the left-hand column with the specific types listed in the right-hand column.

    a. corrugated retinal suface.
    b. shifting fluid.
    c. fixed folds.
    d. concave toward the front of the eye.
    e. smooth, domed appearance.
    f. convex toward the front of the eye.
    g. retina moves with eye movements.

    1. exudative retinal detachment (RD).
    2. traction RD.
    3. rhegmatogenous RD.
    4. 1 and 3.
    5. 2 and 3.

191. T or F -- Because prepapillary vascular loops of the retina are remnants of the hyaloid artery, they never cause any retinal vascular complications.

192. Features differentiating persistent hyperplastic primary vitreous (PHPV) from retinoblastoma include:

       1. age of onset of leukocoria.
       2. presence of microphthalmos.
       3. calcification.
       4. presence of cataract.

  a. 1, 2, and 3.
  b. 1 and 3.
  c. 2 and 4.
  d. 4 only.
  e. 1, 2, 3, and 4.

193. Features differentiating Wagner's disease from Stickler's syndrome include:

       1. cataract.
       2. mid-facial flattening.
       3. high myopia.
       4. high incidence of retinal detachment.

  a. 1, 2, and 3.
  b. 1 and 3.
  c. 2 and 4.
  d. 4 only.
  e. 1, 2, 3, and 4.

194. T or F -- The best way of differentiating familial exudative vitreoretinopathy from retinopathy of prematurity is careful examination of family members.

195. Which one of the following concerning asteroid hyalosis is false?

  a. It is more common with aging.
  b. It is more commonly bilateral.
  c. It is generally associated with no decrease in visual acuity.
  d. The vitreous is otherwise normal.
  e. The particulate matter seen clinically consists of calcium soaps.

196. T or F -- The deposits of synchysis scintillans are more likely to settle inferiorly than those of asteroid hyalosis.

197. The most common cause of vitreous hemorrhage in the American adult population is:

  a. trauma.
  b. retinal tear.
  c. PVD.
  d. diabetic retinopathy.
  e. retinal neovascularization secondary to retinal vein occlusion.

198. What conditions mandate repair with pars plana vitrectomy rather than conventional scleral buckling?

      1. retinal dialysis.
      2. traumatic retinal detachment with accompanying vitreous hemorrhage.
      3. aphakic retinal detachment.
      4. retinal detachment associated with marked proliferative vitreoretinopathy.

a. 1, 2, and 3.
b. 1 and 3.
c. 2 and 4.
d. 4 only.
e. 1, 2, 3, and 4.

199. Advantages of early vitrectomy surgery in a diabetic with vitreous hemorrhage include:

      1. an opportunity to remove the vitreous scaffold which fosters neovascularization.
      2. a lower incidence of complete blindness following vitrectomy surgery in diabetics, compared to nondiabetics.
      3. an opportunity to treat retinal ischemia intensively with endolaser.
      4. an opportunity to remove the lens surgically and improve visualization of the retina for subsequent treatment.

a. 1, 2, and 3.
b. 1 and 3.
c. 2 and 4.
d. 4 only.
e. 1, 2, 3, and 4.

200. Indications for emergent pars plana vitrectomy surgery on an eye with an acute (i.e., unrepaired) rupture or laceration include:

      1. vitreous hemorrhage and associated retinal detachment.
      2. intraocular foreign body.
      3. traumatic endophthalmitis.
      4. vitreous hemorrhage.

a. 1, 2, and 3.
b. 1 and 3.
c. 2 and 4.
d. 4 only.
e. 1, 2, 3, and 4.

201. Which of the following conditions is likely to lead to permanently decreased visual acuity following trauma?

    1. commotio retinae.
    2. subretinal hemorrhage under the fovea.
    3. Valsalva retinopathy involving the fovea.
    4. traumatic macular hole.

    a. 1, 2, and 3.
    b. 1 and 3.
    c. 2 and 4.
    d. 4 only.
    e. 1, 2, 3, and 4.

202. Purtscher's retinopathy has characteristic fundus findings that may be seen in association with:

    1. vigorous chest compression.
    2. acute pancreatitis.
    3. long bone fracture.
    4. systemic lupus erythematosus (SLE).

    a. 1, 2, and 3.
    b. 1 and 3.
    c. 2 and 4.
    d. 4 only.
    e. 1, 2, 3, and 4.

203. A 33-year-old male physician presents to an ophthalmologist complaining of several days of blurry vision in his left eye. He denies any pain, Uhtoff's symptom, or phosphenes. His uncorrected acuity is 20/15 OD and 20/25 OS. Retinoscopy reveals +0.25 +0.25 X 180 OD (giving 20/15) and +1.75 OS (giving 20/20 minus). The external, neuromuscular, and slit-lamp examinations are normal, except for bilateral dyschromatopsia. The right fundus is normal; the left macula is shown in color plates 20 and 21. Which of the following regarding this condition is/are true?

    1. A significant minority of patients will have bilateral involvement.
    2. The patient's refractive error in his left eye was probably different 1 week earlier.
    3. A distinctive form of this disorder is seen in pregnant women.
    4. Laser therapy is effective in preventing recurrences.

    a. 1, 2, and 3.
    b. 1 and 3.
    c. 2 and 4.
    d. 4 only.
    e. 1, 2, 3, and 4.

204. A 69-year-old woman presents to an ophthalmologist complaining of sudden loss of vision in her left eye on the previous day. She denies any pain or phosphenes. Visual acuity is 20/25 OD and 20/400 OS. Examination of the anterior segment is normal. The right fundus is normal, with the exception of mildly dilated retinal veins. The left fundus is shown in color plate 22. All of the following should be part of the initial diagnostic workup except:

a. serum immunoelectrophoresis.
b. FTA-ABS.
c. blood pressure measurement.
d. blood glucose measurement.
e. sensitive thyrotropin (TSH) assay.

205. Color plates 23 and 24 show the left fundus of a 74-year-old man who has noted gradual loss of vision in both eyes. Acuity is 20/40 OD and 20/70 OS. Nuclear/cortical cataract is felt to explain approximately 20/40 acuity bilaterally. The right fundus is normal, except for scattered drusen. Which one of the following regarding this situation is true?

a. Peripheral retinal examination is likely to reveal vascular sheathing.
b. The hemorrhage seen around the optic nerve is derived from the retinal circulation.
c. The process responsible for diminished acuity is probably infectious.
d. Laser photocoagulation has been shown to reduce the incidence of severe visual loss in this condition.
e. The drusen are unrelated to the cause of diminished acuity.

25% of Pts c̄ DM have NPDR

5% of " " " " PDR

At 7 yrs of Duration of IDDM 50% have Retinopathy

At 25 yrs " " " " 90% " "

25% have PDR.

HTN GRADES

0

1 Mild Arteriolar Narrowing

2 Significant Narrowing, c̄ focal areas

3 2+ Retinal Hemorrhages & Edema

4 3+ Disc edema

ARTERIOLAR Sclerosis Grades

0

1 Mild ↑ Reflex

2 Marked

3 copper

4 Silver.

Answers

1. c.   There is thickening of arteriolar walls that leads to nicking of venules, not vice versa.

2. d.   <u>Acute</u> hypertensive episodes can lead to fibrinoid necrosis of choroidal arterioles. The choroid responds to chronic systemic hypertension in a complex fashion that is usually clinically silent.

3. e.   Of course, the type and severity of the disease strongly influence these estimates.

4. c.   The early stages of diabetic retinopathy involve primarily vascular changes. Trouble with photopigment recycling and catabolism is not a factor in the pathogenesis of diabetic retinal disease.

5. True.   Vitreous fluorophotometry may reaveal leakage of fluorescein into the vitreous from abnormally permeable retinal vessels before any clinically detectable changes have occurred.

6. False.   Loss of retinal vascular endothelial tight junctions have been implicated, but the barrier function of the retinal pigment epithelium is generally intact.

7. a.   Pericyte loss occurs early in diabetic retinopathy. Capillary closure may also be seen. Basement membrane thickening is found not just in the eye, but systemically in diabetics. Medial hyperplasia is a feature of hypertensive vasculopathy.

8. False.   The diffuse pattern is associated with more widespread vascular insult and is more difficult to treat than most cases of focal edema.

9. c.   Retinal thickening within the temporal arcades would encompass all macular edema, much of which does not imminently threaten vision. Extensive foveal and parafoveal nonperfusion would imply that the likelihood of improving vision would be small, even with treatment of any associated edema.

10. c.   Formation of extensive IRMA implies widespread severe injury to small arterioles, with the resulting ischemic state commonly being the immediate predecessor of neovascularization. The other options are features of lower risk, nonproliferative retinopathy, with the exception of disc neovascularization (which is a form of proliferative retinopathy).

11. d.

12. True.   New vessels that have not breached the membrane would be better described as IRMA.

13. False.   Retinal tears can easily occur as a result of vitreo-retinal adhesions formed at areas of neovascularization.

14. e.

15. d.   All of the others are either difficult to treat successfully (cystoid macular edema) or are associated with significant retinal damage from previous insult (foveal nonperfusion and extensive foveal hard exudate).

16. True.

17. False.   The ETDRS found that twice as many untreated patients <u>lost</u> vision. It is not accurate to conclude that laser treatment is likely to improve vision in diabetic macular edema.

18. True.   A 60% reduction in progression to severe visual loss was reported.

19. d.   Disc neovascularization greater than half of one disc area is considered high risk, whether or not it is associated with vitreous hemorrhage. This is in distinction to neovascularization elsewhere, which must be associated with bleeding to qualify as high risk. In the setting of vitreous hemorrhage, moderate to severe neovascularization is considered high risk (any new disc vessels associated with hemorrhage are high risk).

20. e.   Decreased night vision results from destruction of extramacular rods. Angle-closure glaucoma may occur after particularly heavy treatment associated with choroidal effusions. Regression of neovascular fronds may be associated wtih contracture and secondary rhegmatogenous or traction retinal detachment. Central scotoma should not be seen acutely following properly performed PRP, but may be seen days to weeks later, due to aggravation of diabetic macular edema.

21. d.   Though rare, cases of retinopathy have been reported in association with sickle trait only. In addition, sickle cell disease can be associated with angioid streaks and comma-shaped conjunctival capillaries.

22. True.   Both are felt to be caused by a similar mechanism: capillary nonperfusion with subsequent retinal ischemia, leading to the production of a vasogenic, diffusible substance. In sickle cell retinopathy, elevated blood viscosity may occlude venules and arterioles, as well as capillaries.

23. True.

24. a.   Preretinal hemorrhage may rarely be seen in nonproliferative disease but typically heralds neovascularization.

25. e.   All can occur. With SS disease, obstruction of the central macular blood supply may occur due to thrombosis of a cilioretinal or macular branch artery. This complication is very unusual in other forms of sickle hemoglobinopathies. Conversely, neovascularization is a relatively uncommon feature of SS retinopathy. If choroidal neovascularization occurs, it is usually related to angioid streaks. As in diabetes, contracture of neovascular fronds may lead to retinal detachment.

26. True.   A number of systemic disorders are associated with angioid streaks, including both sickle cell disease and sickle cell trait. Others include pseudoxanthoma elasticum, Paget's disease of bone, and Ehlers-Danlos syndrome. About 50% of patients with angioid streaks have no associated systemic condition.

27. True.

28. False. Retinal neovascularization, vitreous hemorrhage, and retinal detachments are more characteristic of SC and SThal than of SS disease. This is presumed to be related to the more severe anemia and, subsequently, lower blood viscosity of SS disease.

29. a. Photocoagulation to close the feeder vessels of neovascular fronds can cause regression of the neovascularization but is associated with a relatively high rate of complications. Scatter photocoagulation to the region involved with the neovascularization can effectively control it, with fewer complications. With dense vitreous hemorrhage, vitrectomy may be necessary to permit laser treatment.

30. b. High-risk infants are defined as less than 36 weeks' gestation or birth weight less than 2000 gm who have received oxygen therapy.

31. False. The nasal retina is usually vascularized prior to the temporal side, usually at 36 weeks' gestation. Vascularization of the temporal retina is generally complete by term.

32. e. Natural history studies estimate an 85% rate of spontaneous regression.

33. e. Stage 5 ROP is defined as a total retinal detachment. Stage 1 is a <u>flat</u> demarcation line. The demarcation line of Stage 2 has three dimensions--that is, it protrudes into the vitreous. Stage 3 features extra retinal fibrovascular proliferation. Stage 4 is a subtotal retinal detachment.

34. False. It is hypothesized that immature vascular precursor tissue is susceptible to oxygen-induced cytotoxicity. Environmental oxygen may be sufficient to induce ROP in some cases.

35. a. Improvement of outcome by treatment with cryopexy was found for stage 3 ROP in zones 1 or 2, in the presence of plus disease, with at least 5 contiguous or 8 interrupted clock hours of involvement. When ROP advances rapidly in severity and extent, typically in severely premature infants, it is termed "rush" disease.

36. d. Exposure of an immature retinal vascular system to <u>some</u> source of oxygen is believed to be responsible for the development of ROP. Prematurity and low birth weight are risk factors for ROP because they are indicators of the presence of an immature retinal vascular system.

37. c. The supertemporal quadrant is most commonly affected in BRVO. The most common systemic disease association with BRVO is systemic hypertension. A <u>clear</u> association with POAG, as shown for CRVO, has not been established, although several small studies claim this is true.

38. a. Complications of BRVO can be divided into acute and chronic categories. Macular edema, macular nonperfusion, and hemorrhage may occur acutely. Macular edema, subretinal fibrosis, and posterior neovascularization and can be delayed causes of visual loss following BRVO. Rubeosis iridis is rare but has been reported.

39. True. The BVOS showed that eyes treated for macular edema with photocoagulation had a 60% chance of recovering 20/40 or better vision, compared to 34% for controls.

	ANY NV	NVD	NVE	NVI	NVG
Ischemic CRVO	66	5	8	60	33
Nonischemic CRVO	3	0	0	3	1.4
Ischemic HRVO	58	29	42	13	3
Major BRVO	28	12	24	2	0

40. a. Treatment should not be undertaken, however, until signs of neovascularization are evident because the long-term visual consequences of vitreous hemorrhage from retinal neovascularization are not particularly common or devastating (only 12% of eyes that suffered a vitreous hemorrhage in the study lost 5 or more lines of acuity). Greater than 5 disc diameters of ischemia was found to be associated with a 31% risk of developing neovascularization.

41. False. All forms of CRVO are caused by thrombosis of the central retinal vein at the level of the lamina cribosa.

42. d. Fluorescein angiography of a nonischemic CRVO should show minimal nonperfusion in contrast to an ischemic CRVO, which will show extensive capillary nonperfusion.

43. True. According to one study, approximately 48% of nonischemic CRVO will resolve completely.

44. e. The most common systemic disease associations for CRVO include atherosclerotic heart disease, hypertension, and diabetes. Less common associations include syphilis, sarcoidosis, increased intraorbital pressure, and hypersensitivity and other vasculitides.

45. True. Extremely high intraocular pressure may occlude a healthy central retinal vein.

46. True. In CRVO, the vitreous swells as transudate seeps out of the congested retinal veins. This may cause narrowing of the angle and precipitate angle closure.

47. c. Any CRVO will have hemorrhage in all quadrants, albeit asymmetrically.

48. b. The retinopathy of carotid artery occlusive disease may feature retinal hemorrhages and venous dilation like CRVO, but the central retinal artery pressure is low In CRVO, the retinal arteriolar pressure should be normal or elevated. Cotton-wool spots should not be seen in simple carotid occlusion.

49. False. Occlusion of precapillary arterioles results in cotton-wool spots. Cherry-red spots may arise due to axonal swelling in central retinal arterial occlusion (CRAO) or due to accumulation of metabolites in storage diseases such as Tay-Sachs disease.

50. e. Retinal artery occlusion is caused by embolization or thrombosis of the involved vessel. Uncommon causes of emboli include fat emboli, cardiac myxoma, and talc emboli in intravenous drug abusers. Mitral valve prolapse, vasculitides, and connective tissue disorders have also been associated with BRAO.

51. True. The visual prognosis for ischemic CRVO is poor, with only 10% of eyes obtaining better than 20/400 vision. CRAO has a better visual prognosis than ischemic CRVO, although it is still devastating. In one study, 66% of eyes with CRAO had final vision of less than 20/400, while 18% recovered vision of at least 20/40.

52. d. Studies in monkeys whose central retinal arteries were ligated established that irreversible damage to the retina occurs after 97 minutes of total ischemia.

53. a.   Type I is probably a forme fruste of Coats' disease, but Types II through IV are bilateral and occur in both sexes. Microscopically, the structural abnormalities are similar to diabetic microangiopathy, rather than a true telangiectasis. Unlike diabetes, there is no stimulus for retinal neovascularization. Choroidal neovascularization is another cause of visual loss.

54. c.   *BEALS Bfr Bilaterality*   Eales' disease is an idiopathic retinal vasculitis that generally involves both eyes of young boys or men. The original syndrome was defined as retinal vasculitis in a young man with associated epistaxis, constipation, and positive reaction to dermal purified protein derivative (PPD). A potentially lethal cerebral vasculitis has also been recognized as an occasional finding.

55. e.   Additional causes of retinal vasculitis include Behçet's disease, temporal arteritis, Wegener's granulomatosis, sarcoidosis, herpes zoster, syphilis, and toxoplasmosis.

56. b.   Other causes of visual loss include subinternal limiting membrane hemorrhage, vitreous hemorrhage, subretinal hemorrhage, and macular edema. Photocoagulation around the macroaneurysm may reduce edema and improve acuity. Focal treatment of the aneurysm is not recommended because hemorrhage is likely.

57. b.   Intraocular lens implantation at the time of extracapsular cataract extraction does not affect incidence of CME.

58. c.   Retinal telangiectasia (Coats' disease, Leber's miliary aneurysms) is defined by the presence of an exudative retinal detachment <u>with associated vascular anomalies</u>. This condition is not hereditary and is not associated with systemic vascular abnormalities. Usually, only one eye is involved and there is a male predominance (85%).

59. False.   The vascular lesion is a capillary hemangioma of the retina. It may also be termed a retinal hemangioblastoma.

60. True.   Despite retinal atrophy (or perhaps because of it), breaks and detachments are rarely occur spontaneously.   *RP ass ē OPtic N DRUSEN & COATS.*

61. a.   Café au lait spots are characteristic of neurofibromatosis and are not seen as part of von Hippel's disease.

62. True.   In fact, treatment may be associated wtih a total exudative detachment (which typically resolves).

63. False.   Both congenital retinal areteriovenous malformations and retinal capillary hemangiomas (von Hippel's disease) are associated with subretinal fluid and exudate. Cavernous hemangiomas bleed but usually do not leak.   *- Wyburn MASOY Does indeed leak exudate!*

64. True.   Retinal cavernous hemangioma can cause vitreous hemorrhage, which is presumed to be secondary to traction.   *The Subhyaloid heme ass ē Battered children is also also ē traction*

65. b.   Clinically, the macula is 5 to 6 mm in diameter, centered between the temporal vascular arcades. In this region, ganglion cells form two or three sublayers within the ganglion cell layer.

66. c.   The retinal vessels supply the nerve fiber layer, the ganglion cell layer, the inner plexiform layer, and the inner third of the inner nuclear layer. The choroidal vasculature supplies the outer two-thirds of the inner nuclear layer, the outer plexiform layer, the outer nuclear layer, the photoreceptors, and the retinal pigment epithelium.

67. a.   The membrane may be thought of as an elastin sandwich--the bread is collagenous zones and basement membrane on either side.

68. True.   RPE continually ingests membranes shed by the outer segments of the photoreceptor cells. RPE phagosomes containing ingested outer segment debris are discharged into Bruch's membrane after being processed. This is seen most prominently in the macula, the most metabolically active portion of the retina.

69. True.   Vitamin A required for vision is delivered to and stored in the RPE (of course, the vast majority of vitamin A stores are in the liver).

70. True.   Metaplasia of the RPE can result in both preretinal and subretinal membranes.

71. e.   In fluorescein angiography, white light from the camera first passes through a <u>blue</u> filter. The blue light (wavelength = 490 nm) is absorbed by the fluorescein molecules in the retinal and choroidal vasculature, stimulating them to emit yellow-green light (530 nm). A yellow-green filter is placed to block the blue light reflected from the eye, allowing the yellow-green light into the camera. Fluorescein particles can pass through the spaces between the endothelial cells of the choriocapillaries but normally cannot leak through the RPE.

72. a.   Leakage appears as an area of early hyperfluorescence that gradually increases in size and intensity throughout the angiogram.

73. a.   A focal defect in the internal limiting membrane is not necessary for retinal neovascularization to progress.

74. e.   Photoreceptor atrophy is unavoidable in the setting of marked RPE dysfunction. This is probably the mechanism of visual loss in severe atrophic aged-related macular degeneration (ARMD).

75. b.   CSR occurs preferentially in males in their fourth and fifth decades of life. The classic "smokestack" pattern is uncommon (10% of cases). It is much more common to see a small focal hyperfluorescent leak from the RPE that appears early in the angiogram and increases in size and intensity with time. Laser treatment shortens the course of each attack, but final visual acuity and rate of recurrence are not affected.

76. True.

77. c.   Treatment is generally reserved for (1) occupational or other demands for rapid recovery of binocular function, (2) persistent serous detachment (greater than 4 months), (3) prior episodes of CSR that have been associated with permanently decreased visual acuity, and (4) permanent visual loss due to CSR in the contralateral eye.

78.   a. 4.
     b. 3.
     c. 1.
     d. 2.

79.   False.   The diagnosis of ARMD is made when eyes with drusen or their associated complications develop a <u>decrease in visual acuity</u> not attributable to other ocular conditions.

80.   d.   Possible risk factors for progressive visual loss in AMD include a positive family history, hyperopia, cigarette smoking, and light iris color. Hypertension has not been directly related.

81.   a.   Findings in the nonexudative form of AMD include pigmentary changes, drusen, and areas of geographic atrophy. Patients with central geographic atrophy generally have a guarded visual prognosis.

82.   True.   A PED in a patient younger than age 50 is generally thought to be a variant of CSR and has a better prognosis. Visual acuity often returns to 20/30.

83.   a.   The Macular Photocoagulation Study (MPS) has documented that argon laser photocoagulation is effective in reducing the rate of severe visual loss for extrafoveal CNV (>200 microns from the center of the foveal avascular zone) and juxtafoveal CNV (1-199 microns). For subfoveal CNV, laser treatment may preserve contrast sensitivity and reading speed, but visual acuity is generally worse immediately after laser treatment. Thus far, there have been no controlled studies in the treatment of PED.

84.   b.   Endemic areas include the states of the Ohio and Mississippi River valleys. Systemic antifungal treatment does not lead to resolution of the ocular findings.

85.   d.   At present, the only effective method for treatment for POHS is argon laser photocoagulation.

86.   a.   The likelihood of contralateral choroidal neovascularization in a patient with a disciform macular scar from POHS is increased if there are focal macular scars in the better eye.

87.   c.   Angioid streaks represent discontinuities in abnormally thickened and calcified Bruch's membrane. They do not always extend in continuity from the optic nerve head, and they appear to radiate <u>from</u> the optic nerve head, rather than forming concentric circles around it. Because the overlying RPE is often atrophic, angioid streaks may appear as window defects on fluorescein angiography.

88.   a.   Sickle cell anemia is another potential systemic disease associated with angioid streaks. Up to 50% of patients with angioid streaks have no identifiable systemic illness. High myopia is not associated with angioid streaks but may feature lacquer cracks, which are similar histopathologically.

89.   b.

90.   True.   Approximately 75% of eyes with idiopathic epiretinal membranes maintain a visual acuity of 20/50 or better.

91. False. With the exception of pathologic myopia, full-thickness macular holes have not been known to result in retinal detachment and do not require treatment. This is a controversial area, but some retinologists feel that vitrectomy with intraocular gas injection can improve visual acuity in certain patients whose macular holes are surrounded by a "cuff" of subretinal fluid. A randomized clinical trial to investigate this question is currently under way.

92. b. The incidence of bilaterality of idiopathic macular holes is approximately 25% to 30%.

93. b. A macular cyst is thought to be a precursor to the development of a full-thickness macular hole, particularly in a patient whose fellow eye has a macular hole.

94. c. Although hydroxychloroquine is thought to be less toxic, both hydroxychloroquine and chloroquine have a significant risk of retinal toxicity. Color vision testing and threshold central visual field testing are thought to be important in elevating subclinical retinopathy. The EOG is not the most sensitive parameter in detecting chloroquine retinopathy, although it does reflect pathophysiology (RPE damage) when abnormal.

ERG -SUPRANORMAL Respons

95. False. Because of their slow excretion, toxic effects of chloroquine and hydroxychloroquine may <u>progress</u> despite cessation of the drug. Any abnormalities caused by these medications are probably permanent, although mild deficits may be reversible.

96. True. Both the phenothiazines and the antimalarials (chloroquine and hydroxychloroquine) may cause ERG abnormalities and peripheral pigmentary retinopathy. Thioridazine is probably the most likely phenothiazine to cause retinal toxicity.

97. True. Chlorpromazine (Thorazine) may lead to abnormal pigmentation of the conjunctiva, cornea, eyelids, anterior lens capsule, and retina. Thioridazine (Mellaril) is more likely to cause retinal pigment stippling or widespread atrophy of the pigment epithelium and choriocapillaris but less likely to affect other ocular structures.

98. False. Type II (Hunter) is X-linked recessive, while the rest of the MPS are autosomal <u>recessive</u>.

99. b. Corneal clouding is common in MPS types I-H (Hurler's), I-S (Scheie's), IV (Morquio's), and VI (Maroteaux-Lamy). It may rarely be seen in type II (Hunter's) but is never seen in III (Sanfilippo's).

100. a. Retinal pigmentary degeneration resembling typical RP is seen in type I-H (Hurler's), I-S (Scheie's), II (Hunter's), and III (Sanfilippo's).

101. a. Optic atrophy can be found in all of the MPS except types VI (mild phenotype) and type VII.

102. True. Gangliosides are found in cerebral gray matter, while cerebrosides are found in cell membranes throughout the body.

103. a. In the sphingolipidoses, a cherry-red spot is caused by accumulation of sphingolipids in the retinal ganglion cell layer. The orange-red color of the RPE and choroid stands out in the central fovea, where the ganglion cell layer is very thin or absent. There is no gross accumulation of lipid in Fabry's or Krabbe's disease; thus, no cherry-red spot is present.

104. False.   Ceramide accumulation in blood vessels leads to diffuse angiopathy, with myocardial infarction or stroke quite common. Still, renal failure is the leading cause of death.

105. a.   Pigmentary retinal changes are not characteristic of Fabry's disease.

106. b.   Deposition of cystine crystals in the conjunctiva and cornea with resultant photophobia occurs in all three types of cystinosis (nephropathic, late onset, and benign). A pigmentary retinopathy with a "salt and pepper" appearance occurs only in the nephropathic type. However, no significant visual disturbance occurs. In addition to its benefits as a topical medication, systemic cysteamine is being investigated as a means of preventing renal failure.

107. c.   Radiation retinopathy may occur with doses of about 3000 rads (30 gray) or greater, although rare cases have been reported after as little as 2400 rads.

108. c.   Visual acuity in solar retinopathy is generally not reduced below 20/200 and is frequently only minimally reduced. Recovery is good.

109. c.   The ratio of rods to cones is at least 12 to 15:1. Some investigators claim a ratio as high as 20:1. Rod density is maximal in a ring 20 to 40 degrees eccentric to the fovea, while cone density is greatest in the fovea. Although the cone density is greater in the macula than in the peripheral retina, the number of rods and cones in the macula is roughly equal, and nearly half of all cones lie outside the macula.

110. a. 1.   Blue cones have a maximum spectral sensitivity at shorter wavelengths, red cones at
b. 4.   longer wavelengths, and green cones at intermediate wavelengths. The maximum
c. 3.   spectral sensitivity of rods is at a wavelength between blue and green cones.
d. 2.

111. a. 2.   The a-wave is initial downward deflection in the ERG, which represents the
b. 4.   photoreceptor response. The early receptor potential can be measured in the
c. 5.   early a-wave and represents bleaching of visual pigment in the outer segments.
d. 3.   The b-wave is generated by cells in the bipolar and Müller cell layer.
e. 1.   Oscillatory potentials found in the b-wave are felt to be inhibitory potentials from amacrine cells. The c-wave is a late (2-4 seconds) positive deflection generated by the RPE.

112. True.   The scotopic ERG represents the ERG with rod input only. It is generated with a dim white or blue flash below the cone threshold in a dark-adapted state.

113. False.   Some rod function is represented even in a light-adapted ERG. Rod input can be minimized or eliminated by using only the longest wavelengths (orange-red), or more practically, by using a flicker stimulus.

114. e.   Rods can respond to flickering stimuli of rates of up to 20 Hz. Only cones can respond at higher frequencies, with a maximum of about 70 Hz.

115. c.   While the b-wave amplitude can be decreased in focal or stationary retinal disease, the b-wave implicit time is increased only in diffuse, progressive retinal disease.

116. False.   With increasing stimulus intensity, the b-wave amplitude increases and the implicit time (the time from stimulus to B wave peak) decreases.

Answers   569

117. b.   Oguchi's disease and fundus albipunctatus are forms of congenital stationary night blindness. Choroideremia is an X-linked recessive form of rod-cone degeneration. Fundus flavimaculatus (Stargardt's disease) is a condition with abnormal lipofuscin deposition in the RPE. Functional problems in this syndrome are not limited to night blindness.

118. a. 2.   The amplitude of the a-wave is very small in the scotopic ERG, since cones
     b. 1.   do not contribute to the waveform. The photopic ERG has an a-wave of
     c. 3.   intermediate amplitude. The dark-adapted bright flash ERG has giant a- and b-waves, since rods and cones both contribute maximally to the waveform.

119. a. 2.   In achromatopsia, the rod ERG is essentially normal. In congenital stationary
     b. 3.   night blindness, the cone ERG is essentially normal. In progressive rod-cone
     c. 1.   degenerations, both the scoptoic and photopic ERGs are markedly attenuated or nonrecordable.

120. b.   In electro-oculography, amplitudes generally <u>increase</u> with light adaption and <u>diminish</u> with dark adaption. The EOG is considered abnormal if the <u>light-peak</u> to <u>dark-trough</u> ratio is less than 1.75.

121. d.   In Best's disease, the ERG is generally normal, while the EOG is abnormal.

122. b.   An abnormally low light-peak to dark-trough ratio on EOG has been found to occur in retinal toxicity from hydroxychloroquine and chloroquine.

123. c.   Rods are about 1000 times more sensitive than cones during dark adaption.

124. a. 3.
     b. 4.
     c. 1.
     d. 1.

125. True.   An off-center on-surround receptive field implies that stimulation of the central photoreceptors is inhibitory (ganglion cell impulses diminish in frequency), while stimulation of surrounding photoreceptors is excitatory (ganglion cell impulses increase in frequency).

126. False.   The Purkinje shift refers to a shift in peak <u>spectral</u> sensitivity, from 555 nm to 505 nm, with dark adaption. Dark adaption does increase light sensitivity by a factor of 1000, but this is not the Purkinje shift.

127. True.   Each cone pigment is capable of absorbing a broad range of wavelengths. Thus, although a cone with a red-sensitive pigment absorbs red light most efficiently, it could produce the same firing ratio if stimulated with a much higher intensity of green light.

128. a. 1.   h. 2.
     b. 2.   i. 2.
     c. 1.   j. 1.
     d. 2.   k. 2.
     e. 2.   l. 1.
     f. 1.   m. 2.
     g. 1.   n. 1.

129. a.   Deuteranomalous trichromats are the most common. It is X-linked recessive and found in 5% of the male population.

130. c.   Rod monochromats typically have nystagmus and acuities in the 20/200 range. Blue monochromats have variable nystagmus and acuities in the 20/40 to 20/200 range.

131. b.   Decreased acuity and nystagmus are seen in both disorders. The ERGs in both disorders are similar in that they show cone dysfunction with relatively normal rod function. Rod monochromatism is an autosomal recessive disorder, while blue cone monochromatism is X-linked recessive.

132. a.   Ishihiara plates detect only red-green defects.

133. a. 3.
    b. 2.
    c. 4.
    d. 1.

134. a. 6.
    b. 3.
    c. 4.
    d. 8.
    e. 7.
    f. 2 (also known as Wolfram syndrome).
    g. 1.
    h. 5.

135. True.   Some patients with RP will develop moderate hearing loss with age, but most cases of severe hearing loss are congenital.

136. e.   Most forms of Leber's congenital amaurosis are autosomal <u>recessive</u>. There is an autosomal dominant infantile-onset RP that behaves like a progressive cone-rod degeneration of very early onset.

137. False.   Usher's syndrome only refers to the association of pigmentary retinopathy and <u>congenital</u> deafness.

138. True.   Types I and III feature vestibular dysfunction. Patients with profound deafness are more likely to have cerebellar atrophy.

139. d.   The other syndromes are autosomal recessive. It should be noted that central acuity is spared until later in life relative to X-linked RP.

140. True.   The retinal findings in choroideremia include scalloped RPE atrophy with <u>no</u> or scanty hyperpigmentation.

141. c.   Gyrate atrophy is an <u>autosomal</u> recessive deficiency in ornithine aminotransferase activity. This deficiency causes an increase in serum ornithine levels and a <u>decrease</u> in serum lysine levels.

142. e.   Although the inheritance in fundus flavimaculatus is usually autosomal recessive, autosomal dominant pedigrees have also been documented.

143. b.   Familial drusen is an autosomal dominant disorder that begins with asymptomatic retinal changes in the third decade, which do not become symptomatic until the fourth or fifth decade. The ERG is usually normal or mildly decreased.

144. c.   This scotopic ERG pattern helps to distinguish fundus albipunctatus from retinitis punctata albescens and other forms of congenital stationary night blindness. Normalization of the scotopic ERG after dark adaption has been shown in two pedigrees.

145. True.   Vision may be 20/30 to 20/60 in the early stages of the disease, despite the prominent central "egg yolk" lesion.

146. False.   To the contrary, patients with Stargardt's disease may have poor vision with barely detectable macular changes.

147. b.   The Mizuo-Nakamura effect occurs in Oguchi's disease and X-linked cone dystrophy. The eponym refers to a relative lightening of the RPE and fundus after 3 to 4 hours of dark adaption.

148. e.   While difficulty driving at night would seem to be more likely with rod degenerations, urban night driving is generally done with background illumination at low <u>photopic</u> intensities. Thus patients with cone degeneration may complain of this.

149. a. 2.
     b. 1.
     c. 1.
     d. 2.
     e. 1.
     f. 2.
     g. 2.
     h. 1.
     i. 2.

150. e.   All may mimic a generalized tapetoretinal degeneration. Harada's disease and toxemia of pregnancy are exudative disorders that may resolve and lead to pseudo-RP.

151. c.   Fundus albipunctatus features multiple, tiny white flecks in the deep retina. Oguchi's disease features the Mizuo phenomenon, a goldish fundus sheen that normalizes after several hours of dark adaption.

152. b.   Persistent hyperplastic primary vitreous (PHPV) has also been associated with foveal hypoplasia.

153. a.   Stargardt's disease is generally inherited on an autosomal recessive basis, but dominant pedigrees have also been described.

154. True.

155. b.   Despite the striking fundus appearance of the egg yolk lesion, visual acuity is usually quite good (20/30 to 20/50) at this stage. The amount of lipofuscin cannot be correlated with the amount of EOG depression.

156. True.

157. False.   So-called "multi-focal Best's" features more than one lesion simultaneously.

158. b.   Pattern dystrophies of the retinal pigment epithelium are better seen on fluorescein angiography than with ophthalmoscopy. As in Best's disease, the EOG is usually abnormal despite a normal ERG.

159. b.   Albinoidism differs from albinism in that the former does not have severe visual consequences. Both share certain clinical features, including photophobia, iris transillumination defects, and fundus hypopigmentation.

160. c.   True albinos have abnormal retinogeniculostriate projections as well as foveal hypoplasia. Temporal hemiretinal fibers that would normally project to the ipsilateral geniculate nucleus decussate abnormally. The lateral geniculate nuclei are grossly normal.

161. True.   In general, albinoidism is inherited as an autosomal dominant trait with incomplete penetrance, while true albinism is inherited as either an autosomal recessive or X-linked recessive trait.

162. c.

163. c.   Hermansky-Pudlak syndrome is characterized by bleeding diatheses, while Chédiak-Higashi is characterized by an immune deficiency and abnormal susceptibility to childhood infections.

164. c.   Xenon arc emits polychromatic white light, which cannot be as precisely focused as monochromatic light. In addition, blue light (harmful to the retina and lens) emission is significant.

165. d.   Krypton red is useful for laser therapy in the presence of vitreous hemorrhage. In addition, because it is poorly absorbed by xanthophyll, it is useful for macular laser treatment.

166. d.   Red light penetrates cataract and vitreous hemorrhage better than other wavelengths.

167. True.   This is in contrast to the xenon arc, in which decreasing the spot size decreases the total energy delivered.

168. a.

169. e.   Other potential complications include vitreous hemorrhage, nerve fiber bundle defects, accidental foveal burns, and retinal vascular occlusions. Angle-closure glaucoma after extensive scatter treatment is due to choroidal effusion.

170. a.   Other areas of firm vitreoretinal attachment include the optic nerve and major blood vessels. The vortex veins represent a firm point of attachment between the choroid and sclera.

171. True.   Removal of the lens allows the hyaluronic acid in the vitreous to diffuse into the anterior chamber and out of the eye.

172. b.

173. e.   Hemorrhage or vitreous cells ("tobacco dust") are suggestive of retinal breaks.

174. True.   Spontaneous and familial dialyses occur inferotemporally. Traumatic dialyses tend to occur supernasally.

175. True.   See answer 174.

176. b.   While 8 to 10% of the general population has lattice degeneration, only a small subset will develop a retinal detachment.

177. c.   Estimates range from 20 to 40%.

178. False.   Important histologic features of lattice degeneration include discontinuity of the internal limiting membrane and a pocket of liquefied vitreous overlying the degeneration. Vitreoretinal condensation and adherence occur at the margin of the lesion. Other features include sclerosis of the vessels and variable degrees of retinal atrophy.

179. b.   Lattice degeneration and meridional complexes (redundant retinal folds usually occurring superonasally) increase the risk of RRD. Cobblestone degeneration has occasionally been observed to limit the spread of retinal detachment and does not predispose to RRD.

180. c.   Approximately 22% of patients over age 20 have cobblestone degeneration, usually in the inferior quadrants.

181. b.   In 97% of RRD, a definite break can be found. In the other 3%, one is presumed to be present. This most frequently occurs in the setting of aphakic or pseudophakic retinal detachment, in which the breaks are frequently tiny.

182. c.   Signs suggestive of RRD include (1) lower IOP compared to the other eye, (2) "tobacco dust"--small clumps of RPE cells floating in the vitreous, and (3) corrugated appearance of the retina that undulates with eye movements. A smooth, domed appearance and shifting fluid are more suggestive of exudative detachment.

183. d.   Proliferative vitreoretinopathy is the most common cause of redetachment after successful repair. RPE, glial, and other cells proliferate and subsequently contract, causing fixed folds, traction, and/or detachment.

184. d.   Nearly 100% reattachment can be achieved with RRD secondary to dialysis or small round holes, detachments with demarcation lines (chronic), or those with minimal subretinal fluid. Giant tears and combined retinal-choroidal detachments have a poor prognosis, while aphakic detachments are intermediate.

185. c.   Degeneration of photoreceptors limits recovery of vision. Seventy-five percent of patients with macular detachment of less than 1 week duration will recover vision greater than 20/70. In contrast, those patients with macular detachment of 8 days or greater duration have only a 50% chance of regaining acuity of at least 20/70.

186. a.   In virtually all cases of typical degenerative retinoschisis, peripheral cystoid degeneration can be found, usually anterior to the schisis cavity.

187. c.   Greater than 70% of patients with retinoschisis are hyperopic, and this condition is bilateral in 50 to 80% of cases. However, in typical retinoschisis, complications such as hole formation and retinal detachment are rare. Also the scotoma associated with retinoschisis is absolute, whereas that associated with RRD is relative.

188. False.   Demarcation lines with retinoschisis indicate current or previous full-thickness retinal detachment.

189. False.   A hole in the outer wall alone is sufficient for formation of RD. Indeed, holes in both inner and outer walls lead the cavity to collapse, making the origin of detachment difficult to locate.

190. a. 3.
     b. 1.
     c. 3.
     d. 2.
     e. 1.
     f. 4.
     g. 3.

191. False.   Prepapillary vascular loops are normal retinal vessels that grow into Bergmeister's papilla before returning to the disc. Complications include branch retinal artery occlusion, amaurosis fugax, and vitreous hemorrhage.

192. c.   PHPV should be included in the differential diagnosis of leukocoria and differentiated from retinoblastoma. PHPV is unilateral in greater than 90% of cases and is associated with microphthalmia. Retinoblastoma is often bilateral and has no significant associations with microphthalmia or cataracts.

193. c.   Classification of hereditary hyaloideoretinopathies into two categories has been suggested: those with ocular manifestations only (Wagner's disease) and those with systemic symptoms (Stickler's syndrome). Wagner's disease consists of high myopia, cataract, and an optically empty vitreous. Stickler's syndrome is Wagner's disease plus (1) increased incidence of retinal detachment, (2) facial anomalies, and (3) musculoskeletal anomalies.

194. True.   Familial exudative vitreoretinopathy is autosomal dominant and occurs in full-term infants with normal respiratory status.

195. b.   Asteroid hyalosis is monocular in 75% of cases.

196. True.   Asteroid hyalosis usually does not settle, suggesting some collagenous support of asteroid bodies within formed vitreous. Synchysis scintillans usually settles inferiorly in liquefied vitreous (or in an eye that has undergone vitrectomy).

197. d.   Estimates of the proportion of vitreous hemorrhage due to diabetic retinopathy have ranged from 39 to 54%.

198. c.   Aphakic retinal detachment and retinal dialysis may be repaired with scleral buckling alone. However, traumatic retinal detachment with vitreous hemorrhage, or with severe proliferative vitreoretinopathy, may require vitrectomy to remove vitreous scaffolds which can promote future neovascularization and contraction.

199. b.   Severe visual loss after vitrectomy seems more common in diabetics. Lens removal may increase the risk of rubeosis, although a concomitant retinal detachment may be the key factor prompting lensectomy.

200. a.   Indications for emergent pars plana vitrectomy in the setting of globe penetration include retinal detachment, intraocular foreign body, and endophthalmitis. Vitreous hemorrhage without retinal detachment may be observed or addressed 7 to 10 days after the initial repair of globe rupture.

201. c.   Traumatic macular hole and subfoveal hemorrhage may lead to a permanent decrease in visual acuity. Commotio retinae and Valsalva retinopathy have a good visual prognosis.

202. e.   Severe compressive injuries of the head and trunk or fractures may lead to patches of retinal whitening and hemorrhages known as Purtscher's retinopathy. The disorder is thought to be mediated by air or fat embolism and consequent acute endothelial damage. Virtually identical fundus findings can result in patients with acute pancreatitis, SLE, dermatomyositis, or scleroderma.

203. a.   In a young person, sensory retinal detachment of the macula with pinpoint RPE leaks on angiography, but no other fundus abnormality, is most often due to central serous retinopathy (CSR). Between one-third and one-half of patients will have bilateral involvement; roughly the same proportion will have recurrences. The retinal elevation often induces an artifactual hyperopia; visual acuity can be improved with low plus lenses. Pregnant women may develop a variant that features prominent subretinal fibrin deposition. Laser therapy has been shown to shorten the natural history of the disorder, with little effect on final visual acuity or incidence of recurrence.

204. e.   This woman has suffered a central retinal vein occlusion (CRVO) in her left eye. The dilated retinal veins of the right eye suggest the same process may occur there as well. The most frequent concomitants of CRVO are ocular hypertension (glaucoma) and systemic hypertension. Diabetes is also seen more frequently in patients with CRVO. Syphilitic retinal vasculitis may induce a CRVO-like picture. Hypercoagulable states, particularly monoclonal gammopathy, are associated with bilateral CRVO. Except in the setting of extremely severe orbital congestion, Graves' disease is not associated with CRVO.

205. d.   The figures are most consistent with an extrafoveal choroidal neovascular membrane (CNVM) associated with age-related macular degeneration (AMD). Any peripheral vascular sheathing would be unrelated to the primary disorder. Subretinal hemorrhage in this disorder leads to visual loss and is derived from the choroidal circulation (the source of the abnormal new vessels). Drusen represent the early, mild manifestation of RPE senescence, which culminates in the ingrowth of choroidal vessels through a weakened Bruch's membrane. The Macular Photocoagulation Study (MPS) showed a clear treatment benefit for CNV in this location associated with AMD or presumed ocular histoplasmosis syndrome, as well as for idiopathic CNV.

References

1. Benson, William. "Section 11: Retina and Vitreous." in F.M. Wilson (ed.). Basic and Clinical Science Course. San Francisco: American Academy of Ophthalmology, 1991-1992.

2. Ryan, Stephen (ed.). Retina. St. Louis: C.V. Mosby Company, 1989.

11: Ocular Motility and Strabismus

1. Match the extraocular muscles listed in the left-hand column with the correct nerve supply in the right-hand column.

    a. levator palpebrae superioris.   1. II.
    b. superior rectus.   2. III--inferior.
    c. lateral rectus.   3. III--superior.
    d. inferior rectus.   4. IV.
    e. inferior oblique.   5. V.
    f. medial rectus.   6. VI.
    g. superior oblique.

2. Which of the following does <u>not</u> arise from the annulus of Zinn?

    1. superior oblique.
    2. levator palpebrae superioris.
    3. inferior oblique.
    4. superior rectus.

    a. 1, 2, and 3.
    b. 1 and 3.
    c. 2 and 4.
    d. 4 only.
    e. 1, 2, 3, and 4.

3. The action(s) of the medial rectus muscle with the eye in primary position is/are:

    a. adduction, elevation, intorsion.
    b. adduction, depression, intorsion.
    c. adduction, and intorsion.
    d. adduction, and extorsion.
    e. adduction.

4. Select the appropriate distance from limbus to muscle insertion for each of the muscles labeled in the diagram.

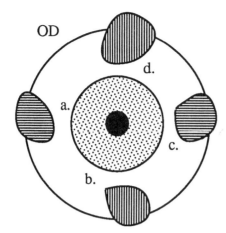

1. 5.5 mm.
2. 6.5 mm.
3. 6.9 mm.
4. 7.7 mm.

5. To maximize the elevation generated by the superior rectus, how must the eye be rotated from primary position?

   a. adducted 51 degrees.
   b. abducted 51 degrees.
   c. adducted 23 degrees.
   d. abducted 23 degrees.
   e. adducted 67 degrees.

6. To maximize the depression generated by the superior oblique, how must the eye be rotated?

   a. adducted 51 degrees.
   b. abducted 51 degrees.
   c. adducted 23 degrees.
   d. abducted 23 degrees.
   e. adducted 67 degrees.

7. T or F -- Both oblique muscles are characterized by a physical distinction between the anatomic origin and the mechanical origin.

8. T or F -- The superior oblique tendon passes between the superior rectus muscle and the globe on the way to its insertion.

9. T or F -- The inferior oblique muscle passes between the inferior rectus muscle and the globe on the way to its insertion.

10. T or F -- The superior oblique muscle becomes tendinous after turning through the trochlea.

11. The primary elevator of the eye in primary position is the:

    a. superior oblique.
    b. superior rectus.
    c. inferior oblique.
    d. inferior rectus.
    e. levator muscle.

12. The primary intorter of the globe in primary position is the:

    a. superior oblique.
    b. superior rectus.
    c. inferior oblique.
    d. inferior rectus.
    e. levator muscle.

13. Match each set of actions from primary position listed in the left-hand column with the appropriate muscle in the right-hand column.

    a. intorsion, depression, abduction.   1. inferior rectus.
    b. extorsion, elevation, abduction.   2. superior rectus.
    c. depression, extorsion, adduction.   3. superior oblique.
    d. elevation, intorsion, adduction   4. inferior oblique.

14. The extraocular muscle with the shortest length of active muscle belly is the:

    a. superior rectus.
    b. inferior rectus.
    c. superior oblique.
    d. inferior oblique.
    e. levator palpebrae superioris.

15. The muscle with the shortest length of tendon is the:

    a. superior rectus.
    b. inferior rectus.
    c. superior oblique.
    d. inferior oblique.
    e. levator palpebrae superioris.

16. Which one of the following concerning the physiology and anatomy of the extraocular muscles is false?

   a. Each of the rectus muscles receives two muscular arteries, which continue on as anterior ciliary arteries.
   b. Each muscle contains both fast (twitch) and slow (tonic) type muscle fibers.
   c. The slow, tonic muscles rely on aerobic metabolism and are innervated by "en grappe" endings.
   d. The fast, twitch type muscle fibers rely on glycolysis and are innervated by "en plaque" nerve endings.
   e. The motor units in extraocular muscle are among the smallest in the human body.

17. T or F -- Of the extraocular muscles, only the inferior oblique fails to penetrate Tenon's capsule.

18. T or F -- Extraconal orbital fat may be encountered as far anterior as 10 mm from the limbus.

19. T or F -- The average point of entry for a motor nerve into its muscle is approximately the junction of the posterior two-thirds and the anterior one-third of the active muscle belly.

20. Which of the following changes in lid position are consistent with the muscle surgery described?

   1. narrowing of palpebral fissure with superior rectus resection.
   2. narrowing of palpebral fissure with inferior rectus recession.
   3. narrowing of the palpebral fissure with inferior rectus resection.
   4. narrowing of the palpebral fissure with superior oblique tenotomy.

   a. 1, 2, and 3.
   b. 1 and 3.
   c. 2 and 4.
   d. 4 only.
   e. 1, 2, 3, and 4.

21. In young healthy eyes, anterior segment ischemia becomes a concern after surgery on how many rectus muscles?

   a. 1.
   b. 2.
   c. 3.
   d. 4.
   e. Anterior segment ischemia may follow unpredictably after any muscle surgery.

22. Each of the following is a correct match of muscular synergist and antagonist except:

    a. medial rectus: synergist--superior rectus; antagonist--lateral rectus.
    b. lateral rectus: synergist--superior oblique; antagonist--medial rectus.
    c. superior rectus: synergist--superior oblique; antagonist--inferior rectus.
    d. inferior rectus: synergist--superior oblique; antagonist--superior rectus.
    e. inferior oblique: synergist--superior rectus; antagonist--superior oblique.

23. In the diagram below, identify by number the muscle responsible for each cardinal position.

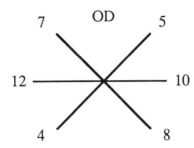
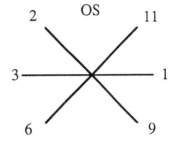

    a. left superior oblique.   g. right inferior oblique.
    b. right lateral rectus.   h. right medial rectus.
    c. left inferior oblique.   i. left lateral rectus.
    d. right inferior rectus.   j. left inferior rectus.
    e. right superior rectus.   k. left medial rectus.
    f. left superior rectus.   l. right superior oblique.

24. T or F -- Hering's law governs binocular motor function while Sherrington's law governs monocular motor function.

25. Which one of the following constitutes a violation of Hering's law?

    a. inhibitional palsy of the contralateral antagonist.
    b. dissociated vertical deviation (DVD).
    c. Brown's syndrome.
    d. cyclic esotropia.
    e. Duane's syndrome.

26. Which one of the following constitutes a violation of Sherrington's law?

    a. inhibitional palsy of the contralateral antagonist.
    b. disassociated vertical divergence (DVD).
    c. Brown's syndrome.
    d. cyclic esotropia.
    e. Duane's syndrome.

27. T or F -- By definition, versions are conjugate binocular movements, while vergences are disconjugate binocular movements.

28. T or F -- In both fusional convergence and fusional divergence, there is an obligatory change in the refractive status of the eye.

29. The site of origin of neural impulses leading to a rightward saccade is the:

   a. right frontal lobe.
   b. left frontal lobe.
   c. right parieto-occipital lobe.
   d. left parieto-occipital lobe.
   e. the site of origin has not been determined.

30. The site of origin of neural impulses leading to a leftward pursuit movement is the:

   a. right frontal lobe.
   b. left frontal lobe.
   c. right parieto-occipital lobe.
   d. left parieto-occipital lobe.
   e. site of origin has not been determined.

31. T or F -- Physiologically, any point not lying on the empirical horopter will be perceived doubly by the human visual system.

32. T or F -- Panum's area of single binocular vision is broader for points in space clustered around the central portion of the empirical horopter and narrower in the periphery.

33. T or F -- If simultaneous stimulation of retinal areas in two eyes leads to the perception of one image, normal retinal correspondence is said to exist.

34. T or F -- Stereopsis only exists for points in space that lie on the empirical horopter.

35. T or F -- For fusion to exist, there must be simultaneous stimulation of corresponding retinal areas with normal retinal correspondence.

36. T or F -- For fusion to exist, the two retinal images must be similar in size and shape.

37. Which one of the following statements concerning motor fusion is false?

   a. Motor fusion is a means of avoiding diplopia.
   b. Motor fusion is the act by which similar retinal images are made to fall on corresponding retinal areas.
   c. A normal convergence amplitude at distance is 14 prism diopters and at near is 38 prism diopters.
   d. A normal divergence amplitude at distance is 14 diopters and at near is 16 diopters.
   e. Normal vertical fusional amplitude varies from 2 to 4 prism diopters and is independent of fixation distance.

38. T or F -- The most important visual clues for depth perception require binocular vision.

39. A vertical slit pattern is projected onto the fovea of the right eye, while a horizontal slit pattern is projected onto the fovea of the left eye. The subject perceives rapidly alternating images of each pattern--first one then the other, never simultaneously. This perception is an example of:

    a. fusion.
    b. stereopsis.
    c. suppression.
    d. retinal rivalry.
    e. normal retinal correspondence.

40. The first cell type in the visual pathway to have receptive fields consisting of circular centers and annular surrounds is the:

    a. photoreceptor.
    b. bipolar cell.
    c. ganglion cell.
    d. lateral geniculate neuron.
    e. occipital cortical neuron.

41. T or F -- The "critical period" for proper development of the visual pathways is longer in humans than in most experimental animals.

42. T or F -- Diplopia occurs when the two foveas of a single patient each contain a distinct retinal image.

43. T or F -- If a patient with manifest strabismus does not complain of diplopia, then suppression must be active.

44. Which of the following regarding amblyopia is/are true?

    1. The incidence in the general population is approximately 2 to 3%.
    2. The presence of an afferent pupillary defect clearly establishes an organic etiology for visual loss, rather than amblyopia.
    3. Patients with amblyopia will frequently perform better with single-symbol acuity test targets than with line targets ("crowded stimuli").
    4. A neutral density filter placed over an amblyopic eye will generally cause a greater decrement in visual acuity than the same filter placed over an eye with maculopathy.

    a. 1, 2, and 3.
    b. 1 and 3.
    c. 2 and 4.
    d. 4 only.
    e. 1, 2, 3, and 4.

45. In which of the following types of strabismus is amblyopia least frequently seen?

    a. infantile esotropia.
    b. esotropia with high accommodative convergence to accommodation ratio (AC/A).
    c. alternating esotropia.
    d. esotropia associated with Duane's syndrome.
    e. exotropia associated with craniosynostosis.

46. T or F -- The proper guideline for intervals between examinations for a child undergoing full-time occlusion therapy is 1 week for every month of age.

47. A 7-year-old patient presents to a pediatric ophthalmologist after failing his school vision test. Visual acuity is 20/20 OD and 20/50 OS, tested with patching and Snellen targets. Motility is full, and there is no apparent tropia on cover-uncover testing. The child has stereoacuity with targets disparate by no less than 60 seconds of arc. Distance Worth four-dot testing reveals fusion. Convergence and divergence amplitudes are normal at distance. The most likely diagnosis is:

    a. cyclic esotropia.
    b. monofixation syndrome.
    c. central fixation with anomalous retinal correspondence.
    d. Duane's syndrome.
    e. factitious visual loss.

48. The patient in question 47 has no history of previous eye surgery. The remainder of his examination is most likely to disclose:

    a. high axial myopia bilaterally.
    b. retraction of the globe on adduction.
    c. anisometropia greater than 2 D.
    d. macular edema.
    e. esotropia developing sometime within the next 24 hours.

49. The most practical and valuable test to perform next on this patient would be:

    a. Lancaster red-green test.
    b. afterimage testing.
    c. Bagolini glass testing.
    d. four prism-diopter base-out test.
    e. fogging refraction.

50. T or F -- The patient in questions 47 through 49 must have abnormal retinal correspondence.

51. A 42-year-old patient presents to the emergency room with a manifest right esotropia. A red glass is placed over the left eye and the patient is asked to fixate at a distant point-light target. In the absence of suppression, and with normal retinal correspondence, the patient should perceive the red light:

a. above the white light.
b. below the white light.
c. to the right of the white light.
d. to the left of the white light.
e. The lights will appear to be superimposed.

52. The patient reports that he sees only the red light. The examiner could conclude that:

          1. the patient must have anomalous retinal correspondence (ARC).
          2. the motility defect is not recent in origin.
          3. the patient will have normal stereoacuity with his distance correction in place.
          4. the patient may be malingering.

a. 1, 2, and 3.
b. 1 and 3.
c. 2 and 4.
d. 4 only.
e. 1, 2, 3, and 4.

53. On further questioning, the patient reports that he actually perceives the white light to be to the right of the red light. These images are superimposed with a 10 prism-diopter prism base-out over the left eye. Simultaneous prism cover test with a distance target and no red glass reveals a 20 prism-diopter right esotropia. These results indicate:

a. normal retinal correspondence (NRC).
b. harmonious anomalous retinal correspondence (ARC).
c. unharmonious anomalous retinal correspondence (ARC).
d. visual confusion on the patient's part.
e. total confusion on the examiner's part--the measurements must be wrong.

54. Which of the following regarding the afterimage test for retinal correspondence is/are true?

    1. It is best to flash the vertical line into the fixating eye.
    2. Regardless of fixation behavior, in the setting of normal retinal correspondence, the patient will perceive a cross with a single central gap.
    3. A patient with a right exotropia, central fixation and harmonious anomalous retinal correspondence will perceive the vertical line flashed into his right eye as being to the left of the horizontal image placed into his fixating left eye (crossed diplopia).
    4. To appropriately interpret this test, the patient's fixation behavior must be determined.

    a. 1, 2, and 3.
    b. 1 and 3.
    c. 2 and 4.
    d. 4 only.
    e. 1, 2, 3, and 4.

55. T or F -- Testing with Bagolini striated glasses for retinal correspondence requires preparation with cover-uncover testing and assessment of fixation behavior.

56. During routine examination, an alternate-cover test reveals outward fixation shifts of each eye as the cover is moved. The cover-uncover test reveals no shift of either eye as the cover is placed over either eye. The correct description of the patient's motility status would be:

    a. orthophoric, orthotropic.
    b. orthophoric, esotropic.
    c. orthotropic, esophoric.
    d. orthotropic, exophoric.
    e. This set of findings is not possible.

57. During a routine examination, the cover-uncover test reveals an outward fixation shift of either eye as the cover is placed over the contralateral eye. The alternate-cover test reveals no shift as the cover is moved back and forth. The correct description of this patient's motility status would be:

    a. orthophoric, orthotropic.
    b. orthophoric, esotropic.
    c. orthotropic, esophoric.
    d. orthotropic, exophoric.
    e. This set of findings is not possible.

58. T or F -- Most of the normal adult population is orthophoric and orthotropic.

59. For a strabismus to be appropriately termed congenital, the disturbance must be documented:

    a. at birth.
    b. within the first 4 weeks of life.
    c. within the first 3 months of life.
    d. within the first 6 months of life.
    e. within the first 12 months of life.

60. The design of effective occlusion therapy for a toddler with strabismus requires careful evaluation of which of the following factors?

    1. age at which the deviation was initially noted.
    2. amount of the day during which the child's eyes are straight.
    3. which eye, if either, the patient prefers fixing with.
    4. a family history of strabismus.

    a. 1, 2, and 3.
    b. 1 and 3.
    c. 2 and 4.
    d. 4 only.
    e. 1, 2, 3, and 4.

61. Of the following acuity tests, which is least likely to lead to an overestimation of actual recognition acuity?

    a. single Snellen letters.
    b. illiterate E.
    c. optotype cards.
    d. Allen cards.
    e. Landolt rings.

62. Which of the following is useful primarily as a screening test for the presence of visual behavior?

    a. Snellen letters.
    b. visual evoked responses.
    c. preferential looking tests.
    d. illiterate E.
    e. optokinetic nystagmus.

63. Which of the following ocular alignment tests require foveal fixation in the deviated eye for quantification of the angle of strabismus?

> 1. the cover-uncover test with prisms.
> 2. the alternate-cover test with prisms.
> 3. the simultaneous prism-cover test.
> 4. the Krimsky test.

a. 1, 2, and 3.
b. 1 and 3.
c. 2 and 4.
d. 4 only.
e. 1, 2, 3, and 4.

64. A patient with strabismus is asked to fixate a penlight held by the examiner. The examiner notes that the corneal reflex in the right eye is central, while that in the left eye is displaced approximately 3 mm temporal to the center of the pupil. Using Hirschberg's method for estimating the angle of strabismus, the examiner concludes that the patient has a:

a. 45 degree esotropia.
b. 45 prism diopter esotropia.
c. 45 degree exotropia.
d. 45 prism diopter exotropia.
e. There is not sufficient information to use Hirschberg's method.

65. To estimate the deviation for the patient in question 64, the examiner chooses to use the Krimsky method. To do this he should:

a. perform simultaneous prism-cover testing until there is no net movement of either eye.
b. he should place prisms over the nonfixing eye until its light reflex appears centered.
c. he should place prisms over the fixing eye until the visuoscope target is foveal in the nonfixing eye.
d. he should place prisms over the fixing eye until the corneal light reflex from the nonfixing eye appears central.
e. he should multiply the distance of the decentered light reflex from the center of the pupil in millimeters by 15 to estimate the deviation in prism diopters.

66. When used with prisms, which of the following is best suited for quantification of a tropia only, with no contribution from a phoria?

a. cover-uncover test.
b. alternate-cover test.
c. Maddox rod testing.
d. simultaneous prism-cover test.
e. double Maddox rod testing.

67. T or F -- The image a subject perceives from a Maddox rod is a real image of a line perpendicular to the orientation of the cylinders in the Maddox rod.

68. T or F -- To test for a vertical deviation, the Maddox rod should be aligned over the eye with its cylinders running vertically.

69. When tested with a Maddox rod held over the affected eye with its cylinders running horizontally, a patient with excyclotropia will perceive:

   a. a horizontal line.
   b. a vertical line.
   c. an oblique line running superotemporal to inferonasal.
   d. an oblique line running superonasal to inferotemporal.
   e. a curved line concave toward the nose.

70. An adult with an acquired right esotropia due to an acquired right abducens paresis is tested with the Lancaster red-green test. He wears the goggles with the red glass over his right eye and the green glass over his left. An examiner holds the green light central on the chart and gives the patient the red light. The patient is then instructed to superimpose his red light on the examiner's green light. To the examiner:

   a. the red light will appear to the left of the green light.
   b. the red light will appear above the green light.
   c. the red light will appear to the right of the green light.
   d. the red light will appear below the green light.
   e. the lights will be superimposed.

71. To the patient:

   a. the red light will appear to the left of the green light.
   b. the red light will appear above the green light.
   c. the red light will appear to the right of the green light.
   d. the red light will appear below the green light.
   e. the lights will be superimposed.

72. The same patient described in question 70 is retested with the goggles reversed--that is, the green lens over the right eye, the red lens over the left eye. The examiner holds the green light as a fixation target centrally, and patient moves the red light. This time, the examiner will observe:

   a. the red light to the left of the green light at the same distance between the two as before.
   b. the red light to the left of the green light at a larger distance between the two than before.
   c. the red light to the right of the green light with the same distance between the two as before.
   d. the red light to the right of the green light at a larger distance than before.
   e. the red light to the right of the green light at a smaller distance than before.

73. If a patient with untreated congenital esotropia is tested with the Lancaster red-green test, when the glasses are reversed and the test is repeated, which one of the following is true?

   a. The position of the lights on the screen will reverse and the distance between them will increase.
   b. The position of the lights on the chart will not reverse and the distance will increase.
   c. The position of the lights on the chart will reverse and the distance will remain the same.
   d. The position of the lights on the chart will remain the same.
   e. none of the above.

74. Broad nasal bridges with abnormally large angle kappa may lead to an error in the diagnosis of strabismus with which of the following methods?

   1. alternate-cover tests.
   2. Maddox rod testing.
   3. cover-uncover testing.
   4. Hirschberg testing.

   a. 1, 2, and 3.
   b. 1 and 3.
   c. 2 and 4.
   d. 4 only.
   e. 1, 2, 3, and 4.

75. T or F -- Temporal displacement of the macula will lead to positive angle kappa.

76. T or F -- Negative angle kappa simulates esotropia.

77. To accurately quantify an esodeviation, prism is most appropriately placed over either eye:

   a. base up.
   b. base out.
   c. base down.
   d. base in.
   e. apex out.

78. To quantify a hyperdeviation accurately, prism is most appropriately placed in front of the deviated eye:

   a. base up.
   b. base out.
   c. base down.
   d. base in.
   e. apex down.

79. T or F -- A patient whose distance esotropia increases by more than 10 prism diopters at near is said to have a clinically high accommodative convergence to accommodation ratio (AC/A).

80. A 31-year-old man with moderate hyperopia presents for routine examination. There is a 10 prism diopter alternating esotropia at distance. While reading through his distance correction at 20 cm, there is a 35 prism diopter esotropia. Eye movements are full, and he denies any history of prior surgery. You conclude that:

a. he has the sequelae of pure, classic infantile esotropia.
b. he must have amblyopia in one eye.
c. he probably has restrictive strabismus.
d. he probably will note double vision if questioned appropriately.
e. he has a high AC/A ratio.

81. The examiner elects to calculate the patient's AC/A ratio. His interpupillary distance is 60 mm, and his near deviation increases to 50 prism diopters when he views an acuity target through a -1.00 diopter sphere over each eye. By the gradient method, his AC/A ratio measures:

a. 5:1.
b. 11:1.
c. 15:1.
d. 25:1.
e. 50:1.

82. By the heterophoria method, the AC/A ratio measures:

a. 5:1.
b. 11:1.
c. 15:1.
d. 25:1.
e. 50:1.

83. In the setting of a heterophoria, fusional vergence amplitudes may be diminished by which of the following?

1. intercurrent illness.
2. fatigue.
3. alcohol consumption.
4. improvement in visual acuity.

a. 1, 2, and 3.
b. 1 and 3.
c. 2 and 4.
d. 4 only.
e. 1, 2, 3, and 4.

84. T or F -- Suppression with the distance Worth four-dot test, but fusion on near Worth four-dot testing indicates peripheral fusion with no central fusion.

85. A 27-year-old man presents to an ophthamologist complaining of double vision and difficulty descending stairs since an automobile accident 1 week earlier. The examiner notes that the patient has a left head tilt and concludes that he must have a right superior oblique paresis. Which one of the following findings could not possibly be present if the examiner is correct?

a. right hypertropia in primary position.
b. left hypertropia in right gaze.
c. right hypertropia aggravated by left gaze.
d. right hypertropia aggravated by right gaze.
e. V pattern esotropia.

86. The muscle that is most likely responsible for aggravation of the right hypertropia seen upon right head tilt with a right superior oblique paresis is the:

a. right superior rectus.
b. right inferior rectus.
c. right inferior oblique.
d. right superior oblique.
e. left inferior rectus.

87. A patient undergoes left orbital exploration for biopsy of a suspicious infiltrate on computed tomography (CT) scanning. Postoperatively the patient is noted to have a widely dilated pupil and poor vision at near in the left eye. He also complains of binocular diplopia. You note an inability to elevate the eye when it is adducted. What findings would you expect on the three-step test?

a. a right hypertropia worse in right gaze and left head tilt.
b. a left hypertropia worse in left gaze and right head tilt.
c. a right hypertropia worse in right gaze and right head tilt.
d. a left hypertropia worse in right gaze and left head tilt.
e. a right hypertropia worse in left gaze and right head tilt.

88. Atropine is relatively contraindicated as a cycloplegic agent in:

1. albinos.
2. neonates.
3. patients with Down's syndrome.
4. patients with heart block.

a. 1, 2, and 3.
b. 1 and 3.
c. 2 and 4.
d. 4 only.
e. 1, 2, 3, and 4.

89. Systemic manifestations of cycloplegic intoxication include:

    1. flushing.
    2. agitation.
    3. tachycardia.
    4. somnolence.

    a. 1, 2, and 3.
    b. 1 and 3.
    c. 2 and 4.
    d. 4 only.
    e. 1, 2, 3, and 4.

90. T or F -- The purpose of the prism adaptation test is to demonstrate whether the patient's deviation is stable over time.

91. Match the mechanism of esotropia in the right column with the clinical findings listed in the left column.

    a. cycloplegic refraction: + 1.50 D OU; distance deviation: 5 prism diopter esophoria; near deviation: 25 prism diopter esotropia; comitant deviation.

    b. cycloplegic refraction + 0.50 D OU; distance deviation: 30 prism diopter esotropia; near deviation: 10 prism diopter esotropia; noncomitant--deviation increases with attempted abduction of the esotropic eye.

    c. cycloplegic refraction: + 1.50 D OU; distance deviation: 45 prism diopter esotropia; near deviation: greater than 60 prism diopter esotropia; comitant deviation.

    d. cycloplegic refraction: + 5.50 D OU; distance deviation: 35 prism diopter esotropia; near deviation: 40 prism diopter esotropia; comitant deviation.

    e. cycloplegic refraction: + 1.00 D OU; distance deviation: 50 prism diopter esotropia; near deviation: 50 prism diopter esotropia; comitant deviation.

    1. refractive accommodative esotropia.
    2. nonrefractive accommodative esotropia.
    3. basic (simple) esotropia.
    4. mixed mechanism esotropia.
    5. paretic esotropia.

92. Which of the following concerning infantile esotropia is/are true?

    1. Although it is typically seen in isolation, it may be associated with neurologic abnormalities.
    2. Amblyopia develops as the child cross-fixates.
    3. Characteristically the esotropia is large (greater than 30 prism diopters).
    4. There is never an accommodative component.

    a. 1, 2, and 3.
    b. 1 and 3.
    c. 2 and 4.
    d. 4 only.
    e. 1, 2, 3, and 4.

93. Findings commonly associated with infantile esotropia on examination include:

    1. latent nystagmus.
    2. overaction of the inferior obliques.
    3. disassociated vertical divergence (DVD).
    4. high AC/A ratio.

    a. 1, 2, and 3.
    b. 1 and 3.
    c. 2 and 4.
    d. 4 only.
    e. 1, 2, 3, and 4.

94. Appropriate options for initial surgical intervention in infantile esotropia include:

    1. bimedial recession.
    2. bilateral resection.
    3. ipsilateral medial rectus recession and lateral rectus resection.
    4. bimedial resection.

    a. 1, 2, and 3.
    b. 1 and 3.
    c. 2 and 4.
    d. 4 only.
    e. 1, 2, 3, and 4.

95. T or F -- A monofixation syndrome with peripheral fusion, good cosmesis, and limited stereopsis is a fairly common outcome of successful management of infantile esotropia.

96. T or F -- Nystagmus blockage syndrome develops purposefully as the patient seeks his or her null point.

97. Parents bring their 3-year-old boy for examination after they note the development of "cross-eyes." Upon closer review, the parents report that they originally noted the deviation to be present throughout the day at age 2 years. A brief "glance" at the child makes a constant moderate-angle esotropia obvious. Which of the following is/are true?

1. Amblyopia is highly unlikely.
2. With further careful questioning, it may be possible to document that the deviation was originally intermittent.
3. The child should be able to perceive the wings of the Titmus fly in three dimensions.
4. It would not be surprising to find a family history of a similar disorder.

a. 1, 2, and 3.
b. 1 and 3.
c. 2 and 4.
d. 4 only.
e. 1, 2, 3, and 4.

98. As part of the comprehensive examination of the patient in question 97, a cycloplegic refraction is performed and reveals +8.50 D OU. Which of the following is/are true?

1. There may be bilateral amblyopia.
2. The deviation will certainly be greater at near than at distance.
3. +3.00 D lenses are likely to have little effect on the distance deviation.
4. The deviation at distance is likely to measure greater than 50 prism diopters.

a. 1, 2, and 3.
b. 1 and 3.
c. 2 and 4.
d. 4 only.
e. 1, 2, 3, and 4.

99. The initial step in management of this patient must be:

a. penalization with atropine bilaterally.
b. alternate occlusion therapy if the visual acuity is normal bilaterally.
c. full correction of the cycloplegic refractive error.
d. bifocals.
e. bimedial recession.

100. Parents bring their child to the ophthalmologist after noting "cross-eyes." On further questioning, they report that they noted the deviation to be present throughout the day since approximately age 2 years. A quick glance at the child reveals an obvious intermittent moderate-angle esotropia. It seems to be larger when the child plays with an object in his hands. Cycloplegic refraction reveals + 1.50 D OU. Which of the following are true?

    1. The deviation at distance is not likely to be large.
    2. The deviation at near is likely to be moderate (20-30 prism diopters).
    3. The deviation at near is likely to be lessened with + 3.00 D lenses over each eye.
    4. The AC/A ratio is likely to be less than 5.

    a. 1, 2, and 3.
    b. 1 and 3.
    c. 2 and 4.
    d. 4 only.
    e. 1, 2, 3, and 4.

101. Which of the following regarding the treatment of esotropia is/are true?

    1. Accommodative esotropia is more likely to require surgical intervention than infantile esotropia.
    2. Bifocals are most helpful in the management of patients with refractive accommodative esotropia.
    3. If refractive correction fails to solve the problem, the only solution is surgical.
    4. Accommodative esotropia may progress over the first 5 to 7 years of life and should be monitored carefully.

    a. 1, 2, and 3.
    b. 2 and 4.
    c. 1 and 3.
    d. 4 only.
    e. 1, 2, 3, and 4.

102. Clinical features of esotropia that are predictive of the need for future surgical intervention include all of the following except:

    a. presence of overaction of the inferior obliques.
    b. equal vision.
    c. large-angle esotropia (greater than 50 prism diopters).
    d. age of onset between 2 and 3 years.
    e. low hyperopia or myopia.

103. Which of the following regarding the treatment of accommodative esotropia is/are true?

1. No improvement of esotropia with miotic therapy rules out the possibility of an accommodative component.
2. Delay in refractive correction of an accommodative esotropia increases the probability of a permanent residual esotropia after full correction is given.
3. It is important to attempt surgical realignment before prolonged occlusion therapy.
4. Surgical realignment resulting in a residual esotropia less than 10 prism diopters may permit the development of peripheral fusion.

a. 1, 2, and 3.
b. 1 and 3.
c. 2 and 4.
d. 4 only.
e. 1, 2, 3, and 4.

104. T or F -- In accommodative esotropia, patients with fully corrected esotropia due to high hyperopia are more likely to develop stress-induced decompensation in their esotropia than patients with a high AC/A ratio.

105. In intermittent accommodative esotropia, some ophthalmologists do not prescribe full hyperopic correction because:

a. distance vision will be blurred.
b. the greater deviation at near will not be fully compensated.
c. the patient may be converted to a constant esotropia without glasses.
d. the patient may become exotropic with full hyperopic correction.
e. the problem never becomes constant.

106. Which one of the following regarding cyclic esotropia is false?

a. The cycle consists of 1 week of orthotropia and 1 week of esotropia.
b. The angle of deviation is generally moderate.
c. The time of onset is similar to accommodative esotropia.
d. Full hyperopic correction may correct the esotropia.
e. Amblyopia is possible, but relatively uncommon.

107. Divergence insufficiency resembles lateral rectus palsy except:

a. there is a typically an esodeviation.
b. the deviation is generally worse at distance.
c. there are commonly no associated neurologic abnormalities.
d. the deviation is comitant.
e. therapy for nonresolving cases includes surgical intervention.

108. Findings that favor the diagnosis of spasm of the near reflex rather than accommodative esotropia include:

  1. new myopia.
  2. esotropia worse at near than distance.
  3. miosis on attempted lateral gaze.
  4. no vertical component.

a. 1, 2, and 3.
b. 1 and 3.
c. 2 and 4.
d. 4 only.
e. 1, 2, 3, and 4.

109. T or F -- Isolated abducens paresis in a child is a neurologic emergency demanding immediate neuroimaging and lumbar puncture.

110. The feature <u>least</u> consistent with acquired abducens paresis include all of the following except:

a. esotropia.
b. deviation greater at distance than near.
c. amblyopia.
d. head turn toward the side of the paretic muscle.
e. noncomitant deviation.

111. Treatment alternatives in acquired abducens paresis include:

  1. patching.
  2. base-in fresnel prisms.
  3. botulinum toxin injections.
  4. ipsilateral medial rectus resection.

a. 1, 2, and 3.
b. 1 and 3.
c. 2 and 4.
d. 4 only.
e. 1, 2, 3, and 4.

112. T or F -- Consecutive exotropia should be repaired immediately, as spontaneous recovery is highly unlikely.

113. T or F -- Sensory deprivation in a child less than 6 years is more likely to lead to esotropia, while that occurring in adults is more likely to lead to exotropia.

114. An exodeviation that is greater at distance than at near is known as:

    a. basic exotropia.
    b. divergence excess exotropia.
    c. true divergence excess exotropia.
    d. simulated divergence excess exotropia.
    e. convergence insufficiency exotropia.

115. To distinguish true divergence excess exotropia from "simulated divergence excess" exotropia:

    a. the deviations are remeasured after cycloplegia.
    b. the AC/A ratio is calculated by the heterophoria method.
    c. the AC/A ratio is calculated by the gradient method.
    d. the deviations are remeasured after prolonged (30-45 minutes) monocular occlusion.
    e. the deviations are remeasured with - 1.00 D lenses over the patient's distance correction.

116. A patient with constant exotropia has a deviation of 35 prism diopters at distance and 15 prism diopters at near. After wearing + 3.00 D lenses over his distance correction for 1 hour, the deviations are remeasured and found to be 35 prism diopters at distance and 30 prism diopters at near. The classification of his strabismus is:

    a. basic exotropia.
    b. divergence excess exotropia.
    c. true divergence excess exotropia.
    d. simulated divergence excess exotropia.
    e. convergence insufficiency exotropia.

117. A patient presents for ophthalmic examination that discloses a comitant exotropia. At distance, his deviation measures 5 prism diopters of exotropia and at near 15 prism diopters of exotropia. His strabismus is best classified as a:

    a. basic exotropia.
    b. divergence excess exotropia.
    c. true divergence excess exotropia.
    d. simulated divergence excess exotropia.
    e. convergence insufficiency exotropia.

118. T or F -- Congenital exotropia is equally as common as congenital esotropia.

119. The most common etiology for constant exotropia is:

    a. decompensated intermittent exotropia.
    b. sensory exotropia.
    c. third nerve palsy.
    d. Duane's syndrome type II.
    e. exotropia associated with craniofacial anomalies.

120. T of F -- Intermittent exotropia, like accommodative esotropia, usually fades away as the child progresses through early adolescence.

121. Clinical features frequently associated with intermittent exotropia include:

        1. variable angle of deviation.
        2. high AC/A ratio.
        3. reflex closure of one eye in bright light.
        4. amblyopia.

a. 1, 2, and 3.
b. 1 and 3.
c. 2 and 4.
d. 4 only.
e. 1, 2, 3, and 4.

122. T of F -- Patients with intermittent exotropia generally have reduced stereoacuity.

123. Useful treatment modalities for intermittent exotropia include:

        1. minus lenses.
        2. phospholine iodide.
        3. base-in prism.
        4. bilateral rectus resections.

a. 1, 2, and 3.
b. 1 and 3.
c. 2 and 4.
d. 4 only.
e. 1, 2, 3, and 4.

124. T or F - Virtually all cases of intermittent exotropia will progress to constant exotropia over time.

125. T or F -- The exotropia associated with Duane's syndrome type II is frequently noncomitant.

126. Clinical features of convergence insufficiency include all of the following except:

a. asthenopia.
b. blurry reading vision.
c. diplopia while reading.
d. exophoria at near.
e. brow ache.

127. T or F -- Treatment of convergence insufficiency may include the use of either base-out or base-in prisms.

128. T or F -- Convergence insufficiency may occur with normal accommodation.

129. T or F -- Innervational vertical deviations are as common as innervational horizontal deviations.

130. A patient presents for evaluation of "wandering eyes." On alternate-cover testing, with the left eye covered, the right eye fixes a distance target. As the cover is shifted to the right eye, the left eye moves down to pick up fixation. As the cover is moved back over the left eye, the right eye moves upward to reassume fixation. This set of findings is consistent with:

   a. right hyperdeviation.
   b. left hyperdeviation.
   c. overaction of the inferior obliques.
   d. dissociated vertical deviation.
   e. overaction of the superior obliques.

131. A patient presents for evaluation of "wandering eyes." On alternate-cover testing, with the left eye covered, the right eye fixes a distance target. As the cover is shifted to the right eye, the left eye moves down to pick up fixation. As the cover is shifted back over the left eye, the right does not move in order to reassume fixation. This set of findings is most consistent with:

   a. right hyperdeviation.
   b. left hyperdeviation.
   c. overaction of the inferior obliques.
   d. dissociated vertical deviation.
   e. overaction of the superior obliques.

132. Which of the following regarding dissociated vertical deviation is/are true?

        1. It is frequently associated with congenital esotropia.
        2. It is often bilateral.
        3. It can be made manifest by monocular visual loss of organic etiology.
        4. The deviation is typically reproducible and measurable.

   a. 1, 2, and 3.
   b. 1 and 3.
   c. 2 and 4.
   d. 4 only.
   e. 1, 2, 3, and 4.

133. A 4-year-old child with a moderate-angle esotropia is noted to have a left hypertropia on right gaze and a right hypertropia on left gaze. When fixing with the left eye in right gaze, there is a right hypotropia, and when fixing with the right eye in left gaze, there is a left hypotropia. The most likely clinical diagnosis is:

    a. right hypotropia.
    b. left hypotropia.
    c. esotropia associated with overaction of the inferior oblique muscles.
    d. bilateral trochlear palsy.
    e. esotropia with DVD.

134. Which one of the following regarding overaction of the superior oblique muscle(s) is false?

    a. Some cases are secondary to weakness of the ipsilateral inferior oblique muscle.
    b. It may be associated with an exotropia in primary gaze.
    c. It is frequently associated with exotropia in downgaze.
    d. Unilateral cases may develop an ipsilateral hypotropia in primary gaze.
    e. The hallmark is depression on attempted adduction.

135. Which of the following features argue for a bilateral rather than a unilateral superior oblique paresis?

    1. head tilt.
    2. symptomatic excyclotorsion.
    3. A pattern esotropia.
    4. aggravation of diplopia with right or left head tilt.

    a. 1, 2, and 3.
    b. 1 and 3.
    c. 2 and 4.
    d. 4 only.
    e. 1, 2, 3, and 4.

136. Indications for surgical treatment of superior oblique paresis include:

    1. significant head tilt.
    2. large hypertropia in primary position.
    3. symptomatic diplopia.
    4. V pattern esotropia.

    a. 1, 2, and 3.
    b. 1 and 3.
    c. 2 and 4.
    d. 4 only.
    e. 1, 2, 3, and 4.

137. T or F -- In long-standing superior oblique paresis, the hypertropia may be greatest in all directions of downgaze.

138. T or F -- Each millimeter of recession of a vertical rectus muscle will result in approximately 8 prism diopters of vertical correction.

139. Surgical strategies for the management of a right superior oblique paresis with symptomatic diplopia include all of the following except:

a. right inferior oblique myectomy.
b. right superior oblique tuck.
c. right inferior rectus recession.
d. right superior rectus recession.
e. left superior oblique tenectomy.

140. The procedure of choice in acquired bilateral superior oblique pareses with symptomatic diplopia is the:

a. bilateral inferior oblique myectomy.
b. bilateral superior oblique tuck.
c. bilateral inferior rectus recession.
d. right superior rectus recession and right inferior rectus resection.
e. left superior oblique tenectomy.

141. The surgical procedure of choice in a superior oblique paresis with excyclotorsion only (no vertical diplopia) is the:

a. ipsilateral superior oblique tuck.
b. ipsilateral inferior oblique myectomy.
c. recession of the ipsilateral superior rectus muscle.
d. lateral transposition of the superior oblique tendon.
e. recession of the contralateral inferior rectus.

142. All of the following are features consistent with double elevator palsy except:

a. ipsilateral hypotropia with large secondary deviation.
b. ptosis.
c. forced ductions indicating inferior rectus restriction.
d. chin-down head position.
e. poor Bell's phenomenon on the side of the palsy.

143. Which one of the following regarding Brown's syndrome is false?

a. Both congenital and acquired forms exist.
b. A common manifestation is hypotropia of the involved eye in adduction.
c. Duction and version testing mimic weakness of the ipsilateral superior oblique muscle.
d. Forced duction testing is necessary to confirm the diagnosis.
e. Acquired cases should be observed for a period of time, since many spontaneously improve.

144. Late clinical findings consistent with an inferior blowout fracture of the orbit include all of the following except:

a. proptosis.
b. paresthesia or hypesthesia of the infraorbital region.
c. ipsilateral hypotropia on upgaze.
d. ipsilateral hypertropia on downgaze.
e. positive forced ductions.

145. Which of the following regarding A and V patterns of horizontal strabismus is/are true?

1. A patterns must measure at least 15 prism diopters difference between upgaze and downgaze to be considered significant.
2. V patterns must measure at least 10 prism diopters between upgaze and downgaze to be considered significant.
3. These forms of noncomitance are seen in fewer than 5% of horizontal strabismus.
4. All the extraocular muscles (in varying combinations) have been implicated as responsible for these patterns.

a. 1, 2, and 3.
b. 1 and 3.
c. 2 and 4.
d. 4 only.
e. 1, 2, 3, and 4.

146. T or F -- Oblique muscle dysfunction is uncommon in A or V pattern strabismus.

147. Factors that are critical in the selection of appropriate surgical therapy for A or V pattern strabismus include:

1. measurements and type of deviation in primary position.
2. presence or absence of peripheral fusion.
3. presence and type of oblique muscle dysfunction.
4. presence or absence of head tilt.

a. 1, 2, and 3.
b. 1 and 3.
c. 2 and 4.
d. 4 only.
e. 1, 2, 3, and 4.

148. A patient presents with an exotropia measuring 15 prism diopters in primary position. In downgaze it diminishes to less than 5 prism diopters, and in upgaze it increases to greater than 30 prism diopters. There is no significant oblique muscle dysfunction noted. Appropriate surgical intervention might include:

1. recession of the ipsilateral lateral rectus.
2. resection of the ipsilateral medial rectus.
3. upward transposition of the lateral rectus and downward transposition of the medial rectus.
4. inferior oblique myectomy.

a. 1, 2, and 3.
b. 1 and 3.
c. 2 and 4.
d. 4 only.
e. 1, 2, 3, and 4.

149. A patient presents with a 15 prism diopter exotropia in primary position that diminishes to less than 5 prism diopters in downgaze and increases to greater than 30 prism diopters in upgaze. There is significant elevation of each eye with adduction bilaterally. Appropriate surgical intervention might include:

1. recession of the ipsilateral lateral rectus muscles.
2. recession of the contralateral lateral rectus muscle.
3. bilateral inferior oblique myectomies.
4. upward transposition of the lateral rectus and downward transposition of the medial rectus muscles ipsilaterally.

a. 1, 2, and 3.
b. 1 and 3.
c. 2 and 4.
d. 4 only.
e. 1, 2, 3, and 4.

150. A patient presents with a 20 prism diopter esotropia in primary gaze that increases to 35 prism diopters in downgaze and diminishes to 15 prism diopters in upgaze. There is overaction of the inferior obliques bilaterally. Appropriate surgical intervention might include:

1. recession of ipsilateral medial rectus muscle.
2. resection of the ipsilateral lateral rectus muscle.
3. bilateral inferior oblique myectomies.
4. upward transposition of the lateral rectus and downward transposition of the medial rectus muscles ipsilaterally.

a. 1, 2, and 3.
b. 1 and 3.
c. 2 and 4.
d. 4 only.
e. 1, 2, 3, and 4.

151. A patient presents with a 25 prism diopter esotropia in primary position. The esotropia increases to 45 prism diopters in upgaze and diminishes to 5 prism diopters in downgaze. There is bilateral depression with attempted adduction. Choices for surgical intervention should include:

1. recession of the ipsilateral medial rectus muscle.
2. recession of the contralateral medial rectus muscle.
3. tenotomy of both superior oblique muscles.
4. upward transposition of the ipsilateral medial rectus muscle and downward transposition of the ipsilateral lateral rectus muscle.

a. 1, 2, and 3.
b. 1 and 3.
c. 2 and 4.
d. 4 only.
e. 1, 2, 3, and 4.

152. A patient presents with a 20 prism diopter esotropia in primary position. The esotropia increases to 35 prism diopters in upgaze and diminishes to 15 prism diopters in down-gaze. Appropriate choices for surgical intervention might include:

1. recession of the contralateral medial rectus muscle.
2. recession of the ipsilateral medial rectus muscle.
3. upward transposition of the ipsilateral medial rectus muscle and downward transposition of the ipsilateral lateral rectus muscle.
4. tenotomy of both superior oblique muscles.

a. 1, 2, and 3.
b. 1 and 3.
c. 2 and 4.
d. 4 only.
e. 1, 2, 3, and 4.

153. T or F -- Adjustable suture techniques are useful for nearly every type of strabismus surgery except superior oblique procedures.

154. Superior oblique overaction is most likely to be encountered in:

a. A pattern esotropia.
b. A pattern exotropia.
c. V pattern esotropia.
d. V pattern exotropia.
e. Y pattern exotropia.

155. Match the type of Duane's syndrome listed in the right-hand column with the clinical findings listed in the left-hand column.

a. deficit of both adduction and abduction with orthotropia in primary position.

b. deficit in adduction with exotropia in primary position.

c. deficit in abduction with esotropia in primary position.

d. the most common type.

1. type I.
2. type II.
3. type III.

156. Systemic associations with Duane's syndrome include:

1. sensorineural hearing loss.
2. Goldenhar's syndrome.
3. spinal column anomalies.
4. congenital absence of the pectoral muscle.

a. 1, 2, and 3.
b. 1 and 3.
c. 2 and 4.
d. 4 only.
e. 1, 2, 3, and 4.

157. T or F -- Like sixth nerve palsy, abduction deficit associated with Duane's syndrome leads to progressive contracture of medial rectus muscle.

158. Indications for surgical intervention in Duane's syndrome include:

1. amblyopia.
2. significant head turn.
3. significant globe retraction.
4. significant deviation in primary position.

a. 1, 2, and 3.
b. 1 and 3.
c. 2 and 4.
d. 4 only.
e. 1, 2, 3, and 4.

159. T or F -- An adduction deficit coincident with abducens and facial palsies makes the diagnosis of Möbius' syndrome very unlikely.

160. The most common cause of third nerve palsy in the pediatric population is:

    a. congenital.
    b. traumatic.
    c. inflammatory.
    d. migrainous.
    e. tumor.

161. In adults, the most common cause of third nerve palsy is:

    a. microvascular
    b. traumatic.
    c. inflammatory.
    d. migrainous.
    e. tumor.

162. Strabismus surgery for patients with Graves' ophthalmopathy generally is performed before:

    a. orbital decompression.
    b. orbital radiation.
    c. tarsorrhaphy.
    d. eyelid surgery.
    e. Strabismus surgery is generally performed last.

163. T or F -- Prisms are frequently a permanent solution for strabismus associated with Graves' disease.

164. T or F -- Helpful techniques in the surgical management of patients with Graves' disease and diplopia include muscle resections with adjustable sutures.

165. T or F -- Surgical realignment of the eyes plays a role in the management of strabismus associated with medication-resistant myasthenia gravis.

166. Which of the following conditions is more commonly seen in boys than in girls?

    a. congenital third nerve palsy.
    b. Duane's syndrome.
    c. congenital sixth nerve palsy.
    d. congenital oculomotor apraxia.
    e. Möbius' syndrome.

167. Which of the following conditions is seen more commonly in girls than in boys?

    a. congenital third nerve palsy.
    b. Duane's syndrome.
    c. congenital sixth nerve palsy.
    d. congenital oculomotor apraxia.
    e. Möbius' syndrome.

168. A child's nystagmus is noted to have equal velocity in all directions and to be symmetric in direction, amplitude and frequency in each eye. The nystagmus would most appropriately be described as:

a. uniplanar.
b. pendular, conjugate.
c. jerk, conjugate.
d. pendular, disconjugate.
e. jerk, disconjugate.

169. T or F -- In a neonate or infant, pendular nystagmus is more likely to be sensory than motor nystagmus.

170. T or F -- The hallmark of congenital nystagmus is an exponentially increasing velocity of the slow phase on electronystagmography.

171. T or F -- In congenital motor nystagmus, near visual acuity may be better than distance visual acuity.

172. Sensory nystagmus in an infant may be seen in association with:

1. aniridia.
2. bilateral macular colobomata.
3. bilateral optic nerve hypoplasia.
4. rod monochromatism.

a. 1, 2, and 3.
b. 1 and 3.
c. 2 and 4.
d. 4 only.
e. 1, 2, 3, and 4.

173. Which of the following regarding latent nystagmus is/are true?

1. Its fast phase is toward the uncovered eye.
2. It may become manifest in the setting of monocular visual loss like amblyopia.
3. It is associated with congenital nystagmus and infantile esotropia.
4. It may be the cause of unexpectedly low monocular visual acuity testing.

a. 1, 2, and 3.
b. 1 and 3.
c. 2 and 4.
d. 4 only.
e. 1, 2, 3, and 4.

174. Characteristics considered classic for spasmus nutans include:

        1. head nodding.
        2. a rapid, small-amplitude, conjugate nystagmus.
        3. torticollis.
        4. hypertonia.

    a. 1, 2, and 3.
    b. 1 and 3.
    c. 2 and 4.
    d. 4 only.
    e. 1, 2, 3, and 4.

175. T or F -- Spasmus nutans generally has its onset within the first year of life and resolves within 2 years.

176. The entity in the differential diagnosis with spasmus nutans that must be ruled out is:

    a. optic nerve meningioma.
    b. parasellar glioma.
    c. pontine glioma.
    d. cerebellar astrocytoma.
    e. syringomyelia.

177. Treatment for a patient with congenital nystagmus whose null zone is in right gaze and who has adopted an extreme left head turn might include:

    a. prism base down OU.
    b. prism base in OU.
    c. prism base in OD and base out OS.
    d. prism base out OD and base in OS.
    e. prism base up OU.

178. T or F -- The goal of muscle surgery in congenital nystagmus is to move the null zone to primary position.

179. Surgical intervention for the patient with a null zone in right gaze and severe left head turn might include:

        1. recession of the right lateral rectus.
        2. resection of the right medial rectus.
        3. recession of the left medial rectus.
        4. resection of the left lateral rectus muscle.

    a. 1, 2, and 3.
    b. 1 and 3.
    c. 2 and 4.
    d. 4 only.
    e. 1, 2, 3, and 4.

180. For which of the following procedures might a two-stage adjustable suture technique be advisable?

        1. disassociated vertical divergence.
        2. strabismus associated with Graves' disease.
        3. muscle transposition surgery in A or V pattern horizontal strabismus.
        4. infantile esotropia.

    a. 1, 2, and 3.
    b. 1 and 3.
    c. 2 and 4.
    d. 4 only.
    e. 1, 2, 3, and 4.

181. For which of the following procedures would a rectus muscle transposition procedure be particularly appropriate?

        1. nonresolving sixth nerve palsy.
        2. double elevator palsy.
        3. nonresolving third nerve palsy.
        4. dissociated vertical deviation.

    a. 1, 2, and 3.
    b. 1 and 3.
    c. 2 and 4.
    d. 4 only.
    e. 1, 2, 3, and 4.

182. A 3-year-old child presents to the ophthalmologist with parents complaining of "cross-eyes" for approximately 1 year's duration. Examination discloses visual acuity of 20/30 OD and 20/100 OS with Allen cards. There is a 35 prism diopter esotropia at distance increasing to 45 prism diopters at near. Refraction reveals + 3.50 D OU. Initial steps in managing this patient should include:

    a. bimedial recessions.
    b. bilateral resections.
    c. prescription of + 3.50 OU with add + 3.50 OU (bifocals).
    d. prescription of + 3.50 D OU and patching of the right eye.
    e. a Kestenbaum procedure (bilateral recess/resect procedure).

183. A 7-year-old boy presents with an exotropia. His deviation measures 30 prism diopters in primary position, 20 prism diopters in right gaze, and 40 prism diopters in left gaze. Near deviation is 15 prism diopters in all directions. Fixation appears to alternate, and visual acuity is 20/20 OU. The patient's parents strongly desire some form of correction. You recommend:

    a. addition of - 2.00 D to his current distance refraction.
    b. base-in prism.
    c. bilateral rectus recessions, equal on each side.
    d. bilateral rectus recessions with a greater distance of recession on the left.
    e. bilateral rectus recessions with a greater distance of recession on the right.

184. A patient presents with symptomatic vertical diplopia from a right hypertropia that is greatest in left, left up-, and left downgaze. Appropriate surgical intervention could include all of the following except:

    a. right superior oblique tuck.
    b. left superior oblique tenotomy.
    c. right inferior oblique myectomy.
    d. right superior rectus resection.
    e. left inferior rectus recession.

185. A 1-year-old child is brought to the ophthalmologist by his parents who have noted that "cross-eyes" developed over the previous 6 months. Your examination reveals an approximately 40 prism diopter esotropia at near that does not seem to diminish significantly when the child fixes at longer distances. The child can maintain fixation with either eye easily. Cycloplegic refraction reveals + 1.50 D OU. An appropriate step in the management of this patient might next be:

    a. prescription of + 1.50 D glasses OU.
    b. prescription of + 1.50 D OU with + 3.50 add OU.
    c. alternate patching throughout the day.
    d. bilateral rectus recession of 8 mm OU.
    e. bimedial rectus recession of 5.5 mm OU.

186. After treating a child with mixed mechanism esotropia for 8 months with full hyperopic correction and occlusion therapy, surgery is undertaken to realign his eyes. Visual acuity measures 20/50 OD and 20/25 OS with HOTV cards. There is an esotropia of 30 prism diopters in all directions of gaze. Appropriate surgical intervention would consist of:

    a. bimedial rectus recession of 4.5 mm OU.
    b. bilateral rectus resection of 7 mm OU.
    c. bimedial rectus recession of 7 mm OU.
    d. recession of the right medial rectus 4.5 mm and resection of the right lateral rectus 7 mm.
    e. recession of the left medial rectus 4.5 mm and resection of the left lateral rectus 7 mm.

187. T or F -- It is probably better initially to overcorrect an exodeviation than to undercorrect it.

188. A 6-year-old patient presents to an ophthalmologist for the first time after failing a school eye examination. Complete ophthalmic examination discloses a visual acuity of 20/20 OD and 20/100 OS. There is a comitant left exotropia measuring 30 prism diopters. Cycloplegic refraction reveals + 0.50 D OU. A year of occlusion therapy of the right eye is undertaken, with little improvement in acuity OS. The next step in the management of this patient might be:

a. prescription of -1.50 D OU.
b. base-in prism.
c. bilateral rectus recession of 7 mm.
d. recession of the left lateral rectus 6 mm and resection of the left medial rectus 7 mm.
e. recession of the left lateral rectus 7 mm and resection of the left medial rectus 6 mm.

189. The maximal advisable recession of the medial rectus muscle in the initial surgical management for esotropia is:

a. 3 mm.
b. 4 mm.
c. 5 mm.
d. 5.5 mm.
e. 6 mm.

190. The maximal advisable resection of the lateral rectus muscle in the initial surgical management of esotropia is:

a. 6 mm.
b. 7 mm.
c. 8 mm.
d. 9 mm.
e. 10 mm.

191. The maximal advisable recession of the lateral rectus muscle in the initial surgical management of exotropia is:

a. 5 mm.
b. 6 mm.
c. 7 mm.
d. 10 mm.
e. 12 mm.

192. The maximal advisable resection of the medial rectus muscle in the initial surgical management of exotropia is:

a. 6 mm.
b. 8 mm.
c. 10 mm.
d. 12 mm.
e. 15 mm.

193. Inferior oblique myectomy, performed to correct either primary overaction of the inferior obliques or to correct a V pattern exotropia, came be expected to yield how much correction of hyperdeviation in adduction or how much esodeviation in upgaze?

    a. 5 prism diopters.
    b. 10 prism diopters.
    c. 25 prism diopters.
    d. 40 prism diopters.
    e. 50 prism diopters.

194. Bilateral superior oblique tenotomies, as part of the treatment for A pattern exotropia, can be expected to cause how much of an esodeviation in downgaze?

    a. 5 prism diopters.
    b. 15 prism diopters.
    c. 25 prism diopters.
    d. 40 prism diopters.
    e. 50 prism diopters.

195. Manifestations of ischemia following excessive rectus muscle surgery include:

    1. corneal edema.
    2. anterior chamber reaction.
    3. hypotony.
    4. retinal neovascularization.

    a. 1, 2, and 3.
    b. 1 and 3.
    c. 2 and 4.
    d. 4 only.
    e. 1, 2, 3, and 4.

196. T or F -- Surgery on the superior rectus muscle is more likely to lead to lid malposition postoperatively than surgery on the inferior rectus muscle.

197. Which of the following regarding diplopia after surgery for esotropia is/are true?

1. Adults with acquired strabismus are more likely to suffer from symptoms than children.
2. Postoperative diplopia is most likely to develop in undercorrection of intermittent exotropia.
3. A trial of preoperative prisms may be helpful in predicting who is likely to suffer from this complication.
4. The complication, if persistent, must be managed with a second surgical procedure.

a. 1, 2, and 3.
b. 1 and 3.
c. 2 and 4.
d. 4 only.
e. 1, 2, 3, and 4.

198. A 2-year-old child undergoes bimedial recession for infantile esotropia. On the first postoperative day, the deviation is measured as less than 10 prism diopters of residual esotropia, with fairly good versions. At the 1 week visit, there is a prominent right exotropia, which increases in left gaze. Duction testing reveals an inability to adduct the right eye past the mid-line. The most likely diagnosis is:

a. surgical undercorrection.
b. consecutive exotropia due to surgical overcorrection.
c. postoperative third nerve palsy.
d. lost or slipped right medial rectus.
e. restriction of the right medial rectus due to orbital fat prolapse.

199. Early signs in the development of malignant hyperthermia include all of the following except:

a. tachycardia.
b. arrhythmia.
c. elevated body temperature.
d. darkening of the blood in the operative field.
e. trismus.

200. The mechanism by which botulinum toxin (oculinum) works is:

a. sarcoplasmic capture of extracellular calcium.
b. direct blockage of post-synaptic acetylcholine receptors.
c. inhibition of the formation of actin-myosin complexes.
d. inhibition of release of acetylcholine from presynaptic nerve terminals.
e. direct blockage of muscle cell membrane calcium channels.

201. Oculinum has been shown to be affective for which of the following conditions?

      1. congenital nystagmus.
      2. acute lateral rectus palsy.
      3. dissociated vertical deviation.
      4. essential blepharospasm.

    a. 1, 2, and 3.
    b. 1 and 3.
    c. 2 and 4.
    d. 4 only.
    e. 1, 2, 3, and 4.

202. The most common complication of botulinum injections is:

    a. vertical strabismus.
    b. Adie's pupil.
    c. ptosis.
    d. perforation of the globe.
    e. retrobulbar hemorrhage.

Answers

1. a. 3. Cranial nerve II is the optic nerve and has no role in muscle innervation. Cranial
    b. 3. nerve V, the trigeminal nerve, does not provide motor innervation within the orbit. It
    c. 6. does supply motor innervation to the muscles of mastication.
    d. 2.
    e. 2.
    f. 2.
    g. 4.

2. a. The superior oblique and the levator muscles each arise posteriorly, above the annulus. The inferior oblique arises from the anteromedial orbital floor. The annulus gives rise to the four rectus muscles.

3. e. The horizontal rectus muscles have no torsional or vertical action in primary gaze. In upgaze, they are elevators (weak); in downgaze, they are depressors (weak).

4. a. 3. The spiral of Tillaux describes the ever-increasing distance from limbus to
    b. 2. muscle insertion with rotation from the medial rectus inferiorly around to the
    c. 1. superior rectus muscle (clockwise OD, counterclockwise OS).
    d. 4.

5. d. With the eye abducted 23 degrees, the superior rectus is parallel to the visual axis, and its contraction will result in maximal elevation. For the same reason, in this position, the inferior rectus is maximized as a depressor. In primary gaze, contraction of the superior rectus not only elevates the eye, but also intorts and adducts the eye. (The inferior rectus will extort and adduct the eye, as well as depress it, in primary gaze.)

6. a. With the eye adducted 51 degrees, the tendon of the superior oblique is parallel to the visual axis, and its contraction will result in maximal depression. For the same reason, in this postion, the inferior oblique will be maximized as an elevator. In primary gaze, contraction of the superior oblique not only depresses the eye, but also intorts and abducts the eye. (The inferior oblique will extort and abduct the eye, as well as elevate it, in primary gaze.)

7. False. The inferior oblique's anatomic and mechanical origins are the same--from the anteromedial orbital floor. The superior oblique has its anatomic origin at the orbital apex. Its mechanical origin is at the trochlea, since this is where its effective force is generated.

8. True. The oblique muscles always run <u>below</u> the corresponding rectus muscle.

9. False. See question 8. The inferior rectus lies between the globe and the inferior oblique (the obliques pass <u>below</u> the recti).

10. False. By the time it reaches the trochlea, the superior oblique is already tendinous.

11. b. The inferior oblique also contributes to elevation in primary gaze.

12. a. The superior muscles act as intorters, while the inferior muscles act as extorters. The oblique muscles are more important for torsion than the vertical recti. Thus, the primary intorter of the globe in primary gaze is the superior oblique.

13. a. 3. See answer 12. The vertical recti are both adductors in primary gaze, while the
    b. 4. obliques are abductors. The vertical recti are the important vertically acting
    c. 1. muscles, and the obliques the important torters.
    d. 2.

14. c. The belly of the superior oblique is approximately 32 mm (the others are 37 to 40 mm).

15. d. The inferior oblique is muscle virtually all the way to its insertion over the posterior sclera.

16. a. The lateral rectus muscle contributes only <u>one</u> anterior ciliary artery to the major arterial circle. Thus, there are a total of seven anterior ciliary arteries.

17. False. All six extraocular muscles that attach to the globe must penetrate Tenon's capsule. The levator muscle does not.

18. True.

19. False. Typically, the motor nerve penetrates each muscle at the junction of the posterior one-third and anterior two-thirds of the belly.

20. b. Since the superior rectus is loosely attached to the levator complex, recession will pull the levator <u>back</u> and widen the fissure, while resection will pull the levator <u>forward</u> and narrow the fissure. The same relationships apply for the inferior rectus, since its sheath gives rise to the capsulopalpebral fascia. Operation on the superior oblique should not affect the palpebral fissure.

21. c. Two muscles may nearly always be safely removed. Removal of four muscles is certain to cause ischemia. Removal of three muscles is likely to lead to some degree of ischemia.

22. c. The main synergist of the superior rectus is the <u>inferior</u> oblique (both <u>elevate</u> the globe).

23.
   a. 6.   g. 5.
   b. 12.   h. 10.
   c. 2.   i. 1.
   d. 4.   j. 9.
   e. 7.   k. 3.
   f. 11.   l. 8.

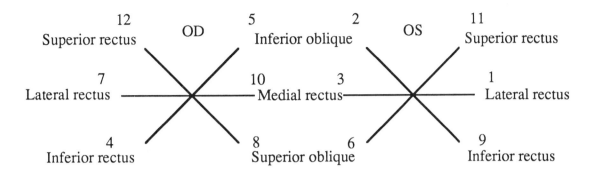

24. **True.** Hering's law of yoke muscles states that "yoked" muscles (contralateral) muscles must always receive equal innervational input. Sherrington's law states that innervation to an (ipsilateral) antagonist decreases as innervation to the agonist increases.

25. **b.** In DVD, the affected eye drifts up under cover. When the cover is shifted to the other eye, if Hering's law is followed, yoke innervation should generate a contralateral hypotropia. This is <u>not</u> seen in DVD for reasons that are unclear.

26. **e.** In Duane's syndrome, innervational impulses to the medial rectus are <u>not</u> associated with decreased innervation of the ipsilateral lateral rectus muscles, as Sherrington's law demands. This is because of anomalous innervation of the lateral rectus, in this case from the oculomotor (III) nerve, which leads to co-innervation of the horizontal rectus muscles, with globe retraction on adduction.

27. **True.** Conjugate binocular movements imply both eyes move a similar amount in a similar direction (right, left, up, down) at the same time.

28. **False.** Fusional convergence is always accompanied by accommodation, but divergence is <u>not</u> always accompanied by relaxation of accommodation.

29. **b.**

30. **d.** Note that saccades are generated contralaterally, while pursuits are generated ipsilaterally.

31. **False.** Within a certain range around the empirical horopter--that is, Panum's space--objects will be perceived as <u>one</u>, with stereopsis. Any point <u>on</u> the horopter must be perceived singly.

32. **False.** Panum's space is broader peripherally and narrower centrally. Again, this range describes the area of object space where an object off the horopter will still be perceived singly and with stereopsis.

33. False. If stimultaneous stimulation of two retinal areas leads to perception of one image, then sensory <u>fusion</u> is said to exist. If the two retinal areas have identical topographic locations relative to the fovea, <u>then</u> normal retinal correspondence exists.

34. False. As described in answers 31 and 32, stereopsis can be generated for points off the horopter, if they lie within Panum's space. Some discrepancy in perception between two eyes <u>must</u> exist for stereopsis to follow. There is <u>no</u> discrepancy for objects located <u>on</u> the horopter!

35. False. In abnormal or anomalous retinal correspondence, simultaneous stimulation of two areas of retina that do <u>not</u> have the same topographic relation to the fovea (noncorresponding) still leads to perception of <u>one</u> image (sensory fusion).

36. True. If the two images are sufficiently different, visual confusion will be created.

37. d. Normal divergence amplitudes at distance is <u>6</u> prism diopters. At near, this increases to 16 prism diopters.

38. False. Monocular clues such as image size, motion, and parallax are probably more important than stereopsis (a higher binocular function) for satisfactory depth perception.

39. d.

40. c.

41. True. In kittens, the critical or sensitive period is probably 6 to 12 weeks. In children, the first 3 to 6 months are particularly important, but the visual system is susceptible to developmental arrest (amblyopia) for the first 6 years of life, perhaps longer.

42. False. Diplopia, or double images of a single object, exists when the two images of the object fall on noncorresponding areas of the retina. When two different objects are simultaneously imaged on the foveas and perceived, visual <u>confusion</u> exists.

43. False. Although suppression is the most common explanation for absence of diplopia with manifest strabismus, marked organic visual loss in the deviating eye will prevent diplopia, requiring no central suppression. In large-angle esotropia, the nasal bridge may "occlude" the deviating eye and prevent diplopia. Anomalous retinal correspondence may also prevent diplopia despite an obvious tropia.

44. b. Approximately 1 in 50 people suffer from amblyopia. The incidence of strabismus, with or without amblyopia, is slightly higher, at 1 in 25 to 30. Afferent pupillary defects may be seen in amblyopia of any cause but should heighten suspicions about an organic lesion. "Crowding" refers to poorer recognition acuities in amblyopia when targets are presented multiply rather than singly. Neutral density filters will not significantly affect vision in amblyopes, unlike patients with maculopathy.

45. c. Amblyopia in Duane's syndrome is uncommon but is more likely than in alternating esotropia, where each eye shares the visual workload.

46. False. One week for every <u>year</u> of age is the typical pattern for follow-up of the patient undergoing treatment for amblyopia.

47.   b.   Cyclic esotropia is rarely accompanied by amblyopia. With full eye movements and no globe retraction, there can be no Duane's syndrome, particularly given amblyopia. Parafoveal fixation is difficult to assign to factitious etiologies. All of the findings described (mild amblyopia, mildly impaired stereopsis, peripheral fusion, eccentric fixation with a central suppression scotoma) are typical of a microtropia (the tropia is either too small to detect or does not exist due to parafoveal fixation and anomalous retinal correspondence).

48.   c.   Microtropia is most commonly seen after successful (or nearly so) strabismus surgery, as well as in the setting of anisometropia.

49.   d.   A weak base-out prism will shift a fixation target nasally. If placed over the microtropic eye, the shift will <u>not</u> move the target out of the suppression scotoma, and <u>no</u> refixation movement is generated. When placed contralaterally, both eyes will shift away from the base of the prism. No fusional convergence will be seen contralaterally because of the central scotoma. In normal eyes, the contralateral eye converges to fuse the fixation images.

50.   False.   A small central scotoma may permit fusion with normal retinal correspondence and without visual confusion.

51.   d.   Esotropia gives uncrossed diplopia on red glass testing. Thus, the left light (red) should appear to the left of the right light (white).

52.   c.   The right image is probably being suppressed. There may be either normal retinal correspondence or ARC. To determine which, the right image is moved out of the central suppression scotoma with a vertical prism. In ARC, the right white light will appear <u>directly</u> below the left red light. On the other hand, it is possible that the patient is malingering (voluntary convergence spasm) and being less than truthful about his perceptions. Findings supportive of this conclusion include a variable and unpredictable amount of esotropia in various gaze positions, as well as noticeable miosis with lateral gaze, particularly to the right.

IN NRC, AFTER MOVING IMAGE OUT OF SCOTOMA LIGHTS WILL NOT BE ONLY VERTICALLY SEPARATED BUT HORIZONTALLY separated as well.

53.   c.   When <u>identical</u> images are projected into each eye, if the angle of the tropia and the angle of subjective image separation are equal, there is normal retinal correspondence. If images are superimposed by a prism whose power is different than that required to neutralize the <u>tropia</u>, there is unharmonious ARC. If ARC is harmonious, there will be fusion with <u>no</u> prism. An amblyoscope is used to project similar images onto each fovea. The angle of deviation between the two targets matches the tropia angle in NRC. If the angle of deviation is less than the tropia, ARC is unharmonious. If the angle is zero in the setting of a tropia, ARC is harmonious.

AS IN ARC c central suppression scotoma.

54.   d.   It is better to flash the vertical line into the <u>deviated</u> eye, since displacement of a horizontal line may be missed with a suppression scotoma. If there is eccentric fixation, the test is more difficult to interpret. In right exotropia and ARC, the image the patients sees with the right eye (vertical) will be displaced to the <u>right</u> (since it lies on the anatomic fovea, nasal to the "pseudofovea" of ARC).

55.   True.   Bagolini-glass testing cannot be interpreted without knowledge of the strabismus findings (tropia present?) and fixation behavior.

56.   c.   There is no <u>manifest</u> deviation (tropia, cover-uncover test) but a latent esodeviation (phoria, alternate-cover test).

57. e.   In the setting of an esotropia (detected by cover-uncover test), the alternate-cover test <u>must</u> disclose some strabismus, since it detects both tropia and phoria. The cover-uncover test detects only tropia.

58. False.   Most of the normal adult population has a small <u>phoria</u>, more often exophoria.

59. d.

60. a.   Decisions regarding occlusion therapy require an assessment of the risk of amblyopia (age of onset, refractive/accommodative components, alternating versus nonalternating) as well as which eye is more at risk. Family history is not critical in determining the actual strategy, as a rule.

61. a.   Snellen figures, particularly presented in rows, are the most challenging, and perhaps most relevant, type of acuity test.

62. e.   Optokinetic nystagmus has been used to <u>quantify</u> acuity, but the procedure is more cumbersome and difficult to score accurately than preferential-looking.

63. a.   The Krimsky test uses prisms over the fixating eye to center the light reflex over the pupil in the devating eye. Foveal fixation is not required.

64. b.   Each millimeter of decentration is 7 degrees of deviation. Each degree is approximately 2 prism diopters. Thus, each millimeter is approximately 15 prism diopters. Three millimeters is 21-plus degrees, or 45 prism diopters. Since the reflex is displaced <u>temporally</u>, the eye must be deviated <u>inward</u> (esotropia).

65. d.   See answer 63.

66. d.   As the fixing eye is covered, a prism is simultaneously placed over the deviated eye. When there is no refixation shift, the prism has neutralized the tropia. The alternate-cover test with prisms will neutralize total phoria <u>plus</u> tropia. The cover-uncover test with prisms will neutralize tropia plus part of the phoria.

67. False.   The real image of a Maddox rod is a line parallel to the axes of the rod, immediately in front of the rod. It requires too much accommodation to be seen. The image that is perceived is a <u>virtual</u> image of a line <u>perpendicular</u> to the rod axes, behind the rod.

68. Truc.   The image formed is a <u>horizontal</u> line that permits perception of vertical image disparity.

69. d.   In excyclotropia, the superonasal retinal quadrant is rotated vertically toward 12 o'clock, and the inferotemporal quadrent is rotated toward 6 o'clock. The vertical line from the Maddox rod will run superonasal to inferotemporal on the retina and be perceived the same way.

70. a. In the Lancaster red-green test, the fovea of each eye is isolated with duochrome glasses. The eye under green glass (left) will not see the red light and the eye under the red glass (right) will not see the green light. By holding the green light centrally, the examiner holds the patient's left fovea centrally. Assuming normal retinal correspondence (NRC), the patient will direct the red light in space along his right visual axis to place the red light on his right fovea and superimpose the foveal images. The patient's right visual axis (in esotropia) crosses his left visual axis, so the right foveal image will fall to the left of the left foveal image (as seen by the examiner). To the patient, the images appear superimposed (assuming NRC).

71. e. See answer 70. This is true because the strabismus is acquired. In that case, we can assume NRC and central fixation.

72. d. In this case, the deviated right eye is fixing centrally (green glass). The larger secondary deviation, a left esotropia of greater magnitude, will cause the red light (left foveal image) appear to the right of the green light (right foveal image).

73. e. Because of suppression, the Lancaster test is not useful for congenital strabismus, but only for acquired cases. In this case, the patient will see only one light!

74. d. The first three tests utilize actual fixation behavior and will not fall victim to large angle kappa or facial anomalies. The Krimsky and Hirschberg methods use apparent eccentricity of pupillary reflexes and may be misguided by these factors.

75. True. The mnemonic that is used is NOTE: Nasal displacement of the light reflex corresponds to pOsitive angle kappa and pseudoexotropia. This occurs with temporal macular ectopia. Temporal displacement of light reflex corresponds to nEgative angle kappa (pseudoesotropia). This occurs with nasal macular ectopia.

76. True. See answer 75.

77. b. The base of the prism is always placed opposite to the direction of the deviation.

78. c. See answer 77.

79. True.

80. e. A 25 prism diopter increase in esotropia from distance to near is almost certainly a high AC/A ratio.

81. c. By the gradient method, AC/A ratio equals the difference in the deviation induced by a lens divided by the specific accommodative gradient (of an extra lens over the distance correction). Minus lenses stimulate accommodation while plus lenses blunt it. Here, 50 - 35 divided by 1 = 15:1.

82. b. By the heterophoria method, the AC/A ratio equals the near deviation minus the distance deviation divided by the accommodative demand at near, plus the pupillary distance (PD) in centimeters. Here this is

$$35 - 10 = 25,$$
divided by 5 (reading at 20 cm) = 5
plus 6 (PD in cm) = 11:1.

Heterophoria method:

$$AC/A = \frac{\text{deviation at near - deviation at distance}}{\text{accommodation (D)}} + PD \text{ (cm)}$$

Gradient method:

$$AC/A = \frac{\text{deviation with lens - deviation without lens}}{\text{lens power (D)}}$$
(AT NEAR) (AT NEAR)

83. a. Factors known to be associated with decompensated latent strabismus include alcohol, fatigue, and illness. Decreased visual acuity (e.g., cataract) may also lead to fusional breakdown, with resultant manifest strabismus.

84. True. When performed at distance, central retinal elements are stimulated, and central fusion is evaluated. When performed at near, more peripheral fusion processes are tested. The test is not capable of detecting small suppression socotomata (i.e., near Worth testing may be normal in the setting of a central scotoma).

85. d. The finding of a left hypertropia indicates that more than a simple right trochlear palsy is present, but does not eliminate this possibility, since the left hypertropia is seen only in right gaze (indicating probable left superior oblique palsy). A right hypertropia in primary gaze that is worsened with left gaze is classic for right trochlear palsy. The V pattern esotropia is convincing evidence of a bilateral superior oblique palsy, but a right hypertopia worse in right gaze, by the three-step test, maps to the right inferior rectus or the left inferior oblique and is thus inconsistent with the diagnosis.

86. a. Right head tilt stimulates intorsion of the right eye to keep the visual field at the proper angle. The intorters are the superior rectus and the superior oblique. In the setting of a superior oblique palsy, the vertical, elevating force generated by the superior rectus is not effectively balanced by the depressing force of the superior oblique, so the eye goes up.

87. c. The clinical findings of mydriasis and accommodative paresis indicate damage to the parasympathetic supply to the globe. These nerves travel with the nerve to the inferior oblique before forming the short root of the ciliary ganglion. The motility findings in this case indicate a probable inferior oblique palsy (inability to elevate the adducted eye). The three-step test should show a left hypotropia (right hypertropia) worsened in right gaze and right head tilt.

88. a. Exaggerated sensitivity to cholinergic blockade has been reported in albinos and patients with Down's syndrome. Infants are also particularly sensitive. Atropine is a treatment for heart block (acutely) and should not cause arrhythmias in patients with this disorder.

89. e. Atropine's central nervous system side effects include both alerting/agitation and somnolence! Flushing and tachycardia are particularly common in infants.

90. False. The prism adaptation test involves prescription of corrective prisms in anticipation of muscle surgery to determine if the patient can achieve sensory fusion with alignment. This test may be associated with an increase in the angle of strabismus, as the patient "eats" the prisms.

91. a. 2. Simple or basic esotropia is generally a large-size deviation with no
    b. 5. increment at near and normal refractive error. Pure refractive accommodative
    c. 4. esotropia is a moderate distance deviation that may be somewhat larger
    d. 1. at near and is always associated with high hyperopia. Nonrefractive
    e. 3. accommodative esotropia is due to a high AC/A ratio. The deviation at distance is small or unmeasurable but increases markedly at near. The refractive error is usually normal. Mixed mechanism esotropia is a combination of simple and accommodative forms with moderate or large distance deviation that increases at near and is associated with a high AC/A ratio (or moderate to high hyperopia).

92. b. With cross-fixation, amblyopia is less likely to develop, since the youngster will use each eye at different times. An accommodative component may be discovered in many cases of infantile esotropia.

93. a. Latent nystagmus, overacting inferior obliques, and DVD are such common concomitants that they should be specifically sought in the examination of a child with infantile esotropia. High AC/A ratio may be seen (see answer 92) but is not typical.

94. a. Surgery for esotropia must provide either weakening of the medial rectus muscles (recession) or strengthening of the lateral rectus muscles (resection). Recession always has a greater effect than a resection of the same amount. Thus, bimedial recession is generally performed before bilateral resection. In some cases, however, bilateral resection may be the first procedure (for instance, in esotropia that is greater at distance). Combined medial and lateral resection is an equally effective alternative.

95. True. Success in surgical management of infantile esotropia is multifaceted, but with reference to the strabismus, the residual turn should be less than 10 prism diopters for the procedure to be termed successful. This amount of residual tropia is frequently cosmetically undetectable. If the residual turn is too small to be detected with typical cover-uncover testing (less than 5-8 prism diopters), a microtropia exists. This situation is stable over time in many cases, and is associated with peripheral fusion and limited stereopsis (see questions 47-50). If there is eccentric fixation near the fovea, visual acuity will be mildly depressed with no tropia evident on cover testing (but no central fusion). •Binocularity with central suppression.

96. True. Congenital motor nystagmus frequently has a point where the amplitude and frequency are dampened (null point). Some experts believe that some children are esotropic in order to hold their null point in eye position. This contention is not universally accepted, however.

97. c.   Amblyopia is certainly possible given the constant esotropia. A large-angle turn might provide cross-fixation, but amblyopia must be ruled out. Given the age of onset, an accommodative component is likely, so an originally intermittent turn is also possible. No patient with manifest strabismus has any stereopsis whatsoever. Certainly, a family history of esotropia of any mechanism is possible.

98. b.   This patient probably has refractive accommodative esotropia. Amblyopia is possible bilaterally, given the high ametropia. The deviation may be greater at near than distance, but this is not highly likely because patients with refractive accommodative esotropia typically have normal AC/A ratios. In this type of esotropia, the turn is usually moderate (20-40 prism diopters), although it may be greater. +3.00 lenses may lessen <u>non</u>refractive accommodative esotropia but typically have little effect on this type (with +3.00 lenses, there would still be a residual 5 D of hyperopia).

99. c.   In all cases of accommodative esotropia, full hyperopic correction is warranted immediately. Penalization with atropine may be useful in cases of noncompliance with spectacles and/or patching therapy. Bifocals may be of value with high AC/A ratio with a residual turn at near after full correction.

100. a.   This is probably a case of nonrefractive accommodative amblyopia (intermittent turn, worse at near, with normal refractive error and high AC/A ratio). +3.00D lenses for near work will relieve the accommodative demand and prevent accommodative convergence from causing an esotropia.

101. d.   Surgery is necessary in virtually all cases of infantile esotropia, while many cases of pure accommodative esotropia will resolve with time and refractive correction. Bifocals are generally most helpful in nonrefractive accommodative esotropia, where high AC/A ratios make the esotropia worse at near. If full refractive correction is not the solution, some experts advocate atropine penalization with full correction or pilocarpine treatment to provide accommodation without convergence. These steps frequently fail, however, and are controversial.

102. d.   Age of onset between 2 and 3 years makes an accommodative mechanism more likely, with better prognosis for refractive correction. The other findings are consistent with a large-angle, congenital esotropia.

103. c.   Persistent esotropia on pilocarpine treatment may be seen in accommodative esotropia, so spectacle correction must always be attempted. Surgical results are much more stable and predictable in the setting of maximal visual acuity (after occlusion therapy).

104. False. The converse is true. That is, with illness or stress, nonrefractive accommodative esotropia (high AC/A ratio) is more likely to decompensate than the refractive variety.

105. c.   Correction with full hyperopic prescription may weaken the patient's fusional divergence, which is the force keeping accommodative esotropia intermittent at its outset. Then, the esotropia may become constant without the "crutch" of the spectacles.

106. a.   The cycle is typically 48 hours long--one day of esotropia, and one day of orthotropia. Many experts believe that this is a variety of accommodative esotropia, with many features similar to it.

107. d.   Divergence insufficiency is indistinguishable from sixth nerve palsy, except it is typically comitant. Sixth nerve palsy is more likely to have an esotropia at near as well.

108. b.   The myopia may be hard to establish if the spasm is intermittent, but the miosis is detectable and the diagnostic "clincher." Also, the angle of turn is highly variable and unpredictable.

109. False.   Although many experts will obtain timely neuroimaging tests (CT/MRI), abducens palsy in a child is a common postviral syndrome and typically resolves uneventfully. The second most common etiology is increased intracranial pressure (central nervous system mass lesions, pseudotumor cerebri).

110. c.   Unless the palsy is acquired early in childhood, goes untreated (with occlusion), and/or does not resolve, amblyopia is highly unlikely. Some children will develop a permanent esotropia after abducens palsy, probably representing a decompensated esophoria. Thus, all cases must be followed to resolution.

111. b.   Medial rectus resection would aggravate the esotropia. The most widely accepted approach in sixth nerve palsy is a muscle-splitting operation utilizing half of the superior and inferior rectus muscles in transposition laterally (Jensen procedure). Prisms may be of temporary assistance, but should be base-<u>out</u> to correct the esotropia.

112. False.   Consecutive exotropia of moderate degree after surgery for esotropia is not uncommon. It commonly resolves within several weeks or months of surgery with no therapy, other than continued occlusion.

113. True.   This is, in general, a useful guideline. It is by no means foolproof, particularly in adults with long-standing esophoria, who may decompensate into esotropia with unilateral visual loss.

114. b.   Exotropia that is equal at distance and near is basic. If the deviation is greater at near, then it is termed convergence insufficiency exotropia. If it is greater at distance than near, it is termed divergence excess exotropia.

115. d.   Divergence excess exotropia may be divided into two subtypes. In some cases of "divergence excess" exotropia, the turn appears larger at a distance because of enhanced fusional convergence at near related to accommodation. Interrupting fusion with prolonged occlusion (greater than 30 minutes) or relaxing accommodation with <u>plus</u> lenses may cause the deviation at near to increase to a measurement similar to the original distance measurement. This is "simulated divergence excess." If these manipulations have no effect (i.e., the distance measurement is still larger), true divergence excess is said to exist.

116. d.   (See answer 115.)

117. e.   (See answer 115.)

118. False.   Congenital exotropia is relatively uncommon. Most exotropias develop during childhood as intermittent deviations.

119. a.   Most constant exotropia is intermittent originally.

120. False. Some cases of exotropia may resolve entirely, but this is much less common than with accommodative esotropia. The majority of cases remain intermittent, becoming manifest with fatigue, stress, illness, or alcohol consumption. Some cases become constant and require surgery.

121. a. High AC/A ratios develop as a fusional mechanism for near work. The turn in intermittent exotropia is highly variable and sensitive to external stimuli (see answer 120). Bright light typically causes reflex closure of the deviating eye. Amblyopia is highly unlikely if the turn is truly intermittent. *The suppression scotoma protects the eye from amblyopia.*

122. False. While this may be occasionally the case, the majority of patients with truly intermittent exotropia have excellent stereoacuity.

123. b. Minus lenses stimulate accommodation and may provide the extra convergence needed for fusion. Base-in prisms may permit fusion but are not advocated by all, since they may weaken fusional convergence and convert an intermittent to a constant deviation. Phospholine plays a role in accommodative esotropia, not exotropia. Lateral rectus resections strengthen the lateral rectus and will exacerbate exotropia.

124. False. Many cases remain intermittent, with decreasing frequency and amount of manifest exotropia.

125. True. It is often larger with attempted adduction. It will also be marked by globe retraction on adduction.

126. c. By definition, convergence insufficiency is a latent deviation, not a manifest one. (This is not the same entity as convergence insufficiency exotropia, which is a manifest deviation.)

127. True. Base-out prisms may be used to stimulate fusional convergence, while base-in prisms may be used to lessen the convergence demand.

128. True.

129. False. Innervational (buzzword for idiopathic) vertical strabismus is far less common than the horizontal varieties.

130. b. The left eye deviates upward under cover, and the right eye deviates downward under cover. This is a left hyper- or a right hypodeviation.

131. d. DVD simulates a hyperphoria but violates Hering's law. When covered, the left eye drifts up. When uncovered, the left eye moves down to assume fixation. By Hering's law, the yoke muscles of the right eye, depressors, should receive equal innervation as the left eye moves down. The right eye should be deviated downward under cover (right "hypo") and move up to reassume fixation when the cover is shifted back to the left eye. This does not occur, consistent with dissociated vertical divergence. (The dissociation refers to the violation of Hering's law with dissociation of yoke muscles.)

132. a. DVD is a frequent concomitant of infantile esotropia and frequently is made manifest only when visual input to the affected eye is interrupted (occlusion, amblyopia, other organic disease). The deviation is highly variable and difficult to measure, making surgery difficult to quantify accurately.

133. c.   This set of findings is not particularly unusual in infantile esotropia. There are two potential explanations for the vertical deviation in lateral gaze. The first is overaction of the inferior obliques. In this condition, on lateral gaze, there is hypotropia of the abducted, nonfixing eye. In DVD, in lateral gaze there is no associated hypotropia, in violation of Hering's law. In fact, if the DVD is bilateral, there may be hyperdeviation of the abducted, nonfixing eye. The distinction between the two is important for surgical planning.

[handwritten margin note: Why is this not A trochlear B.lat palsy?]

134. a.   Overaction of the inferior oblique may be seen as a primary disorder or secondary to underaction of the ipsilateral, antagonist superior oblique. This duality of causes for superior oblique overaction is not seen. Since isolated underaction of the inferior obliques is quite uncommon, secondary overaction of the superior oblique is also uncommon. Only primary mechanisms are recognized.

135. d.   Head tilt and excyclotorsion are not uncommonly seen in unilateral cases and are not useful. V, not A, pattern esotropia results from underaction in downgaze and subsequent unopposed adduction in downgaze by the inferior rectus. In unilateral superior oblique palsies, lateral gaze toward the involved side generally relieves the diplopia. Aggravation of diplopia in both directions argues for bilateral involvement, as does aggravation with head tilt in either direction.

136. a.   If the V pattern esotropia does not cause troublesome diplopia, then surgery is not indicated.

137. True.   Superior oblique pareses are particularly prone to develop "spread of comitance," so that the deviation becomes more difficult to localize. Surgical therapy must also address this.

138. False.   Each millimeter of vertical muscle recession will correct approximately 3 prism diopters of vertical strabismus.

139. c.   Surgical management of superior oblique underaction is generally aimed at weakening the ipsilateral inferior oblique (myectomy) and/or strengthening the ipsilateral superior oblique. If the hyperdeviation is greater than 35 prism diopters in primary gaze, then strengthening the ipsilateral inferior rectus or weakening the ipsilateral superior rectus may be of value. Contralateral superior oblique weakening may also be useful in certain cases.

140. b.

141. d.   This procedure, the Harado-Ito procedure, increases the force vector for incyclotorsion by moving the lateral half of the insertion of the paretic muscle. It has no effect on vertical eye movement or fusion.

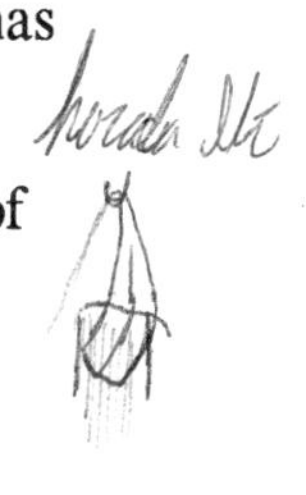

142. d.   Double elevator palsy may be primarily due to elevator weakness or to restriction of the depressors. Ptosis, hypotropia, and poor elevation in any direction are characteristic. A subset will have positive forced ductions for the inferior rectus. Head position is generally an automatic compensation for the hypotropia, with the chin <u>UP</u>.

143. c.   In Brown's syndrome, elevation is limited in adduction, but not in abduction. Duction testing mimics paresis of the ipsilateral <u>inferior</u> oblique.

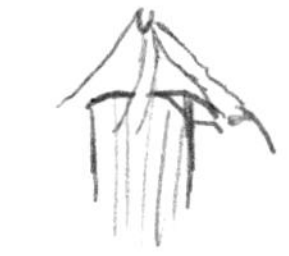

144. a.   Enophthalmos is frequently cosmetically unacceptable. In the acute setting, there may be proptosis, but this usually gives way to enophthalmos as swelling subsides.

145. d.   For an A deviation to be significant, the difference in measurements between upgaze and downgaze must exceed 10 prism diopters. For V patterns, the difference must measure 15 prism diopters. Approximately 15% of horizontal strabismus cases have a significant A or V component.

146. False.   Oblique underaction or overaction is frequently implicated in the pathogenesis of A and V patterns.

147. b.   The basic procedure must address the deviation in primary gaze. If there is no significant oblique dysfunction, then transposition of the rectus insertions may be performed to correct the A or V patterns. If there is oblique dysfunction, then the type and amount must be determined.

148. a.   In V pattern exotropia, one should search of overaction of the inferior obliques or underaction of the superior obliques. If neither is present, then lateral rectus recession and medial rectus resection should be performed with downward transposition (toward the Apex of the V) of the Medial rectus insertion, by one-half the insertion width, and upward transposition (toward the Empty space of the V) of the Lateral rectus insertion, again by one-half the insertion width. The mnemonic for this is MALE:

Medial rectus toward the Apex and Lateral rectus toward the Empty space.

This holds for both A patterns and V patterns.

149. a.   In this case of V pattern exotropia, there is significant overaction of the inferior obliques. Bilateral inferior oblique myectomies will lessen the V pattern by 15 to 25 prism diopters but leave a residual exotropia in primary gaze, necessitating a recess-resect procedure. When oblique muscle surgery has been performed, rectus transpositions are not necessary.

150. a.   In V pattern esotropia with overacting inferior obliques, inferior oblique myectomy will cause 15 to 25 prism diopters of esoshift in upgaze. This only makes the deviation more comitant. Thus, the deviation in primary gaze must be addressed with appropriate medial rectus recession and lateral rectus resection. Since oblique surgery is indicated, rectus transpositions are not.

151. a.   Here, since the A pattern esotropia is greater than 35 prism diopters in upgaze, overaction of the superior obliques may be addressed with superior oblique tenotomies bilaterally. This will create an esoshift of up to 40 prism diopters in downgaze (only). As with V pattern esotropia and inferior oblique myectomy, this only makes the deviation more comitant. Recess/resect (or bimedial recession) procedures must be included.

152. a.   See answer 151. In this case, the A pattern is less than 35 prism diopters, so bilateral superior oblique surgery might leave a residual esotropia in downgaze after horizontal muscle surgery. In this case, the A pattern can be dealt with via transpositions of the rectus insertions (medial rectus toward the apex--up; lateral rectus toward the empty space--down).

153. False.   Quantifying the effect of superior oblique tenotomy is particularly difficult, making adjustable sutures valuable.

154. b.　Remember that the superior oblique muscles are abductors, particularly in downgaze. Thus, overaction will result in overabduction (exotropia) in downgaze (A pattern).

155. a. 3.
     b. 2.
     c. 1.
     d. 1.

156. a.　Klippel-Feil syndrome is one spinal anomaly associated with Duane's syndrome. (Goldenhar's syndrome features cervical vertebral anomalies as well.)

157. False.　This is an important differentiating feature between Duane's and sixth nerve palsy. *why?* The medial rectus muscle nearly always undergoes progressive contracture in the setting of a nonresolving sixth nerve palsy. This virtually never occurs in Duane's syndrome. Forced ductions may help differentiate between the two in puzzling cases of a long-standing abduction deficit.

158. c.　Amblyopia in Duane's syndrome is generally due to anisometropia rather than strabismus. In any case, it must be treated before attempting surgical realignment. Globe retraction may be lessened by lateral rectus recessions but is rarely if ever a solitary indication for surgery.

159. False.　The brainstem nuclei most likely to be involved by Möbius' syndrome are the sixth, seventh, ninth, and twelveth. The third nerve nucleus may also be involved, however, and oculomotor weakness does not make the diagnosis less likely. *POLAND ANOMALY (missing pectorals)*

160. a.　The etiologies for pediatric third nerve palsy, in descending frequency, are congenital, trauma, inflammation, migraine, and neoplasm.

161. a.　The etiologies for adult third nerve palsy, in descending frequency, are microvascular, aneurysm, trauma, and neoplasm.

162. d.　Since muscle surgery, particularly the vertical muscle surgery often indicated in Graves' disease, can affect the position of the eyelids, it is generally wise to perform any strabismus surgery before eyelid repositioning. For instance, some of the lid retraction seen in affected patients may be directly attributable to superior rectus overaction (with subsequent lid retraction) attempting to counter inferior rectus contracture.

163. False.　The deviations of Graves' disease are classically noncomitant and not easily addressed with prisms.

164. False.　Adjustable sutures are very helpful in this condition (which may respond unpredictably to muscle surgery). Resection techniques, however, are generally avoided, since Graves' disease generally causes considerable restriction. Resection would tend to exacerbate this and leave an eye nearly frozen, if overdone.

165. False.　Since the deviations in myasthenia gravis are particularly variable and noncomitant, surgery may cause more difficulties than it relieves.

166. d.　Duane's syndrome is more common in girls, while congenital apraxia is more common in boys.

167. b.　See answer 166.

168. b.　Jerk nystagmus has clearly biphasic velocities--fast in one direction and slow in the other. Disconjugate nystagmus has different amptiude and/or frequency in one eye relative to the other. Uniplanar nystagmus is, as its name implies, present in one plane only, usually horizontal.

169. True.　True motor nystagmus is virtually always of the jerk type. In fact, some "nystagmologists" are reluctant to term any pendular variety as true nystagmus, maintaining that biphasic velocity is part of the definition. Many "pendular" cases of motor nystagmus are actually jerk, with very similar velocities requiring electroculography for differentiation.

170. True.　This is in distinction to latent nystagmus, in which the slow phase shows exponentially decreasing velocity.

171. True.　The hallmarks of congenital motor nystagmus include dampening with convergence and aggravation by fixation. Near work may be associated with convergence and dampening with subsequent improvement in acuity.

172. e.

173. e.　Latent nystagmus becomes manifest with monocular occlusion or visual loss and is probably underdiagnosed. It may be an unsuspected cause of "amblyopia" if acuity testing is performed with total occlusion. Using fogging plus lenses that provide blurred images to the "occluded" eye may circumvent this problem (decreased acuity due to a moving, disorted image).

174. b.　The nystagmus of spasmus nutans is typically small in amplitude but characterized by its disconjugate nature. It may appear to be entirely monocular and raise the spectre of chiasmal or hypothalamic glioma. The third part of the classic triad is head bobbing.

175. True.　The disorder is rarely discovered after the age of 3 years.

176. b.　Many pediatric ophthalmologists will obtain neuroimaging tests of children with monocular nystagmus, unless combined with obvious head bobbing and torticollis. Cases of anterior visual pathway glioma associated with head bobbing have been reported!

177. c.　This combination of prisms will force the child to gaze to the right in order to see objects straight ahead. This will obviate a head turn, which is typically the end point of treatment.

178. True.　This is done by shifting the resting position out of primary position toward the direction opposite to the null zone. Then, to obtain primary gaze, the child will need to innervate ocular muscles as if gaze were toward the null zone!

179. e.　This combination of procedures will shift both eyes to the left in resting position. In order to look straight ahead, the patient will be forced to innervate muscles in a pattern identical to right gaze (null zone) before surgery.

180. a.　In these disorders, the angle of deviation is difficult to quantify or the effects of muscle surgery are hard to predict.

181. a. For cases in which a muscle's force-generating capability is permanently and significantly depressed, resection techniques will offer little. Here, transposition of neighboring, healthy rectus muscles (Jensen procedure) is often helpful.

182. d. This may be a case of partially or totally accommodative esotropia, which will respond nicely to hyperopic correction. Bifocals might be added later if a significant residual esodeviation remains at near with distance correction. Any amblyopia, MUST be treated aggressively with careful follow-up of the treatment effect on each eye.

183. d. Stimulation of accommodative convergence is unlikely to resolve the problem. Since the parents are determined to correct the cosmetic problem, and since the deviation is greater in left gaze, weakening of both lateral recti, more so on the left, should be undertaken.

184. d. Strengthening the ipsilateral superior rectus will aggravate the righ hypertropia. A common approach might be superior oblique tuck alone (if the deviation is less than 25 prism diopters) or combined with inferior oblique tenotomy (if greater than 25 prism diopters).

185. a. Although this probably represents a case of basic esotropia, there may be an accommodative component. There is no way to rule this out without a trial of hyperopic correction. Bifocals might be added later if a significant residual esodeviation remains at near with distance correction. Early surgery might be advocated to maximize the retention of fusion, but only the angle of deviation that remains after refractive correction should be addressed. Close follow-up, as always, is critical.

186. d. Since there is asymmetric vision due to amblyopia, a right-eyed procedure should be chosen (to minimize operative risks on the better-seeing left eye). The guidelines for a 30 prism diopter esotropia are 4.5 mm medial rectus recession and 7 mm lateral rectus resection.

187. True. Undercorrected exodeviations nearly always increase in size until there is total recurrence.

188. e. For the same reason as in answer 186, monocular surgery is preferable. The guidelines for a 30 prism diopter exotropia are 6 mm of medial rectus resection and 7 mm of lateral rectus recession.

189. e. If this results in undercorrection, then additional surgery is necessary.

190. d.

191. d.

192. c.

193. c. The range is 15 to 25 prism diopters.

194. d. This procedure has little eso effect in primary gaze and none in upgaze.

195. a. The ischemia induced by surgery on three or more muscles is entirely anterior.

196. False. The converse is true--inferior rectus surgery nearly always involves manipulation of the lid retractors.

197. b. Acquired forms of strabismus may be associated with troublesome postoperative strabismus, as images are moved closer but not close enough. In congenital cases, suppression will prevent the complication. The prism adaptation test is indeed valuable for predicting postoperative behavior. Undercorrected intermittent exotropia will be associated with suppression and a quick recurrence of large-angle turns. The most annoying diplopia is frequently due to small-angle residual turns, which are manageable with prisms. Many cases will resolve spontaneously over months.

198. d. Consecutive exotropia due to overcorrection alone should not be associated with striking impairment in adduction.

199. c. Elevated body temperature is a relatively late sign. Careful surveillance for the earlier signs is critical.

200. d.

201. c.

202. c. Ptosis is the most common and is seen slightly more frequently in children. Secondary vertical strabismus is the second most common complication.

References

1. Richard, James. "Section 6: Pediatric Ophthalmology and Strabismus." in F.M. Wilson (ed.). Basic and Clinical Science Course. San Francisco: American Academy of Ophthalmology, 1991-1992.

2. Burian, Hermann, and von Noorden, Gunter (eds.). Binocular Vision and Ocular Motility. St. Louis: C.V. Mosby Company, 1974.

Answer sheet--Chapter 1

1. ___	37. ___	73. ___	109. ___	145. ___
2. ___	38. ___	74. ___	110. ___	146. ___
3. ___	39. ___	75. ___	111. ___	147. ___
4. ___	40. ___	76. ___	112. ___	148. ___
5. ___	41. ___	77. ___	113. ___	149. ___
6. ___	42. ___	78. ___	114. ___	150. ___
7. ___	43. ___	79. ___	115. ___	151. ___
8. ___	44. ___	80. ___	116. ___	152. ___
9. ___	45. ___	81. ___	117. ___	153. ___
10. ___	46. ___	82. ___	118. ___	154. ___
11. ___	47. ___	83. ___	119. ___	155. ___
12. ___	48. ___	84. ___	120. ___	156. ___
13. ___	49. ___	85. ___	121. ___	157. ___
14. ___	50. ___	86. ___	122. ___	158. ___
15. ___	51. ___	87. ___	123. ___	159. ___
16. ___	52. ___	88. ___	124. ___	160 ___
17. ___	53. ___	89. ___	125. ___	161. ___
18. ___	54. ___	90. ___	126. ___	162. ___
19. ___	55. ___	91. ___	127. ___	163. ___
20. ___	56. ___	92. ___	128. ___	164. ___
21. ___	57. ___	93. ___	129. ___	165. ___
22. ___	58. ___	94. ___	130. ___	166. ___
23. ___	59. ___	95. ___	131. ___	167. ___
24. ___	60. ___	96. ___	132. ___	168. ___
25. ___	61. ___	97. ___	133. ___	
26. ___	62. ___	98. ___	134. ___	
27. ___	63. ___	99. ___	135. ___	
28. ___	64. ___	100. ___	136. ___	
29. ___	65. ___	101. ___	137. ___	
30. ___	66. ___	102. ___	138. ___	
31. ___	67. ___	103. ___	139. ___	
32. ___	68. ___	104. ___	140. ___	
33. ___	69. ___	105. ___	141. ___	
34. ___	70. ___	106. ___	142. ___	
35. ___	71. ___	107. ___	143. ___	
36. ___	72. ___	108. ___	144. ___	

Answer sheet--Chapter 2

1. ___	37. ___	73. ___	109 ___
2. ___	38. ___	74. ___	110. ___
3. ___	39. ___	75. ___	111. ___
4. ___	40. ___	76. ___	112. ___
5. ___	41. ___	77. ___	113. ___
6. ___	42. ___	78. ___	114. ___
7. ___	43. ___	79. ___	115. ___
8. ___	44. ___	80. ___	116. ___
9. ___	45. ___	81. ___	117. ___
10. ___	46. ___	82. ___	118. ___
11. ___	47. ___	83. ___	119. ___
12. ___	48. ___	84. ___	120. ___
13. ___	49. ___	85. ___	121. ___
14. ___	50. ___	86. ___	122. ___
15. ___	51. ___	87. ___	123. ___
16. ___	52. ___	88. ___	124. ___
17. ___	53. ___	89. ___	125. ___
18. ___	54. ___	90. ___	126. ___
19. ___	55. ___	91. ___	127. ___
20. ___	56. ___	92. ___	128. ___
21. ___	57. ___	93. ___	129. ___
22. ___	58. ___	94. ___	130. ___
23. ___	59. ___	95. ___	
24. ___	60. ___	96. ___	
25. ___	61. ___	97. ___	
26. ___	62. ___	98. ___	
27. ___	63. ___	99. ___	
28. ___	64. ___	100. ___	
29. ___	65. ___	101. ___	
30. ___	66. ___	102. ___	
31. ___	67. ___	103. ___	
32. ___	68. ___	104. ___	
33. ___	69. ___	105. ___	
34. ___	70. ___	106. ___	
35. ___	71. ___	107. ___	
36. ___	72. ___	108. ___	

Answer sheet--Chapter 3

1. ___	37. ___	73. ___	109. ___	145. ___
2. ___	38. ___	74. ___	110. ___	146. ___
3. ___	39. ___	75. ___	111. ___	147. ___
4. ___	40. ___	76. ___	112. ___	148. ___
5. ___	41. ___	77. ___	113. ___	149. ___
6. ___	42. ___	78. ___	114. ___	150. ___
7. ___	43. ___	79. ___	115. ___	
8. ___	44. ___	80. ___	116. ___	
9. ___	45. ___	81. ___	117. ___	
10. ___	46. ___	82. ___	118. ___	
11. ___	47. ___	83. ___	119. ___	
12. ___	48. ___	84. ___	120. ___	
13. ___	49. ___	85. ___	121. ___	
14. ___	50. ___	86. ___	122. ___	
15. ___	51. ___	87. ___	123. ___	
16. ___	52. ___	88. ___	124. ___	
17. ___	53. ___	89. ___	125. ___	
18. ___	54. ___	90. ___	126. ___	
19. ___	55. ___	91. ___	127. ___	
20. ___	56. ___	92. ___	128. ___	
21. ___	57. ___	93. ___	129. ___	
22. ___	58. ___	94. ___	130. ___	
23. ___	59. ___	95. ___	131. ___	
24. ___	60. ___	96. ___	132. ___	
25. ___	61. ___	97. ___	133. ___	
26. ___	62. ___	98. ___	134. ___	
27. ___	63. ___	99. ___	135. ___	
28. ___	64. ___	100. ___	136. ___	
29. ___	65. ___	101. ___	137. ___	
30. ___	66. ___	102. ___	138. ___	
31. ___	67. ___	103. ___	139. ___	
32. ___	68. ___	104. ___	140. ___	
33. ___	69. ___	105. ___	141. ___	
34. ___	70. ___	106. ___	142. ___	
35. ___	71. ___	107. ___	143. ___	
36. ___	72. ___	108. ___	144. ___	

Answer sheet--Chapter 4

1. ___	37. ___	73. ___	109. ___	145. ___
2. ___	38. ___	74. ___	110. ___	146. ___
3. ___	39. ___	75. ___	111. ___	147. ___
4. ___	40. ___	76. ___	112. ___	148. ___
5. ___	41. ___	77. ___	113. ___	149. ___
6. ___	42. ___	78. ___	114. ___	150. ___
7. ___	43. ___	79. ___	115. ___	151. ___
8. ___	44. ___	80. ___	116. ___	152. ___
9. ___	45. ___	81. ___	117. ___	153. ___
10. ___	46. ___	82. ___	118. ___	154. ___
11. ___	47. ___	83. ___	119. ___	155. ___
12. ___	48. ___	84. ___	120. ___	156. ___
13. ___	49. ___	85. ___	121. ___	157. ___
14. ___	50. ___	86. ___	122. ___	158. ___
15. ___	51. ___	87. ___	123. ___	159. ___
16. ___	52. ___	88. ___	124. ___	
17. ___	53. ___	89. ___	125. ___	
18. ___	54. ___	90. ___	126. ___	
19. ___	55. ___	91. ___	127. ___	
20. ___	56. ___	92. ___	128. ___	
21. ___	57. ___	93. ___	129. ___	
22. ___	58. ___	94. ___	130. ___	
23. ___	59. ___	95. ___	131. ___	
24. ___	60. ___	96. ___	132. ___	
25. ___	61. ___	97. ___	133. ___	
26. ___	62. ___	98. ___	134. ___	
27. ___	63. ___	99. ___	135. ___	
28. ___	64. ___	100. ___	136. ___	
29. ___	65. ___	101. ___	137. ___	
30. ___	66. ___	102. ___	138. ___	
31. ___	67. ___	103. ___	139. ___	
32. ___	68. ___	104. ___	140. ___	
33. ___	69. ___	105. ___	141. ___	
34. ___	70. ___	106. ___	142. ___	
35. ___	71. ___	107. ___	143. ___	
36. ___	72. ___	108. ___	144. ___	

Answer sheet--Chapter 5

1. ___	37. ___	73. ___	109. ___	145. ___
2. ___	38. ___	74. ___	110. ___	146. ___
3. ___	39. ___	75. ___	111. ___	147. ___
4. ___	40. ___	76. ___	112. ___	148. ___
5. ___	41. ___	77. ___	113. ___	149. ___
6. ___	42. ___	78. ___	114. ___	150. ___
7. ___	43. ___	79. ___	115. ___	151. ___
8. ___	44. ___	80. ___	116. ___	152. ___
9. ___	45. ___	81. ___	117. ___	153. ___
10. ___	46. ___	82. ___	118. ___	154. ___
11. ___	47. ___	83. ___	119. ___	155. ___
12. ___	48. ___	84. ___	120. ___	156. ___
13. ___	49. ___	85. ___	121. ___	157. ___
14. ___	50. ___	86. ___	122. ___	158. ___
15. ___	51. ___	87. ___	123. ___	159. ___
16. ___	52. ___	88. ___	124. ___	160. ___
17. ___	53. ___	89. ___	125. ___	161. ___
18. ___	54. ___	90. ___	126. ___	162. ___
19. ___	55. ___	91. ___	127. ___	163. ___
20. ___	56. ___	92. ___	128. ___	164. ___
21. ___	57. ___	93. ___	129. ___	165. ___
22. ___	58. ___	94. ___	130. ___	166. ___
23. ___	59. ___	95. ___	131. ___	167. ___
24. ___	60. ___	96. ___	132. ___	168. ___
25. ___	61. ___	97. ___	133. ___	169. ___
26. ___	62. ___	98. ___	134. ___	170. ___
27. ___	63. ___	99. ___	135. ___	171. ___
28. ___	64. ___	100. ___	136. ___	172. ___
29. ___	65. ___	101. ___	137. ___	173. ___
30. ___	66. ___	102. ___	138. ___	174. ___
31. ___	67. ___	103. ___	139. ___	175. ___
32. ___	68. ___	104. ___	140. ___	176. ___
33. ___	69. ___	105. ___	141. ___	177. ___
34. ___	70. ___	106. ___	142. ___	178. ___
35. ___	71. ___	107. ___	143. ___	179. ___
36. ___	72. ___	108. ___	144. ___	180. ___

Answer sheet--Chapter 5

181. ___
182. ___
183. ___
184. ___
185. ___
186. ___
187. ___
188. ___
189. ___
190. ___
191. ___
192. ___
193. ___
194. ___
195. ___
196. ___
197. ___
198. ___
199. ___
200. ___
201. ___
202. ___
203. ___
204. ___
205. ___
206. ___
207. ___
208. ___
209. ___
210. ___
211. ___
212. ___
213. ___
214. ___
215. ___
216. ___

217. ___
218. ___
219. ___
220. ___
221. ___
222. ___
223. ___
224. ___
225. ___
226. ___
227. ___
228. ___
229. ___
230. ___
231. ___
232. ___
233. ___
234. ___
235. ___

Answer sheet--Chapter 6

1. ___	37. ___	73. ___	109. ___	145. ___
2. ___	38. ___	74. ___	110. ___	146. ___
3. ___	39. ___	75. ___	111. ___	147. ___
4. ___	40. ___	76. ___	112. ___	148. ___
5. ___	41. ___	77. ___	113. ___	149. ___
6. ___	42. ___	78. ___	114. ___	150. ___
7. ___	43. ___	79. ___	115. ___	151. ___
8. ___	44. ___	80. ___	116. ___	152. ___
9. ___	45. ___	81. ___	117. ___	153. ___
10. ___	46. ___	82. ___	118. ___	154. ___
11. ___	47. ___	83. ___	119. ___	155. ___
12. ___	48. ___	84. ___	120. ___	156. ___
13. ___	49. ___	85. ___	121. ___	157. ___
14. ___	50. ___	86. ___	122. ___	158. ___
15. ___	51. ___	87. ___	123. ___	159. ___
16. ___	52. ___	88. ___	124. ___	160. ___
17. ___	53. ___	89. ___	125. ___	161. ___
18. ___	54. ___	90. ___	126. ___	162. ___
19. ___	55. ___	91. ___	127. ___	163. ___
20. ___	56. ___	92. ___	128. ___	164. ___
21. ___	57. ___	93. ___	129. ___	165. ___
22. ___	58. ___	94. ___	130. ___	166. ___
23. ___	59. ___	95. ___	131. ___	167. ___
24. ___	60. ___	96. ___	132. ___	168. ___
25. ___	61. ___	97. ___	133. ___	169. ___
26. ___	62. ___	98. ___	134. ___	170. ___
27. ___	63. ___	99. ___	135. ___	171. ___
28. ___	64. ___	100. ___	136. ___	172. ___
29. ___	65. ___	101. ___	137. ___	173. ___
30. ___	66. ___	102. ___	138. ___	174. ___
31. ___	67. ___	103. ___	139. ___	175. ___
32. ___	68. ___	104. ___	140. ___	176. ___
33. ___	69. ___	105. ___	141. ___	177. ___
34. ___	70. ___	106. ___	142. ___	178. ___
35. ___	71. ___	107. ___	143. ___	179. ___
36. ___	72. ___	108. ___	144. ___	180. ___

Answer sheet--Chapter 6

181. ___
182. ___
183. ___
184. ___
185. ___
186. ___
187. ___
188. ___
189. ___
190. ___
191. ___
192. ___
193. ___
194. ___
195. ___
196. ___
197. ___
198. ___
199. ___
200. ___
201. ___
202. ___
203. ___
204. ___
205. ___
206. ___
207. ___
208. ___
209. ___
210. ___
211. ___
212. ___
213. ___
214. ___
215. ___
216. ___

217. ___
218. ___
219. ___
220. ___
221. ___
222. ___
223. ___
224. ___
225. ___
226. ___
227. ___
228. ___
229. ___
230. ___
231. ___
232. ___
233. ___
234. ___
235. ___
236. ___
237. ___
238. ___
239. ___
240. ___
241. ___
242. ___
243. ___
244. ___
245. ___
246. ___
247. ___
248. ___
249. ___
250. ___
251. ___
252. ___

253. ___
254. ___
255. ___
256. ___
257. ___
258. ___
259. ___
260. ___
261. ___
262. ___
263. ___
264. ___
265. ___
266. ___
267. ___

Answer sheet--Chapter 7

1. ___	37. ___	73. ___	109. ___	145. ___
2. ___	38. ___	74. ___	110. ___	146. ___
3. ___	39. ___	75. ___	111. ___	147. ___
4. ___	40. ___	76. ___	112. ___	148. ___
5. ___	41. ___	77. ___	113. ___	149. ___
6. ___	42. ___	78. ___	114. ___	150. ___
7. ___	43. ___	79. ___	115. ___	151. ___
8. ___	44. ___	80. ___	116. ___	152. ___
9. ___	45. ___	81. ___	117. ___	153. ___
10. ___	46. ___	82. ___	118. ___	154. ___
11. ___	47. ___	83. ___	119. ___	155. ___
12. ___	48. ___	84. ___	120. ___	156. ___
13. ___	49. ___	85. ___	121. ___	157. ___
14. ___	50. ___	86. ___	122. ___	158. ___
15. ___	51. ___	87. ___	123. ___	159. ___
16. ___	52. ___	88. ___	124. ___	160. ___
17. ___	53. ___	89. ___	125. ___	161. ___
18. ___	54. ___	90. ___	126. ___	162. ___
19. ___	55. ___	91. ___	127. ___	163. ___
20. ___	56. ___	92. ___	128. ___	164. ___
21. ___	57. ___	93. ___	129. ___	165. ___
22. ___	58. ___	94. ___	130. ___	166. ___
23. ___	59. ___	95. ___	131. ___	167. ___
24. ___	60. ___	96. ___	132. ___	168. ___
25. ___	61. ___	97. ___	133. ___	169. ___
26. ___	62. ___	98. ___	134. ___	170. ___
27. ___	63. ___	99. ___	135. ___	171. ___
28. ___	64. ___	100. ___	136. ___	172. ___
29. ___	65. ___	101. ___	137. ___	173. ___
30. ___	66. ___	102. ___	138. ___	174. ___
31. ___	67. ___	103. ___	139. ___	175. ___
32. ___	68. ___	104. ___	140. ___	176. ___
33. ___	69. ___	105. ___	141. ___	177. ___
34. ___	70. ___	106. ___	142. ___	178. ___
35. ___	71. ___	107. ___	143. ___	179. ___
36. ___	72. ___	108. ___	144. ___	180. ___

Answer sheet--Chapter 7

181. ___	217. ___	253. ___	289. ___	325. ___
182. ___	218. ___	254. ___	290. ___	326. ___
183. ___	219. ___	255. ___	291. ___	327. ___
184. ___	220. ___	256. ___	292. ___	328. ___
185. ___	221. ___	257. ___	293. ___	329. ___
186. ___	222. ___	258. ___	294. ___	330. ___
187. ___	223. ___	259. ___	295. ___	331. ___
188. ___	224. ___	260. ___	296. ___	332. ___
189. ___	225. ___	261. ___	297. ___	333. ___
190. ___	226. ___	262. ___	298. ___	334. ___
191. ___	227. ___	263. ___	299. ___	335. ___
192. ___	228. ___	264. ___	300. ___	336. ___
193. ___	229. ___	265. ___	301. ___	337. ___
194. ___	230. ___	266. ___	302. ___	338. ___
195. ___	231. ___	267. ___	303. ___	339. ___
196. ___	232. ___	268. ___	304. ___	340. ___
197. ___	233. ___	269. ___	305. ___	341. ___
198. ___	234. ___	270. ___	306. ___	342. ___
199. ___	235. ___	271. ___	307. ___	343. ___
200. ___	236. ___	272. ___	308. ___	344. ___
201. ___	237. ___	273. ___	309. ___	345. ___
202. ___	238. ___	274. ___	310. ___	346. ___
203. ___	239. ___	275. ___	311. ___	347. ___
204. ___	240. ___	276. ___	312. ___	348. ___
205. ___	241. ___	277. ___	313. ___	349. ___
206. ___	242. ___	278. ___	314. ___	350. ___
207. ___	243. ___	279. ___	315. ___	351. ___
208. ___	244. ___	280. ___	316. ___	352. ___
209. ___	245. ___	281. ___	317. ___	353. ___
210. ___	246. ___	282. ___	318. ___	354. ___
211. ___	247. ___	283. ___	319. ___	355. ___
212. ___	248. ___	284. ___	320. ___	356. ___
213. ___	249. ___	285. ___	321. ___	357. ___
214. ___	250. ___	286. ___	322. ___	358. ___
215. ___	251. ___	287. ___	323. ___	359. ___
216. ___	252. ___	288. ___	324. ___	360. ___

Answer sheet--Chapter 7

361. ___
362. ___
363. ___
364. ___
365. ___
366. ___
367. ___
368. ___
369. ___
370. ___
371. ___
372. ___
373. ___
374. ___
375. ___
376. ___
377. ___
378. ___
379. ___
380. ___
381. ___
382. ___
383. ___
384. ___

Answer sheet--Chapter 8

1. ___	37. ___	73. ___	109. ___
2. ___	38. ___	74. ___	110. ___
3. ___	39. ___	75. ___	111. ___
4. ___	40. ___	76. ___	112. ___
5. ___	41. ___	77. ___	113. ___
6. ___	42. ___	78. ___	114. ___
7. ___	43. ___	79. ___	115. ___
8. ___	44. ___	80. ___	116. ___
9. ___	45. ___	81. ___	
10. ___	46. ___	82. ___	
11. ___	47. ___	83. ___	
12. ___	48. ___	84. ___	
13. ___	49. ___	85. ___	
14. ___	50. ___	86. ___	
15. ___	51. ___	87. ___	
16. ___	52. ___	88. ___	
17. ___	53. ___	89. ___	
18. ___	54. ___	90. ___	
19. ___	55. ___	91. ___	
20. ___	56. ___	92. ___	
21. ___	57. ___	93. ___	
22. ___	58. ___	94. ___	
23. ___	59. ___	95. ___	
24. ___	60. ___	96. ___	
25. ___	61. ___	97. ___	
26. ___	62. ___	98. ___	
27. ___	63. ___	99. ___	
28. ___	64. ___	100. ___	
29. ___	65. ___	101. ___	
30. ___	66. ___	102. ___	
31. ___	67. ___	103. ___	
32. ___	68. ___	104. ___	
33. ___	69. ___	105. ___	
34. ___	70. ___	106. ___	
35. ___	71. ___	107. ___	
36. ___	72. ___	108. ___	

Answer sheet--Chapter 9

1. ___	37. ___	73. ___	109. ___
2. ___	38. ___	74. ___	110. ___
3. ___	39. ___	75. ___	111. ___
4. ___	40. ___	76. ___	112. ___
5. ___	41. ___	77. ___	113. ___
6. ___	42. ___	78. ___	114. ___
7. ___	43. ___	79. ___	115. ___
8. ___	44. ___	80. ___	116. ___
9. ___	45. ___	81. ___	117. ___
10. ___	46. ___	82. ___	118. ___
11. ___	47. ___	83. ___	119. ___
12. ___	48. ___	84. ___	120. ___
13. ___	49. ___	85. ___	121. ___
14. ___	50. ___	86. ___	122. ___
15. ___	51. ___	87. ___	123. ___
16. ___	52. ___	88. ___	124. ___
17. ___	53. ___	89. ___	125. ___
18. ___	54. ___	90. ___	126. ___
19. ___	55. ___	91. ___	127. ___
20. ___	56. ___	92. ___	128. ___
21. ___	57. ___	93. ___	129. ___
22. ___	58. ___	94. ___	130. ___
23. ___	59. ___	95. ___	131. ___
24. ___	60. ___	96. ___	132. ___
25. ___	61. ___	97. ___	133. ___
26. ___	62. ___	98. ___	134. ___
27. ___	63. ___	99. ___	135. ___
28. ___	64. ___	100. ___	
29. ___	65. ___	101. ___	
30. ___	66. ___	102. ___	
31. ___	67. ___	103. ___	
32. ___	68. ___	104. ___	
33. ___	69. ___	105. ___	
34. ___	70. ___	106. ___	
35. ___	71. ___	107. ___	
36. ___	72. ___	108. ___	

Answer sheet--Chapter 10

1. ___	37. ___	73. ___	109. ___	145. ___
2. ___	38. ___	74. ___	110. ___	146. ___
3. ___	39. ___	75. ___	111. ___	147. ___
4. ___	40. ___	76. ___	112. ___	148. ___
5. ___	41. ___	77. ___	113. ___	149. ___
6. ___	42. ___	78. ___	114. ___	150. ___
7. ___	43. ___	79. ___	115. ___	151. ___
8. ___	44. ___	80. ___	116. ___	152. ___
9. ___	45. ___	81. ___	117. ___	153. ___
10. ___	46. ___	82. ___	118. ___	154. ___
11. ___	47. ___	83. ___	119. ___	155. ___
12. ___	48. ___	84. ___	120. ___	156. ___
13. ___	49. ___	85. ___	121. ___	157. ___
14. ___	50. ___	86. ___	122. ___	158. ___
15. ___	51. ___	87. ___	123. ___	159. ___
16. ___	52. ___	88. ___	124. ___	160. ___
17. ___	53. ___	89. ___	125. ___	161. ___
18. ___	54. ___	90. ___	126. ___	162. ___
19. ___	55. ___	91. ___	127. ___	163. ___
20. ___	56. ___	92. ___	128. ___	164. ___
21. ___	57. ___	93. ___	129. ___	165. ___
22. ___	58. ___	94. ___	130. ___	166. ___
23. ___	59. ___	95. ___	131. ___	167. ___
24. ___	60. ___	96. ___	132. ___	168. ___
25. ___	61. ___	97. ___	133. ___	169. ___
26. ___	62. ___	98. ___	134. ___	170. ___
27. ___	63. ___	99. ___	135. ___	171. ___
28. ___	64. ___	100. ___	136. ___	172. ___
29. ___	65. ___	101. ___	137. ___	173. ___
30. ___	66. ___	102. ___	138. ___	174. ___
31. ___	67. ___	103. ___	139. ___	175. ___
32. ___	68. ___	104. ___	140. ___	176. ___
33. ___	69. ___	105. ___	141. ___	177. ___
34. ___	70. ___	106. ___	142. ___	178. ___
35. ___	71. ___	107. ___	143. ___	179. ___
36. ___	72. ___	108. ___	144. ___	180. ___

Answer sheet--Chapter 10

181. ___
182. ___
183. ___
184. ___
185. ___
186. ___
187. ___
188. ___
189. ___
190. ___
191. ___
192. ___
193. ___
194. ___
195. ___
196. ___
197. ___
198. ___
199. ___
200. ___
201. ___
202. ___
203. ___
204. ___
205. ___

Answer sheet--Chapter 11

1. ___	37. ___	73. ___	109. ___	145. ___
2. ___	38. ___	74. ___	110. ___	146. ___
3. ___	39. ___	75. ___	111. ___	147. ___
4. ___	40. ___	76. ___	112. ___	148. ___
5. ___	41. ___	77. ___	113. ___	149. ___
6. ___	42. ___	78. ___	114. ___	150. ___
7. ___	43. ___	79. ___	115. ___	151. ___
8. ___	44. ___	80. ___	116. ___	152. ___
9. ___	45. ___	81. ___	117. ___	153. ___
10. ___	46. ___	82. ___	118. ___	154. ___
11. ___	47. ___	83. ___	119. ___	155. ___
12. ___	48. ___	84. ___	120. ___	156. ___
13. ___	49. ___	85. ___	121. ___	157. ___
14. ___	50. ___	86. ___	122. ___	158. ___
15. ___	51. ___	87. ___	123. ___	159. ___
16. ___	52. ___	88. ___	124. ___	160. ___
17. ___	53. ___	89. ___	125. ___	161. ___
18. ___	54. ___	90. ___	126. ___	162. ___
19. ___	55. ___	91. ___	127. ___	163. ___
20. ___	56. ___	92. ___	128. ___	164. ___
21. ___	57. ___	93. ___	129. ___	165. ___
22. ___	58. ___	94. ___	130. ___	166. ___
23. ___	59. ___	95. ___	131. ___	167. ___
24. ___	60. ___	96. ___	132. ___	168. ___
25. ___	61. ___	97. ___	133. ___	169. ___
26. ___	62. ___	98. ___	134. ___	170. ___
27. ___	63. ___	99. ___	135. ___	171. ___
28. ___	64. ___	100. ___	136. ___	172. ___
29. ___	65. ___	101. ___	137. ___	173. ___
30. ___	66. ___	102. ___	138. ___	174. ___
31. ___	67. ___	103. ___	139. ___	175. ___
32. ___	68. ___	104. ___	140. ___	176. ___
33. ___	69. ___	105. ___	141. ___	177. ___
34. ___	70. ___	106. ___	142. ___	178. ___
35. ___	71. ___	107. ___	143. ___	179. ___
36. ___	72. ___	108. ___	144. ___	180. ___

181. ___
182. ___
183. ___
184. ___
185. ___
186. ___
187. ___
188. ___
189. ___
190. ___
191. ___
192. ___
193. ___
194. ___
195. ___
196. ___
197. ___
198. ___
199. ___
200. ___
201. ___
202. ___